VISION
REHABILITATION

Multidisciplinary Care of the
Patient Following Brain Injury

VISION REHABILITATION

Multidisciplinary Care of the Patient Following Brain Injury

Edited by
Penelope S. Suter
Lisa H. Harvey

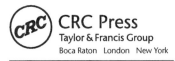

CRC Press
Taylor & Francis Group
Boca Raton London New York

CRC Press is an imprint of the
Taylor & Francis Group, an **informa** business

Cover art by David Linkhart.

CRC Press
Taylor & Francis Group
6000 Broken Sound Parkway NW, Suite 300
Boca Raton, FL 33487-2742

© 2011 by Taylor and Francis Group, LLC
CRC Press is an imprint of Taylor & Francis Group, an Informa business

No claim to original U.S. Government works

Printed in the United States of America on acid-free paper
10 9 8 7 6 5 4 3 2 1

International Standard Book Number: 978-1-4398-3655-2 (Hardback)

Library of Congress Cataloging-in-Publication Data

Vision rehabilitation : multidisciplinary care of the patient following brain injury / [edited by]
Penelope S. Suter and Lisa H. Harvey.
        p. ; cm.
    "CRC title."
    Includes bibliographical references and index.
    Summary: "Providing all of the necessary information required to provide post-acute vision
rehabilitative care following brain injury, this multidisciplinary book bridges the gap between theory
and practice and presents clinical information and scientific literature supporting the diagnostic and
therapeutic strategies applied. It covers all areas of vision care including the structure and function
of the eye, organization of visual perception in the brain, and rehabilitation concepts applied to the
visual system. It offers cutting-edge research, prescribing lenses and prisms, and therapy techniques
that will enable even the experienced clinician to provide enhanced care to the brain injury
patient"--Provided by publisher.
    ISBN 978-1-4398-3655-2 (hardcover : acid-free paper)
    1. Visual agnosia--Patients--Rehabilitation. 2. Vision disorders--Patients--Rehabilitation. 3.
Visual training. 4. Brain damage--Complications. I. Suter, Penelope S., editor. II. Harvey, Lisa H.,
editor.
    [DNLM: 1. Vision Disorders--rehabilitation. 2. Brain Injuries--complications. WW 140]

RC394.V57V57 2011
617.7'503--dc22   2010046266

Visit the Taylor & Francis Web site at
http://www.taylorandfrancis.com

and the CRC Press Web site at
http://www.crcpress.com

Contents

Foreword

One of the most important functions of our brain is to integrate the information from all our senses into a perceptual whole. Only then can we perceive the world as single, integrated, and stable, allowing us to move through it, molding it to our needs and desires. Brain injury shatters this wholeness. Half of one's visual field may be lost or, stranger yet, one may lose awareness of the left side of one's body and everything else to one's left. The eyes may no longer work together resulting in diplopia, visual confusion, and in an impaired spatial sense. Eye movements may not correlate with movements of the head and body, thus, disrupting one's sense that the world is fixed and stable. Balance and coordination may be disturbed, and reading impossible for the words on the page may appear to be written in a foreign alphabet. One may struggle to come up with the right words or to understand their meaning, and the ability to concentrate and work out these problems may be lost. As L. Zazetsky writes in A. R. Luria's book *The Man with a Shattered World,*[1] "Ever since I was wounded, I haven't been able to see a single object as a whole—not one thing…. I've had a hard time understanding and identifying things in my environment. What's more, when I see or imagine things in my mind (physical objects, phenomena, plants, animals, birds, people), I still can't think of the words for these right away. And vice versa— when I hear a sound or a word I can't remember right off what it means." For the past century, conventional wisdom held that the adult human brain is immutable. Most of its circuitry is laid down by early childhood with little possibility, it was thought, of rewiring in adulthood. Great emphasis was placed on the role of "critical periods" in early life for the development of basic perceptual and language skills. Once these critical periods were passed, little neuronal reorganization was possible. A damaged adult brain could not recover. If the brain were injured, the best one could hope for was to develop new strategies to compensate for the functions and skills that were lost.

Despite this mindset, evidence for adult brain plasticity continued to surface and resurface in the scientific and medical literature throughout the last and current centuries. In 1967, Jerzy Konorski in his book, *Integrative Activity of the Brain,*[2] coined the term neuroplasticity, as "the capacity to change its [the brain's] reactive properties as the result of successive activations." Also in the 1960s, Joseph Altman published a series of papers demonstrating a striking form of plasticity, the birth of new neurons in the brains of adult rats.[3] His findings were totally ignored. Fifteen years after Altman's first paper, Michael Kaplan confirmed Altman's discoveries, but he was attacked for his iconoclastic claims and left the research field. Starting in the 1980s, however, scientific investigations confirmed neurogenesis first in the brains of adult birds and later in mammals, including primates. After approximately 30 years, the dogma that no new neurons are born in the adult mammalian brain was finally put to rest. Moreover, recent brain imaging experiments as well as studies revealing the mechanisms of synaptic plasticity have contributed to a new view of the adult brain as dynamic and plastic.

Long before it was accepted by the majority of medical doctors and scientists, optometrists recognized the potential for rehabilitation and recovery in the adult brain. While conventional wisdom suggested that normal binocular vision and stereopsis must develop during a critical period in early life, optometrists, including Frederick Brock and William Ludlam, devised therapies in the mid-1900s that taught adults with infantile strabismus how to fuse and develop stereovision. They recognized that changes in the adult brain require active learning, involving attention, practice, and feedback. While an infant nervous system may change its connections in response to any strong stimulus, an adult brain is pickier. It rewires specifically in response to behaviorally relevant stimuli. The degree of functional improvement or recovery in an adult depends in large part on the motivation of the individual and the design of the therapy.

These insights are critical for the treatment and rehabilitation of the growing number of victims of acquired brain injury, including cerebral vascular accidents, traumatic brain injury, and progressive neurological disease. Most alarmingly, traumatic brain injury is the "signature injury" sustained by servicemen fighting in the current wars in Afghanistan and Iraq. And even a concussion, what has been labeled as mild traumatic brain injury (mTBI), can have serious, long-term consequences.

Up until the 1980s and continuing to a large extent to this day, optometrists and the visual rehabilitation that they provide have not been part of the medical rehabilitation efforts of patients with acquired brain injury. Physical or occupational therapy may proceed without thorough attention to visual skills. This situation results in part because of the covert nature of visual injuries. As discussed throughout this book, visual guidance of movements proceeds largely subconsciously so that we are unaware of vision's role. Thus, problems with maintaining or switching attention may result from difficulties with fixations, saccades, and smooth pursuits. Convergence insufficiency and accommodative dysfunction may manifest themselves as problems with reading. Visual field defects or anomalous egocentric localization (midline shifts) may be disguised as movement and balance problems. Difficulties using escalators or an inability to tolerate crowds may result from a poor spatial sense, which results in turn from impaired binocular function. Zazetsky writes in *The Man with a Shattered World*, "After I was wounded, I just couldn't understand space, I was afraid of it. Even now, when I'm sitting next to a table with certain objects on it, I'm afraid to reach out and touch them."

A publication in 2005 gave optimism that awareness of the crucial role of optometry in the rehabilitation of brain injury was increasing. An entire issue of *Brain Injury Professional*, the official publication of the North American Brain Injury Society, was devoted to neuro-optometric rehabilitation.[4] This signaled that a comprehensive book dedicated solely to the growing body of knowledge in this area was due. A large part of this book is devoted to an explanation of the therapy techniques developed by optometrists to improve binocular vision, visual attention, form perception, spatial awareness, spatial reasoning, speed of information processing, visual memory, multisensory integration, and visual-motor skills. In addition, the use of lenses, prisms, yoked prisms, and partial occluders are discussed for the treatment of photophobia, visual field loss, anomalous egocentric localization, and diplopia—all common consequences of acquired brain injuries. Moreover, this book provides detailed information on the visual and vestibular systems, differential diagnosis, guidelines to the optometrist for working with an interdisciplinary medical team both in a hospital setting and in private practice, and advice for advocating for the patient in the legal system.

Vision Rehabilitation: Multidisciplinary Care of the Patient Following Brain Injury is a call to action. Optometrists trained in vision rehabilitation must play a fundamental role in the treatment of patients with acquired brain injury. And beyond diagnosing visual deficits and prescribing therapies, the optometrist must listen to the subjective experiences of the patient. Acquired brain injury, by disrupting some brain areas and leaving others intact, produces symptoms that are as unique and remarkable as they are tragic. Zazetsky, the patient who is quoted and described in *The Man with a Shattered World*, was wounded by a single bullet that ripped through the parietal-occipital region of his brain. He could write but had great trouble reading his own words or those of others. Thoughts and images appeared to him at random and were lost in the next moment. Yet, with his uninjured frontal lobes, he was keenly aware of his deficits and failures, a situation that tormented him for the rest of his life. Each patient with a brain injury has a unique story that must be heard. Above all, rehabilitation of the brain-injured patient must strive to restore to the individual his or her sense of wholeness, of being a complete and functional human being in a fixed and stable world.

Susan R. Barry, PhD
Author of *Fixing My Gaze*
Professor of Biological Sciences and Neuroscience
Mount Holyoke College
South Hadley, MA

REFERENCES

1. Luria, A. R. (1987). *The Man with a Shattered World*. Cambridge, MA: Harvard University Press.
2. Konorski, J. (1967). *Integrative Activity of the Brain*. Chicago, IL: The University of Chicago Press.
3. Gross, C. G. (2009). Three before their time: neuroscientists whose ideas were ignored by their contemporaries. *Experimental Brain Research, 192,* 321–334.
4. Special Issue on Neuro-Optometry. (2005). *Brain Injury Professional*, 2(3), p. 1–31.

Preface

The purpose of this book is to provide the first textbook in post-brain injury vision rehabilitation for use by both experienced clinicians and students. It was written as a multidisciplinary text. This text should be useful not only for optometrists interested in neuro-optometry, but also for neuro-ophthalmologists, neurologists, physiatrists, occupational therapists, physical therapists, and general rehabilitation professionals such as case managers and life-care planners. Guiding vision rehabilitation following acquired brain injury is a challenging task, requiring knowledge of all areas of vision care, from the structure and function of the eye, to the functional organization of visual perception in the brain. It interacts with other rehabilitation efforts, from the patient's ability to understand the world they see, to fine visual-motor integration, dizziness, balance, and mobility.

There is a wealth of information on vision rehabilitation in the literature. However, it has been difficult for clinicians to access, because it is scattered in pieces, not published in one reference or available from a single source. There is literature for use in the courtroom that provides references to support vision rehabilitation. However, this literature does not tell the doctor how to treat a rehabilitation patient. There are also clinical articles and a few books that give the clinical information for particular aspects of vision rehabilitation, but do not provide a comprehensive overview of the myriad of issues that must be addressed for the patient with brain injury. They also generally do not provide the research that supports intervention. This book was written for both new and experienced clinicians; it brings together the clinical information that will enable them to apply current concepts in vision rehabilitation, and it cites the literature that supports the diagnostic and therapeutic strategies applied.

We have striven to include different points of view. Although the editors are optometrists, the science in vision rehabilitation comes from experimental psychology, medicine, optometry, occupational therapy, physical therapy, and other literatures. Our introductory chapter discusses the extent of vision rehabilitation and presents vignettes of cases demonstrating the need to incorporate vision rehabilitation at every level of rehabilitation. We recruited a neurologist to write the physical substrates of vision chapter, giving a broader perspective from that typically presented in the ophthalmologic or optometric literature. Occupational therapists (OTs) wrote the multidisciplinary treatment chapter. The chapter on spatial vision was initially planned as two chapters written by optometrists (ODs)—one on eye movements/binocular vision, and one on spatial vision. However, both authors agreed that there was no way to decide where one chapter ended and the other began; we interpret space, in large part by how and where we point our eyes, and we point our eyes, in large part based on our interpretation of space. Other chapters were authored or coauthored by ODs, an OD, PhD, a certified vision therapist, an OT, PhD, a physical therapist, and an attorney, all highly respected in the field of rehabilitation following brain injury.

We wanted this book, above all, to be a text for clinicians and people involved in the health-care aspects of rehabilitation to get help to patients in need. We hope that the reader will find it a useful tool, and that rehabilitation centers, case managers, life-care planners, and clinicians, will be encouraged to make certain that the rehabilitation of patients with brain injury includes the entire breadth of vision rehabilitation.

Acknowledgments

I would like to thank all of the chapter authors who gave up practice, leisure, and family time to share their knowledge and experience—and without whom this book would not exist. In particular, thanks to Dr. Neil Margolis for sharing his brilliant clinical insights with me throughout the years; to Dr. Robert Sanet, an amazing teacher who helped me understand many things about vision; and to my coeditor Dr. Lisa H. Harvey for sharing her careful editing, her well-centered perspective, and her friendship. I am grateful for the help and support of my office staff. Thanks are due also to Karen Keeney and Dr. Carl Garbus for contributions, to Steve Suter for library assistance, to Rebecca and Trevor Richards for artistic contributions, to Linda Sanet for selfless support, to David Linkhart for cover art, and *especially* to Katharina Gutcher, without whom this manuscript would never have made it to press.

I am also grateful to the many rehabilitation patients who have taught me so much over the years, and for whom this book was written. Lastly, I would like to thank my son, Andrew, for the love, unwavering support, and chocolate pudding with whipping cream that he provided throughout the long weekends and evenings of working on this book.

Penelope S. Suter

I am immensely grateful to all the gifted authors who have shared their knowledge in this book to advance the field of vision rehabilitation after brain injury.

The book exists because of the heartfelt desire of Dr. Penelope S. Suter, my dear friend and colleague, to get the latest, most evidence-based information into the hands of clinicians who are doing their best to serve those with brain injury from all causes. It has not been an easy task; her dedication and persistence have been extraordinary.

Lisa H. Harvey

Editors

Dr. Penelope S. Suter has been an optometrist in private practice since receiving her OD from the University of California, Berkeley in 1984. She consults for the Centre for Neuro Skills, a comprehensive postacute brain injury rehabilitation center in Bakersfield, California. During optometry school, she was assistant director of the UC-Berkeley Visual Evoked Potentials (VEP) Clinic. She held the position of codirector of the Psychology Department Vision Laboratory at California State University, Bakersfield, from 1984 to 2002, engaging in VEP research. Dr. Suter currently has a specialty practice with a strong emphasis in neuro-optometric rehabilitation, as well as infant vision, vision-related learning problems, and vision care for patients with special needs. Dr. Suter is a Fellow of the College of Optometrists in Vision Development, the American Board of Disability Analysts, and the Neuro-Optometric Rehabilitation Association. Clinically, she publishes and lectures in the area of post-brain injury vision rehabilitation and in applying neural models in the vision rehabilitation therapy room.

Dr. Lisa H. Harvey began her graduate career working in research as a botanist at McGill University in Montreal, Quebec. Feeling the need for more involvement with people in her work, she changed her degree aspirations and received her OD from the University of California, Berkeley in 1983. After 23 years of practicing general optometry with an emphasis on children's vision and vision therapy, Dr. Harvey sold her primary care practice and started a specialty practice in pediatric optometry, vision therapy, and vision rehabilitation. She is also a Fellow of the College of Optometrists in Vision Development.

Contributors

Amy Berryman, OTR, MSHSA
Craig Hospital
Englewood, Colorado

Velda L. Bryan, P.T., CBIS
Department of Clinical Education and
  Research
Centre for Neuro Skills®
Bakersfield, California

Kenneth J. Ciuffreda, OD, PhD
Department of Vision Sciences
State University of New York, College
  of Optometry
New York, New York

Allen H. Cohen, OD, FCOVD
Department of Clinical Sciences
State University of New York, College
  of Optometry
New York, New York

Sidney Groffman, OD, MA
Department of Clinical Sciences
State University of New York, College
  of Optometry
New York, New York

Katharina Gutcher, Dipl.-Ing. (FH)
Augenoptik
Bakersfield, California

Paul A. Harris, OD, FCOVD,
FACBO, FAAO
Baltimore Vision Fitness Center
Baltimore, Maryland

Lisa H. Harvey, OD, FCOVD
Fort Bragg, California

Lynn F. Hellerstein, OD, FCOVD,
FAAO
Hellerstein & Brenner Vision Center,
  P. C.
Englewood, Colorado

Richard Helvie, MD
Centre for Neuro Skills®
Bakersfield, California

Joseph Kiel, LLB
Kiel & Trueax, L.L.C
Denver, Colorado

Diana P. Ludlam, BS, COVT
Department of Vision Sciences
State University of New York, College
  of Optometry
New York, New York

Neil W. Margolis, OD, FCOVD, FAAO
Arlington Heights, Illinois

Thomas Politzer, OD, FCOVD, FAAO
Craig Hospital
Englewood, Colorado

Janet M. Powell, PhD, OTR/L
Department of Rehabilitation Medicine
University of Washington
Seattle, Washington

Leonard J. Press, OD, FCOVD, FAAO
The Vision and Learning Center
Fair Lawn, New Jersey

Karen G. Rasavage, OTR
Craig Hospital
Englewood, Colorado

Robert B. Sanet, OD, FCOVD
San Diego Center for Vision Care
Lemon Grove, California

**Cathy D. Stern, OD, FCOVD,
FCSO, FNORA**
Canton, Massachusetts

**Penelope S. Suter, OD, FCOVD,
   FABDA, FNORA**
Bakersfield, California

Nancy G. Torgerson, OD, FCOVD
Alderwood Vision Therapy Center
Lynnwood, Washington

1 What Is Vision Rehabilitation Following Brain Injury?

*Penelope S. Suter, Lynn F. Hellerstein,
Lisa H. Harvey, and Katharina Gutcher*

CONTENTS

We now have twenty years or more of rapidly accumulating evidence that sensory-perceptual systems, especially at the cortical level, are highly plastic, even in mature mammals. (p. 7622)[1]

As this book nears its completion in 2010, more than 10 years after Kaas' statement above, soldiers are coming home from two wars whose signature injury is brain injury due to widespread use of improvised explosive devices. It is incumbent upon those of us in the rehabilitation field to learn what the new best practices are in diagnosis and treatment of the visual consequences of brain injury. The field of vision rehabilitation following brain injury has been quietly growing and developing over the past two decades. However, full scope vision rehabilitation is still not included in most rehabilitation settings. It is time for vision rehabilitation to become standard of care for patients with acquired brain injury (ABI), whether it be due to stroke, accident, illness, neurological impairment, or trauma.

In this book, we have striven to present the most current, evidence-based practices in the area of vision rehabilitation following brain injury, as well as the critical clinical concepts, and examples of therapies that translate those concepts into treatment. It is important to understand the many aspects of vision to be examined, and to gather quality data on each patient, as the visual system is a *covert* system, where the process and outcome are evidenced not as "visual," but as motor or verbal outputs. Because most patients with brain injury, particularly those with traumatic brain injury (TBI), will present with a myriad of vision deficits, clinicians must be able to step back and synthesize this data so that they can apply their best clinical knowledge, insight and intuition to treat the person before them. The clinical insights and intuitions must be illuminated by a current understanding of the visual system as a whole—eyes, muscles, nerves, brain, and processes, or the overall rehabilitation process will be less effective than that patient deserves.

VISION REHABILITATION (RE)DEFINED

Historically, the term "vision rehabilitation" has been applied to the practice of "low vision" rehabilitation, as well as orientation and mobility training for people who have had either significant loss of visual acuity or visual field. The term has indicated a limited view of vision rehabilitation. However, over the last two decades, researchers have described visual processing pathways in the brain, and clinicians have responded by looking at the visual system as more of a functional whole, with the realization that the visual system is extremely complex, and is integrated with other sensory and output systems. It has become clear that the term vision rehabilitation must be redefined to include rehabilitation of the entire visual system; from rehabilitation of the eye and surrounding structures to rehabilitation and management of sensory processing, integration of visual sensation with input from the other senses, organization of sensory input into visual percepts, and the use of these percepts to support behavioral or cognitive functions. Under the broad umbrella of vision rehabilitation falls rehabilitation of the eye, eyelids, extraocular muscles, surrounding bony structure of the orbit, eye movement and eye teaming disorders, as well as higher order visual functions such as spatial organization, object perception, visual memory, visual thinking, allocation of visual attention, and the ability to integrate visual information with other sensory and output modalities. More than half of our gray matter and multiple subcortical areas are involved in processing vision (see Chapter 3). The complexity is such that multiple professionals must be involved, and vision professionals must work as part of a rehabilitation team to provide the most effective care.

PLASTICITY AND THERAPEUTIC TREATMENT

Plasticity is the basis of all neurorehabilitation, from speech and language to the executive aspects of motor control, cognitive, and vision rehabilitation therapies. All of them rely on the ability of the brain, given the right guidance and experiences, to create new connections and fortify old ones. An amazing example of brain plasticity in adults can be found in the research published by Miltner et al.[2] who demonstrated through magnetic source imaging, that 1 hour following nerve block of medial and radial portions of the hand, the cortical representation of the adjacent structures (representations of the little finger and the skin beneath the lower lip) expanded into the deafferented region. That is, within only 1 hour of diminished input to a portion of the somatomotor cortex, the brain was already rearranging intact receptive networks in what is called the *invasion phenomenon*. These expansions of cortical representation of the little finger and lower lip area were accompanied by functional changes of increased two-point touch discrimination at the lower lip area and mislocalization of touch from the unblocked fourth finger to the neighboring blocked third finger. Other imaging studies on plasticity in adult humans demonstrate changes in brain functional connectivity or size of particular functional brain areas with therapy and practice.[3,4]

The adult brain was initially believed incapable of developing new neural cells. Previous neuroanatomical dogma stated that humans were born with the full complement of brain cells, and that further growth and development was reliant on myelination and formation of connections between already existing neurons. While those two processes are critical (see Chapter 3), research over the last decade has demonstrated that neurogenesis continues throughout the lifetime (reviewed by Qu and Shi, and Ge, Sailor, Ming, & Song).[5,6] Martí-Fàbregas and colleagues,[7] performed histological analysis on autopsied brains of elderly persons (mean age 82 years), who had died an average of 10 days following first-ever middle cerebral artery ischemic stroke. Their findings demonstrated active cell proliferation, in the ipsilateral sub-ventricular zone, but not in the contralateral hemisphere. These findings suggest, as is common knowledge in post-brain injury rehabilitation, that some degree of spontaneous resolution of injury related deficits will occur. However, from a different perspective, these findings also suggest that the sooner one begins rehabilitation therapy, the better chance one has of guiding the structural changes to follow, taking advantage of this new growth in response to injury.

Incredible plasticity in the adult visual system has been demonstrated in psychology experiments by application of inverting prism in normal adults.[8] Initially when wearing these prisms, the world appears upside down and backward. However, after wearing the prisms for several days, the world returns to its normal appearance, demonstrating the amazing plasticity of the visual-perceptual apparatus, as well as the vestibular-ocular reflex, which must also invert. Upon removing the prisms, the world is again, upside down and backward until the visual and vestibular systems reorient.

Further evidence of plasticity in the adult visual system lies in the successful remediation of amblyopia and strabismus in adults. For decades, optometrists who provide vision therapy services have been treating amblyopia and strabismus in adults, restoring visual function and binocularity, in spite of the fact that other vision care providers, including other optometrists continued to advise patients that it was impossible to treat such disorders beyond whatever age they had heard was the end of the "critical period" beyond which plasticity no longer existed. While it is true that in severe deprivation, there is not sufficient experience and brain development to build upon and no amount of therapy can create the cortical reorganization necessary to develop better vision. However, for the vast majority of people who have had some exposure to light and form vision in an amblyopic eye, or some brief period of time when they were young where they had binocular fusion, remediation of amblyopia[9–12] and strabismus,[13] through vision therapy, sometimes with the assistance of surgical intervention, is frequently possible. Dr. Sue Barry is a neurobiologist who had three strabismus surgeries for infantile esotropia, but never attained binocular fusion and never saw in three dimensions until she received vision therapy treatment as an adult. In her book, "Fixing My Gaze; a scientist's journey into seeing in three dimensions,"[14] Dr. Barry documents both the experiential and the neurobiological aspects of first attaining stereopsis in her mid-forties. In short: *In vivo studies have now overturned the dogma that robust plasticity is limited to an early critical period*" (p. 298).[15]

COORDINATING MEDICAL AND FUNCTIONAL REHABILITATIONS

Ophthalmologists, specializing in every aspect of medical vision care are frequently crucial in the early treatment of the patient with brain injury; from surgical care of orbital fractures and muscle entrapment, to retinal tears and detachment, vitrectomy for vitreous bleeding, management for neurotrophic corneas, to surgical intervention for eyelids to protect the cornea in posttraumatic cases of lagophthalmos. As the patient becomes medically stable, much of this care is tapered, and restoration of visual function becomes the focus of rehabilitation.

There are many areas of health care where, because of the limitations of surgical and medical treatment, functional professions have developed side by side with medical specialties to provide restoration of function. Orthopedic surgeons typically refer to physical or occupational therapists to help restore strength and range of motion. Otolaryngologists frequently refer to speech pathologists to help restore auditory perception, speech, and swallowing. Neuro-otologists refer to physical therapists to provide vestibular therapy. Psychiatrists prescribe psychotropic medications, but also refer to psychologists and counselors for cognitive and emotional therapies. Physiatrists and neurologists refer for neuropsychological evaluation. In all of these relationships, the functional practitioner must have a basic understanding of the medical–surgical interventions available, to properly treat and dialogue with the involved medical practitioner. The medical clinician must have a basic understanding of what the functional practitioner is capable of to make good referrals.

In the rehabilitation setting, ophthalmology and optometry must have a similar symbiotic relationship where the interests of full rehabilitation of the patient come first. Frequent referral in both directions should be the rule, with optometrists referring to ophthalmology for advanced medical–surgical intervention, or when there is an unusual neuro-ophthalmic presentation where a neuro-opthalmologist may be able to better diagnose, and ophthalmologists referring to optometrists with special training in vision therapy, low vision rehabilitation, and vision rehabilitation therapy for restoration of visual function. To date, most of these referral relationships have been built between individuals, as it is uncommon for organized ophthalmology or ophthalmological residencies to discuss the functional aspects of the visual system and the fact that optometrists are the vision care professionals who are trained in this area. This is in part due to the fact that most optometrists do not fully utilize their basic training in this area, and so many ophthalmologists are unaware of the extent of the optometric training in functional and rehabilitation vision care.

Because of the practicalities of rehabilitation, optometrists will often provide additional training in vision rehabilitation therapy to occupational therapists who are already in place on a daily basis in the rehabilitation hospitals and centers. The optometrist's role in this case becomes one of diagnosing and guiding/prescribing the necessary vision rehabilitation (see Chapters 2 and 12). Lastly, both ophthalmology and optometry refer to orientation and mobility specialists for patients with severe visual field or visual acuity deficits. Orientation and mobility specialists have in-depth training in teaching those with low vision safe mobility skills and facilitate functional management in the home.

A MODEL FOR ORGANIZING VISION REHABILITATION

Often, models of information processing or reading will begin with a box labeled "sensory input," or "visual input." Exposure to such models may give the nonvision specialist the impression that the processing of the visual system is discrete enough to fit into such a box.

As you read the chapters to follow, there will be a multitude of vision deficits to test for and attend to in the vision rehabilitation patient. There are more than 32 visual areas in the cerebral cortex with over 300 pathways between them, most of them bidirectional,[16] in addition to multiple subcortical areas, and six of the twelve cranial nerves, creating an incredible array of neural networks involved in processing vision. While it is necessary to have a sound understanding of the basic neural underpinnings of vision to formulate appropriate diagnoses, knowing the neural pathways does not provide an adequate basis for guiding vision rehabilitation therapy. A model is required to take what we know about the function of visual neural substrates and translate it into function in the therapy room and daily life.

Working without an overall model may encourage attempts to rehabilitate "splinter" skills, when a more holistic approach to the visual system is required to create a stable reorganization in the visual system. Visual input and processing are pervasive throughout the brain, and individual skills cannot be so easily segregated in therapy. Chapter 4 provides good examples of this, where the authors explain how one must be able to understand space to effectively move and coordinate pointing the two eyes to various positions in space. That chapter is a long one, because it was supposed to be one chapter on eye movements and binocular vision, and a separate chapter on spatial vision. However, and rightfully so, neither of the authors could figure out where the subject matter for one chapter ended and the other began; understanding of space and where and how to point your eyes to process space are inextricably intertwined. The model below (Figure 1.1) is an extreme simplification that serves to remind one about the areas of vision that should be examined and how they relate to other functions.

The model begins with sensory input or reception, which includes optical, ocular motor, accommodative, binocular, and early neural processing up to the level of primary visual cortex, which includes consideration of visual fields, light sensitivity, and early color processing. It must now also include nonimage forming pathways that regulate diurnal rhythms (Chapters 3 and 8). Perception/integration includes organization of both object perception and spatial perception, understanding objects in space not only in relation to the observer, but also in relation to each other; and integrating this with other sensory inputs. Motor output/behavior is the action that we take on the basis of visual input. If the input is threatening, then we use midbrain pathways to take us straight from reception to action. Ordinarily, we work through the longer cortical perception pathways to action. Our motor outputs lead to body orientation, which influences our sensory input. Both our motor output/behavior and our perceptions influence our visual thinking and memory.

Note that all of the arrows are bidirectional, with the major direction of information flow indicated by the closed head arrows. For instance, this means that our perceptions, motor output, body orientation, and, indirectly our thinking and memory affect where we move our eyes next—feeding back to what has traditionally been thought of as reception. They also affect processing of visual input at the level of the lateral geniculate nucleus on the way to primary visual cortex, where only 10%–20% of the connections are afferent from the retina, and the rest are modulating connections, feeding forward from higher processing levels (Chapter 3).

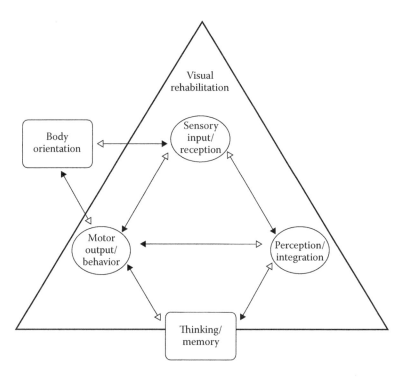

FIGURE 1.1 A model for guiding rehabilitation of the visual system. See text for explanation. (From Ashley, M.J. (Ed.), *Traumatic Brain Injury Rehabilitation,* 2nd ed., CRC Press, Boca Raton, FL, 2004, p. 217. Reprinted with permission.)

PREVALENCE AND IMPACT OF ACQUIRED BRAIN INJURY

MILD TRAUMATIC BRAIN INJURY

According to the U.S. Centers for Disease Control and Prevention, mild traumatic brain injury (mTBI) is

> … the occurrence of injury to the head arising from blunt trauma or acceleration or deceleration forces with one or more of the following conditions attributable to the injury: any period of observed or self-reported transient confusion, disorientation or impaired consciousness; dysfunction of memory around of the time of injury; or loss of consciousness lasting less than 30 minutes.' In addition: observed signs of neurological or neuropsychological dysfunction, such as: seizures acutely following injury to the head; irritability, lethargy, or vomiting following head injury, especially among infants and very young children; headaches, dizziness, irritability, fatigue or poor concentration, especially among older children and adults. (p. 4)[17]

Of the more than 1.5 million people experiencing TBI each year in the United States, it has been estimated that 75% experience mTBI.[18] It is important to note that while the name "Mild" TBI seems to imply that the injury is of little consequence, many studies have demonstrated that mTBI can have severe consequences.

A good example is the study by Vanderploeg et al.,[19] who studied Vietnam era veterans, and compared 254 veterans who had suffered mTBI, to 539 veterans who had suffered motor vehicle accident but no mTBI, and 3,214 controls. The mTBI patient group reported a high percentage of postconcussion syndrome (PCS), between 37% and 41%, dependant on the definition used, as compared to the other two groups that reported between 19% and 25% PCS. PCS includes lingering symptoms such as headache, dizziness, malaise, fatigue, noise intolerance, loss of concentration, memory and intellectual difficulties, and insomnia, as well as affective disorders such as irritability, depression, anxiety, and affective lability. Vanderploeg and colleagues also found that mTBI was associated with peripheral visual imperceptions and impaired tandem (heel to toe) gait. The mTBI group in this study also had poorer psychosocial outcomes, including increased likelihood of self-reported disability, underemployment, low income and marital problems.

Brains Change in Mild Traumatic Brain Injury

Functional Imaging

Because the effects of mTBI on the brain have, until recently, not been reliably imageable with computed tomography (CT) or standard magnetic resonance imaging (MRI) techniques, the existence of mTBI as an entity that can have lasting sequelae has periodically been called into question. However, more recently, functional MRI (fMRI) techniques, such as blood oxygen level dependent (BOLD), and diffusion tensor (DT) MR imaging are able to demonstrate acute changes in the brain following mTBI, often even in patients with Glasgow Coma Scores of 15 (i.e., fully oriented) at the time of the injury. Miles et al.[20] found a relationship between DT imaging measures within days of the injury and neuropsychological tests of executive function 6 months later. Slobounov et al.[21] using BOLD fMRI imaging in normally functioning athletes who had recently suffered mTBI, demonstrated increased area of the brain recruited in multiple locations during a virtual reality spatial encoding and navigation task as compared to controls. Slobounov et al. hypothesized that this expansion of active brain matter may be the beginning of permanent brain reorganization to allow the participant to continue to perform at a high level in spite of damage. They called for longitudinal imaging studies to further test this hypothesis. Chen et al.[22] used BOLD imaging to evaluate male athletes with and without concussion, who were grouped according to their PCS score. Chen and colleagues found that severity of PCS predicted fMRI BOLD signal changes in cerebral prefrontal regions.

Histopathology

Bigler[23] has reported on a 47-year-old male who sustained an mTBI characterized by a brief loss of consciousness and a Glasgow Coma Score of 14 (see Appendix 12.1, Chapter 12) only 7 months before an unexpected and unrelated cardiac death. Microscopic analysis demonstrated hemosiderin-laden macrophages in the white matter and perivascular spaces in the brain, particularly in the frontal lobe, demonstrating that recovery from trauma was still in progress. He had partially returned to work at the time of his death, but was experiencing cognitive difficulties in his work.

Participants in sports who suffer multiple concussion-type injuries have a higher risk of developing severe brain disease—chronic traumatic encephalopathy, initially described in National Football League players (e.g., Omalu et al. 2005, 2006)[24,25] and, more generally, chronic TBI.[26]

Vision Deficits in Mild Traumatic Brain Injury

Post trauma vision syndrome (PTVS) is the most common visual sequel of mTBI.[27] PTVS is a constellation of signs and symptoms that may include convergence insufficiency, high exophoria or exotropia, accommodative dysfunction, low blink rate, difficulties in attention and concentration, ocular motor deficits, and visual-spatial distortions with associated neuromotor affects. Padula[28] has also hypothesized that PTVS (and the associated visual-spatial dysfunction) results from damage to the midbrain, where the superior colliculi organize and integrate visual sensory information into spatial maps at a very basic level. This makes neuroanatomical sense, as the midbrain contains ocular motor centers for convergence,[29,30] and is anatomically placed such that it is subject to whiplash and rotational forces in traumatic injury.

It is important to remember that the vision system is a covert input system and most patients with vision problems following TBI will demonstrate visual deficits in terms of coordination, balance, veering during mobility, ability to concentrate for nearpoint tasks, inability to tolerate visually crowded or busy places, and difficulty reading that may or may not be related to blur. Although any system in the brain can be affected during mTBI, many of the signs and symptoms of PCS, headache, disorientation, fatigue, and poor concentration are also seen in visual dysfunction. Another symptom of visual dysfunction following mTBI is spatial vision dysfunction or anomalous egocentric localization, which can lead to balance problems and impaired tandem gait (as found in Vanderploeg's study above) (see Chapters 4, 6, and 7). Delayed visual memory deficits are also common following both mTBI and moderate to severe TBI.[31] It is important to include a thorough post-brain injury vision evaluation by a functional vision care provider who can determine which of the signs and symptoms arise from a visual etiology.

Lachapelle et al.[32] evaluated evoked potentials to both low-level visual stimuli and event-related potentials to a cognitive "oddball" paradigm. They found that patients with mTBI who demonstrated increased latency in the event-related potentials to texture and cognitive stimuli were at significantly greater risk of negative vocational outcome than participants with mTBI, but normal event-related potentials. Padula and colleagues found that patients diagnosed with PTVS demonstrated decreased visually evoked potential (VEP) amplitude, and that VEP amplitudes in these patients often normalized with application of binasal patches and low amounts of base in prism.[33] Freed and Hellerstein[34] demonstrated normalization of VEPs in adults with mTBI following a program of vision rehabilitation therapy, where the VEPs of matched control patients with mTBI who did not receive vision rehabilitation therapy did not normalize.

MODERATE TO SEVERE TRAUMATIC BRAIN INJURY

Traumatic brain injury is a significant cause of disability in the United States. As reviewed by Crooks et al.[35] following severe TBI, most survivors are disabled to some degree. More than 90% of people suffering a moderate TBI will be able to live independently, although perhaps in a supported environment where assistance for such things as medications, financial management, accommodations for minor physical impairments, or assisted employment. TBI is remarkable in that with shearing of pathways and diffuse axonal injury, deficits can be widespread and multidimensional. Working with TBI patients is the most challenging aspect in a vision practice, as the clinician must use the full scope of their education to test for pathology of the eye, adnexa and orbit, ocular motor deficits, binocular dysfunction, object perception, visual attention, perception, and memory, as well as spatial vision deficits and the associated effects on balance and mobility.

As Crooks et al.[35] point out, visual function incorporates widespread areas of the central nervous system, including brainstem, subcortical, limbic, cerebellar, and cerebral cortical areas. Thus it is difficult to suffer a significant TBI, without suffering significant visual dysfunction. Goodrich et al.[36] in a sample of polytrauma patients, whose injuries occurred in combat situations, found that 74% complained of vision difficulties, and visual impairment was confirmed in 38% of those patients. The rate of visual impairment in blast-related injury was 52%. They conclude that comprehensive eye examinations should be routinely administered in the polytrauma population. As with mTBI, PTVS, and visual memory loss should be tested for in the more severely injured TBI population. Speed of processing is another common problem following TBI (see Chapter 11).

Lepore, in a study of 60 patients with post-TBI ophthalmoplegia found that 39% had CN IV (trochlear) palsies, 33% had CN III (oculomotor) palsies, 14% had CN VI (abducens) palsies, 10% had combined palsies, and 4% had restrictive ophthalmopathy.[37] Nine of the patients had supranuclear dysfunction (see Chapter 12), seven of whom demonstrated convergence insufficiency. This number is probably significantly underestimated, as Lepore used the "push up" technique in his diagnosis of convergence insufficiency. Krohel et al.[38] found that 6 of 23 TBI patients with convergence insufficiency had normal nearpoint of convergence, but showed abnormal convergence ranges on prism vergence testing. Cohen et al.[39] found convergence insufficiency in approximately 40% of both TBI inpatients with recent injuries, and outpatient follow up patients 3 years postinjury. This implies that TBI-related convergence insufficiency does not spontaneously regress. Convergence insufficiency is associated with asthenopic symptoms, fatigue with nearpoint work, diplopia, difficulty concentrating on nearpoint tasks, and reading difficulty. Cohen and colleagues found that in the follow-up group, convergence insufficiency was positively associated with duration of coma, dysphasia, cognitive disturbances, and failure to find placement in nonsupported work situations. Ciuffreda et al.[40] examined ocular motor dysfunction in a retrospective analysis of 160 patients with TBI and 60 patients with cerebral vascular accident (CVA). Similar to Cohen's findings, Ciuffreda found convergence insufficiency in 42% of the TBI patients and 35% of CVA patients. The percentage of patients demonstrating any type of ocular motor dysfunction was 90% in the TBI patients and 86% in the CVA patients.

Schlageter and colleagues found that 59% of TBI patients in their rehabilitation hospital-based sample were impaired on one or more ocular motor or binocular findings.[41] For patients with deficits in pursuits or saccades, a 2-week no-treatment baseline was followed by a 4-week trial of vision rehabilitation exercises. While some patients demonstrated no improvement during the baseline and good improvement in ocular motor skills during the treatment regimen, the sample size was small, the treatment period brief, and this effect did not reach significance. The authors did note that they found that programming a hierarchy of progressively more difficult exercises required a significant amount of training and that it would be useful to refer to an appropriate eye doctor. Kapoor and colleagues have published protocols for ocular motor testing and training following brain injury.[42,43] This same research group[44] also examined follow-up data on 40 patients with TBI or CVA, who completed vision rehabilitation therapy for their oculomotor dysfunction and found that 90% of patients with TBI and 100% of their sample with CVA were treated successfully with improvements in ocular motor skills and symptom reductions stable at retesting 2–3 months later.

Visual field loss (discussed in Chapter 5) is another common finding following TBI. Visual field loss and visual memory loss has previously been negatively correlated with return to work[45] although with proper vision rehabilitation and aids, most forms of visual field loss should not prohibit return to work (see Chapters 5 and 7). Perceptual impairments are common in patients with severe TBI. In a study of patients hospitalized for TBI, McKenna et al.[46] found that 45% of patients who suffered severe TBI had unilateral neglect, and there were 26% each, who demonstrated impairments of body scheme and constructional skills.

STROKE

Stroke, or CVA, is the second leading cause of death worldwide resulting in 9% of all deaths.[47] Approximately 80% of strokes are ischemic, caused by vessel occlusion. The remainder is hemorrhagic, with the most common mechanism being hypertensive small vessel disease.

CVA results in a more localized pathology than traumatic mechanisms of brain injury. The CVA patient may still exhibit any of the visual deficits that are common in TBI. However, the deficits are frequently more specific, with fewer aspects of visual (and other systems) dysfunction exhibited in any given patient. As discussed above, patients with CVA will suffer ocular motor and binocular dysfunction at close to the rate of patients with TBI. However, they are also much more likely to suffer from unilateral spatial neglect and hemianopia or other visual field loss. Unilateral spatial neglect, is an inability to attend to, and therefore perceive an entire hemispace, most markedly, to the left. It has been reported in up to 70% of hospitalized stroke patients.[48] It is critical to test CVA patients carefully for neglect, in all of its various forms (see Chapter 5), as by definition, the patient will not know they have a problem. Certainly many of these patients recover spontaneously. However, in our clinical experience, many CVA patients are sent home with undiagnosed neglect, which puts them at risk for injury.

CASE PRESENTATIONS

It is well documented through numerous studies, and the following chapters in this book that patients with ABI show many types of visual dysfunction, including accommodative, binocular, ocular motor, refractive error shift, visual field loss, visual-spatial disorientation, visual-motor integration, and visual information processing deficits. These problems can occur with mild, moderate, or severe ABI.

Patients often receive retina surgery for detachments, or glaucoma surgery to reduce intraocular pressures. These surgeries are considered medically necessary and important in managing the disease process, as well as improving quality of life for the patient. The treatment does not necessarily cure the patient, but can make a significant difference in functioning and in the quality of life for the patient. The same analogy is present in the field of vision rehabilitation. Since approximately two-thirds of the sensory input to brain is attributable to vision, it is critical to evaluate and appropriately treat patients who have suffered brain injuries. The cases in this chapter demonstrate significant changes in many visual skill and visual processing parameters resulting in quality of life changes.

The patient case history vignettes that follow demonstrate the types of visual dysfunctions discussed in other chapters in this book and include not only the history, diagnosis, and treatment (referencing the relevant chapters in the book) but also the real-life outcomes for the patients and their families. These cases illustrate both the types of patients and visual deficits that one encounters when working in vision rehabilitation, and the reason that you should be practicing or referring patients for vision rehabilitation therapy.

Each of the following case studies was gleaned from the patient files of the contributing authors in this book. These cases illustrate the breadth of visual rehabilitation patients who come in the door of the post-brain injury vision rehabilitation practitioner, and provide guides to the chapters in which one can find information regarding the clinical entities and treatments discussed.

JK

History

JK is a 32-year-old white female, who hit the back of her head in a fall at a restaurant where she was a waitress. She reportedly did not lose consciousness, but she was confused and disoriented for several minutes. JK was referred for a vision evaluation, by her neurologist, $2^{1}/_{2}$ years postinjury. She had been diagnosed with mTBI, whiplash, and cervical strain, and was still not able to work, drive, or perform many of her activities of daily living such as grocery shopping, cooking, writing, reading, paying bills, or driving. Her medications included Depakote and ibuprofen.[49]

Symptoms

JK's symptoms included frequent frontal headaches (one to two times weekly), intermittent diplopia, blurred vision, light sensitivity, difficulty with motor function, poor balance, as well as difficulty with attention, concentration, and organization.

Findings
- Ocular health: both internal and external ocular health were unremarkable; pupils equal, round, and responsive to light, intraocular pressures normal.
- Visual acuity with correction.
  - Distance: right eye (OD) 20/20, left eye (OS) 20/25.
  - Near: OD 20/30, OS 20/60 (with variability and decompensation of visual acuity with the left eye as the examination continued, to 20/200).
- Refraction.
  - Distance retinoscopy: OD +2.50D, OS +2.00 (dull reflex).
  - Refraction was variable and gave inconsistent results.
- Cover test.
  - Distance: orthophoria (i.e., aligned).
  - Near: 10 prism diopters intermittent alternating exotropia.
- Near point of convergence (NPC): 10 inches break/14 inches recovery—decompensates with multiple trials.
- Vergences: Risley prism testing (blur/diplopia/regain fusion).
  - Distance: base out, X/6/2; Base in, X/12/6.
  - Near: unable to test due to diplopia.
- Fixation disparity: exo deviation with instability and alternating suppression (see Chapter 7).
- Accommodation.
  - Positive relative accommodation (PRA) and negative relative accommodation (NRA): unable to test binocularly due to diplopia.
  - Dynamic near retinoscopy: (see Chapter 12).
    - OD variable reflex from +2.00D to +3.00D.
    - OS +.75 D (dull reflex).
  - Accommodative facility testing.
    - Monocular: unable to clear ±2.00 flipper monocularly.
    - Binocular: unable to test due to diplopia.
- Ocular motilities.
  - Pursuits: concomitant with full excursions in all fields of gaze, but with frequent loss of fixation. The patient demonstrated tearing and discomfort during this testing.
  - Saccades: could not be performed without head movements.
- Goldmann visual field testing: generalized constriction of the peripheral isopters for both eyes. There was a homonymous, incongruous lower right quadrantanopia. There was also baring of the physiological blindspot on the left side (Figure 1.2A).
- Visual midline (spatial localization): egocentric visual midline (see Chapter 6) was variable and inconsistent. JK could not accurately grasp or point at objects within arm's reach. She needed assistance in walking long distances because of fatigue and poor balance. She was unable to walk heel to toe on a straight line.
- Electrodiagnostic evaluation: visual evoked potentials demonstrated normal waveform values for each eye on first trial. The second trial showed P100

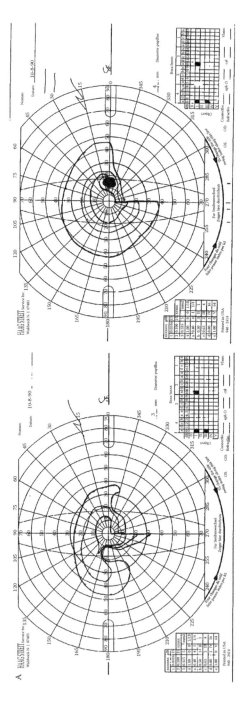

FIGURE 1.2 A: Goldmann visual fields pre-vision rehabilitation therapy. Right eye is represented on the right side. B: Goldmann visual fields post-vision rehabilitation therapy. Right eye is represented on the right side. (From Hellerstein, L.F., and Freed, S., Rehabilitative optometric management of a traumatic brain injury patient. *J. Behav. Optomet.*, 5(6), 143–147, 1994. With permission.)

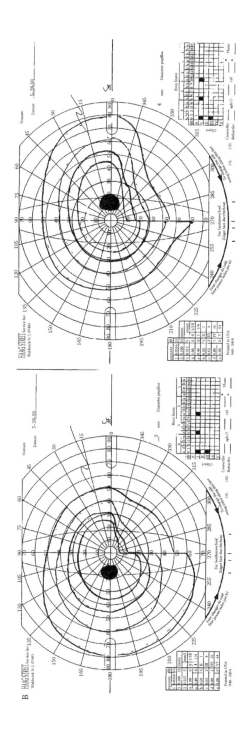

FIGURE 1.2 Continued

latency delays with decreased interwave amplitude responses for the left eye and normal latency values and a decreased interwave amplitude for the right. The third trial demonstrated no consistent or organized waveform responses for the left eye and delays in P100 latency values and further decreased interwave amplitude responses for the right (Figure 1.3A).

Impressions and Diagnoses
- mTBI per JK's neurologist.
- Photophobia.
- Hyperopia.
- Convergence insufficiency intermittent exotropia at near.
- Accommodative dysfunction.
- Ocular motor dysfunctions in pursuits and saccades.
- Photophobia, accommodative insufficiency, convergence insufficiency exotropia, and egocentric visual midline disturbances are consistent with a diagnosis of PTVS (Chapter 6).
- Homonymous incongruous lower right quadrantanopia.
- Abnormal conduction in the anterior visual pathway, greater for the left eye than the right.

Treatment and Management
Two pairs of glasses were prescribed; one pair for distance, +1.00D OU, and a near prescription of +2.00D OU combined with two prism diopters base in OU (see Chapter 6, post trauma vision syndrome). Both glasses included a prescribed tint to decrease light sensitivity (see Chapter 9). Sunglasses and a visor/hat were recommended for outdoors. Rehabilitative vision therapy was prescribed, but delayed for 1 year due to insurance approval difficulties. Weekly vision rehabilitation therapy sessions with home activities were given for a total of 8 months.

The vision therapy plan progressed from equalizing monocular ocular motor skills to improving fusional vergences, increasing accommodative flexibility and eliminating suppression. At the same time, spatial awareness, localization, and balance/movement activities were also emphasized to bring ocular motor, binocular, and spatial perception into balance. Visualization activities, including tachistoscope flash and parquetry block series were utilized to reinforce concepts of spatial relations. Throughout vision rehabilitation, therapeutic yoked prisms (see Chapter 7) were found to be especially useful in developing localization ability and spatial awareness.

Posttreatment Findings
- Visual acuity (wearing refractive correction).
  - Stable 20/20 at distance and near with either eye.
- Refraction.
  - Distance retinoscopy: +2.00 sphere in either eye.
- Cover test.
  - Distance: orthophoria.
  - Near: 8 prism diopters exophoria.
  - NPC: 5 inches break/8 inches recovery.

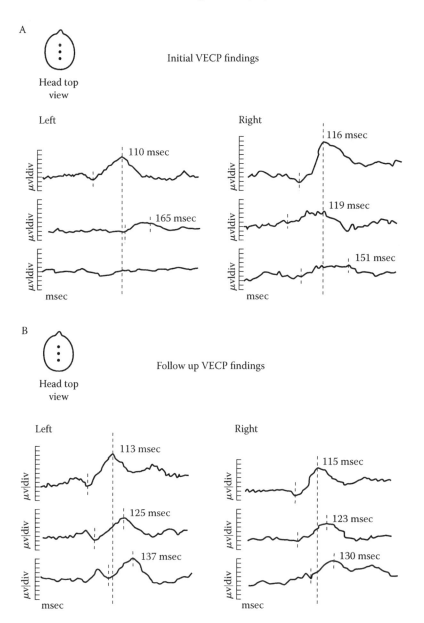

FIGURE 1.3 A: Visually evoked responses pre-vision rehabilitation therapy. B: Visually evoked responses postvision rehabilitation therapy. (From Hellerstein, L.F., and Freed, S., Rehabilitative optometric management of a traumatic brain injury patient. *Journal of Behavioral Optometry*, 5(6), 143–148, 1994. With permission.)

- Vergences: Risley prism testing (blur/diplopia/regain fusion).
  - Distance: base out, 16/20/6; base in, X/10/6.
  - Near: base out, X/14/3; base in, X/24/17.
- Fixation disparity: no deviation.
- Accommodation.
  - PRA +1.00 diopter.
  - NRA −2.00 diopter.
- Ocular motilities.
  - Pursuits: full, unrestricted with good fixation, and no discomfort.
  - Saccades: accurate, with no head movement.
- Goldmann visual field testing: very mild constriction of the peripheral isopters for both eyes in all meridians. The homonymous, incongruous lower right quadrantanopia is much improved. There was no baring of the physiological blindspot on the left as in her initial fields (Figure 1.2B).
- Visual midline (spatial localization): consistent visual midline, which was accurate when wearing glasses. JK was more stable, with better balance when walking.
- Electrodiagnostic evaluation: visual evoked potentials demonstrated normal waveform values for each eye on the first two trials. On the third trial, there was loss of P100 conduction with decreased amplitude responses for P100 for each eye, consistent with loss of both accommodation and attention (Figure 1.3B).

Summary

Subjectively, JK had significant decrease in symptomatology: less double vision; decrease in headache frequency; less visual confusion and blurriness; and improved balance, attention, and organizational skills. She was now able to resume some of her household daily chores such as cooking, cleaning, and shopping. She could read again and started driving. JK could hold a part-time job and was able to shop for herself.

This case is consistent with symptomatology encountered with many patients diagnosed as having a "mild TBI." The term "mild TBI" is very misleading and does not necessarily translate to "mild functional loss" as these injuries can have a devastating impact on function. It is also interesting to note that treatment was initiated over $2^1/_2$ years postinjury, which eliminates "spontaneous recovery" as an explanation for improvement in this patient's visual system deficits. Rehabilitative vision treatment was found to improve not only JK's visual function, but also her overall function in activities of daily living.

VG

History

VG is a 60-year-old male, previously CEO of a thriving company, who suffered an anoxic incident during an elective surgery 4 years before this evaluation. He was referred by his new occupational therapist for neuro-optometric evaluation after having completed all of his formal therapies excepting for occupational therapy for spasticity in his hands. VG had, until the last year, been in the care of an occupational therapist, physical therapist, and orthopedic surgeon. VG had significant difficulty with balance and was transporting in a wheel chair. He had a full-time caretaker to assist with most activities of daily living like bathing, dressing, cooking, driving, reading, writing, and grocery shopping. VG was pleasant and conversant. His visual symptoms were only elicited upon detailed history taking (Chapter 12), as he did not think of them as visual deficits, but as unfortunate consequences of his brain injury, which he would have to accept.

Symptoms

VG's symptoms included headaches while watching TV, blurred vision, double vision, and inability to read due to difficulty with both tracking (Chapter 4) and comprehension, as well as difficulty with memory (Chapter 11). He had severe difficulty with writing, both due to the spasticity in his hands, and the inability to understand how to form the letters (Chapters 4 and 10), even though he could read individual letters and words.

Findings

- Ocular health: unremarkable for his age
- Visual acuity: best corrected
  - Distance: OD 20/20, OS 20/20
  - Near: OD 20/20, OS 20/20

VG neglected to read the letters on the left side of acuity chart (Chapter 5).

- Refraction.
  - Distance: OD +1.25D − 0.75 × 105, OS +0.75D sphere.
- Cover test.
  - Distance: orthophoria.
  - Near: 3 prism diopters left hyperphoria.
  - NPC: 15 inches break/20 inches recovery.
- Dissociated phorias.
  - Distance: orthophoria.
  - Near: 6 prism diopters exophoria.
- Vergences.
  - Near: base out, X/18/6.
- Accommodation: presbyopia.
- Ocular motilities.
  - Pursuits: full and smooth in all fields of gaze.
  - Saccades per DEM testing: extremely poor, scoring 12–22 standard deviations below expectancies for ceiling age; testing was confounded by his poor ability to track print in any direction (these should also have been evaluated qualitatively) (Chapter 12).
- Contrast sensitivity: OD: moderately reduced to low-, mid-, and high-spatial frequencies; OS: moderately reduced to mid-spatial frequencies.
- Visual field testing: visual fields were essentially full to 60 degrees on automated testing, and full to confrontation.
- Sensorimotor testing.
  - Visual midline (spatial localization): VG demonstrated confusion on this test, waiting until the target passed his objective straight ahead point before responding, at any speed, in any direction.

TABLE 1.1
TVPS Results Pre-vision Rehabilitation Therapy

Subtest	Raw Score	Percentile Based on Ceiling Age
Visual discrimination	1	1st
Visual memory	1	1st
Visual-spatial relations	1	1st
Visual form constancy	5	1st
Visual sequential memory	11	5th
Visual figure ground	1	1st

- Line bisection cross-out task (see Chapter 5): VG did not bisect (neglected) most of the lines on the left side of the page, and those that he attempted to bisect were bisected to the far right, particularly on the left side of the page, indicating significant left peripersonal neglect.
- Visual-motor accuracy: poor with either eye or both.
- Visual-motor speed: poor with either eye or both (see Chapter 12).
- Visual-perceptual speed: poor for flashed and moving targets (see Chapter 12).
- Test of visual-perceptual skills-R (TVPS-R): see Table 1.1.

Impressions and Diagnoses
- Hyperopia.
- Astigmatism.
- Presbyopia.
- Convergence insufficiency.
- Left hyperphoria.
- Ocular motor dysfunctions in saccades.
- Severe left peripersonal neglect and associated spatial confusion.
- Severe visual-perceptual deficits as determined by the TVPS-R. His answers tended toward the left side of the test card such that the presentation format was judged to be appropriate, in spite of his left peripersonal neglect.
- Deficits in visual-perceptual speed, visual-motor speed, and visual-motor accuracy.
- Reduced contrast sensitivity.

Treatment and Management
The following bifocal glasses were prescribed: OD: +0.75 – 0.75 × 105 with 1 prism diopter base up OD; OS: +0.50D sphere: add: +2.50D. Once weekly in-office vision rehabilitation therapy with 45 minutes of homework per day was prescribed. VG's vision rehabilitation goals were to be able to read without skipping lines or getting lost, to reduce headaches, and to be able to sign papers.

VG completed 112 vision therapy sessions, 1 session per week. The following deficits were addressed:

- *Binocularity:* close eye stretches, monocular prism jumps, tranaglyphic fusion charts adding base out and base down OD as able.
- *Saccades:* large Hart chart, letter tracking, Space Fixator, line counting.
- *Visual-spatial relations:* Geoboards, Dot-to-Dot construction, Which Stick, Set game, Rush Hour game, Mazes, Perceptual worksheets, Space Matching.
- *Left neglect:* Wall/Pokercard scanning, McGraw card, Acuvision scanning, Tabletop pick-up manipulatives wearing 20 prism diopters yoked bases left, Dot-to-Dot construction, "Complete a picture" drawings, Backspace ball (see Chapters 5 and 7).
- *Visual-perceptual deficits:* Parquetry series, Geoboards with and without memory, Flannelboards with and without memory, Perceptual Worksheets, Where's Waldo, Word search, Hidden Picture's, What's different, Which Stick.
- *Visual-motor accuracy and speed:* Acuvision, VMI series, Kirshner arrows, Slap Taps.
- *Other visual deficits:* while in vision therapy other visual deficits were revealed. VG demonstrated significant difficulty with spatial relations and visual confusion. Concepts like closer or further away, to the right or left, above or below, from a point of reference were very confusing for him. He had no idea that this was true until he started his vision rehabilitation therapy. When asked to simply place a pen above a pencil, which was placed on the table in front of him, he got very frustrated since he knew what above and below meant but was unable to do this task. Other tasks, like staying on the path of a simple maze, were very difficult for him. Even when the pathway was highlighted, VG would get off the path, not because he could not accomplish the motor task, but because he could not understand what it meant to be on or off the path. While there may have been an apraxic element (see Chapter 10), there was clearly also severe spatial confusion.

Posttreatment Findings
- Ocular health: unchanged
- Visual acuity: best corrected
  - Distance: OD 20/20, OS 20/20
  - Near: OD 20/20, OS 20/20

VG was not neglecting the letters on the left side of acuity chart anymore.

- Refraction.
  - Distance: OD +1.25D – 0.50 × 100, OS +0.50D sphere.
- Cover test.
  - Distance: orthophoria.
  - Near: orthophoria.
  - NPC: 4 inches break.

TABLE 1.2
TVPS Results Post-Vision Rehabilitation Therapy

Subtest	Raw Score	Percentile Based on Ceiling Age
Visual discrimination	4	1st
Visual memory	7	1st
Visual-spatial relations	3	1st
Visual form constancy	8	1st
Visual sequential memory	8	1st
Visual figure ground	1	1st

- Dissociated phorias.
  - Distance: 1.5 prism diopters base up OD.
  - Near: 1 prism diopter exophoria.
- Vergences.
  - Near: base out, X/26/16.
- Accommodation: presbyopia.
- Ocular motilities.
  - Pursuits: full and smooth in all fields of gaze.
  - Saccades per DEM testing: improved significantly to only 2–7 standard deviations below age expectancies for ceiling age.
- Visual field testing: unchanged.
- Sensorimotor testing.
  - Line bisection.
  - Visual-motor accuracy: moderate with either eye or both.
  - TVPS-R tested after 45 sessions. Even though the percentile score did not change, improvements can be seen in the raw scores in Table 1.2.

Summary

During his course of vision therapy, VG had significantly improved his balance, due to his improving spatial awareness and diminished peripersonal neglect. He was less dependent on his wheel chair and was able to walk using a four point cane, in spite of the fact that he had been unable to accomplish this task during his years of physical therapy (Chapters 4 through 7). He became interested in reading again and increased reading speed, comprehension, and endurance to where reading was not frustrating anymore. He no longer required help finding the left and right margins of the print. When VG started vision therapy, reading text in columns, as in newspapers, was nearly impossible. Finding things in drawers and cabinets was no longer an overwhelming task. Before coming to vision therapy, VG's world was very confusing and frustrating. Through hard work and dedication, his outlook on life changed significantly. His caretaker, who had become his good friend throughout the process, enjoyed VG's increased independence as well. They were much more able to get out of the house and enjoy going places. VG's case demonstrates two very important points about vision rehabilitation therapy. Had his vision evaluation been performed while he was in active therapy with the rest of his rehabilitation team, he would have walked years earlier and had the advantage of physical therapy helping him with gait, as the vision therapy improved his spatial perception to the point where he could maintain his balance. The second point is that even with extraordinary visual-spatial perception deficits, VG was entirely unaware that he had any sort of visual problem. He assumed that his inability to read was a thinking problem and his inability to stand was a motor problem.

DM

History

DM was referred by a friend for a neuro-optometric evaluation. He was a 41-year-old male who was diagnosed with multiple sclerosis (MS) 20 years previously. He recently experienced a MS flare-up 7 months previous to this vision evaluation. Recently he had been evaluated by a neuro-ophthalmologist who prescribed 4 prism diopters base-down right eye Fresnel prism for vertical diplopia. DM still complained of diplopia (even with his prism glasses). His overall MS symptoms were variable depending on his level of fatigue, stress, and when he had last taken his medications. His visual problems were also part of this variability. DM was currently receiving physical therapy.

His medications included Rebif shots, Aspirin, Baclofen, Lipitor, Plavix, Provigil, and Gabapentin.

Symptoms

His symptoms included diplopia, headaches, decreased balance, and photophobia. Since his flare-up, DM patched or covered an eye with most activities, as the diplopia impacted his balance even more. DM was very angry, wanted to avoid the use of prisms, and just didn't understand the nature of his visual problem.

Findings

- Ocular health: internal and external health was unremarkable for both eyes; pupils equal, round, and responsive to light, intraocular pressures normal.
- Visual acuity with glasses.
  - Distance: OD 20/25, OS 20/20.
  - Near: OD 20/20, OS 20/20 (with +1.50D add).
- Refraction.
  - Distance: OD +1.50D − 1.00 × 115, OS +0.25D sphere.
- Cover test.
  - Distance: 7 prism diopters right hypertropia with 6 prism diopters exotropia.
  - Near: 6 prism diopters right hypertropia with 4 prism diopters exotropia.
- Vergences.
  - Diplopia, unable to obtain fusion.
- Accommodation.
  - Presbyopia, requires +1.50D add.
- Ocular motilities.
  - Pursuits: full excursions in all fields of gaze, but with endpoint nystagmus.
- Visual field testing: visual fields were full with either eye.

Impressions and Diagnoses
- MS by history
- Right hypertropia
- Exotropia
- Diplopia
- Ocular motor dysfunction
- Presbyopia

Treatment and Management

Two pairs of glasses were prescribed. One pair for distance—OD: +1.50 − 1.00 × 115 with 6 prism diopters base down OD, OS: +0.25 sphere. One pair for near—OD: +3.00 − 1.00 × 115 with 6 prism diopters base down OD, OS: +1.75 sphere. A spot patch occluder was prescribed to use when the diplopia became bothersome, therefore eliminating the need to close or cover an eye. Utilizing "magic tape" for the spot patch made it very easy for DM to take the patch on and off his glasses as needed.

Posttreatment Findings
- No significant change

Summary

Patients diagnosed with MS and other neurologic diseases often present with visual dysfunctions effecting visual acuity, eye alignment, ocular motility, balance, and depth perception. These problems may improve with time, only to reappear with other flare ups. Since it already had been 7 months since DM's symptoms increased, spontaneous recovery or remission was more unlikely.

Due to lack of insurance coverage for treatment, DM could only attend four vision therapy sessions. The emphasis of the short-term rehabilitative vision therapy program was to assist DM in understanding his visual deficits, learn to utilize the spot patch (Chapters 4 and 12), learn to utilize the prism appropriately (Chapter 7), and learn to adapt and compensate for tasks such as reading, tracking, and so on. At the completion of the four sessions, DM's attitude had completely shifted. He commented that, "I now have tools to work with. Sometimes I can see singly, but at least I don't get so upset when I have the double vision. I know that I now can deal with it." DM was grateful for the vision help, even though we did not "cure" the vision problem. He left the vision rehabilitative treatment feeling empowered and not nearly as victimized or angry.

ER

History

ER was a 31-year-old female involved in a car versus semitruck motor vehicle accident. She was comatose for 23 months, awoke from coma, and then was diagnosed as being in a vegetative state and "legally blind." Her family found the name of the neuro-optometrist in the phone book, as they were continually looking for resources to help ER. ER was evaluated by the neuro-optometrist 4 years postinjury.

When ER's mother called for the vision appointment, the office triage sheet noted that her mother was not very cooperative with providing information over the telephone. In response to the direct question whether there was any history of ABI, ER's mother stated that the patient was disabled secondary to a TBI due to being hit by a semitruck, the date of injury, and that her eyes went different directions. Her mother did not mention that she was quadriplegic, bedridden, and essentially unable to communicate, for fear that the appointment would be turned down.

ER presented for the vision evaluation in a mobile bed. Her mother said that ER could do yes/no hand squeeze with right hand, although this was not replicated in office. Her mother also worked with ER on flashcards on a regular basis.

ER was completely dependent on her mother for all needs and unable to reliably communicate, fixate objects of interest with either eye, or blink in response to questions. Her mother was persistent in trying to get her daughter's needs met, but all of her physicians insisted that her daughter was "not in there." Nonetheless, 4 years postinjury, ER's mother spent hours talking to her, attending to her needs, and working with flash cards and the yes/no hand squeeze.

Her medications included Baclofen, Dantrium, Reglan, Prevacid, and Tylenol 3.

Symptoms
- Unable to obtain due to lack of communication skills.

Findings
- ER was nonverbal and showed no organized eye movements.
- *Ocular health*: fundi and periphery were unremarkable on dilated evaluation; pupils equal, minimally reactive to light and accommodation; intraocular pressures were 13 mmHg in the right eye and 14 mmHg in the left eye.
- *Visual acuity*: untested. A VEP would have been helpful, but her insurance would not reimburse for this.
- *Refraction*: retinoscopy: OD: −2.00 sphere, OS: +3.00 − 5.00 × 15 scoped on axis as determined by Hirschberg reflexes, using lens bars.
- *Cover test*: unable due to inability to fixate. OD 25–35 prism diopters esotropia at least 90% of time by Krimsky estimation.
- *Accommodation*: MEM, intermittent accommodation to near targets through distance retinoscopy finding.
- *Sensorimotor examination*: able to fixate and follow only intermittently with large black and white infant stimulation checkerboard patterns at approximately 30 cm. She could not fix and follow on faces, lit targets in dim lighting, or other targets presented in normal lighting.
- *Visual field testing*: unable to assess.
- *Visual-perceptual testing*: unable to assess.

Impressions and Diagnoses
- Severe TBI by history
- Quadriplegic
- Nonverbal
- Anisometropia; myopia OD, high hyperopic astigmatism OS, 30 prism diopters right esotropia 90% of time
- Accommodative insufficiency
- Some fixation and following with high contrast infant stimulation checkerboard patterns only

Treatment and Management
Distance refractive prescription for TV watching and other times, when not doing near tasks, were prescribed. Home rehabilitative vision therapy treatment was given. Home therapy techniques include the following:

1. Perform infant stimulation pursuits at 30 cm for 10 minutes, as many times as possible everyday
2. Continue current flash cards

At the 6-month follow-up, longer than usually recommended due to difficulty transporting ER's bed, ER showed good fixations and pursuits for faces or other objects of interest. She demonstrated reliable yes/no nods. ER reported no diplopia, although she now demonstrated alternating esotropia.

Additional home therapy techniques were given to include temporal stretches.

Posttreatment Findings
- Sensorimotor examination: she showed good fixation and pursuits. She was able to look at will at objects of interest.
- Binocularity: ER demonstrated fusion most of the time with intermittent right esotropia. Some accommodative spasm was noted through the glasses and it was advised to emphasize distance viewing only through the glasses.

At the 15 months post-initial evaluation, ER was wearing her distance Rx most of the time. ER was still diagnosed as a quadriplegic, but she was now able to move all four limbs. She was sitting higher, although still transported in a bed. Because of her increased responsiveness, her physiatrist prescribed speech and physical therapy. She was working with a communication device and was able to identify colors and objects. Physical therapy was working with a standing platform to see whether she might be able to use assistive technology to get out of her bed. There was still no speech, but she was working on vocalizations.

At 3 years post-initial evaluation, ER arrived for her evaluation in a wheelchair, able to move all four limbs, and gaining moderate control over her upper extremities, able to (with great effort) generate brief verbal answers, and laughing at jokes. She continues with physical therapy and speech therapy, and is making significant progress in all areas.

Summary

ER improved from no ability to fixate and follow with normal targets and right esotropia 90% of time, to normal fixation and pursuit with binocular fusion most of the time. The rehabilitative vision therapy consisted of utilizing a refractive Rx, infant stimulation pursuits, and temporal stretches, as well as the flashcards that her mother had been using for the past year with ER. Simply listening to the family, applying the refractive correction, and taking time to find a target that her brain was able to "latch onto" and create a fixation and pursuit response, unlocked her ability to create a response. The input from the two eyes comprises about two-thirds of the sensory input to the brain, and with the appropriate stimulus, can be used for enormous leverage into both the normal and damaged brain.

ER's mother was delighted to be able to communicate better with her daughter, and to be able to demonstrate to the outside world that she was "in there." ER, was no doubt delighted to not have to lay, unresponsive in a bed listening to doctors tell her mother that she was not cognizant, and that there was no hope of any recovery. They both continued to work extremely hard on ER's recovery every day. Because ER was now receiving the help she needed to improve, she has regained her status as a member of the community, and both her mother's emotional burden of fighting, unsupported, for her daughter, and her physical burden in terms of caring for her daughter are lightening as ER gains skills.

CONCLUSION

The cases included in this chapter are very varied, and representative of the millions of people who experience visual dysfunctions associated with brain injury. Due to the numerous etiologies of injury, types of dysfunctions, multitrauma involvement, age, medical status of the patients, and other factors, there is not a simple solution in treating these types of patients. It is critical that rehabilitative optometric vision care is included in the evaluation and treatment of patients with brain injury, so that appropriate rehabilitative vision treatment is included early in the healing process. The rehabilitative optometric vision treatment can include one, or many of the strategies presented, including lenses, prisms, occlusion, tints, and rehabilitative vision therapy. Collaborative treatment with other providers is also essential in providing the most effective overall rehabilitation for the patient.

REFERENCES

1. Kaas, J. H. (1999). Is most of neural plasticity in the thalamus cortical? *Proceedings of the National Academy of Sciences, USA, 96*(14), 7622–7623.
2. Miltner, W. T., Liepert, W. H., Meissner, W., & Taub, E. (2004). Rapid functional plasticity in the primary somatomotor cortex and perceptual changes after nerve block. *European Journal of Neuroscience, 12*, 3413–3423.
3. DeGutis, J. M., Bentin, S., Robertson, L. C., & D'Esposito, M. (2007). Functional plasticity in ventral temporal cortex following cognitive rehabilitation of a congenital prosopagnosic. *Journal of Cognitive Neuroscience, 19*(11), 1790–1802.

4. Maguire, E. A., Gadian, D. G., Johnsrude, I. S., Good, C. D., Ashburner, J., Frackowiak, R. S. J., & Frith, C. D. (2000). Navigation-related structural change in the hippocampi of taxi drivers. *Proceedings of the National Academy of Sciences, USA, 97*(8), 4398–4403.

5. Qu, Q., & Shi, Y. (2009). Neural stem cells in the developing and adult brain. *Journal of Cell Physiology, 221*(1), 5–9.

6. Ge, S., Sailor, K. A., Ming, G. L., & Song, H. (2008). Synaptic integration and plasticity of new neurons in the adult hippocampus. *Journal of Physiology, 586*(16), 3759–3765.

7. Martí-Fàbregas, J., Romaguera-Ros, M., Gómez-Pinedo, U., Martínez-Ramírez, S., Jiménez-Xarrié, E., Marín, R., & García-Verdugo, J. M. (2010). Proliferation in the human ipsilateral subventricular zone after ischemic stroke. *Neurology, 74*(5), 357–365.

8. Stratton, G. M. (1896). Some preliminary experiments on vision without inversion of the retinal image. *Psychological Review, 4*, 611–617.

9. Selenow, A., & Ciuffreda, K. J. (1986). Vision function recovery during orthoptic therapy in an adult esotropic amblyope. *Journal of the American Optometric Association, 57*(2), 132–140.

10. Garzia, R. P. (1987). Efficacy of vision therapy in amblyopia: a literature review. *American Journal of Optometry and Physiological Optics, 64*(6), 393–404.

11. Levi, D. M., & Polat, U. (1996). Neural plasticity in adults with amblyopia. *Proceedings of the National Academy of Sciences, USA, 93*(13), 6830–6834.

12. Levi, D. M. (2005). Perceptual learning in adults with amblyopia: a reevaluation of critical periods in human vision. *Developmental Psychobiology, 46*(3), 222–232.

13. Etting, G. L. (1978). Strabismus therapy in private practice: cure rates after three months of therapy. *Journal of the American Optometric Association, 49*(12), 1367–1373.

14. Barry, S. R. (2009). *Fixing my gaze: A scientist's journey into seeing in three dimensions*. New York: Basic Books.

15. McCoy, P. A., Huang, H. S., & Philpot, B. D. (2009). Advances in understanding visual cortex plasticity. *Current Opinions in Neurobiology, 19*(3), 298–304.

16. Felleman, D. J., & Van Essen, D. C. (1991). Distributed hierarchical processing in the primate cerebral cortex. *Cerebral Cortex, 1*(1), 1–47.

17. Department of Health and Human Services, Center for Disease Control and Prevention. (n.d.). Heads up: facts for physicians about mild traumatic brain injury. Retrieved from http://www.cdc.gov/ncipc/pub-res/tbi_toolkit/physicians/mtbi/mtbi.pdf (Accessed February 27, 2010).

18. National Center for Injury Prevention and Control. (2003). Report to Congress on mild traumatic brain injury in the United States: steps to prevent a serious public health problem. Atlanta, GA: Centers for Disease Control and Prevention.

19. Vanderploeg, R. D., Curtiss, G., Luis, C. A., & Salazar, A. M. (2007). Long-term morbidities following self-reported mild traumatic brain injury, *Journal of Clinical and Experimental Neuropsychology, 29*(6), 585–598.

20. Miles, L., Brossman, R. I., Johnson, G., Babb, J. S., Diller, L., & Inglese, M. (2008). Short-term DTI predictors of cognitive dysfunction in mild traumatic brain injury. *Brain Injury, 22*(2), 115–122.

21. Slobounov, S. M., Zhang, K., Pennell, D., Ray, W., Johnson, B., & Sebastianelli, W. (2009). Functional abnormalities in normally appearing athletes following mild traumatic brain injury: a functional MRI study. *Experimental Brain Research,* epub ahead of print. Retrieved from www.springerlink.com (Accessed March 1, 2010) doi: 10.1007/s00221-009-2141-6.

22. Chen, J. K., Johnstion, K. M., Collie, A., McCrory, P., & Ptito, A. (2007). A validation of the post concussion symptom scale in the assessment of complex concussion using cognitive testing and functional MRI. *Journal of Neurology, Neurosurgery, and Psychiatry, 78*(11), 1231–1238.

23. Bigler, E. D. (2004). Neuropsychological results and neuropathological findings at autopsy in a case of mild traumatic brain injury. *Journal of the International Neuropsychological Society, 10*(5), 794–806.
24. Omalu, B. I., DeKosky, S. T., Minster, R. L., Kamboh, M. I., Hamilton, R. L., & Wecht, C. H. (2005). Chronic traumatic encephalopathy in a National Football League player. *Neurosurgery, 57*(1), 128–134.
25. Omalu, B. I., DeKosky, S. T., Hamilton, R. L., Minster, R. L., Kamboh, M. I., Shakir, A. M., & Wecht, C. H. (2006). Chronic traumatic encephalopathy in a National Football League player: part II. *Neurosurgery, 59*(5), 1086–1092.
26. Rabadi, M. H., & Jordan, B. D. (2001). The cumulative effect of repetitive concussion in sports. *Clinical Journal of Sport Medicine, 11*(3), 194–198.
27. O'Dell, M. W., Bell, K. R., & Sandel, M. E. (1998). 1998 Study guide: brain injury rehabilitation, pain rehabilitation. *Supplement to Archives of Physical Medicine and Rehabilitation, 79*(3)(Suppl.1), S10–S14.
28. Padula, W. V., Shapiro, J. B., & Jasin, P. (1988). Head injury causing post trauma vision syndrome. *New England Journal of Optometry, 41*(2), 16–20.
29. Ito, S., Hattori, T., & Katayama, K. (2005). Prominent unilateral convergence palsy in a patient with a tiny dorsal midbrain infarction. *European Neurology, 54*(3), 163–164.
30. Ohtsuka, K., Maeda, S., & Oguri, N. (2002). Accommodation and convergence palsy caused by lesions in the bilateral rostral superior colliculus. *American Journal of Ophthalmology, 133*(3), 425–427.
31. Fisher, D. C., Ledbetter, M. F., Cohen, N. J., Marmor, D., & Tulksy, D. S. (2000). WAIS-III and WMS-III profiles of mildly to severely brain-injured patients. *Applied Neuropsychology, 7*(3), 126–132.
32. Lachapelle, J., Bolduc-Teasdale, J., Ptito, A., & McKerral, M. (2008). Deficits in complex visual information processing after mild TBI: electrophysiological markers and vocational outcome prognosis. *Brain Injury, 22*(3), 265–274.
33. Padula, W. V., Argyris, S., & Ray, J. (1994). Visual evoked potentials (VEP) evaluating treatment for post-trauma vision syndrome (PTVS) in patients with traumatic brain injuries (TBI). *Brain Injury, 8*(4), 125–133.
34. Freed, S., & Hellerstein, L. F. (1997). Visual electrodiagnostic findings in mild traumatic brain injury. *Brain Injury, 11*(1), 25–36.
35. Crooks, C. Y., Zumsteg, J. M., & Bell, K. R. (2007). Traumatic brain injury: a review of practice management and recent advances. *Physical Medicine Rehabilitation Clinics of North America, 18*, 681–710.
36. Goodrich, G. L., Kirby, J., Cockerham, G., Ingalla, S. P., & Lew, H. L. (2007). Visual function in patients of a polytrauma rehabilitation center; a descriptive study. *Journal of Rehabilitation Research & Development, 44*(7), 929–936.
37. Lepore, F. E. (1995). Disorders of ocular motility following head trauma. *Archives of Neurology, 52*, 924–926.
38. Krohel, G. B., Kristan, R. W., Simon, J. W., & Barrows, N. A. (1986). Posttraumatic convergence insufficiency. *Annals of Ophthalmology, 18*(3), 101–102.
39. Cohen, M., Groswasser, Z., Barchadski, R., & Appel, A. (1989). Convergence insufficiency in brain injured patients. *Brain Injury, 3*(2), 187–191.
40. Ciuffreda, K., Kapoor, N., Rutner, D., Suchoff, I. B., Han, M. E., & Craig, S. (2007). Occurrence of oculomotor dysfunctions in acquired brain injury; a retrospective analysis. *Optometry, 78*(4), 155–161.
41. Schlageter, K., Gray, B., Hall, K., Shaw, R., & Sammet, R. (1993). Incidence and treatment of visual dysfunction in traumatic brain injury. *Brain Injury 7*(5), 439–448.
42. Kapoor, N., Ciuffreda, K. J., & Han, Y. (2004). Oculomotor rehabilitation in acquired brain injury: a case series. *Archives of Physical Medicine and Rehabilitation, 85*(10), 1667–1678.

43. Han, Y., Ciuffreda, K. J., & Kapoor, N. (2004). Reading-related oculomotor testing and training protocols for acquired brain injury in humans. *Brain Research Protocols, 14*(1), 1–12.

44. Ciuffreda, K. J., Rutner, D., Kapoor, N., Suchoff, I. B., Craig, S., & Han, Y. (2008). Vision therapy for oculomotor dysfunctions in acquired brain injury; a retrospective analysis. *Optometry, 79*(1), 18–22.

45. Schwab, K., Grafman, J., Salazar, A. M., & Kraft, J. (1993). Residual impairments and work status 15 years after penetrating head injury; report from the Vietnam head injury study. *Neurology, 43*(1), 95–103.

46. McKenna, K., Cooke, D. M., Fleming, J., Jefferson, A., & Ogden, S. (2006). The incidence of visual perceptual impairment in patients with severe traumatic brain injury. *Brain Injury, 20*(5), 507–518.

47. Donnan, G. A., Fisher, M., Macleod, M., & Davis, S. M. (2008). Stroke. *The Lancet, 371*(9624), 1612–1623.

48. Stone, S. P., Halligan, P. W., & Greenwood, R. J. (1993). The incidence of neglect phenomena and related disorders in patients with an acute right or left hemisphere stroke. *Age and Ageing, 22*(1), 46–52.

49. Hellerstein, L. F., & Freed, S. (1994). Rehabilitative optometric management of a traumatic brain injury patient. *Journal of Behavioral Optometry, 5*(6), 143–148.

2 The Interdisciplinary Approach to Vision Rehabilitation Following Brain Injury

Amy Berryman and Karen G. Rasavage

CONTENTS

INTRODUCTION

Chapter 1 discussed the prevalence and extent of visual deficits in people with brain injury and established a clear need for treatment. The purpose of this chapter is to discuss a recommended team approach for meeting this need. Traumatic brain injury (TBI) rehabilitation is a relatively new rehabilitation subspecialty. Interdisciplinary rehabilitation services for people with TBI began in 1978 with the first two National Institute for Disability Rehabilitation and Research (NIDRR) brain injury grants at Rusk Institute in New York and Santa Clara Valley Medical Center in San Jose. The comprehensive services offered by interdisciplinary rehabilitation in these facilities allowed for improved outcomes and expansion of the continuum of care for TBI survivors.[1] As a result of this expansion, Ragnarsson et al. recommended that "A person with TBI, regardless of the source of economic sponsor, requires a comprehensive, interdisciplinary, balanced continuum of services covering all phases of care and rehabilitation from injury through successful long-term community adjustment and reintegration" (p. 4).[2] These services begin with acute care, which can involve trauma units, intensive care units, and acute inpatient rehabilitation. Acute hospitalization alone, however, is not enough to maximize outcomes.[3] When patients become medically stable, postacute rehabilitation is necessary. A variety of postacute rehabilitation settings exist, including hospital-based outpatient rehabilitation, community-based outpatient rehabilitation, community reintegration programs, transitional living programs, vocational rehabilitation, and long-term care.[1,4] This continuum of care is not limited to people with traumatic brain injuries; it is beneficial for people with all types of acquired brain injury (ABI), including TBI, cerebral vascular accident (CVA), and progressive neurological disease. Because the impact of ABI includes physical, cognitive, emotional, and social consequences, the needs of the patients are best met by involvement with multiple medical and allied health specialists throughout the continuum of care.[1,2,5] Providing acute and postacute care within one system is preferred, allowing for continuity of communication. When a consistent system of care is not available, the continuum may become fragmented due to geographical and administrative differences.[1] The ultimate goals of the ABI continuum of care are to maximize potential for recovery, to achieve successful community reentry, and to promote optimal quality of life postinjury.[2,3,5] Many postacute rehabilitation programs utilize an interdisciplinary team approach to achieve these goals.[1,4–6]

The definition of an interdisciplinary team approach is inconsistent in the literature. "Interdisciplinary" is often interchanged with "multidisciplinary."[7] A multidisciplinary team involves members from several disciplines who work to address individual rehabilitation goals. Team members independently perform assessments, develop goals, and provide treatment. They may meet to discuss their respective work with a patient, but do not have a common plan. Comparatively, an interdisciplinary team also involves members from several disciplines. Unlike multidisciplinary teams, interdisciplinary teams formulate a common plan and work together to reach common goals. On an interdisciplinary team, members from each discipline contribute unique interventions toward these goals in collaboration with members from other disciplines. Communication among interdisciplinary team members, including the patient and family, is vital.[8] Because ABI patient care needs are unique, and because patients with ABI require structure and repetition to maximize rehabilitation, ABI rehabilitation is best performed by an interdisciplinary team.[1,4,5] An interdisciplinary approach prevents fragmentation of rehabilitation programming and increases consistency with reinforcing behaviors in treatment. This is particularly important in postacute rehabilitation, as care may be carried out in multiple locations with varied providers.[8] An interdisciplinary approach is also essential when addressing visual impairments because of the extensive impact visual impairments have on the whole person; each team member participates in the common goal of identifying and resolving visual impairments. Most interdisciplinary brain injury rehabilitation teams, however, have a missing participant: an optometrist with special interest and training in the neurological aspects of vision rehabilitation (neuro-optometrist).

Identification and assessment of visual impairments in brain injury is not new to interdisciplinary rehabilitation teams. Traditionally, ophthalmologists have provided consultations for trauma-related ocular issues, eye health, and identification of visual field cuts or visual acuity problems. Ophthalmologists are trained to perform necessary medical and surgical interventions that can improve the quality of life for patients with ABI.[9–11] Occupational therapists have also traditionally played an important role in addressing visual impairments in ABI rehabilitation. They assess and treat visual perception, visual-motor integration, and participation in activities of daily living that involve visual input.[10–12] In addition, they commonly determine potential for return to driving. Occupational therapists are skilled at providing compensatory strategies for visual impairments, but lack comprehensive knowledge regarding remedial visual interventions.[10,13] While these traditional interventions continue to be important in brain injury rehabilitation, additional interventions can be implemented to speed the rehabilitation process. These interventions require the use of lenses and prisms. Neuro-optometrists have expert knowledge of the remedial and compensatory use of lenses and prisms. They also thoroughly evaluate the visual system and identify the extent that impairments impact behavioral performance in rehabilitation.[10,13,14] These specialty optometrists often perform ABI intervention autonomously with patients at different stages of recovery; an evaluation may not be obtained until the patient has exhausted their rehabilitation benefits or has been discharged from active rehabilitation. Many authors suggest, however, that an optometry evaluation should become a standard of care while patients with brain injury are in active rehabilitation.[8–11,13–19] Neuro-optometric evaluation is best applied within an interdisciplinary team approach to holistically address visual impairments and to achieve the common goal of improving the quality of life for people with ABI.

THE INTERDISCIPLINARY TEAM

Successful application of an interdisciplinary team approach to visual impairments in postacute rehabilitation is dependent on the approach used during acute rehabilitation. Interdisciplinary goals for the patient with visual impairments during this phase involve the following: achieving visual comfort while maximizing intact vision and providing compensatory strategies for the patient, caregivers, and treatment team. These goals are appropriate until the patient becomes medically stable. Neuro-optometry can be involved to meet these needs. Neuro-ophthalmology is also involved in the acute phase of rehabilitation to restore ocular integrity and health, and may be of primary importance. Once this happens, functional visual skills become equally as important, and the role of neuro-optometry becomes more salient.[10,17] The postacute interdisciplinary team addresses functional visual goals such as reading, scanning, computer work, and visually mediated balance deficits, while treating the diagnosed impairments directly. The success of this team depends upon the team members involved and their roles in patient care. ABI team members may include, but are not limited to the following:

- Physiatrist
- Neurologist
- General practitioner
- Rehabilitation nurse
- Neuropsychologist
- Neuro-ophthalmologist
- Neuro-optometrist
- Occupational therapist
- Physical therapist
- Speech therapist
- Recreational therapist
- Community reintegration specialist
- Vocational rehabilitation counselor
- Behavioral specialist/counselor
- Family/caregivers
- Case manager
- Social worker
- Respiratory therapist

Each of these team members maintains a distinct role in patient care; each has a role in identifying visual impairments and can initiate recommendations for referral to a vision specialist. Specific team member roles in vision care can include the following.

PHYSIATRIST

The physiatrist acts as the natural leader of the interdisciplinary team and establishes a diagnosis and prognosis for the patient. The physiatrist monitors medical issues and manages medications as needed. The physiatrist communicates with the other team members, makes care recommendations, and writes orders for specialty evaluations such as those performed by neuro-optometrists/neuro-ophthalmologists.

NEUROLOGIST

The neurologist may consult to provide diagnoses and medical interventions that influence overall neurological health, alertness, and attention.

GENERAL PRACTITIONER

Once a patient returns to his or her home community and completes rehabilitation, a general practitioner is identified to continue monitoring and addressing the patient's medical issues. If visual issues were not addressed previously or if visual issues arise, the general practitioner generates referral to the appropriate vision specialist.

REHABILITATION NURSE

The nurse on the postacute interdisciplinary team acts as a liaison between the physician, the patient, and other team members for day to day health questions and concerns. The nurse often coordinates recommended medical appointments, in addition to administering medication and monitoring health status.

NEUROPSYCHOLOGIST

The neuropsychologist provides neuropsychological diagnoses and reports results to the team regarding cognitive abilities, including visual-perceptual skills, visual processing speed, and visual attention. He or she also provides patient prognoses and educates patients and family members throughout the rehabilitation continuum.

NEURO-OPHTHALMOLOGIST

The neuro-ophthalmologist is an ophthalmologist who has special training in the neurological aspects of the visual system. The neuro-ophthalmologist diagnoses problems with the structure, integrity, and health of the eyes, and the neurological aspects of vision, providing medication and lens prescriptions as appropriate. He or she provides medical and surgical support as needed throughout rehabilitation, particularly in the acute phase, and may perform surgery for traumatic strabismus or other impairments when conservative management fails.

NEURO-OPTOMETRIST

The neuro-optometrist is an optometrist who has special training in the neurological aspects of the visual system. The neuro-optometrist not only diagnoses general eye health problems and corrects refractive errors to improve visual acuity but also carefully assess functional binocularity, spatial vision, and visual processing abilities. Neuro-optometrists diagnose injury-related gross ocular and perceptual impairments, provide education regarding functional implications of visual diagnoses, and recommend treatment and compensatory strategies to speed rehabilitation. Treatment often includes prescription of specialty lenses and prisms for improved performance in rehabilitation activities. Many neuro-optometrists work with trained vision therapists in their office to implement in-house vision rehabilitation therapy programs. In addition, some specialize in low vision, and intervene when low vision aids are needed secondary to reduced central vision, blindness, or cortical visual impairment that does not resolve with therapy.

OCCUPATIONAL THERAPIST

The occupational therapist evaluates and treats participation in activities of daily living, sensory-motor integration, and upper extremity functional use. The occupational therapist commonly performs a basic vision screening to assess the patient's gross ocular status, visual-perceptual skills, and the need for formal visual diagnosis. Formal assessments are performed as well as observation during functional activities. The occupational therapist often accompanies the patient to appointments with the optometrist or ophthalmologist, communicates recommendations for treatment with the other team members, and implements recommended treatment.

PHYSICAL THERAPIST

The physical therapist evaluates and treats musculoskeletal impairments, posture, positioning, balance, and ambulation, and identifies functional physical deficits that may be caused by visual or vestibular impairments. The physical therapist performs screenings for vestibular function and communicates findings to the other team members for referral to appropriate specialist(s). He or she incorporates visual recommendations from the vision specialist, including use of prescribed lenses, prisms, or adaptive strategies during treatment sessions for generalization of skill across all disciplines.

SPEECH THERAPIST

The speech therapist evaluates and treats cognition, communication, and typically addresses swallowing. The speech therapist is often the first member of the interdisciplinary team to identify potential visual and perceptual impairments. While physical and occupational therapists generally begin evaluations with motor-sensory assessments, speech therapy begins assessing attention, comprehension, visual processing skills, and other cognitive abilities. The speech therapist communicates findings with the other team members to help identify underlying visual deficits that decrease the patient's cognitive function. The speech therapist applies the recommended compensatory visual strategies in treatment sessions to increase attention, visual-perceptual skills, and visual processing skills for improved cognition.

RECREATIONAL THERAPIST

The recreational therapist works toward home and community reentry through participation in purposeful, meaningful, structured leisure activities. The recreational therapist implements visual recommendations and strategies into these activities.

COMMUNITY REINTEGRATION SPECIALIST/VOCATIONAL REHABILITATION

The community reintegration specialist provides functional opportunities for patients to participate in work-related or community-based productive activity while utilizing vision strategies communicated by the team. This specialist also communicates visual strategies to the patient's vocational rehabilitation counselor as applicable. The vocational rehabilitation counselor incorporates this information at the patient's work site.

BEHAVIOR SPECIALIST/COUNSELOR

Behavioral specialists and counselors provide coping and behavioral management strategies for patients, families, and the treatment team. He or she is particularly interested in the behavioral and emotional impact of visual interventions and can provide structure for increased compliance with visual recommendations.

FAMILY/CAREGIVERS

The patient's family and caregivers are the most important members of the team. They are the experts on the patient and spend the most amount of time with him or her. Family and caregiver involvement is vital to generalization of skill. They provide support for home exercise performance and for implementation of compensatory strategies. They also provide critical feedback to the interdisciplinary team regarding patient performance during nontreatment hours.

CASE MANAGER/SOCIAL WORKER

The social worker or case manager is essential for identifying financial and community resources. He or she often integrates information from team reports to secure funding for rehabilitation, equipment, and specialty evaluations.

OTHER DISCIPLINES

Professionals that may not be on the formal interdisciplinary team, but add to the care of the patient, include chiropractors, osteopathic physicians, massage therapists, acupuncturists, dentists, orthopedic surgeons, independent living skills trainers, spiritual leaders, or other medical specialists. An attempt should be made to communicate visual impairments and recommendations with these specialists as appropriate.

APPLICATION OF INTERDISCIPLINARY TEAM APPROACH

The roles as discussed above clearly indicate the advantage of an interdisciplinary team approach to the treatment of visual impairments in postacute rehabilitation. Interdisciplinary application can include any or all of the aforementioned professionals. A team ideally consists of the professionals necessary to holistically address the patient's specific impairments and functional goals. If interdisciplinary care is not achievable, multidisciplinary care should at least be provided.[7] Models outlining the interdisciplinary relationship between visual specialists and rehabilitation professionals are discussed in the literature.[9,10,12,13] These models generally outline the following process for identifying and addressing visual impairments within an interdisciplinary team: screening, referral, consultation, treatment, and follow-up.

SCREENING

Screening for visual deficits can be performed by any rehabilitation professional working with patients who have ABI, and should be completed early in treatment to best identify and address patient needs. A screening is not diagnostic; it is a method for gathering information and determining the appropriate plan of care. On a formal interdisciplinary rehabilitation team, the occupational therapist commonly performs this screening in conjunction with perceptual testing. Screening should involve the following components:

- Subjective patient and family complaints
- Direct observation by team members
- External ocular observation
- Acuity
- Ocular motility
- Convergence/binocular fusion
- Visual fields

Difficulty noted in any of these areas warrants a referral to a neuro-optometrist. In general, nonsurgical, chronic eye health issues such as dry eyes can be addressed by the neuro-optometrist. Acute, serious eye health issues, however, such as orbital fractures and bleeding indicate referral to an ophthalmologist. Both visual specialists offer important services for patients with brain injury; it is common for a patient to see both specialists throughout the course of rehabilitation.

A neuro-optometrist or neuro-ophthalmologist evaluating a patient with brain injury in his or her office should screen for the following:

- Past or current involvement in rehabilitation
- Gross and fine motor coordination
- Balance
- Speech and communication
- Cognition
- Eye health issues that require referral to another type of specialized eye care professional such as a retinologist

When necessary, vision specialists can make referrals for additional therapies through a patient's primary care physician or insurance case manager.

REFERRAL

An ideal postacute interdisciplinary rehabilitation team should include a consistent optometrist and ophthalmologist with expertise in brain injury rehabilitation for consultation. Many rehabilitation teams maintain a consistent relationship with ophthalmology only, but do not have a relationship with a neuro-optometrist. Four important networks exist for identifying neuro-optometrists: the Neuro-Optometric Rehabilitation Association (NORA), the College of Optometrists in Vision Development (COVD), the Optometric Extension Program Foundation (OEPF), and the American Optometric Association (AOA):

Neuro-Optometric Rehabilitation Association: NORA is an organization comprised of rehabilitation professionals who are committed to advancing the art and science of neurological rehabilitation of visual impairments. A list of these practicing professionals is maintained on the NORA web site: www.nora.cc.

College of Optometrists in Vision Development: COVD is a nonprofit association of eye care professionals, including optometrists, optometry students, and vision therapists. COVD members offer services in behavioral and developmental vision care, vision therapy, and visual rehabilitation. Some COVD members focus primarily on pediatric patients; however, they possess the theoretical foundation for treating patients with brain injury and may be willing to see adult rehabilitation patients. They maintain a member list on their web site: www.covd.org.

Optometric Extension Program Foundation: OEPF is an international nonprofit organization dedicated to the gathering and dissemination of information on vision and vision therapy. A list of optometrist members is maintained on the OEPF web site: www.oepf.org.

American Optometric Association: AOA is a professional association for optometrists and students of optometry. The AOA's goals are to promote the profession of optometry and to improve the public's eye health. AOA optometrists represent the full spectrum of optometric professionals and therefore provide a general starting point for identification of neuro-optometrists. On the web site, www.aoa.org, optometrists are not listed by specialty. Careful inquiry is required when using this list. At the very least, an optometrist on this list who is a general practitioner of optometry may provide information regarding optometrists in the area who specialize in rehabilitation.

When seeking a neuro-optometrist, an interdisciplinary team should consider asking the following questions:

- Do you have experience working with patients who have brain injury?
- Do you have an interest in working with patients who have brain injury?
- Do you have experience in visual rehabilitation separate from low vision?
- What do you include in your evaluation of patients with brain injury?
- What are your views on impacting the visual system postinjury?
- Are you familiar with/have you worked with other rehabilitation disciplines?
- How open are you to working with other rehabilitation professionals?

If an optometrist expresses interest, an initial meeting should be held to discuss patient needs, facility resources, team member roles, rehabilitation philosophy, and a general interdisciplinary model for addressing vision. Further meetings should address consultation method, billing, time frames, and in-service needs. Optometrists expressing interest in rehabilitation do not have to have extensive rehabilitation or ABI experience to participate on an interdisciplinary team. They must, however, agree that visual intervention positively impacts ABI outcomes. They must be willing to work under the rehabilitation umbrella of addressing functional goals in collaboration with other professionals, and they must actively pursue continuing education regarding post-brain injury vision rehabilitation. A background in vision therapy can be quite helpful, as well as consulting with programs that currently include an optometrist on their team.

CONSULTATION

Although this is not discussed directly in the literature, many interdisciplinary brain injury teams are developing "vision clinics" to include optometric evaluation in patient care. These clinics occur at an optometry office, a rehabilitation facility, or a community location depending on the patient needs and on interdisciplinary team resources. A vision clinic is an apportioned amount of time set aside for evaluation of patients with brain injury. At the very least, a vision clinic should include a neuro-optometrist and a liaison from the interdisciplinary team, usually an occupational therapist, to allow for clear communication of findings and recommendations. This therapist is responsible for facilitation of communication between the optometrist and the patient as needed and for conveying findings to the treatment team.[9,13] Members of other disciplines should be invited as appropriate. Family members are encouraged to attend, to provide additional information about the patient, and to receive education.

While vision clinics are a recommended method for consultation, they are not the only option for including neuro-optometric evaluation in rehabilitation. For example, patients can independently participate in evaluations at the optometrist's office. Following the evaluation, the optometrist can provide a report and phone consultation for the therapists involved. The individual needs and resources of the patient, the rehabilitation team, and the neuro-optometrist should be considered when setting up a consultation method.

TREATMENT

Once a clinic or visit model is established, an interdisciplinary rehabilitation team must determine how to effectively implement treatment. This begins with effective communication of diagnoses and recommended intervention.

For patients who are in an active postacute rehabilitation program, regular visual treatment in the optometrist's office may not be feasible.[12] Visual treatment is most effective when carried out across disciplines during therapy, particularly in occupational therapy, under the supervision of an optometrist. This includes ocular motility, convergence, visual field defect, and perceptual interventions. The optometrist can recommend and implement in-house treatment for more complex binocular problems if transportation and funding is available.

Follow-Up

As in any rehabilitation program, regular communication and follow-up are necessary to monitor and continue progress. Optometric follow-up with patients and therapists can be performed in person, over the phone, via e-mail, or through reports sent by therapists. Vision clinics often include specific time for follow-up in addition to evaluation.

Example of How a Site-Based Clinic Is Run: Hospital Program and Dr. P

Hospital Program (HP) is a rehabilitation hospital that offers acute and postacute rehabilitation services for people with ABI. In the acute rehabilitation setting, an ophthalmologist or neuro-ophthalmologist may be involved in surgical reconstruction of the eye, eyelids, and/or orbit area, and in ongoing medical treatment. As early as possible following the acute intervention, the neuro-optometrist evaluates the patient. Dr. P is a neuro-optometrist who participates in a vision clinic that meets in a conference room at HP one afternoon per week. Dr. P brings portable optometric instruments for his examinations. An occupational therapist is designated as the vision clinic facilitator; two or three occupational therapists are trained to perform this role. Upon admission to the inpatient or outpatient programs, occupational therapists perform a vision screening. On the basis of this screening, patients who require a neuro-optometric evaluation receive an order written by the attending physician and are scheduled for a 30-minute session with Dr. P. The vision clinic facilitator assembles all charts necessary for the visit, and attends all vision clinic sessions. In addition, the patient, family members, primary occupational therapist, and other team members attend the visit. Dr. P writes his recommendations and findings in the chart, and the clinic facilitator makes these available to all members of the treatment team. Findings and recommendations are communicated in team meetings by the primary occupational therapist. Dr. P and the primary occupational therapist collaborate regarding follow-up. Dr. P directly bills the insurance and dictates a formal note for the visit. When a current patient discharges to another area, Dr. P researches available optometrists in the patient's community and provides direct communication with that optometrist. If a patient discharges from the rehabilitation program and lives locally, the patient will continue vision treatment in Dr. P's office if needed.

Example of How an Office-Based Clinic Is Run: Transitional Living Facility and Dr. S

Transitional Living Facility (TLF) is a postacute TBI facility with focus on transitional living. Patients live in apartments with daily living assistants and attend a 4–6-hour interdisciplinary rehabilitation program during the day that includes speech therapy, occupational therapy, physical therapy, and counseling. Each patient has an assigned case manager that serves as a liaison between the patient, the treatment team, and the insurance provider. The patients, who are generally 6–9 months postinjury, but may be as much as 10 years postinjury, participate in a 2-week evaluation upon admission. Occupational therapists perform a vision screening and perceptual assessment with each patient. If vision impairment is suspected, the occupational therapists recommend a formal evaluation with Dr. S, a neuro-optometrist, at the initial conference. Case management preapproves the visit with the insurance carriers, and the patient is scheduled to attend the vision clinic held at Dr. S's office. Dr. S apportions one morning per week for patients from TLF. Each evaluation takes approximately 3 hours, and a follow-up takes approximately 1 hour. Dr. S's staff assists in performing portions of the testing. The occupational therapist or family member transports patients and brings assistants from the facility as needed for supervision. The occupational therapist brings copies of the following for the chart: vision screening, results of perceptual assessments, and the completed vision rehabilitation history questionnaire, with signed consent to share information with the TLF and other health-care personnel involved in the patient's rehabilitation. During the appointments, the occupational therapist takes notes regarding findings and recommendations. Dr. S outlines specific recommendations for the interdisciplinary team to incorporate into treatment sessions. Occasionally, Dr. S requests that patients be transported to her office for treatment when complex binocularity problems are present or special equipment is needed for treatment. Dr. S also outlines the mode and time frame for follow-up, which could be a phone consultation or a return to the vision clinic. If glasses are recommended, the patients select frames as appropriate with the in-house optician before returning to TLF to improve the speed of obtainment. Upon return to TLF, the occupational therapist copies the notes and distributes them to members of the treatment team. The findings and recommendations are then reported in staffing meetings. Dr. S is available for phone consultation if the therapists encounter difficulties with execution of the treatment plan. Billing is performed by Dr. S's office; however, the insurance payment should already be preauthorized by the case manager. Dr. S submits a formal report to TLF for case managers and insurance carriers for each visit.

Both, Dr. S and Dr. P provide educational in-services for the interdisciplinary team as needed to improve execution of optometric recommendations and to improve interdisciplinary communication.

CONCLUSION

The examples listed earlier suggest two possible ways to structure inclusion of optometry in rehabilitation; they are not listed as absolutes. When structuring an interdisciplinary team, the needs of the patients and the providers must be considered on an individual basis to create the ideal working relationship. In addition, the examples discussed above have not been successful merely because they reflect solid procedures; they have been successful because the professionals involved demonstrate the interest, passion, professional respect, commitment, and communication to appropriately address visual impairments in patients with brain injury. These professionals are not bound by individual agendas and narrow roles. They are motivated to widen their knowledge about what each profession contributes to an interdisciplinary team, to allow the roles of other team members to inspire their treatment, and to eagerly stretch their boundaries through communication and collaboration for achievement of defined common goals. The common goal of improving vision impairments in postacute brain injury is best met with a comprehensive, skilled interdisciplinary team.

REFERENCES

1. Cope, D. N., Mayer, N. H., & Cervelli, L. (2005). Development of systems of care for persons with traumatic brain injury. *Journal of Head Trauma Rehabilitation, 20*(2), 128–142.
2. Ragnarsson, K. T., Thomas, J. T., & Zasler, N. D. (1993). Model systems of care for individuals with traumatic brain injury. *Journal of Head Trauma Rehabilitation, 8*(2), 1–11.
3. Bigler, E. D., Clark, E., & Farmer, J. (1996). Traumatic brain injury: 1990s update-introduction to the special series. *Journal of Learning Disabilities, 29*(5), 512–513.
4. Khan, F., Baguley, I. J., & Cameron, I. D. (2003). Rehabilitation after traumatic brain injury. *Medical Journal of Australia, 178*, 290–295.
5. American Speech and Hearing Association. (1995, March). Guidelines for the structure and function of an interdisciplinary team for persons with brain injury. *Asha, 37*(Suppl. 14), 23–25.
6. Yagura, H., Miyai, I., Suzuki, T., & Yanagihara, T. (2005). Patients with severe stroke benefit most by interdisciplinary rehabilitation team approach. *Cerebrovascular Diseases, 20*, 258–263.
7. Kaplan, R. M., & Phelps, D. (1976). An interdisciplinary team approach-a case report. *Journal of the American Optometric Association, 47*(9), 1153–1164.
8. Richter, E. F. (2001). Interdisciplinary management and rehabilitation of acquired brain-injured patients. In I. B. Suchoff, K. J. Ciuffreda, & N. Kapoor (Eds.), *Visual and vestibular consequences of acquired brain injury* (pp. 10–31). Santa Ana, CA: Optometric Extension Program Foundation, Inc.
9. Gianutsos, R., Ramsey, G., & Perlin, R. R. (1988). Rehabilitative optometric services for survivors of acquired brain injury. *Archives of Physical Medicine and Rehabilitation, 69*, 573–578.
10. Suchoff, I., & Gianutsos, R. (2000). Rehabilitative optometric interventions for the adult with acquired brain injury. In M. Grabois, S. J. Garrison, K. A. Hart, & L. D. Lehmkuhl (Eds.), *Physical medicine and rehabilitation: The complete approach* (pp. 608–621). Malden, MA: Blackwell Science, Inc.
11. Suter, P. S. (2004). Rehabilitation and management of visual dysfunction following traumatic brain injury. In M. J. Ashley (Ed.), *Traumatic brain injury: Rehabilitative treatment and case management* (pp. 209–249). Boca Raton, FL: CRC Press.
12. Scheiman, M., & Scheiman, M. (2002). Inter-relationship model. In M. Scheiman (Ed.), *Understanding and managing vision deficits: A guide for occupational therapists* (2nd ed., pp. 325–329). Thorofare, NJ: SLACK Incorporated.
13. Gianutsos, R., & Ramsey, G. (1988). Enabling rehabilitation optometrists to help survivors of acquired brain injury. *Journal of Visual Rehabilitation, 2*, 37–58.

14. Cohen, A. H., & Rein, L. D. (1992). The effect of head trauma on the visual system: the doctor of optometry as a member of the rehabilitation team. *Journal of the American Optometric Association, 63*(8), 530–536.

15. Cohen, A. H. (1992). Optometry: the invisible member of the rehabilitation team. *Journal of the American Optometric Association, 63*(8), 529.

16. Kapoor, N., & Ciuffreda, K. J. (2002). Vision disturbances following traumatic brain injury. *Current Treatment Options in Neurology, 4*, 271–280.

17. Hellerstein, L. F. (2002). Visual problems associated with brain injury. In M. Scheiman (Ed.), *Understanding and managing vision deficits: A guide for occupational therapists* (2nd ed., pp. 177–185). Thorofare, NJ: SLACK Incorporated.

18. Hellerstein, L. F., & Fishman, B. I. (2002). Visual rehabilitation for patients with brain injury. In M. Scheiman (Ed.), *Understanding and managing vision deficits: A guide for occupational therapists* (2nd ed., pp. 187–208). Thorofare, NJ: SLACK Incorporated.

19. Politzer, T. (2000). Vision function, examination, and rehabilitation in patients suffering from traumatic brain injury. In G. W. Jay (Ed.), *Minor traumatic brain injury handbook: Diagnosis and treatment* (pp. 311–326). Boca Raton, FL: CRC Press.

3 Neural Substrates of Vision

Richard Helvie

CONTENTS

INTRODUCTION

Vision is one of the most amazing miracles of life—a journey of the light ray being transformed into visual cognition. It is a complex process, requiring continuous evaluation of spatial maps, creating an internal representation of our external world, which allows us to interact with, and navigate through, our environment. We have to stretch our imagination to conceptualize how a small, distorted, upside-down image received at our retina can become the rich visual environment that we perceive. Visual perception is creative, transforming the two-dimensional patterns of light on the retina into a coherent and stable interpretation of a three-dimensional world. These light rays are derived from the physical properties of objects and surfaces. This information is then processed by both serial and parallel systems to produce our internal representation. Objects can be recognized and categorized by various physical attributes of form and color, in addition to movement and location in space. This includes both moving and stationary objects, writing, written language, music, mathematics, and faces. Once processed, this visual information is integrated with other sensory modalities such as touch and sound. Additional integration occurs as visual input is projected by distributed neural networks to higher cortical centers involved with memory, language, emotion, and motor functions. The goal of this chapter is to present a systematic approach to this complex process that can serve as a guide to understanding vision, allowing proper diagnosis and appropriate treatment for visual deficits. It is written from a neurologist's clinical perspective, explaining how the anatomic and functional organization of the brain creates vision, although this reductive approach is not without controversy.

BASIC TERMINOLOGY

It is important to appreciate basic terminology to appreciate the visual system. These terms apply not only to vision but other primary sensory modalities. *Visual reception* refers to receiving the input through the optical and primary afferent visual system. This begins in the eye with the visual stimuli being transmitted through the afferent system to the primary visual cortex. *Visual attention* is a cognitive process of orienting, filtering and selecting inputs, preparing for action, and maintaining thought on a stimulus. This is carried out by inhibitory/excitatory processes, as the brain does not have the processing capacity to attend to the vast stimuli in the environment that are presented to it. *Spatial attention* refers to attending and orienting to the contralateral space (i.e., the space contralateral to the neural substrates mediating it; for instance the left hemisphere generally mediates attention to the right hemispace). *Visual perception* includes filtering of internal/external stimuli as well as higher-order analysis of features in which discrimination and pattern recognition functions are engaged to categorize information. These visual percepts are then integrated with percepts from other sensory modalities and with experiential memories and goals. *Higher visual-cognitive processing* refers to binding together of salient percepts and manipulating them to form concepts and action. The visual system provides major input for the different domains of higher cognitive functioning. *Visual cognition* is the ability to immediately represent, organize, and manipulate the environment or to think, use memory, and make decisions to reach established goals. *Visual social processing* describes the analysis of visual social signaling (smiling, crying, gesturing) in addition to territorial boundaries (interpersonal space).

GENERAL BRAIN ANATOMY

The brain consists of two basic solid components and four anatomical parts. The gray and white matters are the solid core components. The gray matter contains glial cells (astrocytes and oligodendrocytes), neurons (cell bodies), and connections linking neurons (axons and dendrites). Oligodendrocytes produce myelin that envelopes the axons. Oligodendrocytes are unique cells in several important ways that impact both their unique vulnerability and repair ability, including (1) producing all brain cholesterol; (2) having the highest iron content of any cell in the brain; (3) having a high rate of metabolism; and (4) continuing to replicate throughout life. Astrocytes are not only supportive but are neuroprotective, releasing neurotrophic factors and altering glutamate excitoneurotoxicity at synapses, in addition to playing a role in mediating communication between neurons and their neural circuitry.

Gray matter forms the cerebral cortex, a mantel covering the cerebral hemispheres. The neocortex is organized in layers. Each layer has different connections of neurons and cell processes. These layers have specific functions and together assure the overall continuity of the cerebral cortex. This organization is called the *laminar structure* of the neocortex, resulting in geographic areas that have specific function. In 1909, Brodmann described functional areas based on different laminar structures in different parts of the brain, creating a numbered system of "Brodmann areas" that became the predominant system in describing the cerebral cortex for decades.

The neocortex also contains a high percentage of white matter (myelinated cortical/cortical connections). Over 20 billion neurons reside in the neocortex or 70% of the total in the central nervous system, of which 75% are located in the cortical association areas.[1] The Rhesus monkey provides an excellent model for studying the human visual system. Because nearly 70% of the total sensory input to the brain comes from the two eyes, it is not surprising that approximately 50% of the cortex is involved with processing vision.[2] Researchers have identified over 300 intracortical pathways linking over 30 different cortical areas involved from visual function, 7 of which are primary visual association areas, or extrastriate areas.[3] In addition, beneath the neocortex lies the limbic system, which is involved in emotion and memory. The hippocampus and amygdala reside here. Both are located in the anterior temporal lobes. The hippocampus is involved in the acquisition of memory and spatial learning. The amygdala regulates the interaction of the inner self with the external world.

White matter is composed of myelinated nerve cell extensions or processes, called *axons*, which are encased with myelin, carrying signals in the form of nerve impulses between neurons. These axonal pathways interconnect cortical areas, cortical-subcortical areas, and subcortical-subcortical nuclei. They are bidirectional in their transmission capabilities. These are described in different terms, including fasciculus, tract, bundle, peduncle, lemniscus, or funiculus.

FOUR ANATOMICAL COMPONENTS

Cerebral Hemispheres

There are four anatomical components of the brain: the cerebral hemispheres, diencephalon, brainstem, and cerebellum. There are two cerebral hemispheres, the right and the left, and each is divided into four lobes, the frontal, temporal, parietal, and occipital lobes, each involved in a specific role in vision. Figure 3.1 shows a lateral view of the cortex with named parts and can be used as a reference in the subsequent discussion of vision in this chapter. The frontal lobe makes up one-third of cerebral hemisphere volume, is the most complex, phylogenetically the most recent area to develop, and one of the last areas of the brain to myelinate. It is not a single functional unit. There are three major subdivisions, the precentral area, the premotor area, and the prefrontal area. The precentral and premotor areas work as a unit for planning and carrying out motor behavior, including saccadic eye movements, based on incoming sensory inputs. The prefrontal area is a more cognitive sophisticated integrative system, involved in the highest level of visual and other sensory modality processing, resulting in higher action plans, incorporating meaning and intention. There are three subdivisions of the prefrontal cortex based on their locations, the dorsolateral, orbital frontal, and medial frontal areas. The dorsolateral area is primarily involved in working memory and executive functioning, the orbital frontal area in personality and self control, and medial frontal region in motivation for goal-oriented activities. The prefrontal cortex has been described as the "leader of the orchestra." The temporal lobes are involved in object recognition (categorization), memory acquisition, and emotional valance. The parietal lobes are involved in the processing of motion and location, as well as multisensory integration; and the occipital lobe in reception and early visual processing.

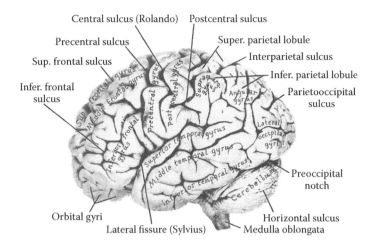

FIGURE 3.1 Lateral view of cortex. (From Carpenter, M. B., and Sutin, J., *Human Neuroanatomy*, 8th ed., Williams & Wilkins, Baltimore, MD, 1983, p. 28. Reprinted with permission.)

Diencephalon

The diencephalon is a region of the brain, including the thalamus and hypothalamus. Pertinent visually related subcortical nuclei located in the thalamus are the pulvinar and the lateral geniculate nucleus (LGN). The pulvinar is located in the posterior thalamus and is considered an association nucleus involved in complex vision. The lateral pulvinar is linked with the posterior parietal, superior temporal,[4] and medial and dorsolateral extrastriate cortices,[5] as well as the superior colliculus.[6] It plays a probable role in integration of somatosensory and visual information. The inferior pulvinar is a strongly represented visual area linked with temporal areas concerned with visual feature discrimination and extra striate areas concerned with the analysis of vision. It also receives visual input from the superior colliculus[6] in addition to direct input from retinal ganglion cells.[5] The LGN is the other thalamic visually related nucleus that is part of the afferent visual system. The LGN also receives projections back from cortically related visual areas, indicating that higher order visual processing can influence visual perception at an early stage. The hypothalamus has many distinct nuclei. It monitors the internal state, is involved in regulating circadian rhythms, and is under the control of the amygdala and prefrontal cortex.

Brainstem

The brainstem has a diverse collection of nuclei related to the alerting-arousal system that helps mediate attention, some associated with specific neurotransmitters. They connect the brainstem with the thalamus, limbic system, and neocortex via the ascending reticular activating system and the median forebrain bundle. These brainstem nuclei include the locus ceruleus (norepinephrine mediated); substantia nigra and ventral tegmental nuclei (dopamine mediated); and the median raphe (serotonin mediated). In addition, the neurotransmitter acetylcholine is involved with transmission in the medial forebrain bundle. The superior colliculus is an important visual nucleus located in the midbrain portion of the brainstem, and will be discussed later in the chapter.

Cerebellum

The cerebellum is involved with spatial organization and memory. It is also involved in refining motor control, and probably motor learning. Although it only makes up about 10% of the total brain volume, it is densely packed with neurons (mostly tiny granule cells). The vestibulocerebellum participates in balance and spatial orientation. It mainly receives vestibular input, along with visual and other sensory input. The spinocerebellum functions to fine-tune body and limb movements. It receives proprioceptive input as well as input from visual and auditory systems, and the trigeminal nerve. It sends fibers to the deep cerebellar nuclei, which project to cerebral cortex and also to brainstem to modulate descending motor systems. The cerebrocerebellum receives input exclusively from cerebral cortex, especially parietal lobe, via the pontine nuclei, and sends outputs to ventrolateral thalamus. The cerebrocerebellum may be involved in planning movement, evaluating sensory information for movement and perhaps some cognitive functions.

BRAIN DEVELOPMENT

The pattern of development varies significantly between gray and white matter. Nearly the entire compliment of brain neurons are formed before birth with development beginning early in gestation.[7] Gray matter remains relatively constant in volume throughout adult life. However, contrary to earlier opinion, neurogenesis does occur throughout life. White matter formation does not begin until the third trimester of gestation and is only partially complete at birth, even at 2 years of age it is only 90% complete.[8] White matter volume fluctuates throughout life. Some myelination requires many years to complete with some studies showing it can continue up to the sixth decade.[9] This myelination process proceeds from caudal to rostral structures or from phylogenetically older to newer areas of the brain, thus the frontal lobes are one of the last areas to myelinate. This postnatal driven myelination is what makes humans unique. Figure 3.2 shows a sequence of myelination in the human brain that reflects the functional maturity not only of vision but also of other systems. The gray matter is like a computer with the white matter being the wiring, and with increased postnatal myelination, there is an increase in speed of neurotransmission or increase in bandwidth. It shows the vulnerability of the developing brain to traumatic brain injury (TBI) and explains why pediatric patients are described as "growing into their deficits" as they grow older.

ANATOMICAL DIVISIONS OF THE VISUAL SYSTEM

OPTIC SYSTEM

The visual system is traditionally divided into two components: the primary and secondary visual systems. However, there is a third component that we sometimes take for granted, the optical system. The purpose of the optical system is to present a clear and undistorted image on the retina. Three primary conditions must be present for this to occur. The first is the refractory system provided by the cornea and the crystalline

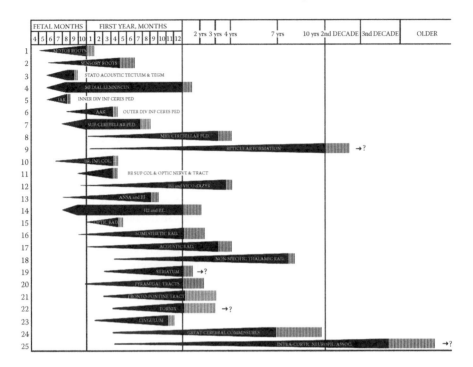

FIGURE 3.2 The sequence of myelination in the human brain. (From M. J. Ashley (Ed.), *Traumatic Brain Injury Rehabilitation,* 3rd ed., p. 284, 2010, CRC Press.)

lens, which converge parallel light rays from distant objects to a specific focus on the retina. The state emmetropia exists when this condition is met. The second involves accommodation that diverges light rays from near objects to the same focus on the retina. The third component is a transparent ocular media, the nonrefractory space occupied by the aqueous and vitreous to project a clear focus on the retina.

Primary Visual System

Retina

Visual function begins in the retina. Unlike other sensory peripheral end organs, the retina is an extension of the central nervous system. Light enters the eye and is focused both by the cornea and the lens, and then passes to the photoreceptors of the retina. There is an area in the retina called the *fovea*, where the cell bodies of the more proximal layers are shifted to the sides, enabling the visual image to be received in its least distorted form. The center of the fovea is called the *foveola*, where the most accurate visual reception occurs. The anatomy of the photoreceptor layer consists of cones and rods. Cones are closely packed in the center of the fovea, reaching 200,000 cones/mm^2. This drops off exponentially from the center of the fovea. The cones are the substrate for day vision, high visual acuity, and color. There are no rods in the fovea as they are distributed bilaterally in the periphery. They are the substrate for night vision, have low visual acuity, and are achromatic.

Thus for the highest resolution of the visual image to occur, it is mandatory that the fovea be targeted on the visual stimuli. The retina has three major functional classes of neurons. The photoreceptors lie in the outer nuclear layer, interneurons, which are the bipolar, horizontal, and amacrine cells, lie in the inner nuclear layer, and ganglion cells lie in the ganglion cell layer. Photoreceptors, bipolar cells, and horizontal cells make synaptic connections with each other in the outer plexiform layer. The bipolar, amacrine, and ganglion cells make contact in the inner plexiform layer. Information flows vertically from photoreceptor to bipolar cells to ganglion cells, as well as laterally from horizontal cells in the outer plexiform layer and amacrine cells in the inner layer. The receptive fields of ganglion cells correspond to patches of receptors lying immediately beneath them; therefore, a lesion within the retina causes a visual field defect, whose shape corresponds exactly to the shape of the lesion. The absorption of light by visual pigments in the photoreceptors triggers a cascade of chemical events that result in the production of electrical energy. This process is called *phototransduction*. This visual information is transmitted in the form of electrical signals by the photoreceptors to the ganglion cells. Modification of the signals occurs as a result of the interneuron cells, altering the electrical signals by incorporating different temporal and spatial patterns of light stimulation in the retina.

Over 22 types of ganglion cells exist in the primate,[10] but only three types appear to be involved in visual perception in that they connect to the lateral geniculate body.[11] These three subsets are termed the magno, parvo, and konio cellular types, the former two being most important in human vision. Ganglion cells have a concentric visual receptive field with a center surround organization with antagonistic excitatory and inhibitory regions. These cells fall into two classes based on their different response to a small spot of light presented at its center creating on-center and off-center cells. A functional segregation of ganglion cells occurs in relationship to the size of the receptive fields and light responsiveness to a small spot of light. The parvo cells have small receptive fields, respond to high spatial and slow temporal frequency, and are involved with perception of detail. The magno cells have large receptive fields, respond to low spatial and fast temporal frequency, and are involved in low contrast and large contour analysis. Of these two subsets of ganglion cells, 80% are parvo cells while the remaining 20% are magno cells. The magno and parvo cells monitor peripheral and central vision, respectively, because of their location in the retina. The axons of these ganglion cells converge toward the optic disk, where they emerge from the eye as the optic nerve. In the superficial retina, between the ganglion cells and optic nerve, the topography turns horizontal, according to the geography of the axons of the retinal cells. Therefore, a lesion involving this area causes a visual field defect whose configuration is based on the configuration of the axonal bundles as they sweep across the retinal surface.

Optic Nerve and Optic Tracts

The nerve fibers pass through the sclera through a sieve-like structure called the *lamina cribrosa*. Since there are no receptor cells (rods or cones) at the optic disk, a blind spot is produced in the field of vision. Each optic nerve contains retinotopic

maps representing both the heminasal and hemitemporal visual space of its compan-
ion eye. The optic nerve passes posteriorly through the orbit and enters the cranial
cavity through the optic foramen and joins its fellow of the opposite side to form the
optic chiasm. At the optic chiasm, a partial decussation of fibers from the two sides
takes place. Fibers from each eye destined for either side of the brain are sorted out
and rebundled forming the optic tracts, which carry visual information from the
contralateral visual fields of each eye. Thus, information from the right hemifield is
routed to the left side of the brain and information from the left hemifield is routed
to the right side of the brain. Each optic tract, in turn, partially encircles the cerebral
peduncle and passes to three significant subcortical structures—the pretectum, the
superior colliculus, and the LGN (see Figure 3.3). The majority of the axons of each

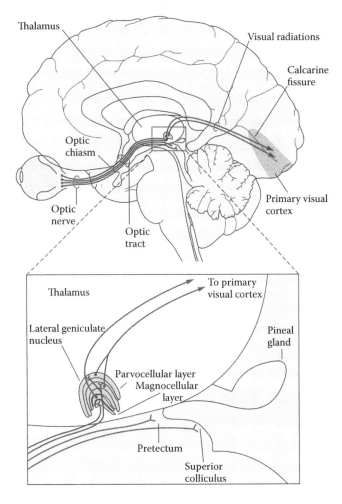

FIGURE 3.3 Route of optic tract to lateral geniculate body, pretectum, and superior colliculus. (From Kandel, E. R. Schwartz, J. H., and Jessell, T. M. (Eds.), *Principles of Neural
Science,* 4th ed., McGraw-Hill, New York, 2000, p. 527. Reprinted with permission.)

optic tract proceed to the LGN located in the thalamus. Within the optic tract, these fibers have not yet approximated each other, thus, a lesion in this area will cause an incongruous visual field defect. Without the retinogeniculate pathway, perception is lost except under limited conditions referred to as blindsight or unconscious vision.

Lateral Geniculate Nucleus

Ninety percent of the retinal axons terminate in the LGN. Conversely, only 10% of the synapses in this nucleus are received from the retina, whereas 90% are received from other areas, predominantly the cerebral cortex. This suggests that while the retinogeniculate connection is the driver, the corticogeniculate link does a great deal of modulation at this very early stage of visual processing. As the optic tract enters the LGN, there is a continuation of the retinotopic representation of the contralateral visual field. In humans, the LGN contains six layers of cell bodies separated by intralaminar layers of white matter or axons. The layers are numbered from 1 to 6, ventral to dorsal. The two most ventral layers of the nucleus are known as the magno cellular layers as their main retinal input is from the M-ganglion cells. The four dorsal layers are known as parvocellular layers and receive input from the P-ganglion cells. Both, the magno cell and parvo cell layers include the same concentric fields with on- and off-center cells that were present in the ganglion cells in the retina. Furthermore, axonal fibers in the ipsilateral and contralateral eyes are segregated in the layers of the lateral geniculate body, layers 1, 4, and 6 of the terminal of axons from the contralateral eye, whereas layers 2, 3, and 5 contain axons from the ipsilateral eye. Although each layer does contain retinotopic maps, the retinal space is not represented isometrically as the foveal region, which occupies less than 10% of the retinal surface, projects to 50% of the surface area of the lateral geniculate body.

Optic Radiations

The axons of the magnocellular and parvocellular cells, exit this structure grouped separately to form the origin of the M and P pathways. Collectively, this white matter tract is called the *optic radiation*. After exiting the LGN, the optic radiation sweeps around the lateral ventricle to terminate in the primary visual cortex, continuing to transmit visual information from the contralateral visual field. The fibers representing the inferior half of the retina are located more ventral than those representing the superior portion of the retina. Those axons representing the inferior retinal input end beneath the calcarine fissure, whereas those representing superior retinal input terminate above the calcarine fissure.

Primary Visual Cortex

Much of the primary visual cortex, V1, occupies the calcarine sulcus, at the posterior pole of the brain. V1 is traditionally discussed as part of the primary visual pathway, as it is the termination site for the optic radiations, and lesions in the optic radiations and V1 result in similar visual field defects. In this chapter, because it is also the *beginning* of visual cortical processing, primary visual cortex will be discussed in the section under Secondary Visual System.

Midbrain Visual Projections

Edinger-Westphal Nucleus

A small portion of fibers of the optic tract continue up to the midbrain, after the majority exit to connect with the LGN. Remaining fibers in the optic tract project to two areas, the pretectum and the superior colliculus. The superior and inferior colliculi together comprise the tectum (see Figure 3.3). The first group of the midbrain destined fibers project to the pretectal nucleus whose cells project both to the ipsilateral Edinger-Westphal nucleus (i.e., accessory oculomotor nucleus) and to the contralateral Edinger-Westphal nucleus via the posterior commissure. Preganglionic neurons in both Edinger-Westphal nuclei send axons out of the brainstem in the oculomotor nerve (CN III) to innervate with the ciliary ganglion. This ganglion contains the postganglionic neurons and innervates the smooth muscles of the pupillary sphincter that constricts the pupil. Pupillary reflexes are clinically important because they indicate the functional state of both the afferent and efferent pathways.

Superior Colliculus

The last portion of the optic tract terminates in the superior colliculus. This is also a nuclear structure of alternating gray and white matter layers. These retinotectal fibers project into its superficial layers conveying, again, a map of the contralateral space. The superficial layers also receive visual input from the visual cortex, whereas cortical input from other sensory modalities project to deeper layers. Under the control of these cortical connections, multisensory and spatial integration occurs. Thus, cortical control is necessary to process more than one modality at any specific time.[12] However, the superior colliculus also operates as a unimodal system for reflexive orienting of the eyes and head using direct retinotectal information. This allows for much quicker response times in survival situations. In everyday situations, the superior colliculus is influenced by control of the frontal eye field in generating and controlling eye and head movements. The superficial layers of the superior colliculus are the origin of the connection linking the pulvinar, which in turn projects to the cerebral parietal cortex, which is the neural network responsible for the orientation of visual attention.

Accessory Optic System: Retinohypothalamic Tract

In addition to the traditional primary visual system, an accessory optic system exists in humans. The accessory optic system is defined as all optic fibers from contralateral retina that do not terminate in the LGN, pretectal nucleus, or superior colliculus. This system involves the processing of retinal, nonvisual (nonimage) information. The retinohypothalamic tract in humans is clinically an important structure in this system.[13] The ganglion cells in this tract, rather than processing light information from rods and cones, are, in themselves, photosensitive. Most retinal ganglion cells that project to the suprachiasmatic nucleus express the photopigment melanopsin,[14] and have come to be called intrinsically photosensitive retinal ganglion cells or ipRGCs (reviewed by Berson).[15] This tract transmits photic information from the retina to the suprachiasmatic nucleus in the hypothalamus where circadian rhythms

are generated. The retinohypothalamic tract leaves the retina via the optic nerve and exits in the optic chiasm en route to the suprachiasmatic nucleus. The clinical significance of other tracts in the accessory optic system in humans have not been precisely delineated.

SECONDARY VISUAL SYSTEM

Neocortical Modules

The secondary visual system is complex, and knowledge of its anatomical and functional organization is required to understand its operation. To appreciate the anatomy and function of the secondary visual system, it is important to think of the brain as a modular unit, although this is an oversimplification. The organizational blueprint of the brain begins in the neocortex, the laminar structure consisting of six layers—a ribbon covering the cerebral hemispheres. Variations in the layers of cells are found in different areas of the cortex, with these areas having similar columns of cells serving a specific function. These areas are called *modules*. An example of such a module is the primary visual cortex in the occipital lobe because of its specific organization of columns of cells serving a specific function, that being vision.

Unimodal Association Cortex

These primary sensory areas in the brain include the primary auditory cortex, the primary somatosensory cortex, and the gustatory and olfactory cortices. Each primary sensory cortex area projects from its specific sensory modality to its surrounding sensory association area, such as the primary visual cortex to the visual association area via a cortical-cortical connection creating a unimodal association cortex. These different sensory association cortices communicate with each other via convergence of the unimodal fibers to form multimodal association cortices.

Multimodal and Supramodal Association Cortex

There are three multimodal association cortices: the posterior, anterior, and limbic association areas, although the last two are also classified as supramodal. Figure 3.4 shows the different primary unimodal and association cortical areas. The posterior multimodal association area allows for the spatial and temporal integration of different sensory modalities and is located in the posterior parietal lobe, especially the angular gyrus. The area is also important for language function. Figure 3.5 shows the connections between the unimodal visual areas with all three multimodal areas. The anterior association area is located in the prefrontal region and allows for visual percepts to be incorporated into various higher cortical functions (concepts) by determining which of the unimodal and multimodal inputs from other parts of the brain should be attended at a specific time. The limbic system serves as a supervisor that processes feeling and emotions that interface between the external world and the internal self in addition to mediating memory. The supramodal areas, the limbic and anterior association areas, help bring our personal past, and the present, into the present. They bring explicit and implicit knowledge gained through past experience to bear on information processing in the here and now. These supramodal systems

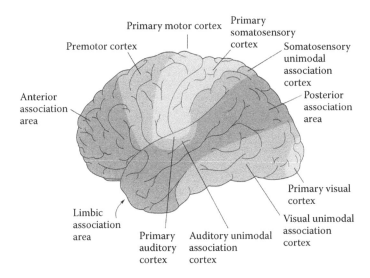

FIGURE 3.4 Different association cortices. (From Kandel, E. R. Schwartz, J. H., and Jessell, T. M. (Eds.), *Principles of Neural Science,* 4th ed., McGraw-Hill, New York, 2000, p. 350. Reprinted with permission.)

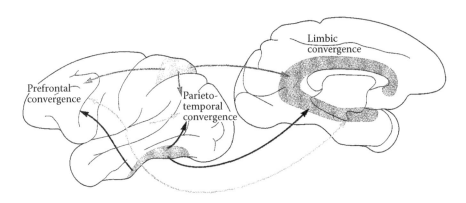

FIGURE 3.5 Visual association cortex connections to the anterior, posterior, and limbic multimodal association cortices. (From Kandel, E. R. Schwartz, J. H., and Jessell, T. M. (Eds.), *Principles of Neural Science*, 4th ed., McGraw-Hill, New York, 2000, p. 355. Reprinted with permission.)

can give rise *de novo* to creativity, ideas, thought, memory, motivation, and free will in the absence of sensory stimulation or action in the immediate present. The supramodal system is paramount to the genesis of our emotions. These higher cortical functions are a process exclusively in the domains of the cerebral cortex. Figure 3.6 shows a schematic of how rudimentary visual information is converted into higher cognitive function.

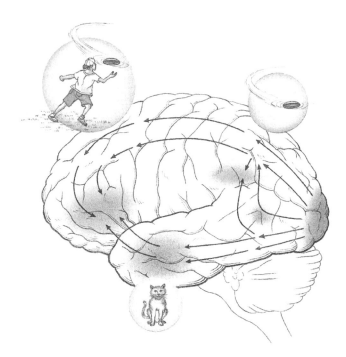

FIGURE 3.6 Major pathways of visual perception; object recognition, motion perception, and motor planning based on visual percepts. (From Devinsky, O. and D'Esposito, M., *Neurology of Cognitive and Behavioral Disorders,* Oxford University Press, New York, 2004, p. 129. By permission of Oxford University Press, Inc.)

Neural Networks

Different cortical nodes, the primary, unimodal, and supramodal cortices, are connected among themselves and with subcortical areas to form distributed neural networks to perform specific functions, including vision. In addition to cortical areas, subcortical structures are involved in both sensory-motor and complex behaviors in a manner determined by both their intrinsic anatomic organization as well as their connections to the cerebral cortex.

These linkages are carried out by numerous axonal pathways located both in the cortex and subcortical white matter. These pathways consist of large groups of axons covered by a myelin coat and are identified as fasciculi, tracts, or bundles. Vision is created by the simultaneous integration of neural networks modulated by attention. These connections are bidirectional and multidirectional. They can converge or diverge from lower to higher centers, higher to lower centers, or can be collateral or spread out at the same level. The organization of the white matter pathways begins in the cerebral cortex. Neurons within a cortical area give rise to three distinct categories of fiber systems that can be distinguished within the white matter immediately beneath the gyrus. These are association fibers, striatal fibers, and subcortically directed fibers. In addition, there are tracts that interconnect subcortical areas.[16] The association fiber tracts can be divided into three categories, the local, neighborhood, and long association fiber systems. The local association fiber system, or the U fiber system, leaves a given area of the cortex and travels to an adjacent gyrus, running in a thin identifiable band immediately beneath the sixth layer of the neocortex. The neighborhood association fiber system arises from a given cortical area and is directed to nearby regions but is distinguished from the local U fiber system that runs immediately beneath the cortex. The long association fiber system emanates from a given cortical region and travels in a distinct bundle leading to other cortical areas in the same hemisphere. The operation of certain long association bundles are mandatory for specific domains of vision. The location of some of the more prominent fasciculi are shown in Figure 3.7 and the role and distributed neural networks shown in Table 3.1. These are outlined in Filley's textbook on behavioral neurology of white matter.[17]

The superior longitudinal fasciculus II connects the angular gyrus and occipital-parietal area with the dorsolateral prefrontal cortex.[16] This is thought to serve as the conduit for the neural systems mediating visual awareness, the maintenance of attention, and provides a means whereby the prefrontal cortex can regulate the focusing of attention within different parts of space. The fronto-occipital fasciculus connects positions in the occipital and parietal lobes with dorsal prefrontal cortex and is an important anatomical substrate involved in peripheral vision and the processing of visuospatial information.[16] The inferior longitudinal fasciculus is a long association fiber system conveying visual information in a bidirectional manner between the occipital and temporal lobes, and its primary visual function is object, color, and face recognition in addition to object memory.[16] The arcuate fasciculus links the caudal superior temporal lobe with the dorsal prefrontal area, mediating language function with input from the visual system. The cingulum bundle connects the caudal cingulate with the

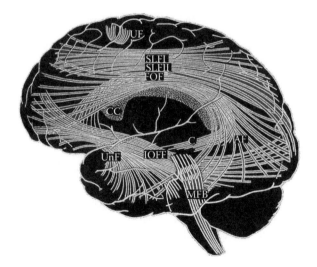

FIGURE 3.7 Major white matter tracts of the brain. AF, Arcuate fasciculus; C, Cingulum; CC, Corpus callosum; FOF, frontal occipital fasciculus; IOFF, inferior occipitofrontal fasciculus; MFB, Medial forebrain bundle which runs to the forebrain; SLF I and II, superior longitudinal fasciculus I and II; UF, U fibers; UnF, Uncinate faciculus. (Modified from Filley, C. M., *The Behavioral Neurology of White Matter*, Oxford University Press, New York, 2001, p. 23. By permission of Oxford University Press, Inc.)

TABLE 3.1
Functional Anatomy of the Attentional Networks

Domain	Gray Matter Structures	Connecting Tracts
Arousal	Reticular activating system	Medial forebrain bundle
	Thalamus	Thalamocortical radiations
	Cerebral cortex	Fronto-occipital (right side of brain)
Visual orientation	Superior colliculus	Collicular-pulvinar
	Pulvinar	Pulvinar-cortical
	Postparietal lobe	
Spatial attention	Parietal lobe (right)	Superior longitudinal fasciculus II
	Prefrontal lobe (right)	(right side of brain)
	Cingulate gyrus (right)	Cingulam (right side of brain)
Visuospatial ability	Parietal lobe (right)	Fronto-occipital fasciculus (right side of
	Frontal lobe (right)	brain)
Higher-order control of body-centered action	Superior parietal lobe	Superior longitudinal fasciculus I
	Premotor areas	
Recognition	Temporal lobes	Inferior longitudinal fasciculus
	Occipital lobes	
Language	Broca's area	Arcuate fasciculus (left side of brain)
	Wernicke's area	Extreme capsule (left side of brain)
Memory	Medial temporal lobe	Fornices
	Diencephalon	Mamillothalamic tracts
	Basal forebrain	Septohippocampal tracts
Emotions and personality	Temporolimbic system	Medial forebrain bundles
	Orbitofrontal cortices	Uncinate fascicli

Source: Filley, C.M., *The Behavioral Neurology of White Matter*, Oxford University Press, New York, 2001, p. 34. With permission.

para-hippocampal and hippocampal areas and is involved in the motivation and emotional aspects of behavior, as well as spatial working memory.[16] The uncinate fasciculus connects the rostral temporal lobe with the prefrontal areas as involved in attaching emotional valance to visual information and recognition memory.[17] An example of this striatal system would be the sagittal stratum, which contains the optic radiation. Besides these cortically derived white matter pathways connecting the cortex with other areas of the same hemisphere, other pathways exist connecting the hemispheres with each other allowing the transfer of visual as well as other information from one hemisphere to the other. These are called *commissural fiber tracks* with the corpus callosum being both the largest and clinically the most important. In summary, there are a multitude of neural assemblies that occur in the brain that are widely anatomically distributed yet functionally anatomically integrated to serve specific domains.[18]

FUNCTIONAL ORGANIZATION OF THE VISUAL SYSTEM

Five principles governing the organization of the visual system in addition to other modalities of sensation and action are outlined in Kandel's book *The Principles of*

Neuroscience.[19] The first states that several brain regions carry out different types of visual processing. The second states that identifiable pathways link different components of the visual system. The third is that each part of the brain projects in an orderly fashion onto the next creating topographical maps. These were discussed in the prior section of Primary Visual System whereas the visual information from the retina was topographically represented throughout successive stages of processing, allowing for neural maps of visual information for the receptive fields to be reformed at sequential levels in the brain. Fourth, in general, the functional visual system is hierarchically organized, transmitting information from lower to higher centers. In addition, because of the complexity of the visual system, parallel circuits also exist to provide interconnections of multiple visually related brain areas. The fifth principle of the visual system is that one side of the brain controls vision for the other side of the body. This means that there is a "seam" down the middle of visual space where the two halves meet.

FUNCTIONAL COMPONENTS OF THE VISUAL SYSTEM

RECEPTION

The optical system, the binocular and accommodative systems, and the primary afferent visual system, provide for the function of visual reception. The optic system and primary afferent system have already been discussed. Visual reception is the ability to see, fixate, fuse, focus, move the eyes to the object of regard, and send the signal in its purest form from the retina to the primary visual cortex. The gaze system is the visual fixation system that allows for bilateral foveation on a desired target. It is dependent on full fields of vision that are selected from the attention system of the brain. The gaze system has two synchronized components (supra- and infranuclear systems).

Supranuclear Gaze Control

The cortical or supranuclear influence on gaze is carried out by six distinct neural networks: (1) the saccadic eye system directs the fovea from one object to another object of interest; (2) smooth pursuits hold the image of a moving target on the fovea; (3) the vergence system acts to move the eyes in opposite directions (i.e., convergent and divergent) so that the image of a single object in space can be placed simultaneously on the fovea; (4) vestibulo-ocular holds images still on the retina during brief head movements driven by signals of the vestibular system; (5) optokinetic system holds the image still insofar as possible during sustained head rotation or watching a sustained stimulus going by, such as a train; and finally (6) the fixation system holds the fovea in place on a stationary target. These complex supranuclear networks result in eye movements coordinating whole muscle groups. With the exception of the vergence system, supranuclear eye networks mediate conjugate eye movements. Thus, other than vergence system disorders, supranuclear damage does not lead to diplopia, but to restrictions of conjugate gaze, as in loss of upgaze or downgaze.

The higher cortical centers that influence gaze specify only a desired change in eye position as determined by visual information of the desired environmental stimulus. These signals are transmitted to various brainstem structures, where motor programming occurs integrating the motor nuclei of cranial nerves (CN) III, IV, and VI with the horizontal and vertical eye centers specifying eye position and velocity. The vertical gaze center is located in the mesencephalic reticular activating system and the horizontal gaze center is in the pontine reticular formation. In addition, through multisensory integration (particularly vestibular and proprioceptive), movements of the head help position the fovea on a target in the visual field. Some of these neural systems for specific gaze function are better delineated than others. Figure 3.8 shows the cortical pathways for saccadic eye movements.

Infranuclear Gaze Control

Misalignment of the two visual axes with complaints of diplopia frequently results with lesions involving the infranuclear portion of the gaze system, including CN III, IV, or VI or the myoneural junction or extraocular muscles they innervate. Intranuclear lesions also result in diplopia. Innervation of extraocular muscles is ipsilateral to the CN nucleus for CN III and VI, and contralateral for CN IV. The infranuclear ocular motor system is a complex motor system requiring the coordination of twelve muscles to move the eyes. These muscles are well known and rotate the eye in the orbit by

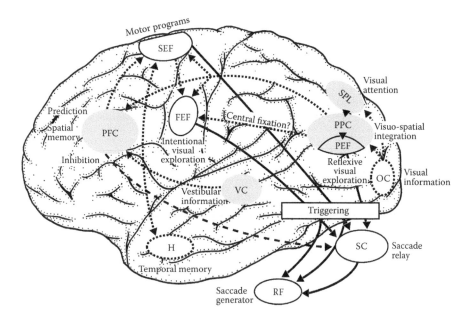

FIGURE 3.8 Cortical pathways for saccadic eye movements. Note that some of the arrows are bidirectional. FEF, frontal eye field; H, hippocampus; OC, occipital cortex; PEF parietal eye field; PFC, prefrontal cortex; PPC, posterior parietal cortex; RF, reticular formation; SC, superior colliculus; SEF, supplemental eye field; SPL, superior parietal lobule; VC, vestibular complex. (Adapted from Boller, F., Grafman, J., and Behrmann, M. (Eds.), *Handbook of Neuropsychology: Volume 4 Disorders of Visual Behavior,* 2nd ed., Elsevier, New York, 2001, p. 22.)

abduction, adduction, elevation, depression, intorsion, and extorsion. CN III supplies four of the six extraocular muscles, the medial rectus, superior rectus, inferior rectus, and inferior oblique. CN III also supplies the levator muscle of the eyelid and carries parasympathetic fibers that supply the smooth muscle of the ciliary body for accommodation and the iris sphincter for pupillary constriction. CN IV innervates the superior oblique muscle, which is frequently palsied in TBI, as CN IV leaves the dorsal aspect of the brainstem in fine rootlets. CN VI supplies innervation to the lateral rectus.

Accommodation

The innervation for accommodation has both premotor and cortical neural components. The premotor neural component for accommodation is the autonomic nervous system with the parasympathetic system initiating the accommodative response to focus closer and the sympathetic system assisting in the relaxation for more distant viewing. The cortical connection for accommodation begins with fibers from the primary visual cortex then extends to the parietal temporal areas and the cerebellum. The circuit continues to the Edinger-Westphal nucleus in the pretectum, where input is received and processed to form a motor command by the oculomotor nerve.

ATTENTION

Attention is a modular process allowing us to be aware of our environment. It serves as both a filter and a binder. The brain's capacity for processing sensory information is more limited, again, than its receptor capacity for evaluation of the environment. Thus, attention serves as a filter selecting salient signals for further processing. Humans have the ability to hold more than one stimulus at a time, thus attention can be described as a variety of phenomena such as simple, sustained, or divided attention. Selective attention is a powerful factor in perception, action, and memory, and in the unity of the conscious experience. The latter function is performed by binding together inputs from all sensory modalities, and then generating a complex internal representation of the external world. This is carried out by attending to only a small number of stimuli, and ignoring the remainder. This binds together perceptual features with spatial maps to form a unified whole. Attention is mediated by both cortical and subcortical components and at the subcortical level is termed preattention.

In their textbook *Neurology of Cognitive and Behavioral Disorders*,[20] Devinsky and D'Esposito provide a reductionalistic anatomical approach to attention, describing three neural networks that mediate this cognitive domain. Figure 3.9 illustrates these neural networks: (1) the arousal alerting system; (2) the orienting system; and (3) the selective attentional networks all of which function and interconnect in a seamless fashion.

The Arousal Alerting Network

The arousal alerting network is a diffusely distributed attentional system that awakens us to survey our internal and external environment for relevant novel or change in visual or other sensory stimuli. It is a total subcortical unit involved in bottom-up processing. Its components consist of the ascending reticular activating system in the

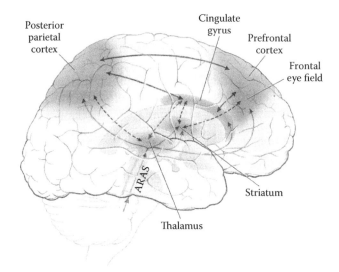

FIGURE 3.9   Functional anatomical networks of attention. The arousal and alerting network, a predominantly subcortical projection system, includes the reticular structures. The orienting network, a mixed cortical-subcortical system, includes the superior colliculus, pulvinar, and posterior parietal cortex. The selective attentional network, a predominantly cortical system, includes the frontal cortex. The three networks interact with each other and with the cingulate cortex to function as a unit. ARAS, ascending reticular activating system. (From Devinsky, O. and D'Esposito, M., *Neurology of Cognitive and Behavioral Disorders,* Oxford University Press, New York, 2004, p. 104. By permission of Oxford University Press, Inc.)

brainstem and its white matter connections to the thalamus and subcortical areas in the limbic system. This activity is mediated by various neural transmitters, including dopamine, acetylcholine, norepinephrine, serotonin, and glutamate.

The Orienting Network

The orienting network is a mixed cortical–subcortical system, whose gray matter parts consist of the superior colliculus in the midbrain, the pulvinar in the thalamus, and the posterior parietal lobe in addition to interlocking white matter connections. The major function of this system is to orient toward a visual stimulus, with each component having specific functions. The superior colliculus attends to novel stimuli, computes target location for attentional shifts, and is involved in hyperreflexive orienting to the ipsilateral field. The pulvinar restricts input to selective sensory regions, filters irrelevant stimuli, facilitates response to include target, and assists in covert orienting.

The Selective Attention Network

The selective attentional network, of which the superior longitudinal fasciculus II is the major component, is a total cortical network involved in voluntary top-down processing. This system has various components. Disengaging attention from the present focus is mediated by the posterior parietal cortex. The left posterior parietal lobe disengages from objects whereas the right posterior parietal lobe disengages from location. The superior parietal lobule allows for voluntary shifts of attention, whereas the frontal eye fields generate saccadic eye movements.

The functional organization of the attentional system is complex and not fully understood. It, again, is the binding or the ability to simultaneously bring online neural circuits that mediate form and spatial representation. The selective attentional system allows this internal representation to enter the realm of consciousness and to proceed as a unified whole. An example of this would be to see a beautiful purple lilac bush with its wonderful color and fragrance. However, the conscious experience is much more unique and different to each individual as this internal representation is connected with other memory and emotional centers giving different meaning to each individual based on past experience, and thus a different subjective conscious experience.

The cognitive control of the anatomical functional system of attention is carried out via either endogenous, voluntary, top-down cortically controlled processing, or endogenous, automatic, reflex bottom-up control, which is stimulus driven. The master switch or cortically represented selective attention of the cortical attention system is unknown but it has been suggested that the prefrontal cortex is an important area. There is, however, controversy as to whether there is likely to be a more widely distributed system of master control throughout the cortex and thalamus or a smaller set of neurons acting as a "spotlight of attention." Crick suggested that the claustrum is a likely candidate for the master switch.[21] To further complicate the issue, attention can not only be a focus but also diffuse with flexibility existing in regards to the attentional focus. If a master switch does exist, where does it report to? What turns the switch off and on, creating a subconscious to a conscious experience? Switching definitely occurs as demonstrated by a simple exercise in studying binocular rivalry. Two different images, one vertical stripes and the other horizontal stripes, can be presented to an individual simultaneously in such a manner that each eye can only see one set of stripes. The person may see the plaid design or alternate back and forth seeing the horizontal or vertical stripes. This is an example of both binocular competition and the switch of attention.

HIGHER VISUAL PROCESSING

PRIMARY VISUAL CORTEX

When visual inputs are projected onto the retina, early and rudimentary visual analysis begins. These signals are transmitted in a spatially, temporally ordered manner with specific receptive fields throughout the afferent system to the primary visual cortex. Higher cortical processing begins in the primary visual cortex and becomes more complex as information travels to extra striate and to higher cortical areas. The primary visual cortex (V1) occupies the medial occipital lobe and is called the *striate cortex*. It contains 250 million neurons connecting with 1.25 million lateral geniculate neurons. It has a laminar organization with special column organization. It contains alternating vertical columns of cells, the orientation and the ocular dominance columns with blobs in peg-shaped patches in the upper layers. Each cell type has a specific function. The orientation cells respond to specific axis of orientation, the blobs with initial color processing, and ocular dominance cells with binocular integration. Stereopsis processing begins in the primary visual cortex as this area is the first in the primary visual system to receive input from both eyes. As a consequence of the separation of the eyes, objects in the environment give rise to a two-dimensional projection that differs slightly in their location on each retina (i.e., retinal disparity). Cells in V1 are responsive to stereoscopic input and exhibit disparity tuning. The thick stripes in V2 and higher visual areas are involved in the higher visual processing for stereopsis.

The magno- and parvocellular pathways remain anatomically segregated as they enter the primary visual cortex through sublayers 4Ca and 4Cb and spread out and connect with simple and more complex cells in more superficial and inferior layers of V1. A major change in receptive field configuration of the orientation cells occurs outside layer 4 becoming elongated rather than concentric. This changes the maximum response from a spot of light to a bar of light. Despite this change of configuration, the receptive fields of the orientation cells remain similar to that of the ganglion cells in the retina still specifying retinal position with antagonistic, excitatory, and inhibitory zones. Simple cells respond to the orientation in a specific axis in its visual field whereas complex cells monitor several simple cells and react to a specific axis of orientation without regard to its visual field location. These complex cells project to hypercolumns of cells both within and outside the primary visual cortex, which respond to lines of orientation from a represented area in the visual field. Lateral networks connect these cells and bring together the data from the visual field or, in other words, put all the pieces together to create an internal representation. Amazingly, a poorly outlined visual image, based on change of contrast, color, texture, and retinal disparity, projected by the afferent visual system from the retina to V1, where it is de-constructed into lines of various orientation by simple and complex cells and then reconstructed by hypercolumns of cells, becomes the three-dimensional picture of the world that we call vision. V1 has extensive connections not only with extrastriate areas and higher cortical areas but also subcortical areas, including the superior colliculus, pons, pulvinar, and lateral geniculate body. The parvocellular pathway exits layers two and three as the ventral stream and the magnocellular layer forms the dorsal stream as it exits layer 4.

EXTRASTRIATE VISUAL ASSOCIATION AREAS

There are seven identifiable visual association areas (extrastriate) in addition to an area involved in the perception of faces. Figure 3.10 shows these visual association areas. Again, there are extensive interconnections between these areas. V2 is located adjacent to V1 and responds to all major visual modalities and is the largest visual association area in the occipital lobe. V3 surrounds V2 and some of its functions include early processing of motion and depth perception in addition to form analysis at lower contrast. The ventral area of V4 is involved in analysis of color whereas its dorsal area is involved with size estimation. V5 is located in the lateral convexity near the junction of the temporal, parietal, and occipital lobes responding maximally to motion detection. V6 has not been precisely localized in humans and it is thought to be involved in self-motion, three-dimensional features, target selection, and visual search analysis. V8 is involved in the higher analysis of color. Facial perception is mediated in the area shown in Figure 3.8, which shows these visual association areas.

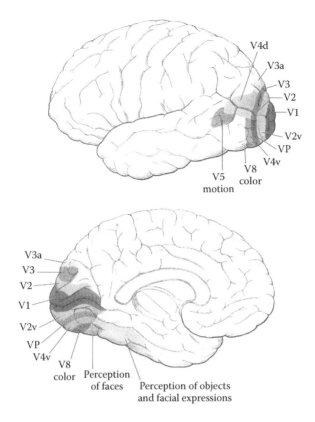

FIGURE 3.10   Principal visual areas in humans. (From Devinsky, O. and D'Esposito, M., *Neurology of Cognitive and Behavioral Disorders,* Oxford University Press, New York, 2004, p. 125. By permission of Oxford University Press, Inc.)

The Ventral "What" Stream

Anatomy of the Ventral Stream

After processing in the occipital lobe, visual information is subjected to additional processing in two discrete but interacting streams or pathways, the ventral (parvocellular) or the "What" system, and the dorsal (magnocellular) or the "Where and How to" system.[22] The inferior longitudinal fasciculus is a long association fiber system and is a major component of the ventral stream connecting the primary visual cortex with V4 and specific areas in the temporal lobe. It is, therefore, the pre-eminent fiber track conveying visual information in a bidirectional manner between the occipital and temporal lobes mediating recognition of objects and faces. The inferior longitudinal fasciculus has two limbs; the horizontal limb, and the vertical limb.[16] The horizontal limb connects rostrally with the temporal lobe at the level of the uncinate fasciculus. The horizontal limb connects with memory (hippocampal and amygdala), as well as other emotional centers, giving additional meaning to the object or face. The uncinate fasciculus provides strong connections between the inferior longitudinal fasciculus and the prefrontal cortex for additional modulation.[16] The vertical limb of the inferior longitudinal fasciculus terminates in the cortex in the lower bank of the superior temporal sulcus with connections to the language system.

Function of the Ventral Stream

In considering how we create recognizable representations of faces and objects, Marr[23] suggests three stages of symbolic representation. The first stage is the primal sketch or the primitive representation comprising brightness or intensity change that is seen by the viewer. These changes in brightness allow one to form the shape of the viewed object. The second stage is a viewer-centered sketch or two-dimensional sketch, representing the viewed object from a viewer-centered frame of reference, with the features presented in relation to where they fall in the retina. The highest level or the object-center reference frame coordinates the shapes and features as they are related to one another rather than how they are related to the viewer. In the latter, no matter which way the object is rotated, they continue to be represented as the same object and recognized.

THE DORSAL "WHERE" OR "HOW TO" STREAM

Anatomy of the Dorsal Stream

The dorsal stream also originates in V1 and projects to V2 to V3 to V5, and then on to additional areas in the parietal and superior temporal cortex. The dorsal stream connection between early visual processing cortices (V1–V3) and V5 (which processes motion) as well as parietal areas (which are involved in the mediation of visuospatial processing) explain why this processing stream has been considered the "Where" system. It also connects these areas to the anterior motor association areas including the prefrontal eye fields, to allow us to plan and execute eye movements and other behaviors, based on our visual input, which is why it is considered the "How to" system. Again, two major components of the dorsal stream include the superior longitudinal fasciculus II and the frontal occipital fasciculus.[16] The superior longitudinal fasciculus II connects the posterior parietal cortex in multisensory integration with the prefrontal cortex and is involved in spatial awareness playing a role in the visual and oculomotor aspects of spatial function. The frontal occipital fasciculus links the parietal occipital areas with the dorsolateral premotor and prefrontal areas and is involved in the processing of visual information regarding the peripheral visual field and therefore visuospatial processing. (The superior longitudinal fasciculus I is not part of the dorsal stream, but connects the superior parietal region and adjacent medial parietal cortex in a reciprocal manner with the frontal lobe, supplemental, eye, and motor areas.)[16] The superior parietal lobule codes movement and position-related activities of the limbs in a body-centered coordinate system, conveying higher-order somatosensory and kinesthetic information regarding the trunk and limbs to the frontal lobe. In the prefrontal cortex, there is an articulation that occurs from these three different long association fiber tracks helping to explain visual-motor integration.

Function of the Dorsal Stream

To understand the visuospatial function of the dorsal stream, or its ability to identify the location of objects, it is important to understand the sensory modality of space. It is a sensory modality without a single end organ, and space representation is the most complex of all sensory modalities. The dorsal stream is specialized for spatial representation in several ways. First, the visual representation in individual dorsal stream areas is uniformly broader than that found in the ventral stream. The latter represents only the central 35–45 degrees of the visual angle, whereas areas of the dorsal stream represent the entire visual field out to 90 degrees. Second, single neurons and several dorsal stream areas are specialized for detection and analysis of moving visual stimuli, including speed and direction. Thirdly, neurons in several dorsal stream areas are sensitive to the depth at which a stimulus appears relative to the viewer. The parietal cortex is the preeminent cortical area responsible for spatial perception. However, there is no evidence of an existence of a single explicit topographical representation of space. Further evidence points to multiple representations of space in a variety of coordinate frames that link separate output systems designated to guide specific motor effectors.

Frames of Reference

There are both viewer-centered reference frames, in which locations are related to the viewer, and allocentric reference frames in which location represent reference frames independent of the observer. The viewer-centered reference frame is the traditional approach of describing the structure involved in vision. Allocentric reference frames include both object-centered and environmental-centered coordinates. Space is represented in a three-dimensional fashion having vertical, horizontal, and radial axis. The parietal lobe houses a structural body map that refers to a representation of the shape and contours of the human body, in general, to one's own body in particular. This representation defines a detailed map of the body surface and its boundaries between body parts that are coded. These spatial maps are divided into hand-centered, body-centered, eye-centered, and retinal coordinates. The visual attentional system then binds together the ventral (what) and the dorsal (where) systems representing the object and its location in space to form a unity conscious experience.

Visual Integration

Visual-motor integration involves not only the above-mentioned neural circuitry but also subcortical circuitry for gait and posture. The body schema refers to an active online representation of one's own body in space that is derived from multisensorial input and its articulation with the motor effector system.[24] The visual control of walking is controlled by inputs of the sensory system to the body schema. This involves multisensorial integration occurring in the posterior association area, anterior association area, superior colliculus, and pulvinar, which directs the motor system to control the extremities, trunk, and ocular motor systems. It involves integration of sensory inputs from the visual, proprioceptive, and vestibular systems. Approximately 20% of neural signals from the eyes interact with the vestibular system. When information from the various sensory systems does not match up, a mismatch occurs between egocentric visual space and the actual visual space resulting in abnormal egocentric localization, also known as visual midline shift.

Pertinent to the visual control of walking involves optic flow. A person perceives the visual pathway of the destination with respect to the body schema and walks in that direction. Steering is based on optic flow, the pattern of visual motion as the patient's focus expands in the direction of the walk. Optic flow is measured by motion sensor neurons in the dorsal stream in the medial superior temporal lobe. Visual cognition is the highest form of processing contributing toward our ability to think, reason, and make decisions by binding together the different brain circuitry simultaneously to accomplish our desired goal. This is carried out in the supramodal areas.

MIRROR NEURONS

Another neural circuitry recently discovered in humans is the mirror-neuron system. Mirror neurons have been described in the inferior frontal gyrus, the adjacent premotor cortex, and the rostral part of the inferior parietal lobule.[25] The mirror-neuron system is connected with the superior temporal sulcus that provides a higher-order visual description of observed action. There are probably other connections to the prefrontal cortex that are involved in visual social processing. This is an observation-execution/emotional analysis system that has been implicated in knowing not only the motor intention of others but also motor imagery and empathy. This system allows us to achieve the very subtle understanding of others that helps explain the complex forms of social cognition and interaction.

SUMMARY OF HIGHER VISUAL PROCESSING

The complexity of the interconnection between brain areas and their numerous diffuse distributions is apparent. There are two types of linkages for processing this visual information: a serial or hierarchical system and a parallel or nonhierarchical system. The hierarchical system is based on the sequential transfers of visual information from lower to higher centers of perception in an orderly fashion, with information being reorganized at each level with more advanced analysis occurring in higher levels. The parallel, or nonhierarchical system, is a system of feed forward and feed back, or collateral connections. The connections are bidirectional. Top-down control refers to the processing of higher to lower centers in a nonduplicated manner for detail and awareness. This includes the influence of the supramodal and multimodal areas of the cortex on bottom-up visual information. Bottom-up processing refers to construction of a visual representation from tiny pieces of information that are perceived at the retina and then transferred by the afferent visual system to the primary visual cortex. Again, this occurs by binding together certain neural networks and excluding others to accomplish the desired behavior, incorporating experiential memories and emotions to the representation. Visual imagery, or imagination, uses the same neural circuitry as visual perception, except that there is no object or event stimulating the visual center; the stimulus is generated in the memory centers, which then in turn stimulate the visual areas.[26] Visual cognition, again, is the result of the binding of multimodal sensory areas with the supramodal association areas for visual manipulation, organization, concept formation, and decision making.

CLASSIFICATION OF VISUAL DEFECTS

The functional anatomic organization of vision is multifaceted, with extensive inter-digitated networks modulated by attention. TBI inflicts diffuse damage to the central nervous system as opposed to a stroke, which is more focal; therefore, it is not surprising that a variety of deficits are noted as sequelae of TBI. Humans are highly reliant on vision for spatial orientation for environment interaction and these deficits can cause functional limitations, sometimes subtle and difficult to diagnosis. Patients with neurological disorders affecting vision present frequently with the characteristic visual field defects and/or decreased visual acuity. In these patients, localization is relatively straight forward, leading to an easy and appropriate diagnosis. However, patients presenting with syndromes of higher cortical dysfunction related to involvement of higher association visual areas have more challenging presentations and require more expertise in diagnosis to ensure proper treatment. Defects will be discussed in relationship to the categorization of the components of the functional visual system—reception, attention, and higher cortical processing.

DISORDERS OF RECEPTION

Any impairment in visual input will result in decreased visual sensory ability. Conditions affecting the optical system of the eye will prevent a clear and undistorted image from being presented to the retina. Conditions interfering with visual fixation, binocular fusion, and focusing will result in decreased visual function in everyday life. This includes abnormalities in the supranuclear and infranuclear neural networks, which are widely distributed, but are predominantly represented in the upper brainstem, which is the most frequent site of diffuse axonal injury secondary to TBI. Common sequelae of TBI, therefore, include abnormalities of eye movement secondary to gaze palsies and CN palsies, in addition to other abnormalities of binocular dysfunction, including accommodation and other nonstrabismic disorders. Ciuffreda et al. [27] review the high frequency of visual ocular abnormalities following TBI.

Lesions involving the primary visual pathway and higher visual association areas impair perception, resulting in absolute or partial defects. This can result in decreased visual acuity to blindness to visual field defects, either homonymous hemianopsia or scotoma, impairment of color vision (achromatopsia), depth perception (astereognosis), and motion perception (cerebral akinetopsia). Color vision is processed by areas V1, V2, V3, V4, and V8 motion by V5 and stereopsis and depth perception by V1 and V2.

DISORDERS OF ATTENTION

The prototype visuospatial defect arising from damage in the attentional system is hemispatial neglect or the inability to orient or attend to the contralateral space. The right hemisphere is dominant for visuospatial function and mediates attention for both the right and the left hemispace, whereas the left hemisphere mediates only the right hemispace. This explains the more favorable prognosis for right-sided neglect. The neural networks involved in attention are widely distributed and neglect can result from lesions involving different anatomical areas of the brain. These areas include the right and left parietal area, the right and left dorsolateral frontal areas, right and left medial frontal areas, right and left striatum, right thalamus, and white matter of the internal capsule and cerebral hemisphere.[28–30] Neglect is not a result of a direct impairment of the primary sensory modality of vision so patients having neglect do not always demonstrate homonymous visual field defects. It can be difficult to separate out unilateral neglect from homonymous hemianopsia. Common tests used in making this differential include line bisection, line cancellation, letter cancellation, copy figures, picture interpretation, and presentation of simultaneous bilateral visual stimuli. The last test, however, is only helpful if a visual field defect is not present. More unusual disturbances of hemispatial neglect involve limits of the size of the object that can be perceived and, in some instances, impairment in the number of objects that can be identified at any given time. The disorder resulting in the perception related to the size of the stimulus is rare and thought to be related to the restriction in the "spotlight of attention." Simultanagnosia is the name of a disorder characterized by an impaired ability to see more than one object at a time. This is explained by the inability to shift attention, narrowing effective visual fields resulting from bilateral posterior parietal lesions. The Navon letter test is a simple screening test to evaluate this function.

DISORDERS OF HIGHER VISUAL PROCESSING

Ventral Stream Disconnections

Although an oversimplification, the easiest approach to conceptualize disorders of higher visual-perceptual and visuospatial processing is to think of disconnections involving either the ventral or dorsal stream. Disconnections involving the ventral stream can be classified as visual–visual, visual–verbal, and visual–limbic. Visual–visual disconnects result in agnosia. Agnosia refers to the clinical condition in which the patient is able to perceive visual stimuli and has preserved language capacity to name the visual representation but recognition is lost. These conditions include the loss of recognition of object feature, object identity, faces, places, and color. These conditions are named, respectively, visual apperceptive and visual associative agnosia, prosopagnosia, topographagnosia, and color agnosia. Apperceptive visual agnosia is the condition in which patients cannot distinguish one form from another, whereas visual associative agnosia is a disturbance of visual recognition with intact visual perception. Loss of connectivity between visual–verbal systems result in pure alexia, color, and object anomia. Visual anomia indicates recognition is intact, but the ability to name is impaired. Impaired linkages between visual–limbic areas result in visual amnesia and hypoemotionality.

Dorsal Stream Disconnections

Disconnects in the dorsal stream can result in malfunction of either the "where" or "how to" systems. Impaired connectivity with V5 can result in abnormal motion perception (akinetopsia) as discussed earlier. Visuospatial processing defects occur when there is a disconnect between the dorsal stream and spatial representation resulting in visual hemineglect, which can be partial or complete, based on viewer-, object-, or environmental-centered references. Optic ataxia or misreaching to a visualized target is a possible example of a disconnect to the dorsal stream and motor areas, although recent data suggest that this is more complicated in its mechanism. Psychic paralysis of gaze, the latter termed *ocular motor apraxia*, is caused by bilateral posterior parietal lesions implying a disconnect between the dorsal stream and the frontal eye fields, as this defect cannot be attributed to an impairment in the brainstem mechanisms controlling eye movements because these patients exhibit normal oculocephalic reflexes and preserved exogenous clued saccadic eye movements.

POSITIVE VISUAL PHENOMENA

The negative visual phenomena, or deficits in vision, have been discussed in relationship to disruption in different parts of the visual system. There are also positive visual phenomena that occur with abnormalities in either the primary visual system or secondary visual system. These are illusions and hallucinations. Three pathophysiological mechanisms are thought to be responsible for these positive visual phenomena. The first is secondary to deafferentation resulting in a secondary release of cortical inhibition. The second is related to direct damage or irritation to the retina, optic nerve, primary visual cortex, or parietal or temporal visually related cortex.[31] The third mechanism is related to disequilibrium between the neurotransmitters acetylcholine and serotonin. A relative excess of serotonergic input or relative deficiency of cholinergic input to the LGN inhibits the latter's ability to transmit visual information to the parietal or temporal visually related cortex.

Visual illusions are distortions of objects in current view. These include micropsia, where an actual object appears smaller; macropsia, where an object appears larger; or metamorphopsia, where an object is distorted. Visual hallucinations are visual images that a person sees, when in reality they are not present in the environment. They can occur with defects of either the primary visual system or secondary visual system. They are classified as unformed or formed, simple or complex. They are caused by a spontaneous activation of a visual related brain area. In general, this activation in a cortical area tends to spread over time leading to more complex hallucinations. Hallucinations are not stored memories as their content is not related to one's past personal experience. It is important in the clinical evaluation of hallucinations to determine if they are monocular, involve one hemifield, or an entire visual field. Monocular hallucinations would indicate unilateral retinopathy or optic neuropathy. Visual hallucinations involving one hemifield would indicate dysfunction in corresponding a unilateral visually related cortex. Visual hallucinations involving entire visual fields would indicate either a deafferentation state or a bilateral retinopathy, optic neuropathy, or visually related cortical dysfunction.[31]

VISION AND TRAUMATIC BRAIN INJURY

Traumatic brain injury is an unrecognized epidemic occurring in the United States. Between 180 and 250 persons per 100,000 suffer from TBI each year. Approximately, 230,000 are hospitalized and released and 50,000 die. It is the leading cause of death and disability among young adults. Children are particularly vulnerable to TBI because during childhood, portions of the brain are still myelinating and so patients

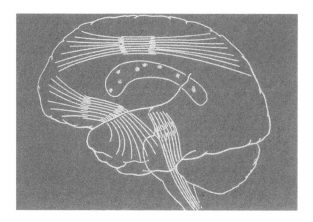

FIGURE 3.11   Schematic drawing of white matter regions in the brain that are most susceptible to diffuse axonal injury in TBI: the brainstem, cerebral hemispheres, and corpus callosum. (From Filley, C. M., *The Behavioral Neurology of White Matter,* Oxford University Press, New York, 2001, p. 167. By permission of Oxford University Press, Inc.)

not only have to recover from the deficit but be able to layer on additional learning to ensure normal development. TBI is many times a catastrophic injury resulting in life-long physical, cognitive, and emotional deficits resulting in a huge emotional burden on families and a financial burden on society. Visual input accounts for approximately two-thirds of all sensory information being processed by the brain. Therefore, visuospatial and visual-perceptual deficits are common sequelae of TBI. The frontal and anterior temporal pole are most frequently damaged because of the way the brain is positioned in the skull, butting up against the jagged bony edges of the anterior and middle fossa. The hallmark pathophysiological abnormality of TBI is diffuse axonal injury, resulting from the shearing forces. The supramodal areas, that is the anterior and limbic association cortices, are of utmost importance because all of the major fasciculi terminate in them. Because of their location in the brain, they are prone to shearing injuries and contusions. Midline brain structures are most vulnerable to diffuse axonal injury, including the subcortical white matter, corpus callosum, and rostral brainstem, the latter explaining the vulnerability of the midbrain systems (see Figure 3.11). Other structures such as CN III, IV, and VI and the eye can be damaged. This is a very simple explanation of the frequent occurrence of visuospatial and visual-perceptual deficits following TBI, in addition to other cognitive problems in the area of memory, attention, and executive function. It is imperative that residual disorders of primary and secondary visual system be diagnosed early and treated both appropriately and aggressively to promote proper brain plasticity that will result in the maximal recovery of visual function.

REFERENCES

1. Nauta, W. H. H., & Feritag M. (1986). *Fundamental neuroanatomy.* New York: W. H. Freeman Publishing.

2. Van Essen, D. C. (1985). Functional organization of the primate visual cortex. In A. Peters, & E. G. Jones (Eds.), *Cerebral cortex* (Vol. 3, pp. 259–329), New York: Plenum Press.

3. Felleman, D. J., & Van Essen, D. C. (1991). Distributed hierarchical processing in the primate cerebral cortex. *Cerebral Cortex, 1,* 1–47.

4. Yeterian E. H., & Pandya D. N. (1997). Corticothalamic connections of extrastriate visual areas in Rhesus monkeys. *The Journal of Comparative Neurology, 378*(4), 562–585.

5. Bowey, A., Stoerig, P., & Bannister, M. (1994). Retinal ganglion cells labeled from the pulvinar nucleus in Macaque monkeys. *Neuroscience, 61,* 691–705.

6. Robinson, D. L., & Cowie, R. J. (1997). The primate pulvinar structural, functional and behavioral environments of visual salience. In M. Steriade., E. G. James, & D. J. McCormick (Eds.), *Thalamus: Experimental and clinical aspects* (Vol. 2, pp. 53–92). New York: Elsevier.

7. Notle, J. (1998). *The human brain: An introduction to its functional anatomy* (4th ed.). St. Louis, MO: Mosby.

8. Bryd, S. E., Darling, C. F., & Wilczymski, M. A. (1993). White matter of the brain: maturation and myelination on magnetic resonance in infants and children. *Neuroimaging Clinics of North America, 3,* 247–266.

9. Benes, F. M., Turtle, M., Khan, Y., & Farol, P. (1994). Myelination of a key relay zone in the hippocampal formation occurs in the human brain during childhood, adolescence, and adulthood. *Archives of General Psychiatry, 51*(6), 477–484.

10. Rodieck, R. W., & Watanabe, M. (1998). Survey of the morphology of macaque retinal ganglion cells that project to the pretectum, superior colliculus, and parvicellular laminae of the lateral geniculate nucleus. *The Journal of Comparative Neurology, 397*(3), 357–370.

11. Dacey, D. M. (1994). Physiology, morphology, and spatial densities of identified ganglion cell types in primate retina. *Ciba Foundation Symposium, 184,* 12–28.

12. Holmes, N. P., & Spence, C. (2005). Multisensory integration: Space, time, and super-additivity. *Current Biology, 15*(18), R762–R764.

13. Dai, J., Van der Vliet, J., Swaab, D. F., & Buijs, R. M. (1998). Human retinohypothalamic tract as revealed by in vitro postmortem tracing. *The Journal of Comparative Neurology, 397*(3), 357–370.

14. Cooley, J. J., Lu, J., Chou, T. C., Scammell, T. E., & Saper, C. B. (2001). Melanopsin in cells of origin of the retinohypothalamic tract. *Nature Neuroscience, 4*(12), 1165.

15. Berson, D. M. (2003). Strange vision: ganglion cells as circadian photoreceptors. *Trends in Neurosciences, 26*(6), 314–320.

16. Scmahmann, J. D., & Pandya, D. N. (2006). *Fiber pathways of the brain.* New York: Oxford University Press.

17. Filley, C. M. (2001). *The behavioral neurology of white matter.* New York: Oxford University Press.

18. Mesulam, M. M. (1990). Large scale neurocognitive networks and distributed processing for attention, language, and memory. *Annals of Neurology, 28*(5), 597–613.

19. Kandel, E. R., Schwartz, J. H., & Jessell, T. M. (2000). *Principles of neural science* (4th ed.). New York: McGraw-Hill.

20. Devinsky, O., & D'Esposito, M. (2004). *Neurology of cognitive and behavioral disorders.* New York: Oxford University Press.

21. Crick, F. C., & Koch, C. (2005). What is the function of the claustrum. *Philosophical transactions of the Royal Society of London. Series B, Biological Sciences, 360,* 1271–1279.

22. Ungerleider, L. G., & Miskin, M. (1982). Two cortical visual systems. In D. J. Ingle, M. A. Goodale, & R. J. W. Mansfield (Eds.), *Analysis of visual behavior* (pp. 549–586). Cambridge, MA: MIT Press.

23. Marr, D. (1982). *Vision: A computational investigation into the human representation and processing of visual information.* New York: WH Freeman and Co.
24. Gallanger, S. (1995). Body schema and intentionality. In J. L. Bermudez, A. J. Marcel, & N. Eilan (Eds.), *The body and the self* (pp. 225–244). Cambridge, MA: MIT Press.
25. Rocea, M. A., Tortorella, P., Ceccarelli, A., Falini, A., Tango, D., Seviti, G., Filippi, M. (2008). The mirror-neuron system in Ms. *Neurology, 70,* 255–262.
26. Kosslyn, S. M., Pascual-Leone, A., Felician, O., Camposano, S., Keenan, J. P., Thompson, W. L., Alpert, N. M. (1999). The role of area 17 in visual imagery: convergent evidence from PET and rTMS. *Science, 284*(5411), 167–170.
27. Ciuffreda, K. J., Kapoor, N., Rutner, D., Suchoff, I. B., Han, M. E., & Craig, S. (2007) Occurrence of oculomotor dysfunctions in acquired brain injury: a retrospective analysis. *Optometry, 78*(4), 155–161.
28. Heilman, K. M., Watson, R. T., & Valenstein, E. (1993). Neglect and related disorders. In K. M. Heilman, & E. Valenstein (Eds.), *Clinical neuropsychology* (3rd ed., pp. 279–336). New York: Oxford University Press.
29. Healton, E. B., Navarro, C., Bressman, S., & Brust, J. C. (1982). Subcortical neglect. *Neurology, 32*(7), 776–778.
30. Heilman, K. M., & Valenstein, E. (1972). Frontal lobe neglect in man. *Neurology, 22*(6), 660–664.
31. Trobe, J. D. (2001). *The neurology of vision* (pp. 71–72). New York: Oxford University Press.

4 Spatial Vision

Robert B. Sanet and Leonard J. Press

CONTENTS

The authors would like to thank Dr. Dan Press, Elliot Press, and Linda Sanet, COVT, for their assistance and technical support in the preparation of this chapter.

INTRODUCTION

Vision is the brain's way of touching the world.

(Merleau-Ponty 1964, p. 177)[1]

We have the subjective impression of an immediate, full detail, pictorial view of the world. However, we are prone to forget that the impression is, in a very real sense an illusion. The illusion is created through our incredible ability to direct our eyes effortlessly to any desired location.

(Findlay and Gilchrist 2003, p. 2)[2]

The visual world, seeming to present itself effortlessly to us, is largely a mental construction. What happens automatically does not happen without learning. Constructing a visual world requires a significant amount of effort and energy, with half of the cerebral cortex devoted to this task. And, seeing, as we now understand it, is at least as much a mental process as a physiological one.[3] Vision is an intelligent process of active construction, with information that is potentially available in the environment obtained at any location or any direction by directing our eyes there, enabling us to continually update information about our environment.[4] The visual system does not simply record images passively, but transforms light patterns processed at the level of the retina into a stable and coherent three-dimensional representation of our visual space world. These concepts, useful in helping us understand how we build visual-spatial knowledge from birth, become absolutely essential for understanding how acquired brain injury (ABI) destabilizes or deconstructs the visual space world we have assembled.

Spatial and temporal aspects of vision convey a sense of the individual's relationship with the environment. These two aspects of the visual system, while separable in the laboratory, become inseparable in the real world as an individual interacts with the environment through sequences of motor actions. We therefore conceptualize spatial vision (adapted from Bullier)[5] as encompassing:

- Understanding the position of our bodies in space
- Computing the relationships between objects and oneself
- Assessing and computing the spatial relationships between objects
- Understanding the visual-spatial features of objects in the environment
- Effective use of vision to guide movement through space
- Visually directed reaching, grasping, and manipulating of objects
- Major contributions to overall cognitive function

Imagine what the resultant cost might be in terms of an individual's ability to function normally in the world if, after an ABI, their eyes were "clumsy" and they could not, as Findlay and Gilchrist stated, "accurately and effortlessly direct their eyes to any desired location in space" (p. 18).[2] We will explore a series of questions to arrive at our understanding of some of the visual sequelae of ABI: What might result if an individual could see clearly, but couldn't perceptually interpret what was being seen? How does an individual deal with and efficiently move through the world if he is not able to accurately locate objects in space, to judge the space between objects, or to understand the relationship of the objects to oneself? How does difficulty directing the eyes to a desired location or seeing double impact a person's ability to navigate space? What problems might arise from a lack of coherence not only within visual pathways, but also between vision and other sensory systems, specifically auditory, vestibular, and somatosensory? How would these alterations affect not only a person's sense of the world, but also the individual's sense of self?

Spatial vision is intimately involved with the prediction, preparation, and control of motor movements. To effectively interact with and move through our world, spatial vision must be dynamic, flexible, anticipatory, and adaptable. The implications of visual-spatial dysfunction after ABI are vast and far reaching, not only in the physical sense but also in the personal and psychological sense. It is no wonder that patients with ABI are insecure, both in relation to the world and ultimately with respect to themselves.

Understanding spatial vision problems associated with ABI enables the clinician to perform an in-depth neuro-optometric diagnostic evaluation to identify problems in visual-spatial performance. Subsequent neuro-optometric rehabilitative care linked to visual-spatial dysfunction reaches beyond the visual problem, to engage the person as a whole. The use of therapeutic lenses, prisms, filters, and optometric rehabilitative procedures can often be the key aspects of an overall treatment plan in helping to restore a more accurate, stable, coherent, and unified visual world.

VISION DIRECTING ACTION

> All I have to do to figure out how much to move my body … is to duplicate with my body the movement specified by my eye.

(Berthoz 2000, p. 148)[6]

To effectively live in and move through our world, vision, in concert with other sensory systems, must efficiently and effectively guide many aspects of human behavior, including motor movements. This holds true not only for general body movement, but also for eye movements as well. Fine ocular movement is part and parcel of visual processing to the point that images of the world will fade from consciousness if eye movements are totally immobilized.[7]

The action systems of eye movements, binocular coordination, and accommodation are crucial for locating objects relative to oneself and to each other, which is the essence of spatial vision, and for interpreting objects, which is referred to as object vision. These systems are in turn affected by our cognitive interpretation of space. The execution of eye movement (ocular motor), vergence (binocular), and focusing (accommodative) movements are dependent upon our internal representations of space. These are the experiential maps that function as global positioning systems for the body.

We typically speak of sensation, perception, and cognition as stages of vision, but it is the reciprocal interweaving of top-down and bottom-up processes that propel and guide movement. Top-down visual processes include attentional mechanisms, internal maps, and cognitive controls. Bottom-up processes include the sensory cues of blur and retinal disparity. The entire process, including pursuit and saccadic eye movements, accommodative control, binocular alignment, and stereopsis, requires a significant number of brain structures working together in a coordinated and efficient manner. These visual structures communicate through neural networks, involving the retina, striate visual cortex, portions of the parietal, temporal, and frontal lobes, thalamic structures, including the LGN and pulvinar, tectum of the midbrain, superior colliculus, brainstem, vestibular system, and no less than 6 of the 12 cranial nerves. There are at least 32 separate visual areas of the brain, with 25 primarily or totally involved with the processing of visual information, and an additional 7 areas that are visual association areas, with more than 305 intracortical connections between these areas (Figure 4.1). Altogether, visual processing contains 14 levels and the great majority of pathways involve reciprocal connections between areas. Within this hierarchy, there are multiple, intertwined processing streams, which, at a low level, are related to the compartmental organization of areas V1 and V2 and, at a high level, are related to the distinction between processing centers in the temporal and parietal lobes.[8]

It is important to note that primary visual cortex, area V1, is only the third level from the origin of external visual input, which begins at the retinal ganglion cell (RGC) layer and passes through the lateral geniculate nucleus (LGN). Area V1 is the principal site for eyesight. The massive and reciprocal interconnections between V1 and the multiple areas beyond clearly demonstrate the difference between sight and the remarkably complex visual process.

The complex neurology of the visual system is comprehensively detailed in Chapter 3. A brief, and not necessarily complete review, is included here only as

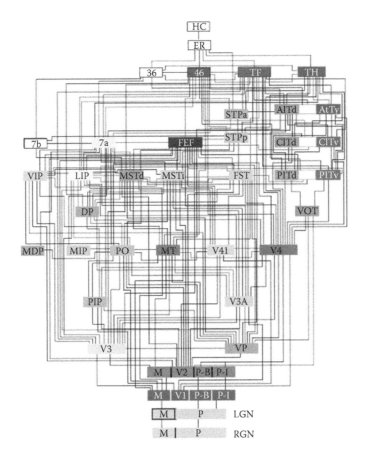

FIGURE 4.1 (**See color insert following page 270.**) Hierarchy of visual areas. This hierarchy shows 32 visual areas. These areas are connected by linkages, most of which have been demonstrated to be reciprocal pathways. (From Felleman, D. J. and Van Essen, D. C., Distributed hierarchial processing in the primate cerebral cortex. *Cerebral Cortex*, 1, 30, 1991. Reprinted with permission.)

it relates to some of the pathways fundamental to our understanding of the visual processes serving spatial vision.

MULTIPLE VISUAL PATHWAYS

Multisensory convergence and integration of information is generally the rule in the brain and most actions involve simultaneous, complex interactions. Actions thought of as simple, such as searching for a cup and then guiding the hand to reach it and then bringing it up to the lips to drink, involve many distinct functions requiring neural integration mediated by numerous visual pathways and brain centers.

Although many professionals tend to discuss the eyes as distinct from the brain, the retina is actually a thin sheet of brain tissue that grows into the eye to provide neural processing for photoreceptor signals.[9] In both structure and concept, the retina is essentially the outermost portion of the brain, converting light into a neural image, prompting the quote from Merleau-Ponty that opened this chapter. Damage to the retina is, therefore, just one of the numerous visual types of ABI.

There are multiple pathways that bring information from the eyes through the optic nerve and into various areas of the brain and the rest of the body. The largest is the geniculostriate pathway, which goes directly to the LGN, then into area V1 of the striate visual cortex in the occipital lobe, and then onward to other areas of the brain for processing and integrating the visual information. The extrastriate tectop-ulvinar pathway goes to the superior colliculus in the midbrain, and to the pulvinar, contributing to spatial orientation and eye movement control and integration of spa-tial information with vestibular, tactile, and auditory information. These extrastri-ate pathways intermingle with the geniculostriate pathways in the visual association areas of the cortex. The remainder of the visual pathways are involved with other visual functions such as optic flow, visual reflexes, and circadian rhythms. A dis-cussion of optic flow appears later in this chapter. A discussion of the other visual pathways is outside the scope of this chapter.

Major partitioning of the neural image begins in the RGCs, dividing information into M and P channels, named for the magnocellular and parvocellular layers of the LGN onto which they project.

Magno cells account for approximately 20% of the RGCs. They are mostly periph-eral retinal cells, although they are distributed throughout the retina, even in the fovea, the most central area of vision.[10] These cells have large receptive fields and they are not designed to resolve fine detail. However, they respond rapidly and transiently so that they can sample a large number of temporal inputs over a short period of time. This allows M cells to provide good temporal resolution when conveying movement and spa-tial information along the retino-geniculo-striate pathway. Functionally, the result is that instead of seeing space as a series of individual snapshots of space separated in time, space can then be perceived as a continual and uninterrupted flow of movement.

After arriving in area V1 of the occipital cortex, the M pathway takes a dorsal route, first to visual association areas V2 and V3, then to the middle temporal (area MT) and middle superior temporal (area MST) regions for motion processing and then forward to the posterior parietal cortex (PPC). This dorsal visual stream of information is involved in the "where is it" and "how to" aspects of the visual pro-cess. Visual areas in the PPC, among other functions, maintain spatial coordinates that allow for the determination of the position and localization of objects in space and are used as a guide to direct ourselves through space. This occurs through sensorimotor transformation of motion and depth detection and stereopsis, serving to interpret and organize space. The posterior parietal lobe contains functionally separate areas: area LIP, which is activated when the individual makes a saccade or attention is directed toward a visual stimulus, and area VIP, where visual and somatosensory information are integrated.

Primary functions of the PPC include the awareness of the movement and direc-tion of movement of objects, localizing objects in space in relation to our bodies, between objects in space, and organizing and preparing our bodies for action. The PPC is essential for the perception of spatial relationships, accurate body image, and the learning of tasks involving coordination of the body in space.[11] The parietal cortex is also the center of multisensory convergence where visual, proprioceptive, and vestibular information are combined.[12,13]

Parvo cells account for approximately 80% of the RGCs. They are also distributed throughout the retina, with heaviest concentration in the fovea centralis and macular regions. They respond slowly compared to magnocellular cells. Each P ganglion cell receives input from a relatively small number of photoreceptors, which allows P cells to provide good spatial resolution, carrying detail-oriented and color information along the retino-geniculo-striate pathway from the retina to the LGN and then into area V1. From area V1, the P pathway goes to V2 and V3, then takes a ventral route forward to area V4 and then into the inferior temporal lobe (area IT). The ventral visual stream is involved with object recognition and has strong connections with the limbic system, which controls emotions, and the medial temporal lobe, where long-term memories are stored. Thus, the ventral visual stream not only provides information about object identification but also provides information in judging the significance of the information (Figure 4.2).

In short, the ventral visual processing stream is a substrate for "What?" properties such as identifying details, properties, and the significance of objects, whereas dorsal visual processing stream specialize in spatiotemporal properties, or "Where" properties of an object in space.[14] Recent literature also terms the dorsal pathway the "How to" system because this system provides crucial information on "how to" act on the objects identified by the ventral visual processing stream.[15] In an undamaged and well-functioning visual system, object localization typically precedes object identification.

There is a clear separation of many visual pathways, and in many of the brain centers used for processing visual information. However, this hypothesis is probably an oversimplification for the complex nature of what is truly occurring. It is important

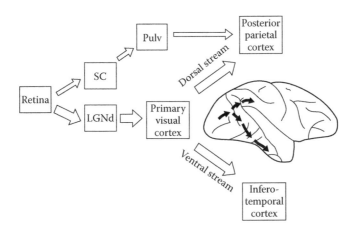

FIGURE 4.2 Diagram of the dorsal and ventral visual pathways. The dorsal pathway travels from retina to the lateral geniculate nucleus (LGN) then to areas V1, V2, V3, V5, and the posterior parietal lobe. The ventral pathway travels from retina to the LGN then to areas V1, V2, V4, and the inferior temporal lobe. (From Milner, A. D. and Goodale, M. A., *The Visual Brain in Action,* 2nd ed., Oxford University Press, New York, 2006, p. 68. By permission of Oxford University Press, Inc.)

to understand that various visual pathways, even though segregated, are also heavily interconnected. They must share, coordinate, and integrate information with one another, and with information from the other senses and brain areas as well.[16,17] Therefore, both in theory and when performing an evaluation and administering therapeutic procedures, it is crucial to remember that in everyday life these visual pathways are intimately bound together. Only when they are well integrated can we function efficiently in our visual space world; sadly, and all too frequently, we see the unfortunate consequences of these visual subsystems not operating and integrating properly and the negative impact that this has on the ABI patient's activities for daily living.

VISION AS AN EMERGENT PROCESS

Vision is actually a cluster of interrelated subsenses that work together to create the visual world we experience. Motion, depth, color, texture, and other properties of the visual world derive from specialized process that work relentlessly, quickly, and in parallel to create a stable visual world from the shifting light that reaches the retinas.

(Freidhoff and Peercy 2000, p. 7)[18]

Dr. A. M. Skeffington, the brilliant theoretician and founding father of modern developmental/behavioral optometry, proposed a model of the visual process that anticipated much of what was to follow in contemporary visual neuroscience. Rather than viewing vision in a bottom-up linear fashion, Skeffington conceptualized vision as emerging from four intimately related and integrated processes or system components:

A. Antigravity: "Where am I?"
B. Centering: "Where is it?"
C. Identification: "What is it?"
D. Speech-Auditory: "How can I communicate it?"

Just as the more recent neuroscience literature shows strong interconnections between the dorsal and ventral streams, Ralph Schrock elaborated Skeffington's model (Figure 4.3) to show the reciprocal interweaving, or reentrant connections that occur between these systems.[19]

The core concept in this model is that understanding vision requires more than looking at isolated processes, or individual structure-function pieces. In essence, Skeffington moved the field away from the camera-like notion of eyesight toward the framework for multiple, distributed, parallel, and reintegrated processing. Speaking of emergence is now commonplace in understanding human behavior, and is recognized as the whole of a system being greater than the sum of its parts.[20]

In postulating vision as an emergent process, Skeffington used terminology distinct from the more familiar visual subcomponents of convergence and accommodation. The terms of centering and identification anticipated, by more than 30 years, research confirming the distinction between spatial vision and object vision.[21,22] Skeffington also conceptualized that "centering" included attentional aspects of vision. Spatial vision, the equivalent of Skeffingtonian "centering," plays a crucial

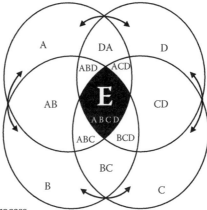

A: The Antigravity Process
B: The Centering Process
C: The Identification Process
D: The Speech-Audition Process
E: The Emergent: Vision

FIGURE 4.3 Skeffington's model of vision, modified by Schrock, demonstrating how he conceptualized the intersections and integrated reciprocal nature of the visual process. (Adapted from Wold, R. M., *Vision, its Impact on Learning*, Special Child Publications Seattle, WA, 1978, p. 32.)

role in the cognitive aspects of localizing objects and motor planning. Object vision, the equivalent of Skeffingtonian "identification," plays a crucial role in recognizing objects through their properties such as form, weight, color, and texture. Skeffington's paradigm remains relevant as a theoretical framework for understanding component processes of spatial vision. Marshall and Fink,[23] applying a similar approach, framed these concepts as follows:

For all embodied creatures that move in an extensive three-dimensional environment, brain circuits devoted to spatial cognition must compute answers to the following types of questions:

- Where am I, and how are my body parts currently oriented?
- Where are important environmental objects in relation to me?
- Where are those objects in relation to each other?
- What do I need to do about these objects?
- How should I go about doing what should be done?

THE ANTIGRAVITY PROCESS: "WHERE AM I?"

Vision is a mode of exploration of the world that is mediated by knowledge of sensorimotor contingencies.

(O'Regan and Noe 2001, p. 940)[24]

Vision is a dynamic system that is intimately involved with an ongoing, adaptive relationship between the body and the environment. To organize things spatially we must first know where we are. Vision plays a key and very active role in the control of posture, locomotion, and manipulatory function, and when vision plays this role it is called *visual proprioception.*[25]

Accurate motor behavior, such as fixating an object or reaching to grasp it requires, as a basis, the correct perception of the target's location in space relative to the body. The antigravity system includes all of the neural structures and resulting information used to answer and continually update the fundamental question: *Where am I?* particularly, as related to movement. Visual, vestibular, and proprioceptive information converge to generate an egocentric, body-centered coordinate system that allows us to determine our body position with respect to visual space.[26,27] To obtain these body-centered coordinates of visual targets, input from the retina must be combined with signals regarding eye position and head position. Three sensory systems are used to generate the coordinates: visual information,[28] vestibular information,[29,30] and proprioceptive information.[31]

Kawar refers to these interactions as multisensory, multidirectional central nervous system (CNS) communications.[32] This can be modeled as a triad consisting of a vestibulocochlear bridge, an ocular motor bridge, and cervical levels 1–5 integrating together with the rest of cervical, thoracic, and lumbar-sacral spinal levels of the body. This triad supports spatiotemporal orientation and organization of the body in space.

The intrinsic role of vision in counterbalancing gravitational forces and in visually guided movement is reflected in clinical tests of standing and walking balance.[33] Separate scores for times executed with eyes open and eyes closed help differentiate the contributions of the visual input from the somatosensory and vestibular input. Under normal circumstances, the ability to offset postural sway is significantly better with eyes open as compared with eyes closed. A patient with ABI who has compromised antigravity processing due to visual imbalance will have little difference in their ability to maintain balance with eyes open versus eyes closed. When vision is interfering with, rather than supporting balance, a patient may even initially exhibit better balance with eyes closed as compared with eyes open.

While walking, patients with ABI may demonstrate a shift in visual midline and altered gravitational sense termed *visual midline shift syndrome* (VMSS). These patients demonstrate balance impairment and associated motor dysfunction, including leaning, falling, or veering to one side during mobility.[34] (For a comprehensive discussion of VMSS see Chapter 6.) Traditional treatment of gravitational imbalance includes occupational therapy and physical therapy.[35] However, due to the multiple systems involved, including the important role of vision, treatment of patients with ABI can greatly benefit from interdisciplinary collaboration, including optometric intervention, as the use of ophthalmic approaches such as lenses and prisms for VMSS can have an immediate and dramatic effect on the motor dysfunction.[36]

The sense of awareness of one's position in space is predicated on what has been referred to as "the invariant."[37–39] Without having a stable frame of reference of self, it is impossible to organize space efficiently and accurately. As an example, consider what it would be like to find the location of a specific place on a map using only the coordinates "two miles west and one mile to the north." One cannot derive the answer without knowing the initial piece of information: "From where?"

The invariant provides a stable frame of reference upon which we build spatial constructs. The mental representation of space, and perception of straight-ahead body orientation, are related to a number of internal reference frames, including visual, vestibular, proprioceptive, and tactile information that allow us to build accurate spatial maps.[40–42] That is to say, the brain orchestrates movement using a series of internal models, maps, or schemes of external reality. Even *before* initiating the movement, the brain has already taken the visual information, anticipated the consequences of the movement, and formulated a series of motor actions to accomplish the goal.

The antigravity system, therefore, relies on the integration of many neurological processes, principally as follows:

- Visual system input that aids in the determination of vertical and horizontal frames of reference, and the perception of self-motion that comes from optic flow patterns across the retina.
- Vestibular system input through the otolith and semicircular canal systems of the inner ear give information about head position relative to gravity, and changes in acceleration and deceleration.
- Proprioception system input from the stretch receptors in the muscles that give information on body position.

Visual input to the vestibular and proprioceptive systems that direct movement, such as when adjusting balance or moving the body and hand to grasp an object or to catch a ball, is due in large part to subcortical "unconscious" visual pathways. The automatic, unconscious visual prediction and computation that supports motor planning and execution of accurate motor movement is often disrupted when patients experience ABI. This results in visual-spatial confusion and inaccurate visual guidance of motor movement.

Visual ambiguity is normally minimized by the effective coupling of visual and vestibular pathways. Vestibular receptors sense head movement and, just as importantly, provide information that movement has stopped. But vestibular receptors cannot easily distinguish between acceleration in one direction and deceleration in the opposite direction. To compound matters, ambiguous information is also given when the head is simultaneously accelerated and tilted. The vestibular system is therefore dependent upon visual information to resolve the ambiguity.[6] How is this accomplished? The intimate relationship between the visual and vestibular system begins early in the sensorimotor process and continues along the neural pathway. All along this pathway, called the *accessory optic pathway*, there are retinal ganglion neurons that fire preferentially when visual movement is in the plane of the semicircular canals.[43] The planes of movement of the extraocular muscles are also very close to being in parallel alignment with the planes of the semicircular canals (Figure 4.4), so that the mechanics of head and eye movements can be smoothly integrated.[44] In addition, the cerebellum contains neurons whose preferential planes of activation are aligned with the following:

a. The orientation preferences of neurons in accessory optic pathways
b. The planes of movement of the extraocular muscles
c. The semicircular canals of the vestibular apparatus

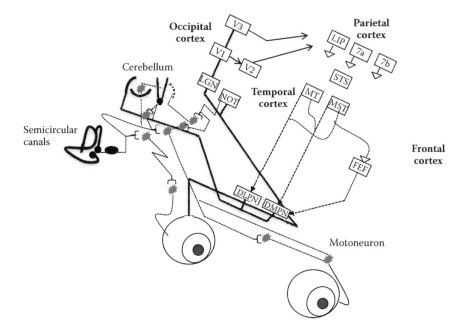

FIGURE 4.4 The main centers involved in processing information about visual movement. (A) The accessory optic system. In this system the movement is broken down into three planes that are aligned with those of the semicircular canals. The nucleus of the optic tract (NOT) encodes horizontal movement of the visual world. (B) Pathways for visual pursuit of objects in motion is transmitted to the lateral geniculate nucleus (LGN) by retinal neurons sensitive to movement, and from there to the visual cortex areas (V1, V2, and V3) then movement information is transmitted to the parietal cortex (7a, 7b, LIP, the areas of the middle temporal cortex [MT and MST] and the frontal oculomotor field [FOF]). From the cortex, control and pursuit signals are sent to the dorsolateral and dorsomedial pontine nuclei (DLPN and DMPN). (Adapted from Berthoz, A., *The Brain's Sense of Movement*, Harvard University Press, Cambridge, MA, 2000, p. 63.)

When objects move in the world, or we move through the environment, there is movement of image information across the retina. This displacement is called *optic flow*, and is detected mainly through changes in the retinal periphery via magnocellular neurons sensitive to movement. Motor components of the antigravity process are informed by the visual perception of motion through optic flow complementing vestibular cues to self-motion.

Optic flow information is conducted subcortically through the accessory optic pathways to the superior colliculus, or directly through the LGN to area V1, the primary visual cortex. The cortical route of optic flow information passes to V2, V3, and to areas MT and MST, where optic flow interpretation occurs. Visual data is combined with vestibular information in MST to solve the very important issue of whether[45,46]:

1. The individual is moving or stationary
2. The object is moving or stationary
3. Both the object and the individual are moving
4. Whether the object and individual are moving at the same or different speeds

Lastly, optic flow patterns are analyzed in the PPC, area 7a, MT, and MST, for spatial orientation during self-movement and for representing the three-dimensional structure of the visual environment[47] thus integrating postural mechanisms and visually guiding movement through space to stabilize and cohere: "Where am I?"

THE CENTERING PROCESS: "WHERE IS IT?"

Visual orienting refers to the coordinated movement of eyes, head and body to explore the environment surrounding the animal or person, and is a response crucial to the development and survival of the individual and species.

(Sprague 1996, p. 1)[48]

The centering process can be defined as the utilization of information from many sources to localize objects in space in relation to oneself.[19] Depending on the location of the object of attention, the process may utilize eyes, head, neck, body, or any combination in a coordinated and integrated fashion.

It would be deceptively simple to say that we direct our eyes to look toward what we aim to see. It must be emphasized that the ocular motor movements that reposition our eyes, that is, saccades and vergence movements, are involved in much more than moving our eyes from one place to another. These ocular motor movements are used as rulers, measuring distances from object to object, or from ourselves to an object. These measurements are part of the spatial computations that are crucial components in the shifting of attention and object vision. They are also used as a guide for the "How to" system in accomplishing complex motor movements of the hands and body. Let's illustrate this with an example: You make a decision to take a drink of coffee from the cup on your desk. While we might think of this as simple "visual-motor" task, complex steps lay beneath the surface. First, attention must be disengaged from whatever you were doing before the decision to move. Then a motor act of the body follows in the form of an ocular saccade, or series of saccades, to locate and fixate the place in space that the coffee cup occupies which aids in reestablishing attention in the new location. A second motor act follows, the vergence movement of the eyes to binocularly realign, which supports locating the object in three-dimensional space. The computations are then put into the system estimating the distance and direction of the hand and body movement necessary to grasp the cup, the directional positioning of the hand and size and opening of the hand and fingers, and the muscular effort needed to lift the cup the desired amount. Under normal circumstances, only *after* these two visual-motor acts are accurately accomplished, can there be the more readily observable visually directed motor movements of opening the hand the correct amount and moving the hand to the correct place in space to grasp the cup movements predicated upon the accuracy of visual information. Only after accurate and efficient saccades and vergence movements are made, can the motor act of reaching for, grasping, and lifting the cup occur in the most accurate and efficient manner. It is crucial when working with patients who have an ABI to understand and remember the fundamental visual processes underlying these basic motor activities of daily living (ADLs). Otherwise, treatment may not be directed at the true cause of the problem, delaying or impeding the overall rehabilitation process.

Localizing objects in space relative to oneself and then acting on them occurs through a multimodal combination of factors in which vision plays the dominant role. In accordance with our earlier discussion on parallel visual pathways, the dorsal processing stream is heavily involved in this aspect of spatial vision. Some of the essential components of spatial vision relating to the "Where is it?" process are classified as ocular motility, vergence, and accommodation. In the balance of this section we will address the role of ocular motility and vergence as centering, and in the following section we will address the role of accommodation in identification. Bear in mind, however, that under normal conditions all three of these interrelated processes are linked together for effective spatial localization and accurate identification.

Depth-movement-sensitive (DMS) neurons, related to vergence, are found in the parietal cortex and are sensitive to change in depth, disparity, or a combination of both.[49] Visual fixation (VF) neurons, related to ocular motility, vergence, and accommodation, are also depth selective and prefer a near target. Their activity increases as the angle of convergence and the degree of accommodation increases, signaling closer distance to the eyes. It is also likely that depth selective neurons receive an efferent copy or corollary discharge from both the accommodative and vergence systems.

Earlier we posed several questions that the brain must solve, and we will reiterate them as follows: Where am I? Where are the important spatial objects in relation to me? What is the relationship between objects? What is it that I need to do about these objects? How can I accomplish what I need to do? Let's explore how these questions are solved through the visual abilities of ocular motility and vergence, keeping in mind that accommodation will be discussed as part of object identification in the next section.

Ocular Motility

Supranuclear eye movements are those that involve coordination of extraocular muscle groups and are mediated by the cerebral hemispheres, cerebellum, and brainstem. They include shifts in direction of gaze (pursuits, saccades, and perhaps fixation), vergence, optokinetic nystagmus, and the vestibular ocular reflex (VOR).

There are three functional classes of eye movements that may occur under either monocular or binocular conditions: fixations, saccades, and pursuits. Fixation holds the image of a stationary object on the fovea by minimizing ocular drifts. Pursuit holds the image of a target on the fovea, when either self, the target, or both are moving, to keep the dynamic image from blurring. Saccades are a jump movement from one place in space to another to bring images of objects of interest onto the fovea. Also, as we move through the environment, vestibulo-ocular movements, using labyrinthine receptors to sense head acceleration, help stabilize gaze by keeping the fovea in line with head movements.[50]

Examples of fixation might be inspecting whether there is a splinter in your finger or keeping your eyes stable on a word when reading, thus allowing for accurate decoding. Pursuits would be used to watch a tennis ball so as to position our hands, body, and racquet properly to hit it, or to follow the runner in baseball as he moves from first to second base. Saccades are the type of eye movements that are used for visual search when trying to locate an object, when reading as we move our eyes from one word to another or from the end of one line to the beginning of the next.

Fixations

There is a separate VF system that is important in keeping our eyes steadily engaged on a target.[51] The primary function of this system is to maintain a steady image on the retina. Destabilized images moving across the retina would cause blur, even at very slow velocities of movement.[52] Accurate fixation and fixation stability are important in keeping our world clear so that objects can be more easily identified. Accurate accommodative function, which is involved with object vision, is highly dependent upon the ability to maintain fixation stability. Importantly, fixation maintenance is a key factor in sustaining visual attention. Equally important is the ability to disengage fixation so that the eyes can be moved to fixate a new location in space.

The parietal cortex is intimately involved with fixation and pursuits and there are two types of pursuit and fixation found there. Visual tracking neurons are activated when tracking a target with pursuit eye movements.[49] VF neurons are activated during fixation of a static target. When we fixate on an object, information is conveyed very rapidly by the magnocellular pathway to the PPC and the lateral intraparietal cortex (LIP), creating an initial spatial attentional window enabling us to identify behaviorally relevant locations.[53] The LIP then encodes the locations of these behaviorally relevant features, then integrates and uses these retinotopic spatial features to control the spatial focus of attention and fixation,[54] thus supporting "What is it?" or, to use other terms, identification, or object vision.

Saccades

The saccadic system is an action system, a visually controlled motor response. In addition, saccades are an integral part of the attentional loop. Typically, the object to be attended to is brought into awareness peripherally. Cognitive and attentional mechanisms direct shifting of attention, which must synchronize with the ocular motor system that computes how to move the eyes so that the image of the object to be attended falls on the fovea, allowing for detailed inspection, identification, and sustained attention. Thus, an inability to move the eyes accurately to the object of attention will interfere with the accurate shifting of attention. Saccadic involvement with vision takes the form of a continually cycling loop, so that vision and cognition can integrate in an intimate way.[55,56] In most normal viewing situations, saccades have a latency of 200–220 msec. In addition, irrespective of the nature of the stimulus a moving or stationary target, of normal or reduced intensity, viewed either directly or eccentrically, saccadic latency remains remarkably invariant with respect to target angular displacement.[57] Parietal areas contribute information important to shifting attention and initiating saccades as well as encoding spatial location of objects and motor errors. The pulvinar projects to the parietal cortex and also contributes to shifts in eye position and attention.

Saccades may be divided into several major subtypes[58]; the most common are listed below:

- Predictive saccades: voluntarily generated in search of, or in the anticipation of, a target appearing in a specific location.
- Remembered saccades: voluntarily generated to the location in space where a target has been previously viewed.

- Reflex saccades: generated in response to unexpected novel stimuli in the environment. The novel stimuli may be visual, auditory, or tactile.

Saccades are frequently affected in brain injury because of the complex nature and significant number of areas scattered throughout the brain involved with the control and monitoring of saccadic eye movements. Interference with the optimal functioning of any one of these areas can have an effect on the generation of appropriate and accurate saccades. The areas involved with saccades include the frontal eye fields (FEF), supplementary eye fields (SEF) of the posterior parietal and frontal lobes, pre-SEF, dorsomedial supplementary motor cortex, dorsolateral prefrontal motor cortex, middle temporal lobe (MT), pulvinar, superior colliculus, brainstem reticular formation, pontine nuclei pathway to the cerebellum, eye field of the anterior cingulate cortex, caudate nucleus, substantia nigra, and the parahippocampal cortex (Figure 4.5).[59,63] The frontal cortex alone contains three areas that contribute to the programming of saccades. The FEF are involved in generating visually guided purposeful saccades. The dorsomedial supplementary motor area is involved in the control of learned ocular motor behaviors. The dorsolateral prefrontal motor cortex contributes to saccades and shifts of attention to remembered target locations. The FEF project to the superior colliculus, brainstem reticular formation, and via pontine nuclei to the cerebellum. Indirect pathways involve caudate nucleus and substantia nigra.

There is another crucial aspect of saccades with respect to spatial vision and spatial constancy, which cannot be overlooked. Whenever the position of the eye is shifted, the image of the environment on the retina moves to a new position. Even though the image is moved we must maintain the sense of straight-ahead and the visual perception of the world must remain stable although the image on the retina is rapidly changing as we move our eye from one place to another. This is accomplished through corollary discharge. A copy of the signal sent to the motor system to move the eyes is simultaneously sent to the sensory motion system and integrated with the new sensory input from the retina. In this way our sensory system can adjust for the image shift and thus maintain our sense of visual stability. The functional result is that even though the images on the retina are shifting, we perceive the world as stable. This can be demonstrated by a simple experiment. If we shift the images on the retina by passively pushing on the eye there is no corollary discharge available to be compared with the sensory input, therefore, as the images move across the retina in this instance, we perceive motion of the visual environment rather than visual stability.[64,65]

Pursuits

Smooth pursuits are the types of eye movements made when following a moving target. These movements are slower than voluntary saccades, with latency around 100 msec after a target has begun to move.[66] Smooth pursuit eye movements function to keep images of moving objects of interest stabilized on the fovea, where visual acuity is the most precise. Smooth pursuit involves multiple areas within the brainstem, cerebellum, and cerebral hemispheres.[67–69]

The primary stimulus to smooth pursuit is motion of images on the retina,[71] but retinal-position errors also can elicit and modify smooth pursuit movement.[72] The

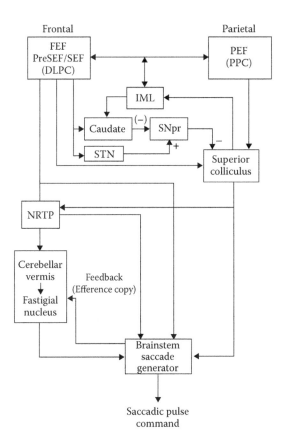

FIGURE 4.5 Block diagram of the major structures that project to the brainstem saccade generator (premotor burst neurons in PPRF and riMLF). Also shown are projections from cortical eye fields to superior colliculus. DLPC, dorsolateral prefrontal cortex; FEF, frontal eye fields; IML, intramedullary lamina of thalamus; NRTP, nucleus reticularis tegmenti pontis; PEF, parietal eye fields; PPC, posterior parietal cortex; SEF, supplementary eye fields; SNpr, substantia nigra, pars reticulata; STN, subthalamic nucleus. Not shown are the pulvinar, which has connections with the superior colliculus and both the frontal and parietal lobes, projections from the caudate nucleus to the subthalamic nucleus via globus pallidus, and the pathway that conveys efference copy from brainstem and cerebellum, via thalamus, to cerebral cortex. −, inhibition; +, excitation. (From Leigh, R. J. and Zee, D. S., *The Neurology of Eye Movements*, 4th ed., Oxford University Press, New York, 2006, p. 130. By permission of Oxford University Press, Inc.)

accurate maintenance of fixation on a moving object is accomplished by a combination of smooth pursuits and saccades. When the object is moving faster than the pursuit system can keep pace, the faster saccade system is activated to reduce retinal slip and reposition the object of regard on the fovea.[73]

There is evidence that complementary processes are involved in the initiation and termination of smooth pursuit movements. When the object stops moving, fixation serves to dampen pursuit, slowing the eye down to foveate.[74] According to Pola and

Wyatt there are two mechanisms involved in pursuit termination: an attentionally controlled change and a change in the spatial distribution of visual signal processing relative to the fovea. It is therefore understandable that patients with ABI may demonstrate difficulty with smooth pursuit eye movements and have difficulty attending to moving stimuli, in attaining stability when shifting gaze, or both.[75]

Leigh and Zee[58] proposed the following anatomical model for smooth pursuit eye movements (Figure 4.6). Signals encoding retinal image motion pass via the LGN to V1 and extrastriate areas MT (V5), MST, PPC, and to the frontal areas FEF and SEF. The nucleus of the optic tract (NOT) and accessory optic system (AOS) receive visual motion signals not only from the retina but also from extrastriate cortical areas. The NOT feeds back to LGN, thereby gating the forward flow of signals. Signals from the frontal, extrastriate, and NOT all converge on the pontine nuclei, which project smooth pursuit information to the cerebellum that feeds forward to the ocular motor neurons of CN III, IV, and VI to generate smooth pursuit eye movement.

Seeing where we look, therefore, requires essential coordination and functional interdependence of higher-order optical and ocular motor information.[76] Primary visual cortex provides visual information as a basis for generating smooth pursuits. The occipital-parietal-temporal lobe junction provides important information for detecting the speed and direction of moving targets and generating tracking responses. In addition, the cranial nerve nuclei of CN III, IV, and VI in the brainstem along with numerous connections with various cortical, subcortical, and peripheral retinal areas and the pathways to the ocular muscles themselves are involved with the control of eye movements.[77]

Saccadic eye movements are initiated in the frontal lobe, as distinct from pursuits and fixations. The fact that pursuits and saccades are initiated in different regions of the brain, and each function has different functional pathways, accounts for why an individual may have accurate pursuits yet inaccurate saccades, or vice-versa after an ABI.

Vergence Movements

Vergence can be subdivided into five subclasses:

1. Tonic vergence: normal vergence tone of the neuromuscular system.
2. Fusional vergence: disparity driven vergence when images fall on noncorresponding retinal points.
3. Voluntary vergence: vergence under volitional control.
4. Accommodative vergence: vergence stimulated by changes in accommodation.
5. Proximal vergence: vergence stimulated by the nearness of an object.

The centers for controlling the various types of vergence are located in separate areas of the brain. There are premotor neurons involved in vergence found in the mesencephalic reticular formation.[78,79] Motor commands for vergence are found near, and possibly within, the ocular motor nucleus.[80,81] Disparity driven vergence movements have substrates in area MT[82,83] and area 7a in the parietal cortex.[84,85] Cerebral control of vergence may be analogous to saccadic driven eye movements with more

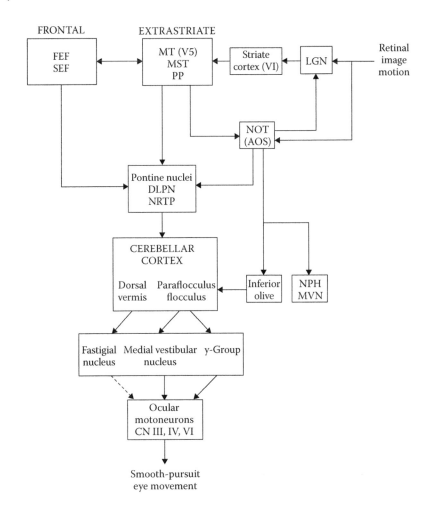

FIGURE 4.6 A hypothetical anatomic scheme for smooth pursuit eye movements. Signals encoding retinal image motion pass via the lateral geniculate nucleus (LGN) to striate cortex (V1) and extrastriate areas. MT (V5), middle temporal visual area; MST, medial superior temporal visual area; PP, posterior parietal cortex; FEF, frontal eye fields; SEF, supplementary eye fields. The nucleus of the optic tract (NOT) and accessory optic system (AOS) receive visual motion signals from the retina but also from extrastriate cortical areas. Cortical areas concerned with smooth pursuit project to the cerebellum via pontine nuclei, including the dorsolateral pontine nuclei (DLPN) and nucleus reticularis tegmenti pontis (NRTP). The cerebellar areas concerned with smooth pursuit project to ocular motor neurons via fastigial, vestibular, and y-group nuclei; the pursuit pathway for fastigial nucleus efferents has not yet been defined. The NOT projects back to LGN. The NOT and AOS may influence smooth pursuit through their projections to the pontine nuclei, and indirectly, via the inferior olive and the nucleus prepositus (NPH)-medial vestibular nucleus (MVN) region. (From Leigh, R. J. and Zee, D. S., *The Neurology of Eye Movements*, 4th ed., Oxford University Press, New York, 2006, p. 203. By permission of Oxford University Press, Inc.)

reflexive stimulus bound movements being generated by the posterior hemispheres and volitional, self-initiated movements by the frontal lobes.[58] The cerebellum has also been implicated in vergence movements, as lesions in the cerebellum lead to transient paralysis of convergence.[86–88] However, the exact role of the cerebellum in vergence movements is not currently known.[58]

All of the various components of vergence must be integrated so that binocular fusion is effortless. This frees attention from the act of vergence, allowing attention to be allocated toward other aspects of visual information processing.[89]

Individuals with ABI often lose coherence of the multiple components contributing to vergence. The distribution of multiple vergence centers in various areas of the brain makes vergence highly susceptible to injuries in many different locations. This may be one of the reasons that vergence dysfunctions, especially convergence insufficiency, are so frequent following brain injury. Multiple vergence centers may also be the reason that vergence problems are so readily remediated with vision rehabilitation therapy procedures in patients with convergence deficits following ABI. The loss of coherence of the multiple components of vergence contribute to the high percentage of individuals who have difficulty with convergence and experience difficulty in sustaining attention after ABI. Convergence insufficiency and difficulty sustaining visual attention are two of the principal signs of post trauma vision syndrome or PTVS.[90]

THE IDENTIFICATION PROCESS: "WHAT IS IT?"

> Think of the months, perhaps the years of work that it would take for a physicist to define just the color tones of a landscape seen only one time, which our eye apprehends with a single look.

(H. von Helmholtz, as cited in Berthoz 2000, p. 25)[6]

Identification, or object vision, occurs through the recognition of objects through their specific attributes such as shape, color, size, and texture. Multiple processes are involved, including attention, prior experience with the object, storage of information, conversion to memory, memory retrieval, association, generalization, and classification. Object vision normally has as its basis stable visual fixation, aided by the ability to attain and maintain a clear image through visual focusing or accommodation.

As with vergence, accommodation can be subdivided into five basic components[91]:

1. Tonic accommodation: normal accommodative tone of the neuromuscular system.
2. Reflex accommodation: reflex driven accommodation to clear an object.
3. Voluntary accommodation: accommodation under volitional control.
4. Convergence accommodation (CA): accommodation stimulated by changes in vergence.
5. Proximal accommodation: accommodation stimulated by the nearness of an object.

Tonic accommodation, or dark focus, is considered to reflect baseline neural innervation from the midbrain, indicative of the "resting state" of accommodation, or default level when no accommodative stimulus is present. Reflex accommodation is the automatic component for minimizing blur. Voluntary accommodation can be developed with training, and small scanning eye movements, or microsaccades, may assist in this process.[92–94] As with the vergence system, voluntary accommodation may be used to compensate for the disruption in neural substrates for other types of accommodation during vision rehabilitation.

Convergence accommodation (typically expressed as the CA/C) interacts with accommodation mediated by convergence (AC/A), but is not often factored into clinical analysis. The CA/C ratio is the amount of convergence-driven accommodation divided by the amount of convergence necessary to converge to the target distance. The AC/A ratio is the commonly taught and computed amount of accommodation-driven convergence divided by the amount of accommodation necessary to clear a target at a specific distance. Typically, because the convergence mediated by accommodation has the greater impact on where the eyes are focused and aligned, the AC/A ratio is taught in clinical analysis of binocularity. However, one must remember that the CA/C is also active and contributing to the binocular alignment.[95]

Proximal accommodation occurs in response to the sensation of a region of space being close to the observer. As with vergence, perceptual factors are involved in the psychophysical nature of nonoptical cues to proximal accommodation,[96] and visual imagery has been shown to influence accommodative response in the appropriate direction for an individual who has been asked to imagine looking near or far.[97]

Ciuffreda[98] presented a model of neurophysiologic correlates of accommodation and vergence (Table 4.1). The clinical utility of this model is that it associates components of accommodative vergence with their probable neural site of origin. Being able

TABLE 4.1

Neurophysiological Correlates of Accommodation and Vergence

Model Component	Possible Neural Sites
Depth of focus	Areas V1, V2 visual cortex
	• Sensory: Contrast Detectors
Panum's fusional areas	Areas V1, V2 visual cortex
	• Sensory: Disparity Detectors
Controller gain	Midbrain
	• Motor: Near Response Cells
Crosslink gain	Midbrain
Adaptive gain	Cerebellum
	• Sensorimotor: Neuroreceptors of ciliary body
Tonic innervation	Midbrain

Source: Adapted from Ciuffreda, K. J., The scientific basis for and efficacy of optometric vision therapy in nonstrabismic accomodative and vergence disorders. *Optometry,* 73, 756, 2002.

to pinpoint the region of damage in ABI has direct clinical implications. Ciuffreda notes, for example, that in most instances accommodative controller gain function in the midbrain is amenable to therapy through blur discrimination techniques, such as sequential sorting of lenses, to sensitize and normalize depth of focus responses.

The model is another reminder of the intimate interactions between accommodation and vergence systems under normal conditions. In everyday life, vergence almost always precedes accommodation. In other words, we decide where to look and then identify what we see. Oftentimes, ABI patients have symptoms such as blur, visual fatigue, or headaches that signal an imbalance between these systems, and sustained visual tasks become stressful. Although beyond the scope of this chapter, it is important to note that generalized stress heightens the imbalance between accommodation and vergence in particular.[99,100]

As it does with the vergence system, attention plays an important role in spatial vision for identifying objects. The feature-integration theory of attention conceptualizes that we identify objects in two different ways that, under normal conditions, work in conjunction.[101] The first route is based on focal attention and is highly correlated with foveal fixation and accommodation. The second route is through top-down flow. These two processes can become disengaged and act independently of one another.[102] When this occurs in ABI, the tight weave we normally hold onto for object identification is loosened, causing a form of visual agnosia.

SPEECH-AUDITORY: ANALYSIS AND COMMUNICATION

Identification of objects is incomplete until a person is able to label and communicate that which is seen. The communication may be internal, in the generation of visual images or more in the form of auditory analysis to tell ourselves what we are seeing, or speech in terms of conveying what is seen. Converting information about the object into symbolic representation provides the freedom of no longer needing the object in front of us. A picture is not worth a thousand words until we have defined, classified, and generalized what is being seen. The speech-auditory domain is therefore a bridge in moving from images to concepts. As we have seen with other bridges in this chapter, multiple pathways are involved in coding, storage, and retrieval of information.

It has long been known that patients with ABI frequently encounter alterations in auditory processing.[103,104] Vision and the auditory-language systems are intimately related. Vision has an impact on the development of audition and language from an early age. John Ratey, MD, reports that researchers have found that linguistic clues, such as the shape of the lips, activate the auditory cortex, suggesting that visual signs impact the perception of heard speech even before the sounds themselves are processed as phonemes.[105] In addition, it has been shown that auditory representation of space in the superior colliculus shifts with changes in eye position,[106] so that any interference with the neural mechanisms monitoring and controlling eye position may also potentially have an impact on the auditory representation of space.

It is outside of the scope of this chapter on spatial vision to have an in-depth discussion of the auditory and language components to overall performance. However, the clinician working in a rehabilitative environment should be conversant not only with traditional indications for speech therapy but also recognize that interferences in the visual process can have an effect on the perception of heard speech and the auditory representation of space.

VISUAL GUIDANCE OF HAND MOVEMENT

> The hands, working under the guidance of the visual system, are the two most important instruments in the rise of human intellect.
>
> **(Elliot, as cited in Sakata et al. 1997, p. 350)[49]**

Spatial vision is a vital underpinning for success at tasks requiring eye-hand coordination. Vision is intimately involved in directing and guiding the action of the hand, judging location, distance, and motor planning. It is essential for everyday tasks from the simple act of picking of a cup to complex motor activities such as writing, driving a car, and participation in sports activities. (See Chapter 10.) Vision not only plays a vital role in motor planning, it also provides the feedback necessary for accurate termination of movement.[107,108] Any eye-hand coordination task requires accurate transformation of visual information from the dorsal stream in the PPC into motor commands in the frontal motor cortex. It is essential to have the correct visual-spatial location of an object relative to the body for accurate reaching and grasping to occur.[27,109,110] There is also strong evidence that the parietal lobe processes depth perception cues to aid in the visual guidance of hand movement.[49]

As discussed previously, vision is involved in directing motor action even before an action is initiated so that the correct motor movement is made to achieve a goal. Dr. Myron Weinstein, a functional optometrist from New York, encapsulated these thoughts by stating: "Vision writes spatial equations for muscles to solve."[111] Vision also presets the tactile system to anticipate the sensory perception. For instance, if one views an object through a minifying lens, while simultaneously holding the object in a covered hand (so that one cannot see the size of the hand), one will judge the object to be the size that they view it, rather than the size that they feel it.[112] As Bach-y-Rita stated, "Vision is not only the analog of tactile perception, it anticipates it" (as cited in Berthoz, p. 85).[6] Neuroanatomical routes involving dorsal pathways projecting to motor areas of the frontal cortex support visually guided actions. Cells in the dorsal-motor route show a gradual transformation from visual sensory signals to motor output signals.[49]

For an individual to be successful in performing eye-hand coordination tasks, whether the relatively less complex one of picking up an object, or complex ones like learning to write or returning a 125 mile/h tennis serve with topspin, vision must orchestrate and direct the correct motor movements. However, for patients with ABI, even the task of accurately locating and then visually guiding their hand to pick up a cup to drink may no longer be simple because the seamless integration of neurological actions involving numerous brain regions has unraveled.

To summarize: Once attention on an object has been engaged, we can use the model previously discussed to quickly retrace the steps. The act begins with the motor planning necessary to make a saccadic eye movement to foveate the object. VF on the object is engaged for identification, combined as necessary with ocular motor scanning of key features. Convergence and stereopsis then provide for accurate localization in preparation for reach, while motor planning for grasp incorporates the visual object features such as size, texture, and weight. Computation continues as the hand grasps and tactile sensation provides confirmation of the visual plan.

ATTENTION

> We tend to prefer sight to all other senses ... a preference explained to the greater degree to which sight promotes knowledge by revealing so many differences among things.
>
> **(Aristotle, *The Metaphysics*, Book I, 1951, p. 67)**[113]

Much of what we have alluded to thus far, but have not yet elaborated on, is the role of attention in spatial vision. There are two distinct processes in visual attention. The *preattentive* process, also known as bottom-up processing, is concerned only with the detection of objects. This process rapidly scans an object's global texture or features, and focuses on the distinction between figure and ground. This is done in parallel rather than serial fashion, looking for properties of the scene such as size, color, orientation, and direction of movement. The *attentive* process then begins to process the information in a serial manner. It is considered top-down, because what is selected must be identified independent of the individual elements of the scene.[114] Dr. Lawrence Macdonald summarized the top-down visual aspects of attention in the simple sentence: "Eyes don't tell people what to see; people tell eyes what to look for."[115]

The size of the attentional window is dynamic, and there is a natural competition between spatial attention and object attention,[116] mediated through competitive interactions from top-down cognitive influences and bottom-up stimulus information. Working memory for objects can bias competition for one object, while other objects are suppressed.[117] Although there is biased competition, there are also shared attentional resources that flexibly move the window of attention between spatial and feature components.[118]

The cognitive act of shifting attention requires three distinct but integrated mental operations[119–122]:

1. Disengagement of attention from present focus
2. Shifting from one location to a different location
3. Engaging attention to the new location or task

From a neuroanatomical perspective, the parietal lobe plays a critical role in selective attention, and the superior colliculus is primed to detect the unusual or unexpected, then projecting to the brainstem reticular formation to stimulate ocular saccades toward the object or location of regard.[123]

Damage to the parietal lobe has been shown to produce deficits in engagement and disengagement with a target.[124] A significant number of optometric vision therapy procedures were intuitively developed to capitalize on the significance of attention to spatial vision, far predating neuroscientific understanding. Procedures like Hart Chart Fixations, Schrock Space Fixator (Figure 4.7), Wayne Saccadic Fixator, and other saccadic procedures using a metronome or other timing device work

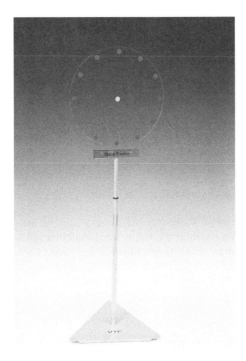

FIGURE 4.7 **(See color insert following page 270.)** Space fixator. The transparent background and swiveling head allows for excellent feedback regarding localization in three-dimentional space when the patient attempts to touch each of the dots in a programmed therapy regimen.

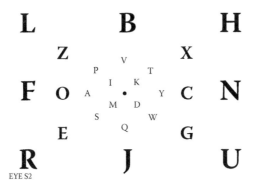

FIGURE 4.8 The adaptation by Lora McGraw of the original form field card developed by Lawrence Macdonald, O.D.

directly on facilitating the initial speed and accuracy of focusing attention, disengagement of attention; movement to a new location, then reengaging attention.

Other vision therapy procedures, such as the McGraw modification of the Macdonald peripheral awareness form field card (Figure 4.8), work on the ability to direct covert attention.

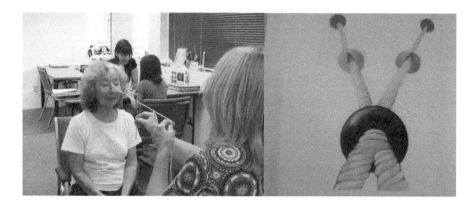

FIGURE 4.9 Stroke patient working on the Brock String and artist's rendition of how the string will appear to the patient if there is correct spatial localization when converging to the first bead, and no suppression. (From Press, L. J., *Applied Concepts in Vision Therapy*, OEP Foundation, Santa Ana, CA, 2008, p. 192a-Plate 4. Reprinted with permission from the Optometric Extension Program Foundation (www.oepf.org).)

MODIFICATION

In a developmental hierarchy, these procedures all work on the principles of engagement, disengagement, movement, and reengagement, while maintaining covert attention. Similarly, a seemingly simple procedure such as the Brock String (Figure 4.9) requires divided attention, as the patient is asked to engage the activity at particular point in space, while simultaneously maintaining awareness of the visual field in a different region of visual space.

It is no wonder, then, that patients with ABI find that their ability to execute these procedures transfers to a variety of ADL skills predicated on fluid attention.

SENSORY COHERENCE

Sensory coherence, or how spatial knowledge is bound together, is predicated on the emergent properties of vision. The superior colliculus receives visual, proprioceptive, auditory, and sensory information from more than 20 different areas of the cerebral cortex.[125]

Although there is no singular structure that binds together visual information, the superior colliculus, located in the midbrain, is both a sensory and motor site. The upper region of the colliculus functioning as a sensory map, while the middle and deep regions appear to embody a motor map.[126] Although many neuroanatomical areas play a role in binding the subcomponents of spatial vision, it may be useful to think of the superior colliculus as a signature area for sensory coherence. The colliculus uses multisensory information to aid in the recognition of moving objects, in the recognition of distinctive features, and in anticipation or prediction of motor movement. The superior and inferior colliculi help combine multimodal information in both spatial and temporal domains from visual, auditory, tactile, and kinesthetic inputs.

Consider the process of combining the sight of an object with its associated sounds in real time. The classic example is listening to a news reporter on television while watching her lips move. The timing of vision and audition are coordinated and unified, despite the fact that the sensory information is coming from two distinct sensory systems, with the speed of light and sound traveling at different temporal frequencies. The same sensory coherence operates for the integration of vision and touch. If you were to watch someone touch your hand, the impression is that the two events happen simultaneously, while in fact the sensory signals from the stimuli arrive to the brain at different times.

The colliculi coordinate both the temporal and spatial aspects of the multimedia presentation, so that our impression is that the visual, auditory, and tactile events are occurring in exactly the same place and at the same time. In spatial vision, the colliculi are also involved in the coordination necessary for the synchronized movement of the eyes, head, and body to center on a single object. Although multiple, distributed neuroanatomical sites participate in the complex match of space and time that results in sensory coherence, the PPC is prominent among the areas that integrate vision with other senses. The PPC receives input from proprioceptive, vestibular, auditory, and somatosensory areas, unifying this with visual input from the occipital lobe and midbrain areas we have reviewed, such as pulvinar and SC.[127]

Herein lies the paradox of coherence. The pattern of raw data sent to the brain is a shaky, fragmented picture.[128] The brain processes the data, combining input from both eyes, and filling in gaps in spatial vision with parallel streams of multisensory information. The result is a happy and competent human being living under the compelling illusion that vision is clear, single, simultaneous, and stable. Compelling, that is, until brain injury shatters the illusion.

VISUAL-SPATIAL DYSFUNCTION AFTER ACQUIRED BRAIN INJURY

The pervasive nature of visual processing throughout the brain makes it very sensitive and vulnerable to injury and accounts for the frequency of deficits in spatial vision evident after ABI. Moreover, injuries causing widespread changes in effective synaptic weighting of these recurrent visual networks can degrade behavior, as small errors can quickly become magnified in nonlinear ways.

(Churchland 1995, p. 172)[129]

Our perception of the world is a creative and personal process. The perception of position in space, distance, and relationship between objects, as well as the size, shape, and color of objects are derived from patterns of light falling on the retina. Perceptions are not precise copies or replicas of the world around us, even though we may perceive them as such. Instead, our brains construct an internal representation of external physical objects and events after analyzing various features of those visual events. Therefore, the more accurate is our ability to visually analyze and interpret those objects and events, the more potential there is for constructing accurate internal visual-spatial representations.

Many of the problems encountered by patients with a brain injury are consequences of errors or disparity between the physical reality of the world and the internal representations, or misrepresentations, of the physical reality constructed in the injured mind and brain. As Churchland[129] stated, these errors can be magnified and degrade behaviors in significant and often devastating ways such that an individual can no longer function in a coherent and efficient manner in the world.

PATIENT SYMPTOMS

After an ABI, patients frequently report many and varied symptoms suggestive of interruption to, or dysfunction of, optimal visual-spatial function. Connections between symptoms or behavior and underlying visual-spatial dysfunction may be obvious and overt, such as double vision, bumping into objects, or difficulty locating and grasping objects in space. Or, the connections to the underlying visual-spatial dysfunction may be less obvious and covert with disturbances such as insecurity when riding on an escalator, discomfort in crowded areas with lots of visual movement such as supermarket aisles, not being able to work comfortably under fluorescent lighting or difficulty with memory. Also, the patient with ABI may experience these, or many other types of disturbances, but not complain about them, because of impaired cognitive or metacognitive function. Very often, the patient or caregiver does not make the connection that the problems encountered in daily life are visually based. Because of this, all clinicians working with patients having ABI must take careful histories, be excellent observers, and be alert to behaviors suggestive of visual-spatial dysfunction. Table 4.2 summarizes some of the visual deficits, signs, and symptoms that may result after an ABI.

INTERFERENCE WITH OPTIMAL FUNCTION OF THE "WHERE AM I?" SYSTEM

Disturbances to the "Where am I?" system may include conditions such as hemiparesis, paralysis, or neglect. Neglect is discussed in detail in Chapter 5 and a discussion of hemiparesis and paralysis is outside the scope of this book. Neglect is often associated with right parietal lobe lesions, however, it may be caused by lesions in a number of different locations in the brain. In addition, the specific way, and area of space, in which the neglect manifests may take on different forms.

One form of neglect, personal neglect, or the neglect of one part or side of the body, is of particular interest to us here. That is because even if the neglect is personal, it can profoundly impact on visual-spatial judgments in peripersonal or close external space. This is predicated on the fact that the "Where Am I?" system serves as the foundation for spatial knowledge of the world around us. Neglect, in fact, may be the tip of an iceberg. A variety of less overt alterations in spatial awareness, such as disorientation or difficulties in movement or balance, or shifts in weight bearing, may indicate an underlying problem in the "Where Am I?" system.

A shift in personal space alters egocentric localization. This means that spatial coordinates are no longer aligned with body projections into space in the same manner they were prior to the ABI. If eye movement and coordination systems have altered in one eye or between both eyes, oculocentric localization (the current or anticipated position of the center of gaze) will also change. This increases the mismatch between egocentric and oculocentric localization. In Piagetian terms, the invariant has become variable, and spatial uncertainty is compounded. How is this seen clinically? Primary shifts in visual midline to adapt to post-ABI binocular dysfunction may result in

TABLE 4.2
Potential Visual Symptoms and Performance Deficits Frequently Reported Secondary to Brain Injury

Visual Ability	Deficit	Potential Patient Symptoms
Ocular motor dysfunction	• Limitations of gaze • Nystagmus • Speed and quality of pursuits and saccades	• Inability to follow objects smoothly • Reading problems • Skipping words • Rereading words • Word/letter reversals
Accommodative dysfunction	• Accommodative insufficiency • Pseudo-myopia • Speed and quality of accommodative response	• Blur • Headaches • Pain • Double vision • Squinting • Closing one eye • Reading problems • Ocular discomfort • Tired eyes • Watery eyes • Falling asleep when reading • Task avoidance
Binocular dysfunction	• Strabismus • Muscle paresis/paralysis • Convergence insufficiency • Reduced or slow fusional ability	• Head tilt or head turn • Diplopia • Depth/spatial judgments • Closing one eye • Headaches • Asthenopia • Reading difficulty • Tired eyes • Watery eyes • Fall asleep when reading • Task avoidance
Visual-spatial/visual information processing dysfunctions	• Visual-vestibular integration problems • Visual-motor integration problems • Difficulty understanding spatial coordinates • Disturbances in body image • Disturbances in spatial relationships • Difficulty sustaining visual attention	• Balance • Distance judgment • Motor coordination problems • Eye-hand coordination • Left-right confusion • Objects appear to move • Agnosia—difficulty in object recognition • Apraxia—difficulty in manipulation of objects • Differentiating, analyzing, categorizing, sequencing, etc. • Inattentive • Visual closure-recognizing faces

continued

TABLE 4.2 (continued)
Potential Visual Symptoms and Performance Deficits Frequently Reported Secondary to Brain Injury

Visual Ability	Deficit	Potential Patient Symptoms
		• Visual memory
		• Figure-ground analysis
		• Reading difficulty and difficulty sustaining reading
		• Writing difficulty and difficulty sustaining writing
Visual field loss/visual-spatial neglect	• Visual field cuts—especially homonymous hemianopsia • Visual-spatial attention/neglect	• Ocular motor-related symptoms • Difficulty locating objects • Difficulty with gait • Difficulty with balance • Bumping into chairs, objects, etc. • Difficulty seeing at night • Spatial insecurity—holding on to walls, other people, etc. • Driving • Disturbances in body image • Disturbances in spatial relations
Other	• Low blink rate • Staring	• Dry eyes

Source: Adapted from Sanet, R. B., Neuro-optometric care of patients with acquired brain injury, Seminar Outline, 2008, September, p. 35, San Diego, CA.

secondary shifts in weight bearing function and movement. Alternatively, primary shifts in weight bearing function may result in secondary shifts in visual midline.

INTERFERENCE WITH OPTIMAL FUNCTION OF THE "WHERE IS IT?" SYSTEM

Supranuclear Dysfunction

Supranuclear dysfunction results from damage to the cerebral hemispheres, cerebellum, or brainstem, resulting in gaze palsies, as well as deficits in gaze stability, pursuits, saccades, vergences, VOR, or optokinetic nystagmus. This can cause a whole host of performance and ADL deficits affecting level of independence, such as insecurity when navigating through space, inaccurately locating and grasping objects, trouble maintaining stable fixation, and difficulty with reading and driving.

Gaze Palsy

Because supranuclear dysfunction involves coordinated actions of groups of muscles, these deficits may appear as gaze palsies (i.e., loss of ability to move the eyes in a particular direction) loss of either right or left gaze, or frequently, in ABI, loss of upgaze and/or downgaze.

Fixation Dysfunction

A stable visual world is predicated on being able to hold steady fixation when looking at a particular point or region in space to localize objects. The maintenance of steady fixation is also crucial in the ability to hold attention in place in space long enough to get the object features analyzed. Equally critical, and frequently disrupted following brain injury, is the ability to disengage attention and fixation so that the eyes can be moved to another location in space.[130]

The ultimate loss of steady fixation is nystagmus, an involuntary rhythmic oscillation of the eyes. Nystagmus can be seen as part of the normal vestibulo-ocular reflex (VOR), or acquired as a result of disease or injury. It is characterized by alternating smooth pursuit in one direction and saccadic movement in the opposite direction.

Pathological nystagmus is the result of damage to one or more components of the vestibular system, including the semicircular canals, otolyths, and the vestibulocerebellum. Nystagmus acquired through brain injury may cause blurred vision, or apparent movement of the world, which may be constant or intermittent, but this varies greatly from patient to patient.

Pursuits and Saccade Dysfunction

As discussed earlier in the chapter, multiple areas throughout the brain mediate ocular motor control. Lesions to the superior colliculus cause increased saccadic latencies, decreased saccadic speed, and decreased saccadic accuracy.[131–133] Lesions to the FEF cause deficits in anticipatory saccades and saccades going to remembered locations.[134,135] Parietal lobe lesions affect fixation,[62] smooth pursuits,[136] and saccadic eye movements.[137,138]

Although there may be full ocular movements and no limitations in gaze, there may still be significant impairment to optimal ocular motor function regarding the accuracy and speed of eye movements. Since, in most cases, navigation through space and accurate reaching (eye-hand) activities rely on the speed and accuracy of ocular motor control, both of these critical functions will be compromised when ocular motor dysfunction persists.[135,139–143]

Binocular Dysfunction

Disturbances in binocular vision are common secondary to ABI.[144–149] Brain injury can impair fusion reflexes at the cortical level, which is postulated as a disruption in the psycho-optical reflexes for central fusion to guide bifoveal fixation.[150] Binocular vision disturbances can be severely disabling to the individual's ability and performance in many areas of life. A small sampling of these affected activities includes posture, balance, ability to move through space, reading, driving, and playing ball sports. As noted for residual eye movement disorders, unresolved binocular disturbances can be a significant impediment to the therapeutic processes provided by both occupational and physical therapists.

Phoric Posture

Increases in exophoria or intermittent exotropia are commonly encountered after ABI.[151–153] Phoric posture, or the binocular position of the eyes, is related to spatial judgments. As previously noted, alterations in habitual visual posture may disrupt the prior match between egocentric and oculocentric localization, adding to difficulty in navigating through space, or in reaching behavior. In addition, acquired high or decompensated phorias frequently produce symptoms such as visual fatigue, intermittent diplopia, and reduced reading comprehension.[154]

Convergence Insufficiency

Underconvergence or increase in exophoria, particularly at near, is extremely common after ABI, even in milder cases. Since accurate vergence is predicated on a match between where the patient looks and where both eyes meet, convergence insufficiency is a state in which the patient is figuratively and literally "spaced out" relative to the actual location of the object of regard. This is suggestive of the association that has been reported in children diagnosed as having attention deficit disorder, who have a significantly higher prevalence of convergence insufficiency.[155] All tasks at near, particularly reading and reaching, may be impacted when there is vergence inaccuracy. Also, convergence may initially be accurate but difficult to sustain. This weakness in stamina frequently results in double vision, fatigue, words running together, reduced comprehension, and falling asleep while reading.

Eye Muscle Paresis or Paralysis

Partial or total damage to the pathways controlling eye muscle movement are common after ABI. Cranial nerve networks of CN III, IV, and VI are particularly susceptible to damage. Disturbance to these pathways may cause strabismus, diplopia, loss of stereopsis, and spatial confusion.

Strabismus in infancy or early childhood results in suppression or other sensory adaptations because the brain is so highly plastic. While there is residual visual plasticity through the lifespan, strabismus resulting from ABI has too sudden an onset to permit rapid adaptation through suppression. While the strabismus and resultant diplopia is visually disturbing, and may negatively affect both performance in life skills and the therapeutic process in many ways, it provides a rehabilitative advantage in being able to tap into the preserved underlying fusion reflex, making the restoration of good binocular vision with stereopsis highly probable using prisms and active optometric vision rehabilitation therapy (OVRT).

Paresis or paralysis of the extra ocular muscles nearly always results in noncomitant strabismus, meaning that the angle or amount of strabismus varies considerably in different positions of gaze. It is therefore important to investigate eye muscle alignment in each of the nine principal positions of gaze for each eye and then again under binocular conditions (Figure 4.10).

As mentioned in our section on eye movements, this often results in a head turn or tilt in an attempt to find the greatest range of residual fusion. When the strabismus is noncomitant, management with prisms alone is challenging since the amount of prism required to attain single vision is variable at different viewing angles.

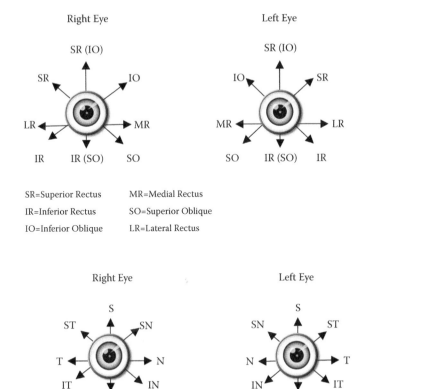

FIGURE 4.10   Diagram showing the extraocular eye muscles and their fields of action.

Patching is frequently used to eliminate the diplopia. While this is an expedient way to block double vision, it comes with a host of tradeoffs and significant drawbacks such as loss of half of the visual field, spatial insecurity, shifts in weight bearing, head turns, and other body warps. OVRT positions the patient to achieve greater success in restoring normal visual function. Patients with acquired double vision who have not as yet been helped through OVRT may even report that they are less bothered by the presence of a second image, than they are by the visual-spatial disruption in covering one eye. After a sufficient period of time, the patient may learn to de-tune or neglect the second image, however, at the expense of valuable cortical resources.

Noncomitant Deviations

Internuclear palsies result from damage to the pathways that run between the oculomotor nerve nuclei in the brainstem, for coordinating actions of the eye muscles. Lesions here will result in loss of smooth coordination of the ocular motor system and frequently result in deficits of horizontal gaze. Nuclear and infranuclear damage tend to result in more localized restriction of ocular motor control.

Noncomitant limitations of gaze are frequently seen after an ABI and are due to either an altered signal to the muscle that moves the eye, or damage to the muscle or orbital wall itself. When trying to move the eyes into the restricted field of gaze using the same reflex patterns before the ABI, the patient will experience diplopia or visual confusion. This can cause warps, or alterations of head, body position, or both to eliminate the diplopic image. As a last resort, the patient can be trained to move the head or body sufficiently to limit the need for eye movements into the field of restricted gaze. However, single vision may oftentimes be restored through OVRT, extending the range of motion of the affected muscle(s). When this is not possible, sectoral, spot, or graded occlusion may be of great benefit as it can eliminate the diplopia only in the affected area or field while allowing for good peripheral vision and motion detection and without resultant postural warps such as alterations in head or body posture. Head or body warps secondary to the visual problem make it more difficult for the patient with ABI to navigate through space. Therefore, when the underlying visual problem is managed with prisms and OVRT, the other therapeutic interventions involving physical, occupational, and cognitive therapies can proceed more easily.

INTERFERENCE WITH OPTIMAL FUNCTION OF THE "WHAT IS IT?" SYSTEM

Refractive Shifts

Changes in refractive measurements, most commonly increases in myopia and astigmatism, have been reported in the literature.[156–158] It should therefore be presumed, until established otherwise, that the patient's distance prescription may have changed after ABI, even if the patient got new glasses shortly before the injury. Changes in optical clarity, especially if significant, will cause disturbances to object vision, making it more difficult for the patient to identify salient information.

Accommodative Dysfunction

Accommodative amplitude normally shows a decline with age, requiring many people in their forties and beyond to need a prescription for near that is different from their distance power. However, insufficiency of accommodation is common after ABI, even with young people.[144,159,160] This will result in blur when attempting near tasks such as reading. Symptoms may include blur, watery eyes, difficulty seeing print clearly, and reduced comprehension. On occasion, a young patient will have sufficiently impaired accommodation to the point of functioning like a 75 year old with absolute presbyopia. Particularly, for a young patient who enjoyed near activities before the ABI and now avoids them, accommodative insufficiency must be presumed to exist until established otherwise. In some instances, the patient will exhibit normal accommodative responses when initially looking at near, but not be able to sustain near point tasks (such as reading and writing) for any appreciable length of time. This may be misperceived as lack of interest of motivation. In reality, these patients have sufficient cognition and vision to identify single words in isolation at near briefly, but cannot sustain focus for any length of time. They experience rapid accommodative fatigue, or loss of stamina, and may even fall asleep when attempting to read, yet be very attentive when listening to someone else read the same material.

Disturbances to Visual Guidance of Hand Movement

This topic is reviewed in Chapter 10, so only a brief discussion will be made here. As previously discussed in this chapter, vision plays a crucial role in locating objects in space and then guiding the hand to grasp or manipulate the object. Trauma causing interference to any one of the significant number of neural structures and pathways involved in visual abilities, including saccades, pursuits, fixation, vergence, stereopsis, and object perception, as well as any of the sites that integrate vision and motor abilities can have a profound impact on the accuracy of eye-hand coordination.

NEURO-OPTOMETRIC EVALUATION

There is a wealth of in-depth evaluation procedures that have been developed to assess various aspects of visual processing. Only those tests specific to spatial vision, as we have approached it in this chapter, will be discussed.

Evaluation of the "Where Am I?" System

There are many testing batteries that have been developed to evaluate the "Where Am I?" system. These tests survey and measure everything from awareness of body position and muscle strength and integration, to finger dexterity, and fine motor control. However, most of these tests were designed for a knowledgeable occupational or physical therapist to administer. For vision care and other professionals who are not familiar with these testing batteries, it is clinically useful to use a simpler and more rapid assessment of the "Where Am I?" system as a basis for an appropriate referral to an OT or PT. The general movement subtest of the Wachs Analysis of Cognitive Structures (WACS),* developed by Dr. Harry Wachs, is easy to administer and provides important insights into body awareness and control, balance, bilateral integration, motor control, timing, and spatial localization.[161] Once the clinician becomes familiar with the test, it takes only 15–20 minutes to administer and score.

Patients with ABI, particularly if recovering from coma, in many ways recapitulate infant development. Goddard reports that lower level primitive survival reflexes exhibited by the newborn and infant, if retained longer than they should, can have a profound effect on slowing the emergence of high-level functions.[162] It has also been observed and reported by many clinicians that primitive survival reflexes, even those that were previously completely integrated, can often reemerge after an ABI. Therefore, clinicians should also strongly consider performing an evaluation of primitive survival reflexes.

---

* *Wachs Analysis of Cognitive Structures*, Harry Wachs, OD, and Lawrence J. Vaughan, MA. Originally published by Western Psychological Services (1977). Now available through www.bernell.com

EVALUATION OF THE "WHERE IS IT?" SYSTEM

The accuracy of the centering system responses is a major contributor to the quality and accuracy of overall spatial vision and the guidance of motor movement. It is important to conduct an in-depth evaluation of as many aspects of ocular motor control as possible, including ductions, versions, saccades, phoria/tropia, vergence, fixation disparity (FD), stereopsis, and spatial localization and awareness.

There are a significant number of optometric tests that have been developed to assess the accuracy, flexibility, and sustaining ability of the "Where Is It?" system. Only those tests that the authors feel are more clinically appropriate and yield the most valuable data for the ABI population will be discussed.

Evaluating Ocular Motor Control

The majority of ABI patients have ocular motor dysfunctions, with accommodative and vergence deficits most common in traumatic brain injury (TBI), and strabismus and cranial nerve palsy most common in cerebral vascular accident (CVA) patients.[151] Ocular motor control should be evaluated on both monocular and binocular bases and both while the patient is sitting and standing, which gives valuable information on the effect of eye movements on balance and posture.

Pursuits, or tracking a moving stimulus, are called *ductions* when conducted under monocular conditions and versions when conducted under binocular conditions. The patient is asked to fixate a target, such as a Wolff Wand, held on the midline, at a distance of approximately 40 cm from the patient's eyes. We refer to this as visually grasping the target, and indeed the patient may need to touch the target to confirm where he is looking. In a well-functioning individual without an ABI, vision typically educates touch. Subsequent to ABI, and before OVRT, the patient may need to use touch to inform vision. We also presume at this stage that the patient has adequate convergence ability to maintain fixation at near, though this may not be the case and is dealt with below. Once the patient has visually engaged, the target is slowly moved laterally from side to side. Proceed from lateral eye movements to vertical eye movements and then to oblique movements. The procedure should be performed for at least one minute so that the effect of time on performance can be assessed.

Look for lack of smooth pursuit, fatigue, or any limitations in gaze that may involve the following:

• Muscle restriction
• Difficulty tracking the target due to attentional loss of fixation
• Difficulty crossing the midline
• Needing to use head movement to support eye movement
• Fatigue, lack of stamina, and reduced performance over time
• Saccadic intrusions
• Nystagmus in specific directions of gaze

Aside from asking a patient to follow the target, two additional reflex techniques may be used to document integrity of pursuits: head turn with fixation maintenance and optokinetic nystagmus stimuli. The examiner can ask the patient to maintain fixation on a stationary target while rotating her head in various directions. This will activate the VOR system more than pure pursuits, but it does let the examiner determine the patency of muscle movement in all directions. However, before doing this, the clinician must ascertain that there are no neck problems that would be exacerbated by moving the head. Optokinetic nystagmus (OKN) is the eye movement response obtained to a repetitive stimulus such as a grating pattern on a rotating drum that the patient is asked to fixate. Thus, the patient makes pursuits in the direction of the target movement, and corrective saccades back to center. The clinician can ascertain integrity of the pursuit pathways horizontally and vertically.

After noting responses on fixation and pursuit, proceed to investigate saccadic function. We use the same Wolff Wand target as for pursuits, this time holding two wands (or other targets such as two small tongue depressors with stickers on them as targets). The examiner holds the two wands equidistant from the midline, separated by about 4 inches (10 cm). The examiner sits directly opposite the patient, directing the patient to look at one of the targets and then to the other. The saccade should be repeated a minimum of five cycles in right and left gaze with each eye.

The clinician should note any of the following behaviors:

- Difficulty disengaging from the target to saccade to the next.
- Hypometric saccades (undershooting)—the saccade lands noticeably short, requiring a secondary movement to look directly at the target.
- Hypermetric (overshooting) of the target—the saccade lands beyond the actual location, requiring a secondary eye movement to look back to the target.
- Needing to use head movement to support eye movement.
- Fatigue or lack of stamina and reduced performance over time.

In some cases, the examiner may find it necessary to ask the patient to point toward or touch the target, or to use more reflexive targets such as alternately lit penlights to drive accurate eye movements. When pursuit or saccadic testing is done on a binocular basis, care should be taken to note the effects of difficulties with binocularity or a noncomitant strabismus. In these instances, observations may change when the patient looks into the field of gaze where the binocular alignment varies considerably from the patient's alignment in primary or habitual gaze. Normative data for the quality of pursuits and saccades are available.[163,164]

To supplement in-space testing of stimulus-generated saccades, objective measures can be obtained for tracking printed material, such as numbers, having limited cognitive demand. Examples are the NYSOA King-Devick (K-D) test and the Developmental Eye Movement Test[†] (DEM). Newer techniques involve computerized activities to assess and rehabilitate eye movement abilities. Computerized reading analysis devices such as the Readalyzer[‡] and Visagraph III[§] are available to use for objective recording tracking eye movements, while the patient is reading. The ocular motor functions measured by these devices include the following:

- Fixations—the number of stops per line
- Span—the number of spaces/letters per stop (perceptual window)

[†] Available from Bernell VTP, 4016 N. Home St., Mishawaka, IN, 46545, www.bernell.com

[‡] Available from Optometric Extension Program Foundation, 1921 E. Carnegie Ave., Suite 3-L, Santa Ana, CA, 92705, www.oepf.org

[§] Available from Taylor Associates/Communications, Inc., 200-2 E. Second St., Huntington Station, NY. 11746, www.readingplus.com

- Regressions—the frequency of backtracking movements
- Duration of fixation—speed of eye movement tracking

The two most common goals for patients seeking our services in ABI rehabilitation seem to center on reacquiring driving skills and being able to read effectively. The evaluation of ocular motilities should involve the type of scanning and tracking patterns essential for both tasks. Data derived from testing using measures such as the DEM, Visagraph, and Readalyzer are very useful in relationship to reading. They measure gaze directions such as left to right and the return sweep to the left, as occurs in reading. These tests, however, cannot substitute for eye movement analysis of scanning related to tasks other than reading. Therefore testing in free space of vectors such as down left (driver's mirror) and up right (rearview mirror), as well as limitations of gaze and excessive head movement should also be carefully evaluated in free space. Although beyond the scope of this chapter, bear in mind that when the patient has a compromised visual field, the nature of habitual scan paths will frequently be altered.[165]

Evaluating Binocularity

Numerous tests are available to evaluate the quality of binocularity as related to spatial vision, including the quality, comfort, and accuracy of vergence, object localization, and stereopsis. Some of these tests, such as phoria measurements, are routinely performed by optometrists with the patient behind a phoroptor. For patients with ABI, these tests should be conducted in free space outside the phoroptor so that they can be evaluated in all fields of gaze.

Phoria

A phoria is classically defined as the neuromuscular deviation of the eyes.[77] Functionally, a phoria measurement is an ocular alignment, or misalignment, relating to the difference between the reality of where the object of regard is physically in space, as compared to where the individual subjectively perceives it to be.

There are several ways to measure the magnitude and comitance of the phoria. Owing to damage in neurological control or muscle response, it is not uncommon for patients with ABI to have different phoria values in different positions of gaze. This should be assumed to be true until clinically established otherwise, rather than the reverse. The patient may also have diplopia in specific positions of gaze, which by definition is a tropia rather than a phoria. There may be positions of gaze in which the patient exhibits a phoria and others in which the patient exhibits a tropia. This is why it is crucial to evaluate visual alignment or posture in each of the nine cardinal positions of gaze (see Figure 4.10). This may either help explain a patient's habitual head tilt or turn, or help counsel a patient who experiences variability in binocular control without realizing why. The literature defines noncomitancy as a difference in measurement of at least five prism diopters in different fields of gaze. The authors would like to take strong issue with this definition as a patient with a subtle fourth cranial nerve palsy demonstrating no deviation in primary gaze, and a two diopter deviation in downward gaze, would not qualify as having a noncomitant deviation; yet, the patient would most definitely experience symptoms, including visual fatigue, diplopia, and significantly reduced performance when reading.

There are several ways to measure a phoria in free space:

a. Cover test with loose prisms or prism bar (Figure 4.11)
b. Maddox rod with a modified Thorington card (Figure 4.12)
c. Maddox rod with Risley prism (Figure 4.13)

The advantage of the cover test is that it provides an objective measure of phoria. A disadvantage, when working with an ABI population, is that many patients have difficulty spatially picking up fixation as the eye is uncovered, leading to false findings. In addition, the test using loose prisms or prism bar is tiring for the patient as it takes a very long time to accurately determine both the vertical and horizontal deviation in all nine positions of gaze. Maddox rod measurements have the advantage that the patient is viewing with both eyes simultaneously, neither eye is covered, and it is much more quickly and easily performed. The disadvantage is that it is a subjective test. However, since we are primarily interested in the relative differences in different positions of gaze, and in results at near versus far, when the patient is capable of responding we much prefer the information gained through Maddox rod testing. The measurements can also be used as a starting point, and later refined using loose prisms, before deciding the exact amount to prescribe and in which field of gaze it might be needed. Clearly when measuring vertical phoria or cyclophoria, which can be subtle, the Maddox rod is easier to use and also much more sensitive than a cover test in detecting small, but significant, amounts of deviation.

Vergence Testing
Patients with ABI may exhibit poor vergence control even when there is minimal phoria, or even orthophoria. This can result in asthenopia, blur, or frequently double

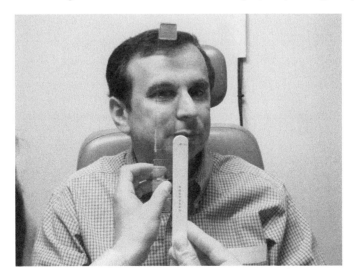

FIGURE 4.11 Neutralizing double vision with a prism bar, a measure of the subjective angle of strabismus. When there is extraocular muscle paresis, the magnitude and sometimes the direction of strabismus will vary in different positions of gaze.

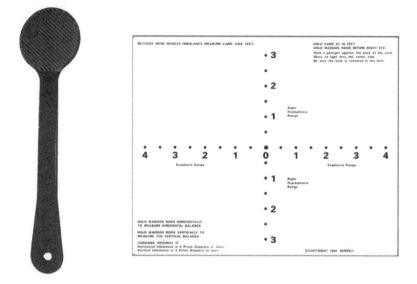

FIGURE 4.12   **(See color insert following page 270.)** Maddox rod and phoria card (modified Thorington method) for assessing phoria in a two-dimensional plane. (Reprinted with permission from Bernell, V. T. P. www.bernell.com, 4016 N. Home St. Mishawaka, IN 46545.)

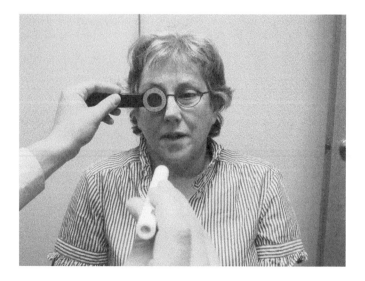

FIGURE 4.13   Handheld Maddox rod-Risley prism combination, measuring angle of phoria in three-dimensional space. (Reprinted with permission from Bernell, V. T. P. www.bernell.com, 4016 N. Home St. Mishawaka, IN 46545.)

vision when the patient is under stress or fatigued. It is therefore important to measure fusional vergence ranges in both directions, base-in and base-out, regardless of the magnitude or even in the absence of a phoria.

When it is possible for the patient, the easiest way to measure fusional vergences is in a phoropter. If this is not possible, the preferred method of measuring vergence ranges in free space, both vertical and horizontal, is with a prism bar. When the patient is capable of responding accurately, a column of small letters on a stick can be used as the fixation target at near, vertical for horizontal ranges and horizontal for vertical ranges. For distance, either a projected column of letters or a strip of letters can be used. If the patient is incapable of responding verbally the clinician may note the break point by observing when the patient begins to alternate looking laterally between the two images for horizontal ranges, or vertically for vertical ranges. Another method is to use a penlight or transilluminator as the fixation target, and observe when the corneal reflexes indicate that the patient has gone into diplopia, and when recovery occurs as the prism demand is lessened.

Nearpoint of Convergence and Nearpoint of Discomfort for Convergence

The nearpoint of convergence (NPC) and particularly the nearpoint of discomfort for convergence (NPDC) are often receded in patients with ABI. While the NPC is a point in space frequently measured, the NPDC is often more indicative of the patient's symptomology. As defined here, the NPDC is the point in space where the patient reports discomfort in sustaining fixation as the target approaches. We conduct the test in the same way that we look for blur, break, and recovery with NPC, but very importantly we ask the patient to first report when the target becomes uncomfortable to look at. This will typically occur at a point further away than when the patient perceives blur or doubling, and will many times account for the patient's subjective symptoms or avoidance of tasks at or within the NPDC, even at times when the NPC is found to be within normal limits.

Stamina is challenging for patients most with ABI, within both a physical and cognitive framework. From that standpoint, it is important to do repeated measures of NPC and NPDC. We recommend repeating these spatial points for three successive trials to assess visual sustaining abilities. The break point should be approximately 2–3 inches (5–7.5 cm) and the recovery point approximately 3–4 inches (7.5–10 cm) with only a mild, if any, reduction in performance on successive trials.[95,165–168] Abnormalities should be noted from either the established normative data or qualitatively in a decrease in performance on successive measures. This is, in essence, a type of visual stress test.[169]

Clinicians often use a penlight or transilluminator as a fixation target for convergence, but we suggest this be avoided. Since photosensitivity is problematic for many patients with ABI, it may be difficult to sustain fixation on the target as the light approaches, not because there is a problem with convergence but because of the increasing light intensity. We prefer to use a target such as the Wolff Wand or the same target used for vergence testing such as a fixation stick with letters. In cases where the patient is not photosensitive, but the NPC is highly receded (e.g., 16 inches, or 40 cm or greater), a penlight pointed well below the patient's eyes may be used as a stronger stimulus to fixation and convergence.

Fixation Disparity

As suggested by the terminology, FD is the amount of misalignment between bifoveal fixation of the eyes under fused conditions. Neutralizing the amount of misalignment, in the manner in which one measures a phoria, is known as the associated phoria. The associated phoria may be in the same or opposite direction as the conventional phoria (see the previous section).

Testing for FD can be very useful in patients with ABI, not as a global sense of spatial projection as the conventional phoria, but as another metric useful when other tests do not uncover the reason for the patient's symptoms. FD is consistent with the concepts expressed previously of repeated measures and visual stress.[169] We use this clinically by inspecting the slope of the fixation disparity curve (FDC).

Fixation disparity curves are generated first by measuring the amount of disparity in primary gaze with no added prism. The disparometer was initially developed for use on the nearpoint rod in the phoropter, but we prefer to use the Wesson or Saladin cards for measurement of FD in real space. After the amount in primary gaze is measured with zero added prism, loose prism is introduced incrementally, alternating between base-in and base-out directions. With each change in prism, note the change in minutes of arc of FD. The values are typically plotted on a grid. The zero added prism condition represents the center of the FDC, and a minimum of three prism demand values (3^Δ, 6^Δ, and 10^Δ are values readily found in trial prism sets) in each direction, and the resultant minutes of arc FD value are adequate to generate a curve.

There are four basic FDC curve types, but as related to symptomology for patients with FD, we are more interested in the slope of the FDC, which indicates the relationship between the prism demand, or the stressor, and the response of the system, in FD minutes of arc. If the increased prism results in a relatively small change in FD, the patient is able to absorb prismatic demand without having it increase disparity. This results in a relatively flat curve and is what we refer to, in functional optometry, as a flexible binocular system, or one with good degrees of freedom. Conversely, if relatively small changes in prism result in a relatively large shift in FD, the slope of the FDC will appear steep. A steep FDC equates to a patient having a tight or inflexible visual system.

Conventional FD theory holds that when contemplating prescribing prism, the amount that moves the flat portion of the FDC closest to zero is desirable. Through the AC/A ratio, the same approach can be taken when prescribing plus lenses for near.[170] Our approach uses FDC more as an index of the flexibility of the visual system. As the patient rehabilitates, systems that are tight or inflexible, showing a steep FDC at the outset before a program of OVRT, progressively become more flexible and adaptive after the OVRT program is completed.

Stereopsis

The term stereopsis is often used interchangeably with depth perception. However, it is so much more, as it emerges from the confluence of retinal disparity information from the two eyes, resulting in fine depth discrimination and a sense of space that cannot be attained monocularly. Dr. Susan Barry, a neurobiologist, has a beautifully written description of the impact that stereopsis can have on the quality and enjoyment of life in her book, *Fixing My Gaze*.[171] Because stereopsis requires excellent teaming of the eyes, it also serves as a reflection of the quality of binocular vision. Stereopsis is routinely measured with lateral disparity targets, such as the Stereo Fly, Animals and Wirt Circles, though these provide some nonbinocular cues to depth. Random dot stereograms (RDS) require bifoveal fixation, therefore patients with lesser quality binocular vision, particularly those with strabismus, will have more difficulty perceiving these targets.

As useful as RDS are in teasing out strabismus, they are poor targets for simulating spatial projection. Non-RDS targets are better indicators of how well the patient can use disparity cues under natural seeing conditions. Many clinical tests of stereopsis also involve figure-ground perceptual skills, requiring the patient to extract a key figure from its background. Some patients with ABI may have an additional level of difficulty responding to RDS targets because their figure-ground sensitivity has been reduced or compromised.

Given that stereopsis is an index of the quality of binocularity, any reduction below the optimal level of 20 sec of arc represents compromised binocular function. Interferences in binocular processing of depth will often surface when doing OVRT procedure involving stereoscopic judgment. It will also be a factor in a patient's ability to develop accurate and flexible binocular projection with free space fusion targets such as Vectograms, eccentric circles, and lifesaver cards. This surfaces in our discussion below concerning vectograms with regard to "SILO" and motion parallax.

When there is a change in vergence demand, there is a perceptual phenomenon that occurs called "SILO." Two images, one routed to each eye, (which are disparate in a horizontal direction but similar enough to fuse), will be perceived as having depth through stereopsis. When stereoptic targets are moved in a convergent (base-out) direction, the target will appear to become smaller (S) and move inward (I) to the patient (small-in), and as it is moved in a divergent (base-in) direction the patient should perceive the target as getting larger (L) and moving outward (O) or further away (large-out). Thus, the acronym, SILO, meaning small-in, large-out. Vectograms, polarized stereo targets made by the Stereo Optical, can provide very valuable clinical information and can be used to evaluate numerous visual abilities: the patient's range of fusion, flexibility between the vergence and accommodative systems, awareness and appreciation of changes in stereopsis awareness, or just noticeable differences (JND), SILO, visual-spatial localization, motion parallax, and the matching of vergence information with hand localization. The patient is seated in front of the Vectogram with the Vectogram in the ortho demand position. At this setting, both the vergence and accommodative systems are postured in the plane of Vectographic target. The clinician then begins to slowly separate the Vectograms inducing a convergence (base-out) demand on the vergence system. For the target to be fused, convergence must now be postured in front of the plane of the target. This will bring in reflex vergence accommodation. However, to maintain clarity the patient must relax accommodation back to the target as vergence is increased. The flexibility to keep vergence in one plane and accommodation in another plane is a measurement of the degrees of freedom between the two systems. It has been observed that patients with limited degrees of freedom are more likely to be symptomatic. The patient is asked to report any changes she observes. The important observations include the following:

- Whether the target is clear and comfortable to view
- When the target becomes blurred

- When the target becomes double
- When single vision is reestablished
- The level of visual discomfort at any time during the procedure
- Dizziness, headache, nausea, or other physical symptoms induced by the procedure
- Visual discrimination of the changes of perceived size and distance (SILO)

To evaluate the appreciation and awareness of parallax, the patient is asked to move from side to side. When the Vectograms are in a convergent demand, the patient should report a "with" parallax (the target moves in the same direction as the patient's movement). When a divergent demand is introduced, the patient should report an "against" parallax (the target moves in the opposite direction as the patient's movement).

To evaluate the matching of the vergence and the proprioceptive system, we can ask the patient to localize where he perceives the object to be. If there is a match, then the patient will spatially localize the target to be in the same exact location where the vergence system is postured (where the visual axes intersect) at that moment in time. Oftentimes patients will localize in a different place, that is, the visual system is localizing in one place in space while the proprioceptive system is localizing in another, indicating a perceptual mismatch between these two sensory systems.

As the vergence demand is increased the clinician should carefully observe the eyes of the patient to see if they are converging or diverging correctly. It should also be noted how much change there is in vergence demand before the patient notices changes in SILO, which gives an indication of the level of spatial discrimination and awareness of just noticeable differences.

The authors have also noticed a curious phenomenon regarding the viewing of Vectographic targets in patients with traumatic brain injury, even mild ones, especially those that are very symptomatic. When presented with Vectograms, most markedly with the Spirangle Vectogram, the majority of the patients become extremely uncomfortable and symptomatic, and many are unable to view the Vectogram comfortably while it is stationary in the ortho position. Further investigation is necessary; however, it is possible that this test could be used to diagnose visual disturbances in patients who have suffered a mild ABI when other diagnostic tests do not show deficits.

EVALUATION OF OBJECT VISION—THE "WHAT IS IT?" SYSTEM

Evaluation of various aspects of the "What is it?" system (object vision) is discussed in Chapter 11. In-depth evaluation of refraction and accommodation as related to object vision will be briefly touched upon in this chapter because interferences in these functions are common after an ABI, even in young patients, affecting important components of the "What is it?" system. We will touch upon a few key aspects of this system.

Refraction and Spectacle Lenses

As noted previously, changes in refraction are sometimes seen after ABI, warranting careful refraction with each patient. In addition, because of disturbances or interferences to the magnocellular pathway, progressive addition lenses (PALs), which previously produced comfortable and efficient vision may no longer be well-tolerated after ABI.

It is widely recognized that PALs induce peripheral distortion that requires adaptation on the part of every patient for whom they are prescribed.[172] Some patients adapt more readily to these induced peripheral distortions. Patients with ABI who do not receive OVRT will often function poorly with PALs, experiencing disequilibrium, dizziness, spatial insecurity, visual fatigue, and significant ocular discomfort. Untreated ABI patients will do comparatively better with bifocal lenses. However, patients undergoing OVRT, which emphasizes efficient spatial vision, will frequently adapt as well as patients who have not experienced an ABI.

Hypersensitivity to sensory input is a generalized phenomenon for patient experiencing ABI. Intersensory integration may be more challenging for ABI patients as well. In particular, visual-vestibular mismatches contribute to disorientation. The clinician must therefore anticipate that even when changing prescription lenses to improve clarity, the patient may have difficulty adapting to the change due to the new gain introduced in the VOR.[172] Because of the effects of eye movements scanning through different parts of the spectacle lens, the patient must recalibrate the gain of the VOR when a new Rx is received. For most patients this occurs readily and seamlessly, but patients with ABI may not adapt as readily.

Accommodation

Some of the many reasons why sight may be blurred following an ABI are interference with retinal function, disturbance in the primary visual pathway, or accommodative system dysfunction secondary to damage to CN III, Edinger-Westphal nucleus, or the crystalline lens network. Because accommodative dysfunctions, including difficulty in latency, amplitude, facility, and sustaining ability are so common after ABI, clinical testing of accommodation is critical for the ABI population, even in young children. Consider the following analogy: One individual can lift no more than a 20 lb weight, but can do so repeatedly. When fatiguing, the patient only needs to rest for a minute before being able to lift the 20 lb weight repeatedly again. A second individual can lift a 40 lb weight, but after doing so repeatedly is depleted to the extent that she has to rest for 10 minutes before being able to lift the weight again. The second individual has more amplitude, or strength, but the first individual has greater stamina. Fortunately, all of these functions can be evaluated and successfully treated with lenses and OVRT.[93,98,142,152,153,173,174]

- Monocular "Push-Up" amplitude of accommodation

The patient should be wearing best spectacle Rx for distance, and one eye is covered. The target can be the same 20/40 size letters on a stick used for vergence and NPC testing. Depending on the age or state of the patient, the target may be initially blurred at 16 inches or 40 cm, and plus lenses added to attain clarity. Assuming the target is clear at 16 inches with the distance refraction in place, the target is moved inward toward the face, directly along the line of sight. As with convergence, the patient is asked to report the initial point of discomfort for accommodation, this is recorded as the NPDA. As the examiner proceeds to move the target inward, the patient is asked to report when he first perceives any discernable blur and then when it is difficult to read. The procedure is then repeated with the fellow eye. Any responses that are less than normative data for age, or any significant asymmetry between the two eyes, are indicative of an accommodative problem.

- Facility and sustaining ability

Accommodative lens flippers (e.g., ±2.00) can be used to evaluate both accommodative facility and sustaining ability in pre-presbyopic patients. Variables recorded are the number of cycles cleared in 1 minute and whether one side, plus or minus, is more difficult to clear than the other. Difficulty may be encountered in either blur, or in the time taken to attain clarity. The patient should then rest for 1 minute and repeat the test. Difficulty with stamina is sometimes not noted on the first round, but noted after the patient tries to repeat the cycle.

- Nearpoint retinoscopy

This is an outstanding tool for evaluating accommodative function of patients with ABI. Most tests require subjective responses from a cooperative, alert, and observant patient. However, nearpoint retinoscopy can be used to evaluate accommodative responses even when the patient is not responsive, and is predicated only on the patient being able to look at the target.

There are several different forms of nearpoint retinoscopy, and we tend to favor MEM (Figure 4.14), Stresspoint, Book, and Bell. Each has relative strengths, and the examiner selects whichever form provides the type of accommodative probe desired.

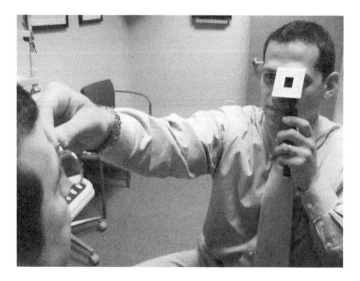

FIGURE 4.14 Monocular estimate method nearpoint retinoscopy being performed on a patient to estimate the lag of accommodation.

A detailed review of all of these retinoscopic procedures can be found in a monograph by Valenti.[175]

REHABILITATION THERAPY AND MANAGEMENT PROCEDURES

> To change the wiring in one skill, you must engage in some activity that is unfamiliar, novel to you but related to that skill, because simply repeating the same activity only maintains already established connections … Intellectually stimulating activity stimulates neurological growth … In living human subjects, skill acquisition recruits more neurons to master the skill, and as the skill becomes more automatic, less of the recruited cortex is used. Thus, the brain has a tremendous ability to compensate and rewire with practice … Our brains are wonderfully plastic throughout adulthood.
>
> **(Ratey, *A User's Guide to the Brian*, 2002, pp. 21, 36)**[105]

There are many optical tools and vision rehabilitation procedures that may be beneficial to compensate for, or to fully remediate, dysfunctions in spatial vision. These modalities may include the use of filters, prisms (compensatory, micro, and yoked), low vision aids, field expanding devices, and OVRT. Other chapters discuss extensively the use of filters (Chapter 8), prisms (Chapter 7), and field expansion devices (Chapters 5 and 7). In this chapter we will focus our discussion on OVRT procedures.

Optometric vision rehabilitation therapy programs use some orthoptic procedures designed to improve eye muscle function, eye teaming ability, or increase the focusing power of the eye. However, OVRT procedures are, using some of Ratey's terminology, a coordinated and integrated series of "unfamiliar" or "novel" visual tasks designed to produce more cognitive awareness as a means of improving eye movement control, enhanced accommodative and binocular function, finer stereopsis, and most importantly, improved overall spatial function. OVRT procedures have also been developed for a host of other visual deficits encountered after an ABI, but a discussion of them is outside of the scope of this chapter. While conventional orthoptic therapy procedures can be thought of as "bottom-up" exercises to allow one the freedom to fixate, focus, and team the eyes efficiently, OVRT includes more "top-down" cognitively based visual awareness procedures. The procedures are designed to correct spatial misperception, enhance spatial localization, and develop more accurate visual-spatial maps. The paradigm shift from orthoptic therapy to OVRT is one that is more consistent with the neurology of vision. One must have the visual-spatial understanding of where to point and focus the eyes in space to most effectively direct the neuromuscular substrates necessary to perform the mechanics of the task.

Some 50 years ago, one of the pioneers in the area of OVRT, Dr. Ralph Schrock, defined the therapy in terms parallel to those that Dr. Ratey described as needed for new neural growth. Dr. Schrock defined optometric vision therapy as "The art and science of arranging conditions so that an individual can acquire new relationships in his visual world and through these new relationships can learn to utilize processes that allow him to extract and act on a greater amount of information in a more efficient manner" (p. 29).[176]

It needs to be stressed that the OVRT procedures must be practiced frequently and over a sufficient period of time so that they become automatic and can be sustained after the therapy program is completed; literally writing new neural software. The OVRT procedures, as in Ratey's description of how to change neural wiring, are designed to recruit "more neurons to master the skill, and as the skill becomes more automatic, less of the recruited cortex is used" (p. 21).[105] Thus, using the OVRT procedures, "the brain rewires with practice ..." (p. 36).[105] This rewiring improves overall visual-spatial function enabling the individual to sustain visual attention for longer periods of time, better direct motor performance to support more accurate eye-hand coordination, navigate through the world more efficiently and effectively, and with less effort and expenditure of energy.

The judicious use of low power plus lenses can have a positive effect on reestablishing this crucial balance between vergence and accommodation. In addition, numerous studies have shown that both of these functions respond well to optometric vision therapy. [95,98,177–188]

A number of OVRT techniques have also been developed, such as the Wachs Block Sequence, Flipped and Rotated Forms, and Schrock Size Constancy procedures to develop attentional factors involved in object identification of size, shape, position in space and relative position of two or more objects, and rotation of forms.

GUIDELINES FOR WORKING WITH PATIENTS WITH AN ACQUIRED BRAIN INJURY

Optometrists specializing in working with patients who have suffered an ABI frequently find that the patient is highly symptomatic, and that the extent and severity of the symptoms do not necessarily correlate directly with the degree of abnormality in clinical findings. This does not mean that the symptoms are any less real, or that the patient is just being dramatic or overreacting. It may signal that the patient is visually hypersensitive, and that mechanisms existing in other patients to allow them to function efficiently and comfortably have been compromised in patients with ABI.

Clinicians working with patients having experienced ABI will occasionally encounter a patient who may wish to embellish symptoms because of worker's compensation or other medicolegal issues or claims. However, the commonality and frequency of the reports from a multitude of patients,[146] and the behavioral observations of the neuro-optometrists treating them, strongly suggests that post-ABI patients be given the benefit of the doubt unless it can be established that their ocular motor function is not contributing to their symptoms, rather than the reverse.

With these ideas in mind, the following guidelines will be helpful when working clinically with patients who have experienced ABI:

1. Always begin the OVRT procedure in a quiet area.
2. Speak slowly and in a soft voice and reduce peripheral auditory stimuli as much as possible.
3. Do not make rapid movements, especially in the visual periphery, as they may be too visually stimulating or distracting. Keep peripheral visual stimuli to a minimum in area in which you are working.

4. Try to work under full spectrum lighting, and keep fluorescent light flicker to a minimum so that the peripheral magnocellular system is not overstimulated.
5. Be sure that you have engaged the patient's attention before beginning a VT procedure.
6. Speak slowly and confirm that the patient understands what it is you are asking of them prior to beginning the procedure.
7. If the patient cannot tell you what they are going to do prior to the procedure, break it down into smaller components. You may have to begin with something as basic as confirming that the patient understands where to look.
8. As the patient demonstrates competence, increase the demand of the OVRT in very small increments.
9. When a lens or prism prescription is being used, it is important that it be reevaluated frequently. If the patient has been given compensatory prism, the magnitude may decrease as OVRT proceeds. When yoked prism is used, the base direction or magnitude of the prism may need to be adjusted.
10. Integrate OVRT procedures into the patient's ADLs.
11. Patients and caretakers should be advised and reminded that OVRT programs take considerable time, and consistently make the patient aware of gains in performance even if they are relatively small, both in OVRT and in ADLs.

KEY CONCEPTS FOR OPTOMETRIC VISION REHABILITATION THERAPY PROCEDURES

Combining insights from authorities such as Drs. Schrock and Ratey with the authors' personal experiences, we offer the following concepts and principles for enhancing the therapeutic outcome of OVRT procedures:

1. The OVRT procedure must have value in and of itself.
   The therapist should have an in-depth understanding of each specific procedure, including its goals and benefits before beginning each procedure.
2. The patient must be actively engaged and invested in the procedure.
   Conditions must be arranged so that the patient is actively involved.
3. The OVRT procedure must provide a novel stimulus.
   The patient should not be allowed to practice "business as usual."[189]
4. The OVRT procedure should require a visual decision.
   Conditions must be arranged so that the patient is asked to make a visual decision about something that changed as a result of doing the procedure.
5. The OVRT procedure must provide a means of evaluation and feedback.
   The procedure needs to be arranged so that *both* the patient and the therapist have feedback concerning performance, and know how to modify performance when the desired outcome is not being achieved.

6. A specific OVRT procedure should set the stage for subsequent procedures.

   The therapist should understand and be familiar with a logical developmental hierarchy or sequence of the therapy procedures.

7. The OVRT procedure needs to be appropriate for the patient's present level of function.

   The therapist must understand when and how to introduce each procedure, and at what level of difficulty. The therapist must recognize when and how to modify the procedure so that it is attainable.

8. The procedure should be able to sustain the patient's visual attention.

   Irrespective of the specific tasks involved, each procedure should enable the patient to gain visual rapport and sustain visual attention on the task.

9. The OVRT procedure must be mastered and internalized.

   The patient needs to work on the procedure until each newly acquired visual ability is rapid, automatic, and can be sustained over time.

10. Intersensory integration should be introduced into all OVRT procedures.

    Once mastered, the procedure should be integrated with vestibular, auditory, and general motor abilities.

ILLUSTRATIVE OPTOMETRIC VISION REHABILITATION THERAPY PROCEDURES

It is outside the scope of this chapter to discuss all of the possible OVRT procedures that are available to the clinician, and there are many resources available that include an extensive number of procedures.[164,169,190,191]

The authors of this chapter have chosen three procedures as illustrations of OVRT to help the reader understand not just the procedures themselves, but the complexity and remarkable rehabilitative value of what may seem on the surface to be simple procedures.

It is crucial to remember that these procedures are part of a comprehensive program and must be applied in the appropriate order in a sequence of OVRT, specifically designed for the individual patient, so that the patient receives maximum benefit for their efforts. If not, the treatment, rather than being helpful, may lead to frustration and possibly even a worsening of the visual dysfunction. The procedures must be applied under optometric supervision, as they are complex and one must understand the binocular, ocular motor, accommodative, sensory, and spatial implications of the technique to apply them with efficacy. In addition, the clinician should have an in-depth understanding of neglect, suppression, anomalous correspondence, and other visual sensory adaptations that will affect the patients' responses to the therapy procedures.

In an institutionally based brain injury rehabilitation program, it is often the occupational therapist that provides a valuable bridge between the patient and the neuro- or functional optometrist. While it is common, appropriate, and generally beneficial to the patient in an institutionally based rehabilitation program for occupational therapists to carry out OVRT programs under optometric prescription and supervision, it is critical for both the doctor and the therapist to realize that an occupational therapist does not have the background to carry out a comprehensive OVRT program in an effective and safe manner without additional training. Given the complexity of the visual system, especially a compromised one, a weekend seminar or two is insufficient. Initial and ongoing training, along with close patient supervision by the optometrist, is necessary. At best, inappropriately applied vision therapy procedures can be ineffective and result in frustration, making the patient resistant to future appropriately applied OVRT. At worst, *inappropriately applied vision therapy procedures can result in constant, intractable diplopia, or strabismus where there was none before.* The following procedures are included as examples to illustrate the complexity of OVRT procedures and the benefit that they can yield in improved visual-spatial abilities and should not simply be excerpted to use in a general rehabilitation program without optometric consultation and supervision.

Brock String

We opened the chapter by noting that the visual world is largely a construct, requiring learning and effort to attain a level of automaticity. One of the challenges in working with patients with ABI is to set the conditions for creating awareness of what is being seen, and then to make efficient and effective changes as guided by the therapist. Many of the procedures seem deceptively simple on the surface, but should be taken to be complex and effortful for the patient until established otherwise.

This is particularly true of procedures such as the Brock String, appearing to be child's play with a long rope and three colored beads, but which is in fact a biofeedback device for visual-spatial localization and binocularity requiring a high degree of attention to spatial vision.

Phase One

The string is held on the bridge of the nose, slightly below eye level, midway between the two eyes. If the patient is incapable of holding the string, the therapist can assist. The opposite end of the string is tied to the door handle across the room so that the string is taut. Initially only one bead is used so that the patient has a specific fixation target to look at. When the patient is fixating the bead accurately, and has normal binocular vision, two ropes are perceived, appearing to angle inward from the right and left sides. This normal perception of double vision is termed physiological diplopia.

If the patient is having difficulty with fusion, any one of several binocular abnormalities may be perceived:

- Nonphysiological diplopia: the bead toward which the patient aims his eyes appears double. The two ropes do not appear to meet anywhere in space or meet in front of or behind the place in space the patient is attempting to fixate.
- Suppression: the patient perceives only one rope, or one rope fades in and out, and sees one bead, cortically suppressing or de-tuning the image corresponding to the one eye or the other.
- Anomalous correspondence between the two eyes sometimes resulting in the two strings being perceived as one projecting from the midline.

Patients with ABI most commonly have difficulties with this procedure due to underconvergence, or convergence insufficiency, in the form of exophoria or exotropia, encountering double vision. It is precisely because ABI results in a sudden change in spatial vision that the patient isn't typically able to adapt to double vision through the slowly acquired mechanisms of suppression or anomalous correspondence. In addition, these adaptations to binocular misalignment are more readily established when there is a great deal of visual plasticity, typically at a very young age.

An element of complexity here is that we are asking the patient to simultaneously maintain awareness that is relatively focal in terms of the bead being fixated centrally on the visual axis, and relatively ambient in terms of the two ropes appearing to angle inward from the periphery. Patients with ABI who have difficulty simultaneously balancing ambient and focal vision will find it difficult initially to attain accurate spatial localization on the Brock String.

When a patient encounters diplopia of the bead being fixated, there are several options to encourage fusion. One method is to increase the size of the target. This can be done by creating a hole in ping-pong ball and replacing the front bead with the ball. To aid spatial localization, the patient can be directed to touch the target. The kinesthetic feedback can be an effective cue to the object's actual location in space, and an effective support to guide fusion. If the ball or bead is beyond arm's length, a dowel stick can be used for touch. If, despite these measures, the patient is unable to attain or maintain fusion, Base-in prism can be used to enable the patient to merge the targets at the point of fixation. Once attained, the patient tries to extend the range of fusion. This can be done in several ways:

- Doing a cover/uncover procedure to condition the automaticity of the muscle motor memory fusion reflex. The patient covers one eye, which eliminates the normal physiologic diplopia of the second rope. The patient then uncovers the eye and tries to regain the identical appearance of the rope before covering the eye. That is, the two ropes meeting at the bead or ball.
- When the eye is covered briefly, for a second or two, recovery of fusion is normally instantaneous. But for the patient with ABI and underconvergence, even a brief interruption of fusion may be enough to disorient their sense of space and accurate vergence. In some instances, particularly when there is motor weakness on one side of the body, the recovery ability after one eye is covered and then uncovered is noticeably different in comparison to the other eye.
- Once the patient is able to achieve refusion when the eye is covered briefly, a delayed cover/uncover is performed by covering the eye for 10 sec. Typically, the longer the eye is covered, the longer it will take for the patient to overcome the diplopia initially seen when the eye is uncovered. With repeated practice, the patient should be able to increase the recovery time. For patients with ABI, this is also an important component of stamina or sustainability, in being able to do this more than once or twice in succession.
- It is important to move into various fields of gaze as we rarely converge symmetrically. Rather, convergence is usually skewed to the right, left, or up or down from straight ahead. In addition, moving into various fields of

gaze is especially important for patients with ABI because so many have noncomitant deviations. Once the patient is able to stabilize and automatize fusion at a fixed distance, several variations can be performed. One is to have the patient attempt to stand up and sit down, while maintaining gaze at the same distance. Another is to be able to turn the head to the left or right, or moving the chin upward or downward so as to move the string into different fields of gaze. If the patient is sufficiently mobile, the procedure can be done on a balance board with support initially from the therapist.

- Visual-vestibular integration: having the therapist moving the string versus the patient moving the head while fixating the stationary bead.

Comitant Strabismus   If the patient is experiencing esophoria or esotropia (a binocular imbalance in which the strings appear to meet in front of the point in space where the eyes are directed), then the ball should be moved inward to seek a centration point. This is the point at which the visual axes are coincident with where the patient is looking. Low power plus lenses, of +0.50 or so, may assist localization and touch may also aid in localization. Once the centration point is found, the patient attempts to extend this range outward.

Vertical Imbalance   If there is a residual vertical imbalance that the patient cannot overcome, the strings may be perceived as being on two different planes, one slightly higher than the other, so that again the strings do not appear to meet at any point in space. Small amounts of vertical prism can be used to offset this imbalance. A slight head tilt may be needed to orient the strings on the same plane. The patient then, very slowly, reduces the head tilt, while still attempting to maintain the strings in a level plane. When there is noncomitancy (see below), repositioning the string to change the angle of view may locate a position from which the patient can begin, in which there is no vertical imbalance.

Visual Neglect   Although binocular suppression is the usual explanation for why patients cannot perceive both strings in space simultaneously, visual neglect or inattention (discussed in detail in Chapter 5) simulating suppression should be taken into consideration with ABI patients. When looking down the length of string toward a point of fixation, the two strings on the way to the bead being fixated appear to come from opposite sides. The right eye is seeing the string angling inward from the left side and the left eye sees the string angling inward from the right side. If the patient has left neglect, then the patient will be missing the rope that is on the left side, even though there is no suppression of the right eye when binocular testing is conducted to right of midline.

A technique that is useful in overcoming suppression, and also may be helpful in overcoming neglect, is to use the translid binocular integrator as an electronic Brock String. The intermittent photic stimulation of the light bulbs seen in physiologic diplopia facilitates attention. Anaglyphic (red and green) lenses can be used so that the two bulbs seen in physiologic diplopia have distinct colors, in contrast to the fixated bulb, which is seen in one combined color referred to as luster.

Noncomitant Phoria or Tropia   We pointed out earlier that ABI can result in non-comitant binocular misalignment. In these instances the patient may be able to achieve fusion when the Brock String is in one position of gaze, but not in another. Take as an example a patient who has "V" pattern exotropia. By definition, the exotropia or outward drift of the eyes is greater when the patient is looking upward, and normalizes as the patient looks in downgaze. The patient may adopt a chin-upward posture to maintain fusion. In these instances it is important to begin the Brock String procedure with the patient standing, and looking on a downward angle. Conversely, if the patient has unstable postural balance when standing, he can remain seated while doing the procedure, with the end of the string angled so that it is below eye level, facilitating the chin-upward posture.

Aside from altering head posture, when there is noncomitancy, yoked prism can be used to move the point of regard into the region of better fusion. Using the preceding example, if the patient has a "V" pattern exotropia, then using yoked prism with base-up prism direction of the same magnitude in front of both eyes moves the visual field downward into the area where the patient has less exo drift.

Phase Two

Assuming that the patient has been successful in finding a point in space where the strings meet coincident with where the eyes are aimed, and is able to demonstrate reflex fusion and automaticity at that point, we are ready to introduce the second bead. Again, this seemingly simple addition to the task is deceptively complex, and incorporates elements of spatial vision introduced earlier in the chapter.

Divided Attention   When the second bead is introduced, the demand on divided attention increases. For the more common clinical scenario, in which the patient has convergence insufficiency, the first bead is positioned at a distance of 16 inches or 40 cm from the eyes, on the midline. The second bead is positioned at about 5 feet from the eyes, well beyond the front bead and outside arm's length. The patient's attention is directed to the second bead, and the percept should be that of a long "V," with two strings meeting at the second bead. The bead at 16 inches should be seen in physiological diplopia.

Some patients will find it difficult to divide their attention so that they can look at one point in space along the visual axis and simultaneously process what is happening proximal or closer to that point. It is worth reiterating that the concept of physiological diplopia is predicated on dividing attention between the fused visual percept at the point of fixation, and the simultaneously diplopic appearance of points outside the fusible plane of fixation. As noted in phase one above, patients with underconvergence will usually have to move the beads further away before accurate binocular perception is achieved, and patients with overconvergence or eso projection will have to move the beads inward until a region of normal physiologic diplopia and fusion is found. And, as noted in phase one, the balance between relatively focal visual attention to the fixated bead and ambient visual attention to the beads seen in physiological diplopia may be difficult to attain or maintain.

Fluidity in Spatial Vision   After the patient is able to change fixation between the two beads, a third bead is introduced. When the patient has achieved good self-control and command of binocular visual space, he should be able to decide on which of the three beads to fixate and have the two strings intersect at whichever of the beads is fixated. When the patient slowly moves between the beads, self-generated pursuits are made. When the patient visually jumps between beads, a series of saccades and fixations are used. Accommodative and vergence control is required to maintain the fixated bead clear and single.

Vergence-Accommodative Flexibility   Small letters can be printed on the beads to give greater feedback on the accuracy of the accommodative response while the patient is performing the vergence movement. When the patient can fuse the beads into one (fusion accuracy) the letter on the bead may be blurry (accommodative inaccuracy). This response would mean that the patient may not be posturing accommodation accurately.

Eccentric Circles

The free space procedure seen in Figure 4.15 is another valuable tool providing binocular feedback to the patient regarding spatial localization. The target is two separate sets of concentric circles, each having a large outer circle and a smaller inner circle. The center of the inner circle is displaced slightly laterally from the center of the surrounding larger circle. When the two sets of circles are fused, the larger outer circle serves as the reference circle seen "on plane." Since the smaller inner circle is displaced from center, it will be seen either in convergent or divergent disparity, causing it to appear to float either ahead of the plane of regard or beyond the plane of regard. The word "CLEAR" appears in the center of the circles to serve as a feedback to accurate accommodation.

Let us assume again that we are working the more common scenario of a patient with ABI who underconverges in space. Begin by asking the patient to fuse the circles in divergent depth, which should be relatively easier. The patient holds the two sets of circles on the midline. With the letters "B" found on the bottom of the transparent circles as points of overlap, the patient looks at a point in between and through

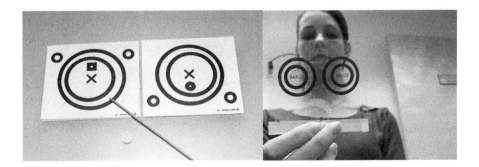

FIGURE 4.15 Eccentric circles on opaque background to facilitate convergence, or on transparent background to facilitate divergence when looking beyond the plane of the circles. (Reprinted with permission from Bernell, V. T. P. www.bernell.com, 4016 N. Home St. Mishawaka, IN 46545.)

the original two circles. A third circle should appear in between the original two circles, which now have become blurred, indistinct, and peripheral. (Some patients may require the use of a pointer to help them localize for this task.) The new third circle, which is a virtual target that is a uniquely fused image, should come into focus. The small circle will appear further away in space from the reference larger outer circle.

Some patients will find their hold on the third, fused circle is tenuous at first. It appears for a moment and then is lost. It is essential that the background against which the circles are held is uniform, preferably blank, and uncluttered. A large blank wall or the blue sky is an ideal backdrop. As with the Brock String, this deceptively simple looking target is a complex spatial task that requires divided visual attention. In this instance, the patient must suspend focal awareness of the original target, and convert focalization to the newly created fused target. The binocular percept occurs uniquely in the patient's brain, but is projected into space based on the fused disparity cues.

After divergence is attained, if the patient previously required use of a pointer to localize in space, the procedure should then be attempted without a pointer. This encourages the development of internal frames of reference. If the appearance of the binocular set of circles is stable, as with the Brock String procedure, the patient can do the cover/uncover procedure to build reflex fusion and automaticity.

Vergence Facility

Once the patient is able to accurately diverge and ultimately to converge, a higher degree of flexibility can be attained by changing from divergence to convergence at will. These changes will be very slow in coming at first, and then with practice more flexibility can be achieved.

The Dynamic Field and Optic Flow

A common complaint of patients with ABI is the inability to deal with visual motion. Part of this is tied to visual-vestibular mismatch as the patient moves through visual space. Visual disorientation is commonly encountered in busy, crowded areas such as supermarket aisles where objects create clutter and optic flow as the patient moves, or even worse, wide busy places such as shopping malls with the cluttered flow of people moving in a direction opposite to the individual.

Earlier we noted that Eccentric Circles should be done with a blank and uncluttered background to facilitate spatial localization. But once this is attained, the patient should use the circles in a visual field that includes other objects. This adds obvious complexity to the figure-ground nature of the task. More importantly, the patient is asked to move the Eccentric Circles in a clockwise and then a counterclockwise direction. This sets up an optic flow of the background relative to the projected fixation plane of the fused circle. The flow changes with convergent or divergent disparity, and with the direction in which the patient moves the target, circling clockwise or counterclockwise.

Acquired brain injury patients who can maintain control of binocular projection in the presence of optic flow with free space targets, such as eccentric circles, help stabilize their visual environment. In addition, when the target is held stationary and the patient is able to pivot his head about the X, Y, and Z axes:

- Tilting the head to the left and right
- Turning the head rightward and leftward
- Moving one's chin upward and downward

There are degrees of freedom attained in the gain of the VOR that further stabilizes spatial vision.

Space Fixator

As previously mentioned in this chapter, many aspects of visual-spatial function are frequently interfered with or compromised after an ABI. The Space Fixator (Figures 4.7 and 4.16), a procedure developed by Dr. Ralph Schrock, is designed to help the patient reestablish some of the visual-spatial function that has been lost. The Space Fixator, as is true for many other OVRT procedures, uses a deceptively simple piece of equipment. However, when used in the proper manner by a trained and knowledgeable vision therapist, the procedure can be very effective in developing lasting improvements in visual-spatial abilities, which then routinely transfer to ADL skills. The abilities that can be improved when using the Space Fixator include steady fixation maintenance; visual-spatial and visual-motor judgments on the X, Y, and Z axes;

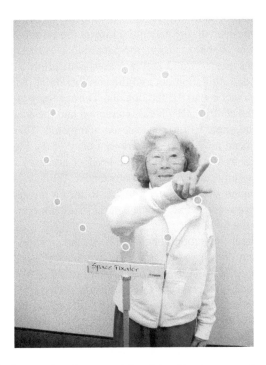

FIGURE 4.16 Patient performing a peripheral localization procedure using the space fixator.

saccadic accuracy; decreased saccadic latency; disengagement and reengagement of attention; integration of central- peripheral localization; motor planning and sequencing; bilateral integration; balance; eye-hand coordination; visual auditory and visual-vestibular integration; self-monitoring/awareness; and both sustained and divided visual attention.

The Space Fixator is a square Plexiglas sheet, approximately 16 × 16 inches (40 × 40 cm) with 12 evenly spaced colored stickers arranged in a circular pattern like the numbers on a clock dial. Critical aspects also include the apparatus being on a stand, which can be easily raised and lowered, and the Plexiglas sheet being attached to the stand in a manner that allows for rotation of the sheet around the vertical axis allowing for feedback on spatial judgments on the Z axis.

Phase I—Central-Peripheral Integration

Among the common symptoms or complaints from patients after an ABI is difficulty with saccadic fixation, accurately locating objects in space, and sustaining visual attention. This phase of the Space Fixator begins to address these functional deficits. The Space Fixator should be positioned within arm's reach, directly in front of the patient on the patient's midline and with the central dot placed approximately at nose level. The procedure is usually done in a standing position; however, if the patient has difficulty standing or if there are balance issues, various stages of the procedure can be performed while the patient is seated. The patient views the Space Fixator with both eyes open; however, if there are problems with double vision, an occluder may be used and the procedure performed with one eye at a time.

The procedure begins with the patient looking at the central dot. Then, using the peripheral component of spatial vision, the patient locates the fixation target to his right in the 3 o'clock position and makes a conscious effort to be simultaneously aware of both the central fixation dot and the peripheral dot. After this is done, the patient then makes a saccade to the fixation dot. The accuracy of the saccade will be directly related to the central–peripheral interaction and the accuracy of the correct peripheral spatial judgment before the saccade is initiated. There should be an eye movement without head movement. The transparency of the Plexiglas sheet allows for easy observation by the therapist of the level of accuracy of the patient's eye movement, as well as any supportive head movement. While looking steadily at this target, the patient again uses peripheral vision to locate the central dot again and subsequently makes a saccade back to the central fixation target. Fixation should be maintained at each dot for 1–3 sec.

In the same manner the patient repeats the sequence for the 9, 6, and 12 o'clock positions. The key to the procedure is the development of good central-peripheral relationships and accurate peripheral spatial localization. After the awareness and localization on the horizontal and vertical axes are mastered, the oblique movements are practiced. The patient strives for a rhythmic shift and accurate eye movements. In the beginning, the therapist can give feedback to the patient so that the patient can become aware of any saccadic inaccuracies or if head movement is being used to support the eye movement. However, as one of the key aspects of the procedure is self-awareness and self-monitoring, the goal is for the patient to become aware of any head movement or inaccuracies in eye movements, and then to self-correct. Patients are encouraged to maintain a steady fixation of the target they are looking at between shifts, and to discipline their eyes to move only on command.

Phase II—Metronome

A metronome is now added to the procedure and the patient is asked to move his eyes to the beat of the metronome. The starting speed is usually 60 beats/min; however, this can be modified up or down as needed. The metronome adds other layers of complexity and integration; both with timing and the integration between vision and audition. The central-peripheral and self-monitoring/awareness aspects of the procedure are still strongly emphasized.

Phase III—Motor Sequence with Visual–Verbal-Motor Integration

Frequently, after an ABI, patients report difficulties with eye-hand coordination, sequencing, memory, and sustaining visual attention. This phase of the procedure begins to address these issues. Subsequent to the patient mastering the peripheral awareness, saccadic eye movement, rhythm and visual-auditory competence in Phases I and II, the patient is now ready to begin the next level of integration which, along with the visual integrative demands of Levels I and II, adds complexity and integration with the addition of motor planning, sequencing, eye-hand coordination, and spatial judgment on the X, Y, and Z axes.

The following sequence of four sequential movements is first demonstrated by the therapist and then practiced by the patient:

1. "Look"—the patient fixates the center dot, while maintaining peripheral awareness of all dots. The patient then makes a saccade from the center dot to the target in the 12 o'clock position. The eyes should move *exactly* at the same time that the patient says "look."
2. "Ready"—patient maintains fixation on the dot and raises dominant hand to right temple in a "salute." The hand should move at *exactly* the same time as they say "ready."
3. "Touch"—maintaining fixation on the dot, the patient touches the target dot with the index finger of his dominant hand.
4. "Down"—and the eye returns to the center dot and the hand returns to the patient's side.

It is important to note that the Plexiglas is moveable around the Y axis. Because of this, the patient must make an appropriate spatial judgment and appropriate motor (eye-hand coordination) response not only on the X and Y axes, but on the Z axis as well or the Plexiglas sheet will rotate giving feedback to both the patient and therapist about the accuracy of eye-hand spatial judgments and accuracy on the Z axis. If this can be performed adequately then the patient continues to the dot in the 1 o'clock position, and repeats the sequence and then continues the sequence through all of the dots.

Phase IV—Motor Sequence with Metronome

When Phase III with the metronome is mastered, the patient executes the sequence starting with 12 o'clock in rhythm with the metronome and he continues with the four-step sequence through all of the dots, one after the other around the circle without pauses or stopping between the individual dots. This level emphasizes motor planning, sequencing, auditory, visual and motor coherence, and sustained visual attention aspects of spatial vision. Central-peripheral integration and self-monitoring/awareness continue to be emphasized at this level and at all subsequent levels as well. All subsequent phases are practiced first without the metronome, and then, once mastered, the metronome is added.

Phase V—Nondominant Hand
The sequence is repeated using the nondominant hand.

Phase VI—Alternate Bilateral Integration
The patient repeats Phase III, but now uses alternating hands, thus in addition to all of the other visual-spatial abilities that are being trained, introducing another level of complexity and demand, that of the reciprocal interweaving of bilateral integration and interhemispheric transmission of motor and other information across the corpus collosum.

Phase VII—Homolateral Integration Using Dominant Hand and Foot
This phase adds the aspect of a "homolateral" pattern that includes top/bottom coordination with foot movement being included adding yet another layer of complexity and integration—that of homolateral coordinated movement and integration of vision with balance demands. At this level, when the dominant hand is used on the "Touch" command, the hand will touch the target and at the same time the right foot will step forward touching the toe to the floor. On the "down" command, the hand, foot, and eye return to the starting position.

Phase VIII—Homolateral Integration Using Nondominant Hand
Repeat Phase VII using the nondominant hand and foot.

Phase IX—Homolateral Bilateral Integration
The patient repeats the sequence using an alternating homolateral pattern, touching the first dot using one side (foot and hand combination) and then the second with the other side and continuing the alternate pattern until all dots are successfully completed.

Phase X—Contralateral Bilateral Integration
Repeat all steps in level IX using a "contralateral pattern." When the right hand is used to "touch," the left foot steps forward and when the left hand is used to "touch," the right foot steps forward.

Phase XI—Change Direction—Homolateral Pattern
The patient begins in a homolateral pattern, alternating hands. When the clicker is sounded the patient completes the sequence for the target he is on. Then, when the patient moves his eyes to the next target, the patient changes the direction of eye movement. That is, if he was moving his eyes in a clockwise manner, upon hearing the clicker, he will finish the sequence for the dot he is on and then, on the next dot,

switches to a counterclockwise pattern. It is important that the clicker be sounded in an unpredictable manner so that the patient must monitor at all times and be prepared to change his visual-motor performance. The patient should practice at this level to obtain mastery of changing without pausing to stop before switching the direction of the saccade. This level further increases the attentional and cognitive demands of the task.

Phase XII—Change Direction—Contralateral Pattern
Repeat Phase XI using the contralateral pattern (e.g., right hand/left foot).

Phase XIII—Motor Planning with Bilateral Integration and Divided Attention
The patient proceeds using the homolateral pattern in a clockwise manner. When the clicker sounds, the patient must complete the sequence for the target he is on. For the very next target he will switch to the contralateral pattern and continue with that until the clicker sounds again, at which point he will change back to the homolateral pattern. The patient *does not* change the direction of eye movements at this level, *only* the pattern of hand and foot from homolateral to contralateral. It is important that the clicker be sounded in an unpredictable manner so that the patient must maintain awareness and be prepared to change at any point. Remember, however, that the patient always completes one previous sequence before changing on the next dot. The patient is to strive to make the required change accurately, working to the beat of the metronome without a decrement in performance. This level requires inhibition to delay the response, and memory aspects.

Phase XIV—Ultimate Integration of Systems with Divided Attention
The patient is instructed to respond to two cues:

1. When the clicker sounds, he is to change the direction of eye movement *only*.
2. When the therapist says "same" the patient uses a homolateral pattern. When the therapist says "opposite" the patient switches to a contralateral pattern. If the therapist says "same" when the patient is performing a homolateral pattern or says "opposite" when the patient is using a contralateral pattern, the patient does not need to make a change. Change is only made when the command is different than what is being performed. In this way the patient must not only monitor whether a command is given but also analyze if the command necessitates a change in performance.

Phase XV—Peripheral Localization
All of the levels outlined above are repeated using a variation of the "Look-Ready-Touch-Down" sequence. The variation is as follows:

1. "Locate"—while maintaining fixation on the center target, the patient locates the 12 o'clock target using peripheral vision.
2. "Touch"—continuing to maintain fixation of the center target, the patient touches the target at the 12 o'clock position. No eye movement is made. The

patient must accurately touch the target dot using only peripheral awareness peripheral and spatial localization to guide the motor movement.
3. "Look"—the patient shifts fixation to the target at the 12 o'clock position to
verify the accuracy of the touch. If it was inaccurate, then the same dot is
repeated until a more accurate peripheral spatial location is made.
4. "Down"—the arm returns to the patient's side and the eye returns to the
center dot.

The patient peripherally locates the 1 o'clock target and continues the sequence
through all of the dots.

Bifocal (Split-Pupil) Rock with Marsden Ball

This procedure is designed to develop awareness and control over the accommodative system as it relates to dorsal/spatial vision and ventral/object vision interaction.
The authors have found it to be one of the most powerful vision training procedures
for building visual-spatial awareness through the accommodative system. When
used in the proper manner by a trained and knowledgeable vision therapist, this
procedure can be very effective in developing lasting improvements in steady fixation maintenance, accurate pursuits and saccades, visual-spatial judgments on the
Z (near-to-far) axis, decreased accommodative latency, increased accommodative
facility, flexibility, and stamina, disengagement and reengagement of attention, integration of central-peripheral localization visual processing, bilateral integration, balance, visual-auditory and visual-vestibular coherence, self-monitoring/awareness,
and both sustained and divided visual attention.

Phase I—Saccadic Eye Movements

The patient stands or sits in a good balanced posture with the Marsden Ball at eye
level approximately 3 feet (1 m) away. The Marsden Ball should have letters on it that
can be seen at 3 feet to give more sensitive feedback as to the accuracy of the accommodative response. The patient should use their habitual prescription if it is needed
to see the ball clearly. If not, then no spectacle prescription should be worn. One eye
is occluded with a translucent occluder, allowing for observation of the occluded eye
by the therapist. The patient holds a −4.00 diopter lens below the uncovered eye and
slowly raises the lens in front of the eye until the lens splits the pupil and two balls
are seen. The patient looks at the image of the ball inside and then outside of the lens.
The demand is for a near-far saccade from peripersonal space to extrapersonal space.
At this level no attempt is made to make one image or the other clear.

Phase II—Accommodative Flexibility

The setup of the procedure is the same as in Phase I with the patient holding a −4.00
diopter lens below the uncovered eye. The patient attempts to make the image in the
lens clear and, if this can be accomplished, then attempts to make the image outside
of the lens clear. If necessary, the power of the lens can be reduced if it is impossible for the patient to make the image of the ball inside the lens clear; however, the
patient should be encouraged to work hard and practice before the therapist settles
for a reduction in the power of the lens.

The therapist then asks: "How do the balls look?"

There are a number of visual tasks that need to be performed and observations to be made by the patient for the patient to perform this procedure including accommodation, visual-spatial awareness, visual discrimination, spatial constancy, and the visual attention aspects of vision.

For patients to make the image clear inside of the lens they must use four diopters of additional accommodation to clear the image. Outside of the lens they must relax accommodation to the distance of the ball.

Do not give the patient any answers. The patient will hopefully discover that they have voluntary control over making the image of the ball outside or inside the lens to be clear and that as one ball becomes clear and the other becomes blurry as they look outside or inside the lens. The goal at this level is to have the patient alternately clear the image of the ball inside the lens and then the one outside the lens easily and rapidly. A metronome can also be added and the patient is asked to rhythmically and rapidly clear first one image and then the other. This will decrease accommodative latency and increase accommodative flexibility. The beauty of using a translucent occluder becomes readily apparent during this phase. When the unoccluded eye accommodates, the reflex convergence movement of the eye under the occluder should be observed. In this way the speed as well as the stability of the accommodative response can be objectively determined through careful observation by the trained vision therapist.

When the procedure has been performed successfully with one eye, it is repeated with the other eye. If there are differences in facility, quality, or spatial awareness then practice more with the eye that needs more experience. This is an important consideration at this level and at all subsequent levels of the procedure.

Phase III—SILO Awareness with Perceptual Discrimination and Constancy

The SILO phenomenon, discussed previously, should also be observed during this procedure using minus lenses. Therefore, during this procedure, if there is good discrimination and accurate spatial localization then the patient should see the virtual image of the ball viewed inside of the lens to be smaller and closer and ball seen outside of the lens to be larger and further. The image of the ball inside of the lens should appear to be behind the lens and the distance should be equal to the reciprocal of the power of the lens. So, in the case of a −4.00 lens the image should appear 10 inches or 25 cm behind the lens.

Frequently, there is a mismatch between the cognitive preset by the patient and the optics of the lens. So, instead of responding accurately to the visual information presented to them (SILO response) the patient sees the smaller image as further and the larger image as closer (SOLI response). If the patient has difficulty achieving the correct perceptual matching of sensory systems there are a number of ways that the therapist can arrange conditions to help the patient to resolve the perceptual mismatch:

1. Jiggling the lens from side to side. The movement of the lens emphasizes magnocellular/ambient visual processing that helps to support the "where system."
2. "Tromboning" the lens, that is, the patient moves the lens rapidly closer and further away from the eye.
3. Having the patient walk closer and further away from the ball.

4. Holding the lens on the midline and performing the procedure with both eyes open.
5. Having the therapist use a dowel stick to localize the place in space where each ball is reported to be seen. Amazingly, sometimes the mismatch is so great that the patient verbally reports that the smaller ball viewed through the lens appears further than the larger ball viewed outside the lens, yet when the therapist hold up the dowel, where the patient instructs them to hold it is actually closer than the big ball.

Birnbaum, commenting on the benefit of SILO stated: "When accommodation or convergence is stimulated with minus lenses, base out prisms, or vectograms, a conflict is thus created. The visual input suggests that the object of regard is smaller and closer (SILO), yet the logic of daily experience tells us that when objects appear smaller, they are further away (SOLI). The logic of daily experience is thus in direct conflict with the visual input. The SILO response indicates that the individual's spatial judgment is based primarily on current visual input, a SOLI response suggests that greater emphasis is placed on logic and past experience. When patients give persistent SOLI responses, it is desirable to create an opportunity to experience SILO. The value of the SILO response is twofold. First, the image viewed through the minus lens is perceived by the SILO responder as both closer and smaller, and thus serves as a more appropriate stimulus for accommodation than the target that is perceived by the SOLI responder to be smaller and further away. Second, the SILO response signals the ability to perceive events in the here and now, rather than through the filters of one's expectations, logic, and past experience" (p. 343).[181]

Phase IV—Internalizing Spatial Projection
When Phase I, II, and III are performed well, then emphasis is placed on the patient becoming cognitively aware of the location in space they need to look to make each of the balls immediately clear. In the example used above, if the patient is accurately localizing and projecting at 4 feet away then the larger ball will be immediately clear. If they are localizing and projecting at 10 inches (25 cm) when looking through the lens, then the image in the lens will be immediately clear. This Phase clearly demonstrates the dependence of the accommodative-focal system using spatial information to get objects in space immediately clear or, in other words, the dependence of the "what" system on the "where" system. The goal of the procedure at this level is for the patient to be able to rapidly change focus between images of the ball inside and outside the lens while being instantaneously aware of the feeling of looking close and far and of SILO.

Phase V—Metronome
A metronome is added to increase the demand for rhythm and auditory-visual integration. In addition, as the patient becomes more adept at the speed of the accommodative changes there is frequently a reduction in accommodative latency.

Phase VI—Increasing Accommodative Amplitude and Flexibility
The power of the minus lens is increased, which increases the accommodative amplitude demand and also the flexibility demand as the patient switches their focusing

demand from the target inside of the lens to the one outside of the lens. The power of the minus lenses that the patient will be able to accommodate is related to the age of the patient; decreasing in a more clinically significant way after 40 years of age. However, at any age the power should be increased to the maximum that is achievable with effort.

Phase VII—Discrimination Just Noticeable Differences

This phase stresses discrimination by reducing the lens power in −0.50 steps. As this is done the differences in size and distance between the ball viewed inside the lens and the ball viewed outside of the lens become less; therefore it is more difficult for the patient to discriminate spatially and perceptually. The therapist should keep reducing the lens power by 0.50 steps until the "Just Noticeable Difference" (JND) is reached. The optimal JND would be to be aware of a difference with −0.25 diopters; however, clinical experience indicates that a difference of −0.50 diopters is usually the minimum JND for most patients.

Phase VIII—Moving Ball

When all other levels have been mastered, the therapist swings the Marsden Ball directly in front of the patient, parallel to the plane of the head and body. This adds another level of complexity and neural integration demand, as the patient must use pursuit eye movements to track the ball, while still making saccadic eye movements from one ball to the other along with the accommodative changes when looking at the image inside and then outside again. The therapist should begin with small lateral excursions of the ball and then increase the size of the movement as the patient is able to integrate pursuit eye movements with accommodative changes. When this is accomplished the ball can be swung in a diagonal or circular motion that will, in itself, cause constantly varying spatial and accommodative demands layered on top of the spatial and accommodative demands induced when looking inside and outside of the lens.

This technique, using the lens with the moving ball, changes the apparent speed of the two balls such that the image of the ball inside the lens appears to move faster than the ball outside the lens.

Phase IX—Balance

For ambulatory patients, when it has been possible for the therapist to establish a good sense of balance, a balance board is introduced adding yet another layer of complexity into the procedure. At this level there is a significant demand for neural integration between areas responsible for the saccadic, pursuit, accommodative, balance, visual-auditory, and visual-vestibular function.

Summary of Procedures

The four deceptively simple but in actuality complex and powerful procedures presented here are but a fraction of the OVRT procedures available to the clinician working with the ABI patient. These procedures can begin to give the reader an idea of the potential OVRT procedures have to produce profound improvements in neurological functioning and thus the resultant quality of life for a patient with ABI. In typically eloquent fashion, Oliver Sacks remarked that instead of seeing the brain as programmed like a computer, there is now a much more powerful and biological notion of experiential selection.[192] That is to say, within genetic, anatomical, and physiological limits, experience literally shapes the connectivity and function of the brain. If this is the case, then ABI is an unanticipated reversal of fortune that shapes the disconnectivities and dysfunctions of the brain, resulting in discontinuities of spatial perception. In essence, a river that ebbs when it should flow.

In selecting a representative sample of optometric rehabilitative vision therapy procedures, we have presented a multiphasic approach to the elements of perception that form the building blocks of spatial vision. Some of these involve deceptively simplistic materials. As evidenced by the phases and levels through which we scaffold these procedures, considerable effort involving the doctor, therapist, and patient is necessary to restore connectivity and fluidity to the spatial visual system. Yet the changes that occur through restoration of a coherent spatial system are, for the individual, profound.

REFERENCES

1. Merleau-Ponty, M. (1964). *Le visible et l'invisible*. Paris, France: Gallimard.
2. Findlay, J. M., & Gilchrist, I. D. (2003). *Active vision: The psychology of looking and seeing*. New York: Oxford University Press.
3. Mitchell, H. B. (2008). *The roots of wisdom*. Belmont, CA: Thomson Higher Education.
4. Hoffman, D. D. (1998). *Visual intelligence: How we create what we see*. New York: WW Norton and Company.
5. Bullier, J. (2004). Hierarchies of cortical areas. In J. H. Kaas, & C. E. Collins. (Eds.), *The primate visual system* (pp. 181–204). Boca Raton, FL: CRC Press
6. Berthoz, A. (2000). *The brain's sense of movement* (translated by G. Weiss). Cambridge, MA: Harvard University Press.
7. Press, L. J. (1990). The application of chaos theory to behavioral optometry. *Journal of Behavioral Optometry, 1*(4), 98–100.
8. Felleman, D. J., & Van Essen, D. C. (1991). Distributed hierarchical processing in the primate cerebral cortex. *Cerebral cortex, 1*(1), 1–47.
9. Sterling, P. (2004). How retinal circuits optimize the transfer of visual information. In L. Chalupa, & J. S. Werner. (Eds.), *The visual neurosciences* (pp. 234–259) Cambridge, MA: The MIT Press.
10. Siminoff, R. (1991). A simulated human fovea: the L-type cells of the magnocellular pathway. *Biological Cybernetics, 66*(2), 191–202.
11. Bear, M. F., Connors, B. W., & Paradiso, M. (2007). *Neuroscience: Exploring the brain*. Hagerstown, MD: Lippincott Williams & Wilkins.
12. Andersen, R. A., Snyder, L. H., Bradley, D. C., & Xing, J. (1997). Multimodal representation of space in the posterior parietal cortex and its use in planning movements. *Annual Review of Neuroscience, 20*, 303–330.
13. Desmurget, M., Epstein, R. S., Turner, C., Prablanc, C., Alexander, G. E., & Grafton, S. T. (1999). Role of the posterior parietal cortex in updating reaching movements to a visual target. *Nature Neuroscience, 2*(6), 563–567.
14. Ungerleider, L. G., & Mishkin, M. (1982). Two cortical visual systems. In D. Ingle, M. A. Goodale, & R. J. W. Mansfield (Eds.), *Analysis of visual behavior* (pp. 549–586). Cambridge, MA: The MIT Press.

15. Goodale, M. A., & Milner, A. D. (1992). Separate visual pathways for perception and action. *Trends in Neurosciences, 15*(1), 20–25.
16. Farah, M. J. (2000). *The cognitive neuroscience of vision.* Oxford, UK: Blackwell Publishers.
17. Farivar, R., Blanke, O., & Chaudhuri, A. (2009). Dorsal–ventral integration in the recognition of motion-defined unfamiliar faces. *Journal of Neurosciences, 29*(16), 5336–5342.
18. Freidhoff, R. M., & Peercy, M. S. (2000). *Visual computing.* New York: Scientific American Library.
19. Schrock, R. E. (1978). Research relating vision and learning. In R. M. Wold (Ed.), *Vision, its impact on learning* (p. 32). Seattle, WA: Special Child Publications.
20. McLaughlin, B. P. (1999). Emergentism. In R. A. Wilson, & F. C. Keil (Eds.), *The MIT encyclopedia of the cognitive sciences.* Cambridge, MA: the MIT Press.
21. Mishkin, M., Ungerleider, L. G., & Macko, K. A. (1983). Object vision and spatial vision: two cortical pathways. *Trends in Neurosciences, 6*, 414–417.
22. Bridgeman, B. (1999, June). Two visual brains in action. *Psyche, 5*(18). Retrieved from psyche.cs.monash.edu.au/v5/psyche-5-18-bridgeman.html
23. Marshall, J. C., & Fink, G. R. (2001). Spatial cognition: where we were and where we are. *Neuroimage, 14*(1), S2–S7.
24. O'Regan, J. K., & Noe, A. (2001). A sensorimotor account of vision and visual consciousness. *Behavioral and brain Sciences, 24*(5), 939–1031.
25. Shumway-Cook, A., & Woollacott, M. H. (2001). *Motor control: Theory and practical application.* Philadelphia, PA: Lippincott Williams & Wilkins.
26. Karnath, H. O. (1994). Subjective body orientation in neglect and the interactive contribution of neck muscle proprioception and vestibular stimulation. *Brain, 117*(5), 1001–1012.
27. Karnath, H. O., Sievering, D., & Fetter, M. (1994). The interactive contribution of neck muscle proprioception and vestibular stimulation to subjective straight ahead orientation in man. *Experimental Brain Research, 101*(1), 140–46.
28. Brecher, G. A., Brecher, M. H., Kommerell, G., Sauter, F. A, & Sellerbeck, J. (1972). Relation of optical and labyrinthian orientation. *Optica Acta, 19*, 467–464.
29. Morant, R. B. (1959). The visual perception of medial plane as influenced by labyrinthian stimulation. *Journal of Psychology, 47*, 25–35.
30. Hamann, K. F., Strauss, K., Kellner, M., & Weiss, U. (1992). Dependence of visual straight ahead on vestibular influences. In H. Krejcova, & J. Jarabek (Eds.), *Proceedings of XVIIth Barany society meeting* (pp. 65–66). New York: Plenum Publishing.
31. Taylor, J. L., & McCloskey, D. I. (1991). Illusions of head and visual target displacement induced by vibrations of neck muscles. *Brain, 114*(2), 755–759.
32. Kawar M. (2007, October). *Optimizing performance through vestibular activation: An occupational therapist's perspective.* Presented at 37th Annual Meeting, College of Optometrists in Vision Development, St. Petersburg, Florida.
33. Ayres, A. J. (2004). *Sensory integration and Praxis test (SIPT)* (updated edition). Los Angeles, CA: Western Psychological Services.
34. Padula, W. V. (2000). *Neuro-optometric rehabilitation.* Santa Ana, CA: Optometric Extension Program.
35. Rosen, S. A., Cohen, A. H., & Trebing, S. (2001). The integration of visual and vestibular systems in balance disorder – A clinical perspective. In I. B. Suchoff, K. J. Ciuffreda, & N. Kapoor (Eds.), *Visual and vestibular consequences of acquired brain injury* (pp. 174–200). Santa Ana, CA: Optometric Extension Program.
36. Connor, M., & Padula, W. V. (2005). Visual rehabilitation of the neurologically involved person. In M. Gentile (Ed.), *Functional visual behavior in adults: An occupational therapy guide to evaluation and treatment options* (2nd ed., pp. 85–103). Bethesda, MD: AOTA Press.

37. Kephart, N. C. (1957). *Optometry, psychology and education* (p. 39). Duncan, OK: Optometric Extension Program.
38. McAnish, M. (1966). Body image as related to perceptual-cognitive-motor disabilities. In J. Hellmuth (Ed.), *Learning disorders* (Vol. 2, p.114). Seattle, WA: Special Child publications.
39. Piaget, J., & Inhelder, B. (1967). *The child's conception of space.* New York: The Norton Library.
40. Biguer, B., Donaldson, I. M. L., Hein, A., & Jennerod, M. (1998). Neck muscle vibration modifies the representation of visual motion and direction in man. *Brain, 111*(6), 1405–1424.
41. Karnath, H. O., Schenkel, P., & Fischer, B. (1991). Trunk orientation as the determining factor of the contralateral deficit in the neglect syndrome and as the physical anchor of the internal representation of body orientation in space. *Brain, 114*(4), 1997–2014.
42. Karnath, H. O., Christ, K., & Hartje, W. (1993). Decrease of contralateral neglect by muscle vibration and spatial orientation of trunk midline. *Brain, 116*(2), 383–396.
43. Simpson, J. (1984). The accessory optic systems. *Annual Review of Neuroscience, 7,* 13–41.
44. Hoffman, K. P. (1988). Responses of single neurons in the pretectum of monkeys to visual stimuli in three-dimensional space. In B. Cohen, & V. Henn (Eds.), *Representation of three-dimensional space in the vestibular, oculomotor, and visual systems* (pp. 1–261). New York: New York Academy of Sciences.
45. Wurtz, R. H., Duffy, C. J., & Roy, J. P. (1993). Motion processing for guiding self-motion. In T. Ono, L. Squire, M. E. Raichle, D. Perett, & M. Fukuda (Eds.), *Brain mechanisms of perception and memory: from neuron to behavior* (pp. 141–165). New York: Oxford University Press.
46. Shadlen, M. N., & Newsome, W. T. (1996). Motion perception: seeing and deciding. *Proceedings of the National Academy of Sciences of the United States of America, 93*(2), 628–633.
47. Prazdny, K. (1980). Egomotion and relative depth from optical flow. *Biological Cybernetics, 36,* 87–102.
48. Sprague, J. M. (1996). In M. Norita, T. Bando, & B. E. Stein (Eds.), *Progress in brain research: Extrageniculostriate mechanisms underlying visually-guided orientation behavior* (Vol. 112, p. 1). Amsterdam, Netherlands: Elsevier.
49. Sakata, H., Taira, M., Kusunoki, M., Murata, A., & Tanaka, Y. (1997). The TINS lecture. The parietal association cortex in depth perception and visual control of hand action. *Trends in Neurosciences, 20*(8), 350–357.
50. Leigh, R. J., & Zee, D. S. (2006). *The neurology of eye movements* (4th ed.). New York: Oxford University Press.
51. Luebke, A. E., & Robinson, D. A. (1988). Transient dynamics between pursuit and fixations suggests different systems. *Vision Research, 28*(8), 941–946.
52. Barnes, G. R., & Smith, R. (1981). The effect of visual discrimination of image movement across the stationary retina. *Aviation, Space, and Environmental Medicine, 52*(8), 466–472.
53. Gottlieb, J. (2007). From thought to action: the parietal cortex as a bridge between perception, action and cognition. *Neuron, 53*(1), 9–16.
54. Culhan, J. C., & Valyear, K. F. (2006). Human parietal cortex in action. *Current Opinion in Neurobiology, 16*(2), 205–212.
55. Neisser, U. (1967). *Cognitive psychology.* New York: Appleton-Century Crofts.
56. Liversedge, P., & Findlay, J. M. (2000). Saccadic eye movements and cognition. *Trends in Cognitive Sciences, 4*(1), 6–14.

57. Darrien, J. H., Herd, L., Starling, L. J., Rosenberg, J. R. & Morrison, J. D. (2001). An analysis of the dependence of saccadic latency on target position and target characteristics in human subjects. *BMC Neuroscience, 2*(13), doi:10.1186/1471–2202-2–13

58. Leigh, R., & Zee, D. (1991). *Neurology of eye movements* (2nd ed.). Philadelphia, PA: FA Davis.

59. Fox, P. T., Fox, J. M., Raichle, M. E., & Burde, R. M. (1985). The role of cerebral cortex in the generation of voluntary saccades: a positron emission tomographic study. *Journal of Neurophysiology, 54*, 348–369.

60. Rodman, H. R., Gross, C. G., & Albright, T. D. (1989). Afferent basis of visual response properties in area MT of the macaque. I. Effects of striate cortex removal. *Journal of Neuroscience, 9*(6), 2033–2050.

61. Gaymard, B., Rivaud, S., Cassarini, J. F., Dubard, T., Rancurel, G., Agid, Y., & Pierrot-Deseilligny, C. (1998). Effects of anterior cingulate cortex lesions on ocular saccades in humans. *Experimental Brain Research, 120*(2), 173–183.

62. Pierrot-Deseilligny, C. H., Ploner, C. J., Muri, R. M., Gaymard, B., Rivaud-Pechoux, S. (2002). Effects of cortical lesions on saccadic eye movements in humans. *Annals of the New York Academy of Science, 956*, 216–229.

63. Herdman, A. T., & Ryan, J. D. (2007). Spatio-temporal brain dynamics underlying saccadic execution, suppression and error-related feedback. *Journal of Cognitive Neuroscience, 19*(3), 420–432.

64. Helmholtz von, H. (1962). *Treatise on physiological optics* (translated by J. P. C. Sothall). New York: Dover Press.

65. Skavenski, A. A., Haddad, G., & Steinman, R. M. (1972). The extraretinal signal for the visual perception of direction. *Perception and Psychophysics, 11*, 287–290.

66. Ciuffreda, K. J., & Tannen, B. (1995). *Eye movement basics for the clinician*. St. Louis, MO: Mosby.

67. Fukushima, K. (2003). Roles of the cerebellum in pursuit–vestibular interactions. *Cerebellum, 2*(3), 223–232.

68. Ilg, J. J. (2002). Commentary: smooth pursuit eye movements from low-level to high-level vision. *Progress in Brain Research, 140*, 279–298.

69. Krauzlis, R. J. (2005). The control of voluntary eye movements: new perspectives. *Neuroscientist, 11*(2), 124–137.

70. Thier, P., & Ilg, U. J. (2005). The neural basis of smooth-pursuit eye movements. *Current Opinion in Neurobiology, 15*(6), 645–652.

71. Rashbass, C. (1961). The relationship between saccadic and smooth tracking eye movements. *Journal of Physiology, 159*(2), 326–338.

72. Carl, J. R., & Gelman, R. S. (1987). Human smooth pursuit: stimulus dependent responses. *Journal of Neurophysiology, 57*(5), 1446–1463.

73. Orban de Xivry, J. J., & Lefevre, P. (2007). Saccades and pursuit: two outcomes of a single sensorimotor process. *Journal of Physiology, 584*(1), 11–23.

74. Pola, J., & Wyatt, H. J. (2002). Target position and velocity: the stimuli for smooth pursuit eye movements. *Annals of the New York Academy of Sciences, 956*, 216–229.

75. Steinman, S. B., & Steinman, B. A. (2007). Applications of visual attention to vision therapy and rehabilitation. *Journal of Behavioral Optometry, 18*(5), 121–126.

76. Owens, D. A., & Reed, E. S. (1994). Seeing where we look. *Behavioral and Brain Sciences, 17*, 271–272.

77. Von Noorden, G. K., & Campos, E. C. (2002). *Binocular vision and ocular motility: Theory and management of strabismus* (6th ed.). St. Louis, MO: Mosby.

78. Judge, S. J., & Cumming, B. G. (1986). Neurons in the monkey midbrain with activity related to vergence eye movement and accommodation. *Journal of Neurophysiology, 55*(5), 915–930.

79. Mays, L. E. (1984). Neural control of vergence eye movements: convergence and divergence neurons in midbrain. *Journal of Neurophysiology, 52*(6), 1091–1108.
80. Keller, E. L., & Robinson, D. A. (1972). Abducens unit behavior in the monkey during vergence movements. *Vision Research, 12*(2), 369–382.
81. Mays, L. E., & Porter, J. D. (1984). Neural control of vergence eye movements: activity of abducens and oculomotor neurons. *Journal of Neurophysiology, 52*(4), 743–761.
82. Maunsell, J. H. R., & Van Essen, D. C. (1983). Functional properties of neurons in middle temporal visual area of the macaque monkey. II. Binocular interactions and sensitivity to binocular disparity. *Journal of Neurophysiology, 49*(5), 1148–1167.
83. Tanaka, K., Saito, H., Fukada, Y., & Moriya, M. (1991). Coding visual images of objects in the inferotemporal cortex of the macaque monkey. *Journal of Neurophysiology, 66*, 170–189.
84. Gnadt, J. W., & Mays, L. E. (1989). Posterior parietal cortex, the oculomotor near response and spatial coding in 3-D space. *Society of Neuroscience Abstracts, 15*, 786.
85. Sakata, H., Shibutani, H., Kawano, K., & Harrington, T. L. (1985). Neural mechanisms of space vision in the parietal association cortex of the monkey. *Vision Research, 25*(3), 453–463.
86. Holmes, G. (1922). Clinical symptoms of cerebellar disease and their interpretation. *The Lancet, 200*(5158), 59–65.
87. Sander, T., Sprenger, A., Neumann, G., Machner, B., Gottschalk, S., Rambold, C., & Helmchen, C. (2009). Vergence deficits in patients with cerebellar lesions. *Brain, 132*(1), 103–115.
88. Westheimer, G., & Blair, G. (1974). Functional organization of primate oculomotor system revealed by cerebellectomy. *Experimental Brain Research, 21*(5), 463–472.
89. Daum, K. M., & McCormack, G. L. (2006). Fusion and binocularity. In W. J. Benjamin (Ed.), *Borish's clinical refraction* (2nd ed., pp. 145–148). St Louis, MO: Butterworth-Heinemann.
90. Padula, W. V. (1992). Neuro-optometric rehabilitation for persons with TBI or CVA. *Journal of Optometric Vision Development, 23*(1), 4–8.
91. Cooper, J. (1987). Accommodative dysfunction. In J. F. Amos (Ed.), *Diagnosis and management in vision care.* Boston, MA: Butterworth-Heinemann.
92. Bobier, W. R. & Sivak, J. G. (1983). Orthoptic treatment of subjects showing slow accommodative responses. *American journal of optometry and physiological optics, 60*, 678–687.
93. Hung, G. K., Ciuffreda, K. J., & Semmlow, J. L. (1986). Static vergence and accommodation: population norms and accommodative effects. *Documenta Ophthalmologica, 62*(2), 165–179.
94. Ciuffreda, K. J. (2006). Accommodation, the pupil, and presbyopia. In W. J. Benjamin (Ed.), *Borish's clinical refraction* (2nd ed.). St. Louis, MO: Butterworth-Heinemann.
95. Scheiman, M., & Wick, B. (2002). *Clinical management of binocular vision: Heterophoric, accommodative, and eye movement disorders* (2nd ed.). Philadelphia, PA: Lippincott Williams and Wilkins.
96. Hennessy, R. T., & Liebowitz, H. W. (1971). The effect of a peripheral stimulus on accommodation. *Perception and Psychophysics, 10*, 129–132.
97. Malmstrom, F. V., & Randle, R. J. (1976). Effects of visual imagery on the accommodative response. *Perception and Psychophysics, 19*, 450–453.
98. Ciuffreda, K. J. (2002). The scientific basis for and efficacy of optometric vision therapy in nonstrabismic accommodative and vergence disorders. *Optometry, 73*(12), 735–762.
99. Forrest, E. B. (1980). Stress: a redefinition. *Journal of the American Optometric Association, 51*(6), 600–604.
100. Birnbaum, M. H. (1985). Nearpoint visual stress: clinical implications. *Journal of the American Optometric Association, 56*(6), 480–490.

101. Treisman, A. M., & Gelade, G. (1980). A feature integration theory of attention. *Cognitive Psychology, 12*(1), 97–136.

102. Hécaen, H., & Albert, M. L. (1978). *Human neuropsychology*. New York: Wiley.

103. Lackner, J. R., & Teuber, H. L. (1973). Alterations in auditory fusion thresholds after cerebral injury in man. *Neuropsychologia, 11*(4), 409–415.

104. Carmon, A., & Nachshon, I. (1971). Effect of unilateral brain damage on perception of temporal order. *Cortex, 7*(4), 410–418.

105. Ratey, J. (2002). *A user's guide to the brain: Perception, attention, and the four theaters of the brain* (p. 95). New York: Vintage Books.

106. Jay, M.F., & Sparks, D. L. (1984). Auditory receptive fields in primate superior colliculus shift with changes in eye position. *Nature, 309*(5966), 345–347.

107. Jeannerod, M. (1981). Specialized channels for cognitive responses. *Cognition, 10*(1–3), 135–137.

108. Biguer, B., Jeannerod, M., & Prablanc, C. (1982). The coordination of eye, head, and arm movements during reaching at a single visual target. *Experimental Brain Research, 46*(2), 301–304.

109. Milner, A. D., & Goodale, M. A. (1993). Visual pathways to perception and action. *Progress in Brain Research, 95*, 317–337.

110. Mountcastle, V. B. (1995). The parietal system and some higher brain functions. *Cerebral Cortex, 5*(**5**), 377–390.

111. Weinstein, M. (1964, July). *Vision and movement*. Personal lecture notes. Lecture to the summer residents at the Optometric Center of New York, New York.

112. Rock, I., & Victor, J. (1964). Vision and touch: an experimentally created conflict between the two senses. *Science, 143*, 594–596.

113. Aristotle. (1951). *The Metaphysics* (translated by P. Wheelwright). New York: Odyssey Press.

114. Treisman, A., Vieira, A., & Hayes, A. (1992). Automaticity and preattentive processing. *American Journal of Psychology, 105*(**2**), 341–362.

115. Macdonald, L. (1965, June). *Visual training*. Personal lecture notes. Optometric extension program foundation graduate clinical seminar, Boston, MA.

116. Deco, G., Pollatos, O., & Zihl, J. (2002). The time course of selective visual attention: theory and experiments. *Vision Research, 42*(**27**), 2925–2945.

117. Chelazzi, L., Miller, E. K., Duncan, J., & Desimone, R. (2001). Responses of neurons in macaque area V4 during memory-guided visual search. *Cerebral Cortex, 11*(**8**), 761–772.

118. Bulakowski, P. F., Bressler, D. W., & Whitney, D. (2007). Shared attentional resources for global and local motion processing. *Journal of Vision, 7*(10), 1–10.

119. Posner, M. I. (1980). Orienting of attention. *Quarterly Journal of Experimental Psychology*, 32(1), 3–25.

120. Broadbent, D. E. (1982). Task combination and selective intake of information. *Acta Psychologica, 50*(**3**), 253–290.

121. Peterson, M. S., Kramer, A. F., & Irwin, D. E. (2004).Covert shifts of attention precede involuntary eye movements. *Perception and Psychophysics, 66*(3), 398–405.

122. Eysenck, M. W., & Keane, M. T. (2005). *Cognitive psychology: A student's handbook* (5th ed.). New York: Psychology Press.

123. Van Opstal, A. J., Hepp, K., Hess, B. J. M., Strauman, D., & Henn, V. (1991). Two-, rather than three-dimensional representation of saccades in monkey superior colliculus. *Science; 252*(5010), 1313–1315.

124. Posner, M. I., Walker, J. A., Friedrich, F. J., & Rafal, R. D. (1984). Effects of parietal injury on covert orienting of attention. *Journal of Neuroscience, 4*(7), 1863–1874.

125. Kandel, E. R., Schwartz, J. H., & Jessell, T. M. (2000). *Principles of neural science* (4th ed., p. 794). New York: McGraw-Hill.

126. Crick, F. (1994). *The astonishing hypothesis.* New York: Charles Scribner's Sons.
127. Goodale, M. A., Milner, A. D., Jakobson, L. S., & Carey, D. P. (1991). A neurological dissociation between perceiving objects and grasping them. *Nature, 349*(6305), 154–156.
128. Mlodinow, L. (2008). *The Drunkard's walk: How randomness rules our lives.* New York: Pantheon Books.
129. Churchland, P. M. (1995). *The engine of reason, the seat of the soul: A philosophical journey into the brain.* Cambridge, MA: the MIT Press.
130. Drew, A. S., Langan, J., Halterman, C., Osternig, L. R., Chou, L. S., & van Donkelaar, P. (2007). Attentional disengagement dysfunction following mob assessed with the gap saccade task. *Neuroscience Letters, 417*(1), 61–65.
131. Albano, J. E., Mishkin, M., Westbrook, L. E., & Wurtz, R. H. (1982). Visuomotor deficits following ablation of monkey superior colliculus. *Journal of Neurophysiology, 48*(2), 338–351.
132. Wurtz, R. H., & Goldberg, M. E. (1974). Activity of superior colliculus in behaving monkey. IV. Effects of lesions on eye movements. *Journal of Neurophysiology, 35*(4), 587–596.
133. Lee, C., Roher, W. H., & Sparks, D. (1988). Population coding of saccadic eye movements by neurons in the superior colliculus. *Nature, 332*(6162), 357–360.
134. Goldberg, M. E., & Bruce, C. J. (1986). The role of the arcuate frontal eye fields in the generation of saccadic eye movements. *Progress in Brain Research, 64*, 143–154.
135. Deng, S-Y., Goldberg, M. E., Segraves, M. A., Ungerleider, L. G., & Mishkin, M. (1986). The effects of unilateral ablation of the frontal eye fields in the monkey. In E. L. Keller, & D. S. Zee (Eds.), *Adaptive processes in visual and oculomotor systems* (pp. 201–208). Oxford, UK: Pergamon Press.
136. Bogousslavsky, J., Miklossy, J., Regli, F., & Janzer, R. (1990). Vertical gaze palsy and selective unilateral infarction of the rostral interstitial nucleus of the medial longitudinal fasciculus (riMLF). *Journal of Neurology, Neurosurgery, and Psychiatry, 53*(1), 67–71.
137. Sharpe, J. A., & Lo, A. W. (1981). Voluntary and visual control of the vestibulo-ocular reflex after cerebral hemidecortication. *Annals of Neurology, 10*(2), 164–172.
138. Sapir, A., Hayes, A., & Rafal, R. (2004). Parietal lobe lesions disrupt saccadic remapping of inhibitory location tagging. *Journal of Cognitive Neuroscience, 16*(4), 503–509.
139. Sharp, J. L. (1986). Adaptation to frontal lobe lesions. In E. L. Keller, & D. S. Zee (Eds.), *Adaptive processes in visual and oculomotor systems* (pp. 239–246). Oxford, UK: Pergamon Press.
140. Collin, N. G., Cowey, A., Latto, R., & Marzi, C. (1982). The role of frontal eye fields and superior colliculi in visual search and non-visual search in rhesus monkeys. *Behavioral Brain Research, 4*(2), 177–193.
141. Guitton, D., Buchtel, H. W., & Douglas, R. M. (1985). Frontal lobe lesions in man causing difficulties in suppressing reflexes glances and in generating goal-directed saccades. *Experimental Brain Research, 58*(3), 455–472.
142. Kapoor, N., Ciuffreda, K. J., & Han, Y. (2004). Oculomotor rehabilitation in acquired brain injury: a case series. *Archives of Physical Medicine and Rehabilitation, 85*(10), 1667–1678.
143. Ciuffreda, K. J., Suchoff, I. B., Marrone, M., & Ahmann, E. (1996). Oculomotor rehabilitation in traumatic brain-injured patients. *Journal of Behavioral Optometry, 7*(2), 31–38.
144. Suchoff, I. B., Kapoor, N., Waxman, R., & Ference, W. (1999). The occurrence of visual and ocular conditions in an acquired brain-injured patient sample. *Journal of the American Optometric Association, 70*(5), 301–308.
145. Suchoff, I. B., Gianutsos, R., Ciuffreda, K. J., & Groffman, S. (2000). Vision impairment related to acquired brain injury. In B. Silverstone, M. A. Lang, B. P. Rosenthal, & E. F. Faye (Eds.), *The lighthouse handbook on vision impairment and vision rehabilitation* (Vol. 1, p. 523). New York: Oxford University Press.

146. Kapoor, N., & Ciuffreda, K. J. (2002). Vision disturbances following traumatic brain injury. *Current Treatment Options in Neurology, 4*(4), 271–280.
147. Suter, P. S. (2004). Rehabilitation and management of visual dysfunction following traumatic brain injury. In M. J. Ashley (Ed.), *Traumatic brain injury: Rehabilitative treatment and case management*. Boca Raton, FL: CRC Press.
148. Padula, W. V., Wu, L., Vicci, V., Thomas, J., Nelson, C., Gottlieb, D., Benabib R. (2007). Evaluating and treating visual dysfunction. In N. D. Zasler, D. I. Katz, & R. D. Zafonte (Eds.), *Brain injury medicine: Principles and practice* (p. 511). New York: Demos.
149. Kapoor, N., & Ciuffreda, K. J. (2009). Vision deficits following acquired brain injury. In A. Cristian (Ed.), *Medical management of the adult with a neurological disability* (pp. 407–425). New York: Demos Medical Publishing.
150. Duke-Elder, S., & Wybar, K. (1973). *System of ophthalmology, Vol.6: Ocular motility and strabismus*. St. Louis, MO: Mosby.
151. Ciuffreda, K. J., Kapoor, N., Rutner, D., Suchoff, I. B., Han, M. E., & Craig, S. (2007). Occurrence of oculomotor dysfunctions in acquired brain injury: a retrospective analysis. *Optometry, 78*(4), 155–161.
152. Ciuffreda, K. J., & Kapoor, N. (2007). Oculomotor dysfunctions, their remediation, and reading-related problems in mild traumatic brain injury. *Journal of Behavioral Optometry, 18*(3), 72–77.
153. Ciuffreda, K. J., Rutner, D., Kapoor, N., Suchoff, I. B., Craig, S., & Han, M. E. (2008). Vision therapy for oculomotor dysfunctions in acquired brain injury: a retrospective analysis. *Optometry, 79*(1), 18–22.
154. Craig, S. B., Kapoor, N., Ciuffreda, K. J., Suchoff, I. B., Han, M. E., & Rutner, D. (2008). Profile of selected aspects of visually symptomatic individuals with acquired brain injury: a retrospective study. *Journal of Behavioral Optometry, 19*(1), 7–10.
155. Granet, D. B., Gomi, C. F., Ventura, R., & Miller-Scholte, A. (2005). The relationship between convergence insufficiency and ADHD. *Strabismus, 13*(4), 163–168.
156. Kowal, L. (1992). Ophthalmic manifestations of head injury. *Australian and New Zealand Journal of Ophthalmology, 20*(1), 35–40.
157. London, R., Wick, B., & Kirschen, D. (2003). Post-traumatic pseudomyopia. *Optometry, 74*(2), 111–120.
158. Leslie, S. (2009). Myopia and accommodative insufficiency associated with moderate head trauma. *Optometry and Vision Development, 40*(1), 25–31.
159. Gianutsos, R., Ramsey, G., & Perlin, R. R. (1988). Rehabilitative optometric services for survivors of acquired brain injury. *Archives of Physical Medicine and Rehabilitation, 69*(8), 573–578.
160. Al-Qurainy, I. A. (1995). Convergence insufficiency and failure of accommodation following midfacial trauma. *The British Journal of Oral & Maxillofacial Surgery, 33*(2), 71–77.
161. Wachs, H., Lawrence, J., & Vaughan, M. A. (1977). *Wachs analysis of cognitive structures*. Los Angeles, CA: Western Psychological Services.
162. Goddard, S. (1995). *A teacher's window into the child's mind* (pp. 1–2). Eugene, OR: Fern Ridge Press.
163. Maples, W. C. (1995). *The NSUCO oculomotor test*. Santa Ana, CA: Optometric Extension Program.
164. Griffin, J. R., & Grisham, J. D. (2002). *Binocular anomalies: Diagnosis and vision therapy* (4th ed., pp. 24–25). Boston, MA: Butterworth-Heinemann.
165. Schuett, S., Heywood, C. A., Kentridge, R. W., & Zihl, J. (2008). The significance of visual information processing in reading: Insights from hemianopic dyslexia. *Neuropsychologia, 46*(10), 2445–2462.
166. Gallaway, M., Scheiman, M., Frantz, K. A., Peters, R. J., Hatch, S., & Cuff, M. (1991). The significance of assessing nearpoint of convergence using different stimuli. *Optometry and Vision Science, 168*(Suppl.), 93.

167. Hayes, G. I., Cohen, B. E., & Rouse, M. W. (1998). Normative data values for the nearpoint of convergence of elementary school children. *Optometry and Vision Science, 75*(7), 506–512.

168. Scheiman, M., Gallaway, M., & Frantz, K. A. (2003). Nearpoint of convergence test procedure, target selection, and normative data. *Optometry and Vision Science, 80*(3), 214–225.

169. Press, L. J. (2008). *Applied concepts in vision therapy.* Santa Ana, CA: Optometric Extension Program.

170. Goss, D.A. (1995). *Ocular accommodation, convergence, and fixation disparity* (2nd ed., pp. 73–74). Boston, MA: Butterworth-Heinemann.

171. Barry, S. (2009). *Fixing my gaze: A scientist's journey into seeing in three dimensions.* New York: Basic Books.

172. Werner, D. L., & Press, L. J. (2002). *Clinical pearls in refractive care.* Boston, MA: Butterworth-Heinemann.

173. Han, Y., Ciuffreda, K. J., & Kapoor, N. (2004). Reading-related oculomotor testing and training protocols for acquired brain injury in humans. *Brain Research Protocols, 14*(1), 1–12.

174. Ciuffreda, K. J., Kapoor, N., & Han, Y. (2005). Reading-related ocular motor deficits in traumatic brain injury. *Brain Injury Professional, 2*(3), 16–20.

175. Valenti, C. A. (1990). *The full scope of retinoscopy.* Santa Ana, CA: Optometric Extension Program.

176. Schrock, R. E., & Heinsen, A. C. (1966). *Schur-Mark out-of-office training system.* Meadville, PA: Keystone View Co.

177. Liu, J. S., Lee, M., Jang, J., Ciuffreda, K. J., Wong J. H., Grisham, D., & Stark, L. (1979). Objective assessment of accommodation orthoptics: dynamic insufficiency. *American Journal of Optometry and Physiological Optics, 56*(5), 285–294.

178. Sterner, B., Abrahamsson, M., & Anders, S. (1999). Accommodative facility training with a long-term follow-up in a sample of school-aged children showing accommodative dysfunction. *Documenta Ophthalmologica, 99*(1), 93–101.

179. Lovasik, J. V., & Wiggins, R. (1984). Cortical indices of impaired ocular accommodation and associated convergence mechanisms. *American Journal of Optometry and Physiological Optics, 61*(3), 150–159.

180. Suchoff, I. B., & Petito, G. T. (1986). The efficacy of visual therapy: accommodative disorders and nonstrabismic anomalies of binocular vision. *Journal of the American Optometric Association, 57*(2), 119–125.

181. Birnbaum, M. H. (1993). *Optometric management of nearpoint vision disorders.* Boston, MA: Butterworth–Heinemann.

182. Cooper, J., Selenow, A., Ciuffreda, K. J., Feldman, J., Faverty, J., Hokoda, S. C., & Silver, J. (1983). Reduction of asthenopia in patients with convergence insufficiency after fusional vergence training. *American Journal of Optometry and Physiological Optics, 60*(12), 982–989.

183. Grisham, J. D., Bowman, M. C., Owyang, L. A., & Chan, C. L. (1991). Vergence orthoptics: validity and persistence of the training effect. *Optometry and Vision Science, 68*(6), 441–451.

184. Wick, B. (1977). Vision training for presbyopes. *American Journal of Optometry and Physiological Optics, 54*(4), 244–247.

185. Cooper, J., & Duckman, R. (1978). Convergence insufficiency: incidence, diagnosis and treatment. *Journal of the American Optometric Association, 49*(6), 673–680.

186. Grisham, J. D. (1988). Visual therapy results for convergence insufficiency: a literature review. *American Journal of Optometry and Physiological Optics, 65*(6), 448–454.

187. Scheiman, M., Mitchell, L., Cotter, S., Cooper, J., Kulp, M., Rouse, M., & Wensveen, J. (2005). A randomized clinical trial of treatments for convergence insufficiency in children. *Archives of Ophthalmology, 123*(1), 14–24.

188. Convergence Insufficiency Treatment Trial (CITT) Study Group. (2008). Randomized clinical trial of treatments for symptomatic convergence insufficiency in children. *Archives of Ophthalmology, 126*(10), 1336–1349.

189. Sanet, L. Z. (2006, October). *Vision therapy 101.* Presented at the meeting of the College of Optometrists in Vision Development, St. Petersburg, FL.

190. Scheiman, M. M., & Rouse, M. W. (1994). *Optometric management of learning-related vision problems.* St. Louis, MO: Mosby.

191. Swartwout, J. B. (1991). *Optometric vision therapy manual—Procedures and forms for in-office and out-of-office training programs.* Santa Ana, CA: Optometric Extension Program.

192. Sacks, O. (2004). In the river of consciousness, *The New York Review of Books, 51*(1), 41–45.

5 Evaluation and Treatment of Visual Field Loss and Visual-Spatial Neglect

Neil W. Margolis

CONTENTS

INTRODUCTION

Homonymous hemianopia, which is the loss of half the visual field on the same side in both eyes, is frequently found concurrently with visual-spatial neglect. Visual field plots of hemianopia are physical representations of the neural insult; they respect the neural anatomy. By contrast visual-spatial neglect is a cognitive phenomenon that can vary subject to cueing and to the type of stimulus presentation. If there is a dense homonymous hemianopia without visual-spatial neglect, patients will usually understand that they have a visual field loss for which they need to compensate. However, they are not necessarily efficient at doing so.

It is extremely common for both optometrists and ophthalmologists to misdiagnose visual-spatial neglect as visual field defect. The pathology education for both professions has largely concentrated on eye disease, and therefore, little attention has been given to cortical aspects of vision, including visual-spatial neglect. This occurs in spite of the fact that more than 70% of patients hospitalized for stroke suffer from visual-spatial neglect[1] and while many spontaneously recover with time, many are sent home undiagnosed. *For this reason, every patient with brain injury should be evaluated by an eye doctor with special expertise in the neurological aspects of vision and rehabilitation.*

VISUAL FIELD LOSS

Visual field loss is extremely common following acquired brain injury and varies from small isolated blind spots, or scotomata, to loss of vision in an entire eye, or an entire homonymous hemifield. The visual consequences are not simply a matter of loss of visual information gathered from the affected areas of the visual field, but include changes in the three-dimensional structure of perceived space[2] and shifts in center of gravity affecting balance.[3] Patients with rightward visual field loss near the fovea, will experience severe difficulty with reading, as they are unable to preview the next word in their periphery to program the next eye movement. Patients with loss of central vision in one eye experience loss of stereopsis, which interferes with fine visual-motor coordination, as required during activities of daily living (ADLs) such as cooking and judging distances during mobility, including driving.[4] Depending on the extent of monocular vision loss, patients may also lose some peripheral visual field on the side of the affected eye; they must learn to turn their head slightly to move their nose out of the way to expand the field covered by the unaffected eye. In cases of homonymous hemianopia, scanning patterns must be entirely retrained. Zhang et al.[5] found that nearly 15% of patients with homonymous hemianopia had diplopia. Further evidence that it is not just loss of vision in the "blind" field that causes difficulty in homonymous hemianopia is provided by Leo et al.,[6] who found that processing of cross-modal auditory-visual localization appears to revert to subcortical mechanisms in the blind field and Paramei and Sabel,[7] who demonstrated that contour-integration deficits are found in the "intact" visual field.

Perimetry or other visual field testing, to the highest level of the patient's capabilities, is critical in assessing the patient's safety, abilities, and responses, as they move through rehabilitation and return to daily life at home and in the community. In a retrospective study of 220 individuals, 160 with traumatic brain injury (TBI) and 60 with cerebral vascular accident (CVA), Suchoff et al.[8] found that 46% of the group had visual field defects on perimetric testing. Of the patients with TBI, 39% demonstrated visual field defects, as compared to 67% of the patients with CVA. They further categorized the vision deficits into scattered defects, restricted visual field, homonymous defects, and nonhomonymous, or unilateral defects. Following CVA, most visual field defects were homonymous (31%), followed by scattered defects (13%), nonhomonymous (13%), and restricted visual field (8%). In the TBI patients, scattered defects were most common (22%), followed by homonymous (9%), restricted visual fields (6%), and nonhomonymous (1%). While most patients with large, dense homonymous visual field defects will notice that they have blind areas, those with less dramatic visual field loss may not. Townend et al.[9] examined CVA patients 9 months poststroke, using both confrontation visual field testing and perimetric testing. Consecutive CVA patients were selected from hospital records, on the basis of the likelihood of them being able to drive if their vision were normal and their ability to participate in perimetric testing. Homonymous visual field defects were found in 16% of these patients—half were partial hemianopia (mostly right hemianopia) and half were partial quadrant defects. Surprisingly, none of the patients with visual field loss were aware of their loss, and only two of these visual field deficits were detected using confrontation fields assessment. Of those with significant perimetric visual field loss, 30% were driving without knowledge of, or rehabilitation for, their visual field loss.

Visual field loss has been negatively correlated with return to work.[10] When closed head injury patients are categorized into mild/moderate or severe head injury groups, patients with visual field defects score lower on neuropsychological testing in both groups 10–19 months postinjury.[11] Many patients with visual field loss are still told, "Go home, you will get used to it," rather than being referred to a rehabilitative specialist. Rehabilitation for patients with visual field loss is necessary, not only to enhance quality of life, but clearly, for safety reasons. Patients with hemianopia and otherwise relatively intact cognition can be rehabilitated back into many different occupations, and in many states are able to drive. Patients with visual field loss should be evaluated on an individual basis. This is necessary to determine if they meet the peripheral field requirements to drive in their state and/or whether they are safe drivers. Some states define the minimum peripheral visual field requirements for all drivers in terms of degrees of peripheral vision relative to a central fixation point. Other states only have field requirements for commercial drivers. Unfortunately many of the peripheral vision field screeners used at state operated driving evaluation centers are not sensitive to visual fixation. This allows candidates to pass erroneously by using compensatory scanning techniques. Standards for passing visual field tests for the purpose of driving with the use of field awareness prisms have not been established. Studies,[12,13] as well as clinical experience, reveal that patients with visual field loss can indeed be safe drivers.

Patients who meet their state's peripheral vision requirements for driving and are otherwise suitable candidates should be trained in efficient scanning techniques to compensate for their individual field deficit. They should then be referred to a driving center affiliated with a rehabilitation clinic for a predriving evaluation. A driving simulator is often used as part of this preroad screening. If appropriate, this screening will be followed by on-road evaluation and training. Finally, if the patient shows appropriate skills and requires reactivation of his license he is referred to the state operated driving center for final on-road testing. These patients may end up with an unrestricted drivers license, a license with the requirement of augmentative wide angle or side mirrors, or license with restricted driving privileges. Driving may be restricted within a geographic zone or to daylight driving only.

NEURAL SUBSTRATES OF VISUAL FIELD LOSS

Visual field loss is best thought of as a physical sight loss or sensory loss that will respect the anatomy of the visual pathways. This can be measured by confrontation field testing, tangent screen, or, preferably if the patient is able, automated or projection perimetry. Field loss that originates from damage to the optic nerve may respect the horizontal meridian of the visual field. Visual field loss, which originates from a chiasmal or retrochiasmal lesion, will tend to respect the vertical meridian, and may respect the horizontal meridian, such that the visual field may be grossly considered in four quadrants.

It is generally true for vision loss anterior to, and including the optic chiasm, that the pattern of visual field loss allows localization of the lesion (Figure 5.1). Monocular vision loss implies a retinal or optic nerve lesion. Bitemporal visual field loss is generally due to compression of ganglion cell axons as they hemidecussate at the chiasm, often due to pituitary tumor. Altitudinal field loss is common in anterior ischemic neuropathy.

Until recently, it has been "common knowledge" that for homonymous (generally retrochiasmal) lesions, a greater congruency in the visual field defects implied a more posterior lesion. Zhang et al.[14] examined visual field loss and brain imaging in 904 cases of homonymous visual field loss without neglect, and found that there was poor correlation between the old assumptions and the actual location of lesions in the visual pathways. For instance, retrochiasmal visual pathway lesions produced unpredictable visual field defects, with the exception of homonymous sectoranopia and unilateral loss of the temporal crescent (Figure 5.2), which were exclusively due to lesions involving the lateral geniculate body and the anterior part of the occipital lobe. Only 52% of the homonymous hemianopias with macular sparing were secondary to occipital lesions. Homonymous hemianopia with macular sparing was also found among lesions involving the optic radiations or optic tract.

DIAGNOSING VISUAL FIELD LOSS

Testing should be performed to the maximum capability of the patient, because the chances of missing scattered scotomas, quadrantanopia, or even bitemporal hemianopia on confrontation testing is relatively high.[15,16] Therefore, if the patient is able,

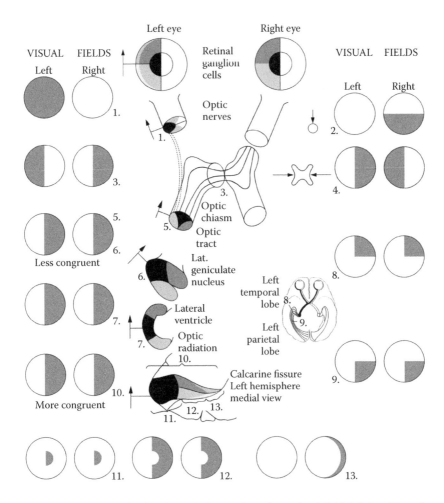

FIGURE 5.1 Primary visual pathway lesions and resultant visual field deficits. (From Suter, P. S., and Margolis, N. W., Managing visual field defects following acquired brain injury. *Brain Inj. Prof.*, 2, 3, 26, 2005. Reprinted with permission.)

it is most appropriate to obtain an automated perimetry field response, which would serve as the most sensitive base line of the visual field loss. The test is only valid if fixation is accurate and the patient does not over or under respond to the stimuli. Additional confrontation fields can then be used temporally to determine the far peripheral extent of the field. Occasionally one will find a patient who demonstrates extremely restricted fields on perimetry and then turns out to have a spared temporal crescent on confrontation testing.

Perimetry
Automated visual field testing should be performed on 60-degree fields, rather than the standard 30-degree visual field. Projection perimetry allows

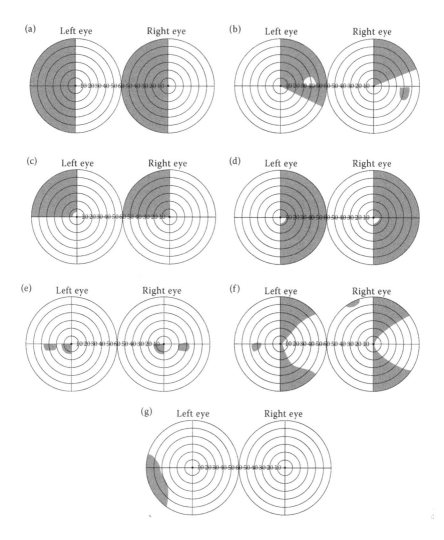

FIGURE 5.2 Classification of visual field defects: (a) Left homonymous hemianopia; (b) Incomplete right homonymous hemianopia, worse superiorly than inferiorly; (c) Left superior homonymous quadrantanopia; (d) right homonymous hemianopia sparing the macula; (e) Left homonymous scotomatous defect; (f) right homonymous sectoranopia; (g) Loss of temporal crescent in the left eye. (Adapted from Zhang, X., Kedar, S., Lynn, M. J., Newman, N. J., and Biousse, V., Homonymous hemianopias; clinical-anatomic correlations in 904 cases. *Neurology*, 66, 6, 907, 2006.)

examination to 90 degrees. The normal visual field extends approximately 60 degrees nasally and 90 degrees temporally. Unfortunately, perimetric testing is not always possible due to the physical, cognitive, attentive, or behavioral status of the patient. Many practitioners screen patient's visual fields with frequency doubling technique (FDT) perimeters. However, FDT is not a reliable way to screen for neurological visual field defects. Fong et al.[17] compared FDT versus Humphrey automated perimetry screenings in 15 eyes of nine patients with complete hemianopias or quadrantanopias, and found that the FDT failed to pick up any abnormality in 3 eyes, and overall, considerably fewer points were picked up as abnormal with FDT. Wall et al.[18] described similar findings with hemianopias, but found that automated perimetry and FDT were equivalent in detecting optic neuropathies.

For patients who cannot be positioned in an automated perimeter or projection instrument, the tangent screen can be used to plot the central 30 degrees. The tangent screen is a manual method by which the examiner moves a small target along meridians on a black felt board to test sensitivity around the visual field. The patient's job is to tell when the target disappears and reappears. The physiological blind spot is plotted, giving the patient an opportunity to see how the target may disappear in the midst of the board. The tangent screen is time intensive, but quite good for plotting scotomata in the central area. An instrument that is no longer manufactured, but which is quite helpful with patients who cannot sit for automated perimetry is the Harrington Flocks visual field tester. It is a series of large cards, each with a fixation target and one to four stimulus dots that appear briefly when the examiner flashes the ultraviolet light on the unit. The patient can respond by saying, showing, or writing the number of stimuli viewed, or by pointing to where they saw the stimuli presented. They have as long to respond as necessary. This provides a fairly quick quantitative assessment of the central 25 degrees.

Amsler Grid

Amsler grids may be used to define small central scotomas, or to better define the border of hemianopias. Test administration is typically as follows. Patch one of the patient's eyes. Holding the Amsler grid at 40 cm (16") from their eye, have the patient fixate the center dot. Then ask if, without moving their eye, they can see all four corners of the grid. If so, again without moving their eye from the center fixation point, they are to tell you if there are any areas of the grid that are distorted, wavy, or missing. If there are areas where the grid is not uniform, they are to mark those areas with a pencil, while keeping their fixation on the central dot. If there is a central scotoma, use a grid that has diagonals drawn from corner to corner in both directions forming an "X" in the middle. The patient can fixate where the diagonals would intersect, and perform the test.

Confrontation Field Testing

Various sorts of confrontation fields may be useful, depending on the patient's abilities to respond.

a. Confrontation testing to determine the peripheral extent of the visual field is carried out to find the full extent of the visual field when 60-degree (or less) perimetry has been performed, or when the patient is unable to respond to perimetric testing. Confrontation fields may be performed with one or two examiners. Two examiner confrontation fields tend to give more reliable results,[19] but are not always practicable in the clinic. Confrontation fields are performed by first patching one of the patient's eyes. Stand 20 inches in front of the patient and have him look at your nose. Introduce your hands randomly, starting from behind the patient's face, at face level from the left and right peripheral vision side of the patient, testing superior to and inferior to the patient's fixation point, so that all four quadrants are tested. Ask the patient to tell you when he first notices your hand. Ensure that the patient does not look away from your nose. For example, the patient with complete left hemianopia will not be aware of the evaluator's hand presentation in the left visual field, either above or below the fixation point, where in a quadrantanopia, they may see it above, but not below the fixation point. The advantage of the second examiner is that the patient cannot follow the direction of the examiner's arm to try to predict where the hand will appear.

b. Place a rectangular sheet of paper (legal pad size) in a clipboard and place it vertically in front of the patient. A cross or obvious fixation point should be placed in the center of the sheet at eye level. Ask the patient to report when the pencil is first seen as it is introduced at different heights from the left or right side from behind the sheet. Be sure the patient is always fixating on the fixation point. Again, for example, the patient with complete left hemianopia will not notice the pencil when it is introduced from the left side until it is at the fixation point. Often, the border of the hemianopia will be somewhat different above versus below the fixation point. If a hemianopia is leftward, patients will have difficulty returning to the proper line of print while reading. If the defect is rightward, patients will have difficulty previewing and saccading to the next word. The Amsler grid may be used in the same way. This technique allows you to assess whether the patient has sufficient macular sparing to preview the next word in reading and to anticipate what sort of difficulty they may have with mobility.

c. Obtain a picture of a face the size of a legal sheet and place it vertically and centered in front of the patient. Ask him to fixate on the nose of the person in the picture. Watch from behind the sheet to ensure fixation is maintained. Ask the patient if he is able to see both eyes of the face, while they are fixating on the nose. The patient with a complete left hemianopia will not be able to see the detail on the left side of the face. This test may be performed with the examiner's face, but the picture allows charting the blind area on the test stimulus.

d. Red cap testing may also be performed as a confrontation test, as sometimes the visual field deficit is relative or small, and while the patient may be unable to detect relative scotomas, the red cap of an eye drop bottle may be used to check all four quadrants for equal red saturation. Relative scotomas tend to desaturate color, and so the cap may appear less red or may even be achromatic, or gray appearing.

In all cases of apparent peripheral visual field loss, except on the red cap test, the differential diagnosis that must be made is visual-spatial neglect, which may mimic visual field defects, or exist concurrently with visual field defects.

INTERVENTION FOR VISUAL FIELD LOSS

Central Vision Loss

Central vision loss causes loss of visual acuity, and these treatment protocols have been delineated in an entire "low vision" literature. This literature has historically been called *vision rehabilitation*, a term dating from before neurovision rehabilitation was established as a subspecialty. There are many fine texts in this area,[20] and it is beyond the purview of this book.

Loss of Vision in One Eye

Loss of vision from one eye causes deficits in stereopsis, or fine depth perception, as well as loss of vision from the temporal visual field on the side of the loss. Patients with deep-set eyes or high bridges can be taught to turn the head slightly toward the visual loss, as this removes the bridge of the nose from the nasal line of sight and expands the visual field immediately. Sometimes, in driving, visual field expanding rearview mirrors or mirrors mounted on the front fender of the car on the side of the loss may be helpful. The loss of stereopsis is probably the most disconcerting, creating safety issues in the kitchen and in driving.[4] While the patient may adapt, if advised to be cautious and left to their own devices, adaptation will be easier if they are prescribed rehabilitative exercises emphasizing spatial judgments and fine visual-motor judgments on the Z axis with both stationary and moving targets.

Space matching is one such exercise. The only equipment necessary is a string, and perhaps a tape measure. The object is to judge the distance to an object and the height or width of the target object. If the patient is able to perform heel to toe walking, they are to guess the number of heel to toe steps it will take them to reach the object from where they are standing. At the same time, grasping the string tightly between the thumb and forefinger of each hand they define the length of string that matches the width of the object, so that they can simply hold the string up to the object to compare when they arrive. If the patient is unable to walk, they may guess the distance in feet and inches or meters, and compare their judgments to the actual measured distance. Objects should be chosen between 2 and 15 feet away, and the location should be varied so that distances to furniture in a room are not simply memorized. This exercise teaches the patient to judge distances with monocular cues and provides feedback regarding these cues and size constancy. The distances can be randomized by tossing a beanbag and judging the distance to the beanbag.

Scattered Scotomas

When there are scattered small scotomas, the visual fields from each eye should be compared to see whether there are any that are congruent so that the loss is not covered by the intact vision from the other eye. If so, then the patient must be made aware of these areas and taught to scan so that the scotoma is not stationary.

Concentric and Altitudinal Vision Loss

Concentric and altitudinal visual field loss generally present the same sort of difficulties in up and down gaze. Patients with superior visual field loss must be educated
to survey spaces for overhead lamps and cabinets that may be dangerous. Also, they
need to be consciously aware of the car trunk lid when it is raised. Patients with
inferior field loss will have difficulty negotiating uneven ground or crowded spaces
where there may be obstacles, small children, or pets underfoot. Education, scanning training, and perhaps bases down yoked prism, or a cane with which to stabilize themselves and assist in judging surfaces are alternatives for inferior field loss
compensation and therapy. If concentric field loss is not severe (e.g., ±30 degrees
residual), it is fairly common with scanning training to see good expansion of the
field. It is possible that this may be a common psychogenic finding, although it can
certainly occur with magnocellular damage.

Cortical Blindness

Patients with cortical blindness, whether congenital or resulting from ABI, should
have appropriate rehabilitation attempted. It is more common than not that when
these individuals who show little or no fixation, or are perhaps "locked in" (cognizant, but unable to respond motorically or verbally), following severe TBI are
provided with visual stimulation, they are able to learn to respond, sometimes in
surprising ways to visual information (see case study, Chapter 1). It is too frequent
that doctors label patients with brain injury who are unable to respond as blind and
in a vegetative state without knowing. The visual system provides well over half of
the input to the brain, and can be a powerful starting point to initiate rudimentary
responses. Further, if the patient is "locked in" then acquiring the ability to fixate
and change fixation provides them the ability to communicate on a two (or more)
alternative forced choice answer board, or perhaps some of the more complex fixation driven computer-based communication devices that allow for many choices.

The initial goal of therapy is simply fixation and pursuit. Two types of targets are
helpful in eliciting this, and both should be attempted. The first is bold black and
white contoured stimuli such as large checks. These stimuli are available as infant
stimulation cards.* Nearpoint retinoscopy should be used to refine a nearpoint prescription. The card should be placed 12–16 inches from the patient's face and slowly
moved laterally rightward and leftward from center six or eight times, looking for
any attempt to fixate or follow. If any attempt is ascertained, or even suggested, then
this should be sent as home therapy, applied as many times daily for up to 10 minutes
at a time as will work into the schedule. Particularly in patients who are "locked in"
or unable to respond, it is important to keep the card at a reasonable distance from
the eyes and make sure there is an appropriate nearpoint prescription if it is called
for; stimuli held too close to the eyes may be aversive. The second type of target to
which responses may be elicited are lit targets (not simply bright beams of light)
in a dim room. Many party shops carry "jelly monster" finger puppets that illumi-
nate well, providing a bright colored lit target when placed on a penlight. The same

* Infant stimulation cards are available from Optometric Extension Program Foundation, Inc.,
  www.OEPF.org

procedure should be followed with this target if no pursuit is elicited with the black and white target. If pursuits are elicited, careful attention should be paid to whether one side is easier to fixate or pursue into than another. Visual-spatial neglect or a definite direction of gaze preference may coexist. In this case, pursuits should be first learned in the easier field of gaze, and then emphasized into the nonpreferred field. The same training pattern should be adopted when the patient advances to the point that saccades are being trained. They should initially be trained in the field of gaze away from the neglected side; that is, train in the field of gaze where it is easiest for the patient to make a movement. *When advancing to training for a two alternative forced choice board, it is critical that the choice pictures must be far enough apart to be able to discern which picture the patient is fixating, but close enough together so that both choice panels are placed well into the easily accessible field of gaze, rather than directly in front of the patient, where one choice is difficult to access.*

If no pursuit at all is demonstrated with either type of target, then blindsight training may be attempted as a home-based therapy. Blindsight is the ability, following damage to the visual cortex, to use residual vision, which does not reach consciousness.[21] More recently, because of the variety of residual visual behaviors blindsight patients demonstrate, Danckert and Rossetti[22] have suggested classifying blindsight into three separate types: (1) action blindsight, where the patient is able to perform an action, such as saccading or pointing to an object in the blind field, (2) attention blindsight, where attentional processes contribute, as in priming perceptual tasks in the intact visual field, without a motor response, and (3) agnosopsia, which includes the ability to guess the correct perceptual aspects, such as form or color of an object in the "blind" field, in spite of not having any conscious awareness of the object. Multiple subcortical tracts have been implicated as possible mediators of blindsight. Leh et al.[23] demonstrated, using diffusion tractography, that hemispherectomized individuals with attentional blindsight showed stronger than normal connectivity of the superior colliculus to the intact hemisphere from both the ipsilateral and contralateral superior colliculi. Tracts were mapped from the superior colliculi to areas close to the frontal eye fields, the parieto-occipital areas, visual association areas, and primary visual areas. Indeed, the contralateral tracts were stronger in the patients with attentional blindsight than in normal control participants. Hemispherectomized individuals without attention blindsight demonstrated only weak ipsilateral connections from the superior colliculus to portions of primary and secondary visual cortices. As reviewed by Leh et al.,[23] the superior colliculus connections do not explain blindsight that involves complete color discrimination, as the superior colliculus does not receive short wavelength (blue cone) input. Danckert and Rossetti[22] suggest the interlaminar layers of the dorsal lateral geniculate nucleus may mediate agnosopsia, while action blindsight may be mediated by a superior colliculus to pulvinar to dorsal stream (posterior parietal cortex) pathway.

Individuals who use blindsight may be able to maneuver around obstacles, but without conscious awareness that the obstacle is there in their path or what it might be. They deny being able to see objects, movement, or color in the blind area of their visual field, but are sometimes able to guess the color or direction of movement of an object at rates much higher than chance. Huxlin et al.[24] and Chokron et al.[25] have demonstrated improvement in blindsight functions with training. The essence of the training is to move lit targets in a dim room, as above, either in a vertical or horizontal direction and have the patient guess which direction the object is moving, vertically or horizontally. The target cannot be an object that casts a beam, or the patient may detect it in areas of residual vision. For each aspect of training, feedback should be given. Then one holds two such objects of different colors and the patient attempts to discriminate which color. The patient attempts to point to target objects held in front of him or her in the blind field. Forced choice shapes can be held, one in each visual field, and the patient states whether they are same or different. Large optotype letter recognition and letter naming can also be attempted. As the patient progresses, training is generalized to lighted conditions, and avoiding obstacles during mobility is added. Boyl et al.[26] studied 541 case records of children between 2 months to 19 years of age with severe visual field loss and found 23 cases of spontaneous evidence of blindsight. They suggest that use of this phenomenon in children is vital to their rehabilitation. However, even in patients who show no spontaneous evidence of blindsight, training should be attempted for a limited time, perhaps 2 months, to see whether a functionally useful blindsight response can be trained.

Homonymous Defects

Homonymous hemianopia will show some spontaneous resolution (greater than 10 degrees horizontally or 15 degrees vertically) in approximately 50%–60% of patients within the first 6 months. Little spontaneous resolution has been demonstrated to occur beyond that point.[5] However, resolution beyond 6 months postinjury has been demonstrated in multiple studies of various rehabilitation techniques. Patients with quadrant deficits (particularly superior defects) will find adaptation and compensation considerably less difficult than those with hemianopic defects. Those with superior quadrant deficits, generally only require warnings about scanning new surrounds as they enter (and being mindful in familiar settings) for overhead lighting and cabinets, which can be hazardous. Those with inferior defects will find that they interfere with reading, and mobility, including driving, and should be treated as hemianopes, with modifications.

Treat Diplopia

Firstly, as diplopia is a significant complaint in many patients with homonymous hemianopia, the diplopia must be resolved. The clinician must assess the cause of diplopia and decide whether the loss of binocularity is potentially useful, as it may provide expansion of visual field, as in the case of moderate to large exotropia, or whether it should be treated and relieved, as in the case of a convergence insufficiency. If one is to "use" the tropia, then cling patches[†] or Bangerter foils[‡] can be applied to one lens of the patient's glasses to decrease the visual acuity in the nondominant eye, reducing visual confusion. Generally, therapies involving visual

---

[†] Cling patches are thin fogging patches that press onto lenses calibrated to 20/100, 20/200, and 20/400 degradations in visual acuity available from Bernell Corporation 4016 N. Home St. Mishawwka, IN, 46545, www.bernell.com

[‡] Bangerter foils are thin fogging or occluding patches that press onto lenses and are calibrated to various degradations in visual acuity available from 20/20 to NLP available from Fresnell Prism and Lens company 6824 Washington Ave.S, Eden Prairie, MN, 55344, www.fresnel-prism.com

motor activities, pointing to, or touching targets moving across the field of view, or during mobility should be applied to help the patient figure out this new way of seeing. If the diplopia is to be treated, routine vision therapy or orthoptic therapy are effective in both the non-ABI and ABI populations.

Perceptual Speed

The existence of a significant peripheral visual field deficit necessitates scanning of the environment. However, the clinician and patient must be mindful that when a hemianope scans into the blind field, they leave the normally sighted field unviewed. For instance, a left hemianope fixating straight ahead, views 90 degrees of visual field from the straight ahead position to the right side. If they swing their eye 45 degrees leftward, to scan 45 degrees to the left of straight ahead, their intact visual field, now only extends 45 degrees rightward of straight ahead.

Because the patient with hemianopia must scan, get the information from the blind field and return to a near primary position, perceptual speed is critical for safety and should be tested and trained if found deficient. Tachistoscopic presentations are available in computer programs, tachistoscopes, and numerous vision therapy or vision rehabilitation instruments, such as the Dynavision.[§]

Scanning

Patients with homonymous hemianopia spend more time scanning in the blind field to compensate for their hemianopia.[27] Without rehabilitation, the majority of hemianopes tend to adapt disorganized scan paths with multiple refixations in the blind field, as well as the "intact" field.[28] Further, Nelles et al.[29] demonstrated using functional magnetic resonance imaging (fMRI) that hemianopic patients show reduced activation in the frontal, parietal, and supplementary eye fields during saccades. Kerkhoff, Münßinger, and Meier[30] found that a three-step process helped increase the hemianopic search field and decrease search times, resulting in lasting improvements in ability to perform ADLs. The initial step was to practice large saccades (30–40 degrees) into the blind field. Head movement was discouraged, and, indeed, frequent head movements were deleterious to performance improvement. The second step in the training process was to have the patient adopt either a horizontal or vertical scanning strategy on tasks involving scanning an array for a target. Lastly, these skills were generalized to ADLs, as in scanning kitchen shelves for particular spices. Patients who participated in these treatments demonstrated expanded search fields. Many patients also demonstrated small, but functionally significant, restitution of their visual field loss. Both scan path efficiency and visual field restitution were demonstrated to progress during scanning training, and were retained, but did not continue to improve after scanning training was stopped, as evidenced by follow-up data (averaging 22 months posttraining). Pambakian et al.[31] have found similar results with improvement in time to execute functional tasks, while many others[32] have also found small extensions of spared visual field following saccadic training which, in studies may be administered in real space situations or via

---

[§] The Dynavision is available from Performance Enterprises, 76 Major Button's Dr. Markham, Ontario, Canada, www.dynavision2.com

computer programs. Nelles et al.[33] compared presaccadic training and postsaccadic training fMRIs. Training was on both a scan board following a horizontal, row-by-row scan strategy, and during ADLs including mobility. The fMRI results showed changes posttraining in extrastriate cortex of the affected hemisphere and peristriate cortex of the unaffected hemisphere, as well as ocular motor areas.

An easy way to set up an array at home is to place cards from a deck randomly across a broad expanse of wall. The patient sits several feet from the wall, so that she can scan the entire width and height of the card array without head movement, and flips cards over from a second deck, scanning as quickly as she can for each card. The time to find all of the cards is a measure of scanning efficiency. In general, large saccades to the edge of the array scanning back toward the intact field, moving from bottom to top, or top to bottom, as the patient scans across, creates fewer refixations and a more efficient scan path.

Scanning must also be practiced during mobility. It is helpful to have the patient practice scanning into the blind field at a certain rhythm with their steps, for instance every fifth or sixth step scan into the blind field with their eyes until they get in the habit. Patients must be taught to look into the blind field each time they make a turn toward the blind side, or when they arise from sitting position, to be sure they are safe to turn that direction and to orient themselves for the next move. *Again, while head movement is necessary for large excursions into the blind field, most scanning should be done without head movement, as head movement is deleterious to efficient scanning.*[30] *Head movement also activates the vestibular system and creates dizziness and disorientation if it is used as a general scanning procedure during mobility.*

Borderzone Stimulation

Another therapeutic concept that has been applied is borderzone stimulation. Most visual field recovery occurs at the blind edge of the sighted field in homonymous hemianopia. Thus, technologies such as the NovaVision** therapy system have been developed to map the edge of the blind field and present stimuli in the blind field near that border. There are studies that demonstrate small increases in visual field resulting from borderzone stimulation, but studies where fixation is tightly controlled have brought these results into question (reviewed by McFadzean).[34] Nonetheless, more research is accumulating that appears to demonstrate the efficacy of this technique. It remains an alternative, particularly for patients who are computer oriented or who have limited mobility. However, Kasten et al.[35] performed cluster analysis on 6 months posttherapy data from patients treated with borderzone therapy, and found three types of patients. The first group improved during therapy and continued to improve after therapy ceased. The second group improved during therapy, but showed visual field regression after cessation of therapy. The final group demonstrated no positive effect of therapy. They hypothesize that the group that continued to improve may have been people who learned to use their regained vision in daily life. From a clinical point of view, the scanning therapies, discussed previously, have been demonstrated to be as efficacious in restoring visual field as borderzone

---

** NovaVision Inc., 3651 FAU Boulevard, Suite 300, Boca Raton, FL, 33431, 1–866–620–2545, www. novavision.com

stimulation, and have the added benefit that they have immediate compensatory effects. Scanning therapies not only restore visual field along the borderzone, they involve patients in their immediate safety and efficiency during mobility and ADLs, rather than requiring daily computer time, which is otherwise nonproductive. It is possible, but has not yet been demonstrated in the literature, that combining scanning and borderzone stimulation treatments might yield results for more patients or overall better results for the patients who do experience visual field recovery.

Peripheral Prism

A frequently successful peripheral prism device for patients with homonymous visual field loss developed by Dr. Daniel Gottlieb is a large dioptric (e.g., 20 pd) bases out prism mounted in the patient's lens—usually on the temporal side in the hemianopic field (Figure 5.3). Fitting kits and training instructions are available from Rekindle™.[††] The prism is out of sight until the patient scans into the blind field, and then, when viewing through the prism, the images of objects more peripheral are imaged closer in toward the midline so that the patient does not have to make such a large saccadic excursion. If the patient is binocular, the view is also diplopic when viewing in the prism, so the patient is taught to scan quickly into the prism and out. If there is an object of interest viewed in the prism, they must then turn their head to look at it without the prism to eliminate the diplopia. Patients wearing this system report improved function and safety with it.[36,37] Gottlieb et al.[38] reported visual field recovery both during the training phase and afterward for some patients wearing the peripheral prism system.

The prism is generally fit temporally (with the margin at the temporal limbus), and decentered slightly downward. Fresnel prisms can be used to trial this lens approach, but degrade easily and must be replaced on a frequent basis. A ground prism button inserted into the lens, with the patient's refractive error ground into the prism is most optimal. One big advantage of this prism system is that it gives the patient a tool that they put on every day, which reminds them to scan. Thus, it reinforces continuation of their scanning therapy. For further discussion of the Gottlieb prism system, see Chapter 7.

Peli Prism

The other major prism system for homonymous visual field deficits developed by Dr. Eli Peli[39] is also extremely useful for some patients. Neither of these two major prism systems for homonymous field loss is going to meet with acceptance from every patient. The good news is that both prism systems can be trialed with stick-on Fresnel prisms, which are relatively inexpensive and can be applied to the patient's existing glasses. Prism placement and patient training are critical to acceptance with either system and the doctor must be careful that the glasses frames have been properly fitted before placing the prism, so that there is no slippage. *Prescription of prism and lenses fall under the licensure of optometrists and physicians alone, and may not be trialed by other rehabilitation personnel, as there are safety and perceptual concerns that must be carefully considered.*

[††]   Rekindle™, Gottlieb Vision Group, 10700 Medlock Bridge Rd. Suite 103, Johns Creek, GA, 30097, 1–678–417–9778, www.rekindlevision.com

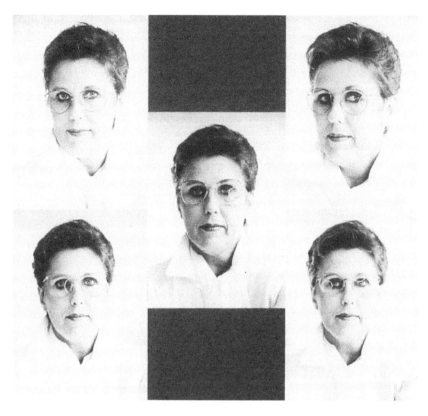

FIGURE 5.3   Patient wearing Gottlieb style peripheral prisms for various visual field deficits. Top left: For optic nerve disease with loss in only one eye in the inferior left visual field; Top right: For retinal detachment; Middle: For left hemianopia; Bottom left: For left hemianopia (blind left eye) nasally mounted Visual Field Awareness System™; Bottom right: For complex visual field loss with only one quarter of vision remaining in the inferior left visual space, using two prisms. (Adapted from Gottlieb, D., Allen, C. H., Eikenberry, J., Ingall-Woodruff, S., and Johnson, M., *Living with Vision Loss: Independence, Driving and Low Vision Solutions*, St. Barthélemy Press, Ltd., Atlanta, GA, 1996, p. 109. Out of press. Reprinted with author's permission.)

The Peli prism system uses a 40-prism diopter Fresnel prism to create peripheral exotropia. It is a simultaneous viewing system where narrow bars of prism cross the visual midline, above and below fixation, with their bases into the visual field defect (Figure 5.4). This means that, unlike the Gottlieb prism system, the Peli prism system impinges on the sighted field, creating constant peripheral diplopia above and below fixation. Typically, it is recommended that these be placed both superiorly and inferiorly. Again, when possible, the prism is placed on the lens of the eye toward the defect. This causes displacement of images from the blind field into the sighted field without eye movement, providing simultaneous awareness, peripherally, of objects from approximately 20 degrees into the blind field. The patient is taught *not* to look into the prism.

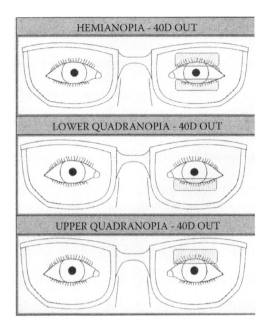

FIGURE 5.4 Examples of Peli Lens™ field expansion prism applications. (Reprinted with permission from Chadwick Optical.)

If the patient or doctor judge that an inferior prism causes too much visual confusion and makes mobility unsafe, then a superior prism may be placed initially. Bowers et al.[40] found that 12 months following fitting, 47% of patients were still wearing the prism glasses at least part time. However, this study makes it clear that proper fitting and training are critical to success, as wear at 1-year rates varied between 27% and 81% for different clinic groups, with the higher rates at the clinics that fit more prisms. Fitting kits and instructions are available from Chadwick Optical.[‡‡] These prisms are further discussed in Chapter 7.

Prism for Balance

Often significant homonymous visual field loss may cause a change in the center of gravity of the patient, and a subsequent veering or loss of balance. Yoked prism may be applied in their glasses to realign the perceived world with the patient's visual midline, as described in Chapters 6 and 7. The doctor must weigh safety issues when applying this prism. For instance, it is possible that a patient may be at significant risk for fall due to imbalance, which can be corrected by application of yoked prism with the bases into the sighted field. However, application of this prism correction actually increases the extent of the blind field, creating a different safety issue. If the improvement in fall risk is sufficient to justify such a prism application, the doctor must be certain that the patient is wearing and efficiently using a compensatory peripheral prism system, or is quite adept at scanning into the blind field.

‡‡Chadwick Optical, P. O. Box 485, White River Junction, VT, 05001, 1–800–410–1618, www.chadwickoptical.com

VISUAL-SPATIAL NEGLECT

Many stroke and head injury survivors have difficulty regaining everyday living skills and independence as a result of their inability to be completely aware of their visual surroundings.[41] This phenomenon of visual unawareness is called *visual-spatial inattention*, unilateral spatial inattention, visual hemi-inattention, visual imperception, or visual-spatial neglect. It is a cognitive deficit that refers to the relative lack of awareness that the survivor exhibits to objects, people, or to any visual stimuli presented in the visual space contralateral to the cerebral lesion. Unawareness of the deficit is a central feature of the condition. Visual-spatial neglect has been reported in up to 82% of assessable right hemispere stroke patients and 65% of assessable left hemisphere patients hospitalized for stroke.[1] These high percentages were found using a modified Behavioral Inattention Test,[42] which included pointing to objects around the room, menu reading, cancellation tasks, copying line drawings from the left side of the page, and reading a newspaper article. In contrast, Becker and Karnath,[43] using only a crossout task, found an incidence of visual-spatial neglect in hospitalized stroke patients of approximately 25% of patients with right brain damage and 2% of patients with left brain damage demonstrated visual-spatial neglect. In this latter study, the researchers also tested for visual extinction, and found similar percentages of patients who exhibited visual extinction, but little concurrence with spatial neglect. These results add to the evidence that visual-spatial neglect has multiple etiologies and the results of Becker and Karnath imply that visual extinction occurs with a type of neglect that may not be demonstrated with cancellation tasks. Interestingly, Stone, Halligan, and Greenwood[1] found almost exactly the same incidence of visual extinction in their patient series as did Becker and Karnath.

CHARACTERISTICS OF VISUAL-SPATIAL NEGLECT

Neglect is frequently found in association with hemianopia, hemiparesis, and other perceptual and sensorimotor deficits. Patients believe that they have an appropriate representation of their environment; consequently, problems of denial and decreased awareness of the need to compensate for the deficit occur. Neglect is found to vary in severity from person to person as well as within the same person depending on the nature of the visual stimulus. Typically, left visual-spatial neglect follows right hemisphere injury and is more frequent and longer lasting with more severe effects than right side visual-spatial neglect.[44]

The presence of moderate to severe visual-spatial neglect can disrupt a variety of daily activities such as dressing, eating, reading, writing, walking, returning to work, and driving. Patients with left visual-spatial neglect will typically veer to the left when walking or bump their left shoulder on the doorframe. When reading they will typically skip words on the left side of the page, skip lines or change the beginning of words. They will frequently lose their spatial orientation and get lost in both familiar and unfamiliar environments. When eating they will often leave the food on the left side of the plate untouched, or be unaware of objects or people on their left sides. They may not groom the left side of their face or comb the hair on the left side of their head.

The characteristics of visual-spatial neglect vary widely between patients. Visual-spatial neglect may be categorized by proximity into personal, peripersonal, and extrapersonal neglect,[45] and/or categorized as premotor and perceptual neglect. Further, in perceptual neglect, it may be divided into object neglect, where parts of objects are neglected, or scene neglect where half of the scene is neglected (reviewed by Medina et al.).[46]

Patients with personal neglect may shave only half of the face, or have difficulty dressing due to unawareness of the left arm or leg. Patients with peripersonal neglect will have difficulty with visual-spatial neglect for space within arm's reach. Interestingly, if given a tool that extends their reach, the peripersonal neglect extends to the end of the physical tool, but not the beam of a laser pointer.[47] Patients with extrapersonal neglect may have intact personal and peripersonal awareness, but neglect one hemifield of space beyond arm's reach.

Tegnér and Levander[48] dissociated premotor and perceptual deficits in neglect by having patients perform a line cancellation test while viewing the lines in a mirror, which flipped the view of the lines and hand right to left. This created a situation where 4 of the18 patients cancelled lines only in right hemispace (i.e., directed their attention leftward, but failed to execute movements toward contralateral hemispace) and 10 of 18 patients cancelled lines only in left hemispace, which is consistent with an attention perceptual deficit for left hemispace. Perceptual neglect may be viewer centered, stimulus centered, or object centered (Figure 5.5). The most common form of perceptual neglect is viewer centered, where one half of the patient's view is unattended. Stimulus-centered neglect is relatively less common.

In viewer-centered neglect, the neglect may be centered on the trunk, or head centered[49–50] or have gaze centered aspects. While it has been noted that left neglect patients show improved awareness of leftward stimuli when the eyes are positioned into right gaze,[51] or when the trunk is rotated leftward,[50] these are functionally impracticable positions for someone having difficulty seeing leftward. Therefore, much of the mainstay of neglect treatment is practice and repetition of leftward scanning. Often patients are taught to scan leftward with their heads. However, this strategy is both disorienting and fatiguing, as the vestibular system comes into play with excessive head movement as the head scanning strategy requires. Scanning with the eyes is a more natural situation and may not only compensate but also help to remediate the neglect. If the neglect is head centric, this means that the edge of the neglected hemifield is determined by where the nose is pointed.

Frequently, visual-spatial neglect also has an altitudinal component such that there are more stimuli missed on crossout tasks in the bottom half of the page (more proximal to the patient).[52]

NEURAL SUBSTRATES OF VISUAL-SPATIAL NEGLECT

Visual-spatial neglect, unlike visual field loss, results from damage to multiple neural substrates outside of the primary visual pathway. This is also probably the reason that the characteristics of the visual-spatial neglect vary so widely. Neural substrates

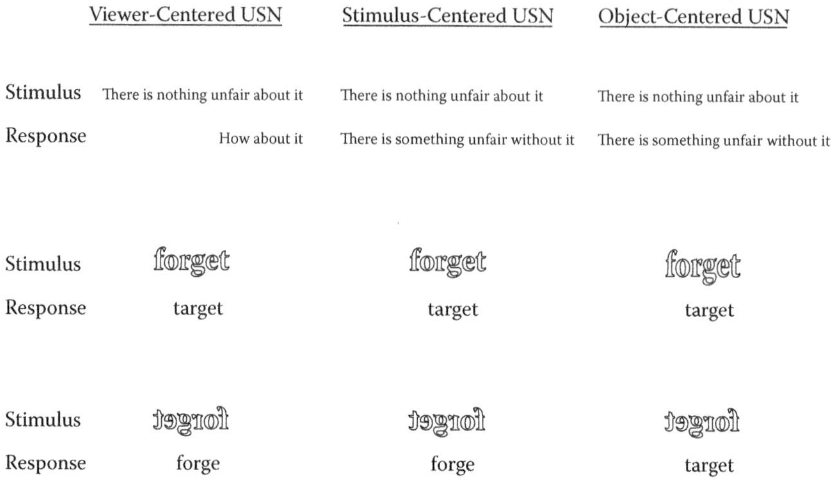

	Viewer-Centered USN	Stimulus-Centered USN	Object-Centered USN
Stimulus	There is nothing unfair about it	There is nothing unfair about it	There is nothing unfair about it
Response	How about it	There is something unfair without it	There is something unfair without it
Stimulus	forget	forget	forget
Response	target	target	target
Stimulus	forget (mirror-reversed)	forget (mirror-reversed)	forget (mirror-reversed)
Response	forge	forge	target

FIGURE 5.5 Examples of errors reading sentences, words in standard print, and words in mirror-reversed print, with different patterns of errors that reflect distinct forms of unilateral spatial neglect (USN). Note that patients with all forms of neglect make errors on the contralesional side of single words in standard print. Viewer-centered USN and stimulus-centered USN can be distinguished by performance in reading sentences, with omission of words on the contralesional side of the sentence in viewer-centered USN versus errors on the contralesional side of individual words, throughout the sentence, in stimulus-centered USN. Stimulus-centered USN and object-centered USN can be distinguished by reading mirror-reversed words, with errors on the contralesional side of the printed stimulus (the final letters) in stimulus-centered USN versus errors on the contralesional sides of the canonical presentation of words (the initial letters), in object-centered USN. (From Hillis, A. E., Neurobiology of unilateral spatial neglect. *Neuroscientist*, 12, 2, 155, 2006. Reprinted with permission.)

for attention are widespread, with differing functions that can be categorized into a subcortical arousal and alerting network, a mixed cortical-subcortical orienting network, and a cortical selective attention network (see Table 5.1). Mesulam,[53] in 1981, wrote a review of the neural substrates of neglect, and concluded that four cerebral regions provided an integrated network for the modulation of extrapersonal directed attention. These four substrates included the posterior parietal area that provides an internal sensory map, the limbic (cingulate gyrus) that regulates spatial distribution of motivational valence, the frontal areas that coordinate motor programming for exploration and reaching, and a reticular component that determines arousal level. In large part this framework still stands, but with additional areas implicated as research accumulates.

Parietal Lobe

The most common location for the lesion causing left spatial inattention is thought to be the right parietal lobe.[54] In most patients, corresponding lesion to the left parietal lobe causes mild or transient visual-spatial neglect of the right space. It has been hypothesized that the right hemisphere modulates attention to both hemifields, where the left hemisphere modulates attention mainly to the right hemifield

TABLE 5.1
Functional Anatomy of the Attentional Networks

Network and Anatomical System	Function
Arousal and Alerting Network (Subcortical)	
Ceruleocortical noradrenergic	Arousal, alerting, selective attention
Mesolimbic and mesostriatal dopaminergic	Behavioral activation and motivation, stimulus salience
Basal forebrain cholinergic	Memory and attention
Nonspecific thalamic glutaminergic	Cortical activation, synchronization
Orienting Network (Mixed Coritical-Subcortical)	
Superior colliculus	Detecting novel stimuli, computing target location for attentional shifts, hyperreflexive orienting to ipsilesional field
Pulvinar	Restricts input to selected sensory region, filters irrelevant stimuli, assists in covert orienting, facilitates responses to a cued target
Posterior parietal cortex	Disengages attention from present focus
Selective Attentional Network (Cortical)	
Posterior parietal cortex	Disengages attention from present focus
Right	Greatest effect: mostly disengaging from locations
Left	Least effect: mostly disengaging from objects
Superior parietal lobule	Voluntary shifts of attention
Frontal eye fields	Generates volitional saccades
Premotor cortex	Motor intention
Dorsolateral frontal cortex	Working memory, self-monitoring
Anterior cingulate cortex	Motivation, exploratory behavior, attention to action

Source: From Devinsky, O., and D'Esposito, M., *Neurology of Cognitive and Behavioral Disorders*, Oxford University Press, New York, 2004, p. 105. By permission of Oxford University Press, Inc.

only.[53] Thus, damage to the left parietal lobe may cause an imbalance in allocation of attention from the preinjury state, but damage to the right parietal lobe, common in middle cerebral artery infarct or aneurysm, causes marked visual-spatial neglect, as this is the major cortical substrate for orienting and allocating selective attention to the left hemifield. In very young children, this hemispheric dominance for spatial attention is not yet fully developed as evidenced by line-bisection tasks at ages 4–5 years. Children show adult-like line bisection with a slight leftward bias in bisection by 7–8 years of age (reviewed by Smith and Chatterjee).[55]

Temporal Lobe

In the last decade, a number of anatomical studies have found the center of lesion overlap to be in the right superior temporal cortex and insula. These studies specifically did not use line bisection to select patients. In their follow-up study, Rorden et al.[56] found that patients who committed line-bisection errors common to neglect more often had damage between the middle occipital and middle temporal gyrus. This is consistent with the findings of Binder et al.[57] who found that patients who performed poorly on line bisection tended to have more posterior lesions, as compared to patients who performed poorly on crossout tasks.

Frontal Lobe

Frontal lobe has been implicated in visual-spatial neglect, both lateral aspects of the frontal lobe and the medial, cingulate gyrus (reviewed by Husain and Kennard).[58] Hussain and Kennard also found, analyzing brain imaging from five patients with focal infarcts of the right frontal lobe and associated visual-spatial neglect, that the common area of lesion overlap was part of the homologue of Broca's area in the right hemisphere, which is considered part of premotor cortex in the human. These patients demonstrated no extinction phenomenon.

Parietofrontal White Matter Tracts

Within each hemisphere there are long-range white matter tracts carrying information to distant processing areas (for details, see Chapter 3). Bartolomeo[59] discusses two patients undergoing electrical stimulation to map functional areas during brain surgery, where inactivation of the second branch of the superior longitudinal fasciculus caused maximal rightward deviation in line bisection. He and others[60] discuss the parietofrontal network for spatial awareness, rather than thinking of the areas as discrete areas causing spatial neglect.

Subcortical

The putamen and caudate nucleus of the basal ganglia, as well as the pulvinar of the thalamus, have been implicated in neglect.[61] All three are directly connected to the superior temporal gyrus, which is also implicated in neglect. Sapir et al.[62] found that directional hypokinesia (i.e., delay in initiating a motor response such as reaching into the neglected hemifield with the "unaffected arm"), in neglect, was correlated with lesions involving the ventral lateral putamen, the claustrum, and the white matter underneath the frontal lobe. None of their patients without directional hypokinesia had a lesion in the same region. They suggest that the association of hypokinesia with basal ganglia lesions may implicate unilateral dopamine depletion as an important factor in neglect with motor involvement.

Dopaminergic

Spatial attention is mediated in part by dopaminergic pathways. Further, in healthy children, dopaminergic genotype has been found to bias spatial attention, with some genotypes exhibiting slower orienting to the left hemispace in children of ages 9–16.[63] Unfortunately, drug trials to increase dopamine levels have met with mixed results. For example, trials with amantadine to increase dopamine levels in patients with neglect demonstrated few positive and almost equal negative results on measurements of neglect in these patients.[64]

DIFFERENTIATING VISUAL-SPATIAL NEGLECT FROM HOMONYMOUS HEMIANOPIA

It is important to differentiate whether patients have only a visual field loss, or field loss and visual-spatial neglect, or only visual-spatial neglect. The differentiation dictates the type of intervention and treatment approaches that will be recommended. There are many tests that can be applied in the clinic. It appears from the literature, that behavioral observation, crossout tasks, line bisection, visual field, and copying tasks each contribute to diagnosis in different patients with different variations of visual-spatial neglect.[65]

The presence of visual-spatial neglect can be determined by using the following tests and questions:

a. Extinction: Present a hand in the patient's right visual field and he will see it. Present it in the left visual field and the patient will see it in the absence of a field defect. Present your hands simultaneously in the right and left field and the patient will often times not be aware of the left side hand. This process of left stimulus suppression with bilateral simultaneous presentation is called "extinction." This examination can be refined for patients with moderate rather than dense neglect, by performing a finger count double simultaneous confrontation. In this modification the examiner holds up both hands in two of the four visual quadrants, and flashes one or two fingers on each hand. In moderate neglect, the patient will be able to see both hands, and when fingers are presented one side at a time, they will be able to accurately finger count in all quadrants. However, extinction will be present when flashing fingers on both hands simultaneously so that they only count the ones in the unaffected field.

b. Number cross: The numbered cross has the center of the cross as zero with numbers extending to the left and right at regular intervals to 28. The card is held vertically and centered 10 inches in front of the patient (Figure 5.6).

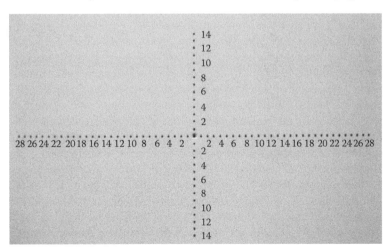

FIGURE 5.6   Number cross test for visual-spatial neglect.

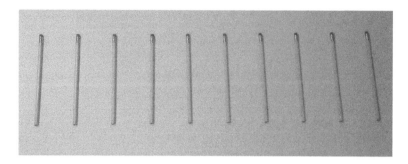

FIGURE 5.7 (See color insert following page 270.) Pencil layout test for visual-spatial neglect.

The patient is then asked to tell the evaluator which number is the farthest to the left on the card, as well as which number is the farthest to the right of the card. Neither the patient's eye movement nor head posture should be restricted as this is not a field test. Typically patients with left visual-spatial neglect will see a number less than 28 on the left, but will identify 28 as the number farthermost to the right on the scale.

  c. Pencil layout: The patient should be centered in front of a rectangular table. Space ten identical pencils evenly, and parallel to each other, in front of the patient. The pencils should be spaced so that the arrangement runs across his midline. Ask the patient to count the pencils. Typically patients with left visual-spatial neglect will miss pencils to the left side of their midline (Figure 5.7).

  d. Line crossout test[66]: On a plain sheet of paper draw generally horizontal lines of various lengths. These lines should be at different positions to the right and left of the center of the page. The patient's attention is drawn to the limits of the array of lines, and then the patient is instructed to work from the top of the page to the bottom of the page and to cross out each of the lines. The patient with moderate to severe left visual-spatial neglect will typically miss crossing the lines on the left side of the page.

  e. Line-bisection crossout task[67]: This task was developed because of the growing literature demonstrating dissociation between performance on line-bisection and crossout tasks in visual-spatial neglect.[56] On a legal size sheet of paper oriented horizontally, draw horizontal, and vertical lines. The paper is taped on the table in front of the patient, centered on the patient's midline. The patient is discouraged from leaning to the side during the task and is instructed to bisect each of the lines in front of them. Lines greater than 5 cm long at a working distance of 40 cm are diagnostic for bisection purposes. The patient with neglect will act as if they fail to perceive the neglected end of the line, and so will bisect the line away from the neglected side. In contrast, the patient with hemianopic visual field defect will most often bisect the line in the opposite direction, toward the defect. Indeed, Kerkhoff and Bucher,[68] have suggested that line bisection is an early method to assess homonymous hemianopia. The patient with both visual neglect and hemianopia will tend to bisect lines accurately.[30] Therefore, the line-bisection test must be combined with visual field testing to correctly interpret the bisection (Figures 5.8A and 5.8B). Patients with overtly more severe neglect will, as in the Albert line crossout test above, miss crossing out lines on one side of the paper or in the lower, or closer, quadrant to the patient. Sometimes, one will see a line-bisection result that implies neglect, but no functional evidence of neglect can be elicited.

In the literature, an off center line bisection has often been interpreted as evidence of neglect. However, it more likely demonstrates a distortion or bias in spatial perception or, perhaps directional inequalities in saccadic efficiency. Indeed, in the normal population, there is a slight bias to cross the line leftward of center and vertical lines slightly above center by about 2% of the length of the line, especially in left-handed subjects or when using the left hand, so one should "eyeball" the result, or take this into account when measuring. Importantly for interpretation, Nielsen et al.[69] also found that bisection is biased toward the central visual field when gaze was fixed so that the bisected line is seen only in one hemifield, including upper or lower. Sometimes on this task, one will see the bisections all biased toward the center of the page.

   f. Letter cancellation: Have the patient search and color all the e's in a paragraph of nonsense words. The patient with left visual-spatial neglect will typically miss a greater than average number of e's, especially on the left side of the page. Different colored pencils may be used at timed intervals to demonstrate the patient's strategy in crossing the e's.
   g. Hart chart: Place a chart containing 100 letters (10 across and 10 down) across the room and have the patient call out the letters. Typically the patient with left neglect will miss letters on the left side of the chart. These patients will also skip letters on the left side of the standard acuity chart when visual acuity is being measured.
   h. Picture scanning: Present a wide-angle detailed picture within 14 inches of the patient in the vertical meridian and ask him to describe objects in the picture. The patient with left neglect will typically ignore detail on the left side of the picture.
   i. Picture drawing: Have the patient draw a picture of a clock or a petalled flower. Typically the clock numbers will be crammed onto the right side of a distorted clock face or the flower will have poor detail on the left side, with petals missing on the left side only.
   j. Visual-spatial midline[70]: Stand first to the patient's right side and present a vertical pencil at eye level, about 16 inches from the patient. Move the pencil laterally in front of the patient, first moving from the patient's right to left side, and then from the left to right side. The patient should be instructed to stop the evaluator when the pencil appears to be in the middle of the patient's nose—straight ahead. The patient should be allowed to move his eyes in an unrestricted manner, but his head should be positioned straight ahead. There should not be any background objects in view ahead

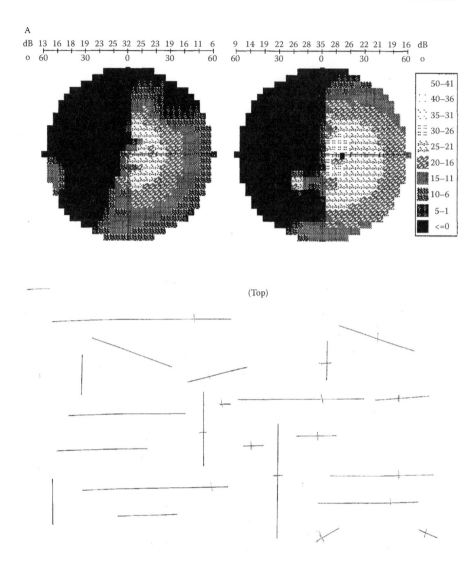

A

(Top)

FIGURE 5.8   A: The line-bisection crossout task must be interpreted in light of the visual fields. In neglect, you may see two patterns that indicate two different aspects of neglect; failure to cross out lines on the neglected side of the page, or bisecting the longer lines markedly off center away from the neglected field. These may appear separately, or in conjunction.

of the patient that might influence his subjective judgment of straight ahead. When the patient stops the examiner at the perceived straight-ahead position, the examiner must move his head around to align in front of the patient—without changing the spatial location of the pencil—to eliminate parallax from the clinician's observation of where the patient judged

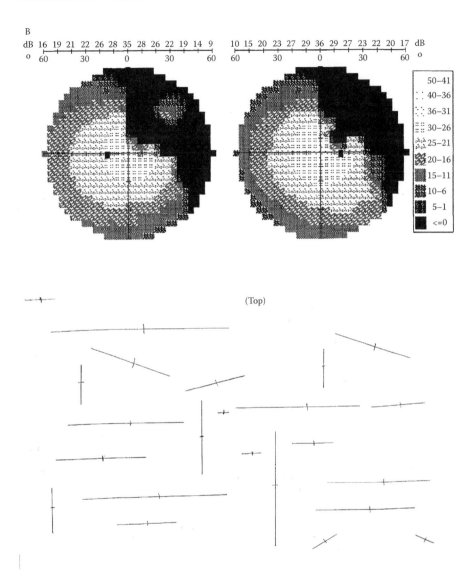

FIGURE 5.8 B: In visual field loss, the lines are bisected toward the affected field. This patient actually also demonstrated an interesting neglect in terms of lack of perceptual awareness of his defect, even following education; however, he showed no other aspects of neglect, was cognitively aware of his field loss, and returned to work and driving.

straight ahead to be. Repeat the test by standing on the patient's left side. The patient with left side visual-spatial neglect will typically respond as if the pencil is centered when it is actually in front of the right eye. The response is usually recorded on a schematic drawing of the face. The test is often repeated holding the pencil laterally and moving it from above and below, having the patient stop the examiner when the pencil is directly in front of the patient's eyes, to test for vertical abnormalities of perceived visual-spatial midline.

k. Observation: An essential part of the evaluation of visual-spatial neglect is observing the patient ambulate through space. Instruct the patient to walk down a hallway and through a doorway staying in the center as much as possible. Observe him walking between furniture obstacles placed close together. Instruct him to walk both forward and backward in that order. Typically, he will be seen veering to the left, often bumping his left shoulder on the doorframe.

l. Distant line bisection using a light pointer can be used to determine the presence of extrapersonal neglect.

m. There are standardized test batteries designed to define the side, severity, and specificity of the visual-spatial neglect such as the Behavioral Inattention Test[42] and the Visual Object and Space Perception Battery.[71] Lindell et al.,[72] in attempting to evaluate various measures of neglect, found that the Behavioral Inattention Test did not diagnose 7 of 24 cases of neglect that were demonstrated by the 11 visual neglect tasks used in their study. Of the tests Lindell et al. used, Random Shape cancellation, Complex Line bisection, and Star cancellation together detected 88% of the neglect cases. To catch all of their neglect cases, Two-part picture, Article reading, and Object finding had to be added.

Patients with left side visual-spatial neglect appear to have a visual-spatial midline shift so that they behave as if their visual midline (visual reference) is at a point to the right of true midline. This results in a reduced awareness of left side visual space. The reduced awareness of the left side of surrounding space is actually referenced against an internal (mental) construct of space rather than against an external geographical location. This can be seen by the affect of the nature of the stimulus presented as well as the affect of cueing on the severity of the neglect response.

INTERVENTION FOR VISUAL-SPATIAL NEGLECT

Numerous studies have demonstrated improvement in visual-spatial neglect related to rehabilitation.[73–78]

Therapy for visual-spatial neglect is divided into activities that address static predictive situations versus nonpredictive dynamic situations.

Compensatory Interventions for Static Presentations

For visual activities that have predictive margins and a static presentation, such as reading, the following compensatory and rehabilitative interventions are recommended:

a. Place a red Velcro strip as a left margin on each page. Encourage the patient to rub one of his left fingers against the velcro. The red strip acts as a visual cue to remind the patient to make a complete left refixation to the beginning of the next line. The Velcro rubbing against a left hand finger serves through proprioception to increase attention to the left visual space.

b. Turn the page 90 degrees to allow the patient to avoid reading left to right across his midline.
c. Have the patient make a pen trail below the sentence that he is reading. This permanent trail assists him in differentiating that which has been read versus that which has not been read.
d. The use of a brightly colored T square can be used. The brightly colored vertical arm serves as the left margin. The horizontal arm is moved down each sentence as it is completed to increase the likelihood of starting the scan at the beginning of each sentence and to avoid skipping any lines.
e. Number sentences on the left margin to serve as a left side guide. This numbering will also help the patient keep track of what he has to read.

Rehabilitation Activities for Static Presentations
a. Tracking the printed words from a book on tape.
b. Calling out the first and last letter of each word on a page of print. Begin the exercise with large print progressing to standard size print as performance allows.
c. Calling out the first and last letter of each line going from large to standard size print.
d. Coloring in specified letters of a word using a pencil. For example, instruct the patient to color in all the "o's" on a page.
e. Finding/counting specified words in paragraphs.
f. Scanning to locate or matching cards from a widely spaced arrangement.

General Mobility and Orientation Strategies
These strategies involve either direct or indirect methods of directing visual attention toward the neglected visual space. The development of full field scanning approaches, visual-spatial judgments, body image in space awareness, laterality and bilaterality concepts are all necessary.

The most classic compensatory technique for left visual-spatial neglect involves encouraging the patient to turn his head toward the left side and to look to the left. As visual-spatial neglect is frequently head centric, learning to turn the head into the neglected field simply imbeds the neglect, as the eyes never cross into the neglected field. A further problem with this technique is that it relies on the patient's ability to understand the magnitude of the leftward eye scan or head turn required to cover left visual space completely. Typically, patients with left visual-spatial neglect have a misconception of left visual space.

A novel technique, the "Margolis Eye Throwing Technique"[79,80] relies on proprioceptive and kinesthetic (as apposed to visual) cueing, to ensure complete scanning of the environment. Patients are first taught to close their lids and to move their eyes as far to the left as they can. This encourages them to rely on nonvisual cues for the eye movement. Once they have moved their eyes to the farthest point that the extra ocular muscles will allow, they are asked to open their eyes. They should then be able to describe objects to their far left. If they do not turn their eyes to the extreme leftward position then tactile reinforcement such as tapping next to the left eye on the temple and verbal coaching are helpful. Typically no sclera should be visible temporal to the iris in the left eye if the patient has turned his eyes far enough to the left. The next step in learning this method is to teach them to "throw their eyes to the left," as far as they can, and then to "scan to the right." The author has found this technique to be effective for a number of reasons: The fact that the patient is not relying on a visual cue to understand how far to the left to look but is relying on a proprioceptive cue results in more consistent and complete scans. The patient is scanning from an extreme leftward position that represents the farthest position for any person to begin a scan. Patients with left visual neglect generally make complete rightward scans, but tend to make incomplete leftward scans.[81] Typically the further the patient looks into the neglect space side the less accurate and complete the scans become. Therefore, the fact that the patient is making a rightward scan from an extreme left starting position increases the likelihood of a more complete awareness of the surrounding visual environment. The "motor" act of throwing the eyes to the left side also serves as a left side arousal mechanism. The visual attention "spotlight" follows the visual axis so that as the eyes are first pointed to extreme left, the "spotlight" of visual attention is directed to this visual field and then follows the eye movements from the left to the right side. The slogan for practicing the technique becomes "throw your eyes to the left, scan to the right." The patient is encouraged to practice the technique until it becomes habitual. Family members are encouraged to remind the patient to carry out the technique in all settings. The author has also used a vibrating pager that is placed against the patient's skin on the left side of their waist to reinforce "throwing" their eyes to the left. The pager is set to oscillate every 10–15 seconds and is worn for a prescribed number of hours every day. The oscillation of the pager should trigger an eye throwing response. Over time the pager is removed and continued habitual eye throwing is the goal.

Body image awareness, a prerequisite for general mobility and orientation, needs to be rehabilitated in these patients. The following are examples of activities that develop body image awareness:

a. The patient is instructed to respond to individual limb tapping. He is told to move the limb that is tapped, in an outward direction from the body and then back to the starting position. Once this has been accomplished he is then required to respond when limbs on the same side of midline (right or left) are tapped simultaneously. The next challenging level of this therapy is when the patient is required to respond when limbs across the midline (such as left arm and right leg) are tapped. Once the patient has successfully completed these exercises, he can be further challenged by requiring him to respond to a lighter tap and eventually responding to the therapist' pointing to a limb or limbs while expecting a shorter response time. Depending on the patient's physical capability, even limited movement may be accepted as an awareness of the response requested. This activity is frequently referred to as "Angels in the Snow."

b. The patient is to stand behind another person who is of similar height and build. The patient is then touched on his back. Initially only extreme points such as shoulder edges and the middle of the neck are touched. Then more random points between these points are touched. The patient should project his appreciation of these points by touching the corresponding points on the person who is standing in front of him. The author refers to this activity as "Mannequin Projections."

c. In a slightly dimmed room, have the patient stand in front of an overhead projector so that a shadow of his body image is cast on the wall. Place a mark on his shadow in the middle of his projected neck. The patient is instructed to walk toward the wall while constantly maintaining the position of the wall mark in the middle of his neck shadow. This requires progressively greater accuracy as his shadow becomes progressively smaller as he gets closer to the wall. The patient gets immediate feedback via his shadow as to his body position relative to the wall mark.

d. A variation on the above approach is to place black tape vertically and centered down the front side of the patient's body. Another piece of black tape is placed vertically down the center of a full-length mirror at the end of a hallway. The patient is required to walk toward the mirror, keeping his body tape in line with the vertical black strip on the mirror.

e. Instruct the patient to bunt a balloon with the limb it is thrown against. The balloon should be thrown at right arm, left leg, right shoulder, chest, and so on.

f. Body image can be further improved by having the patient walk forward and backward down the center of a corridor, through the center of doorways and between obstacles without touching them.

g. The patient should practice picking up dowel rods of varying sizes at the perceived midpoint of each rod. Depending on the tilt of the rod the patient is holding, he will gain feedback as to where the true midpoint is.

The following activities are examples of therapies designed to improve orientation and scanning in physical space:

a. Every patient should have at least a 2-week trial of prism adaptation, as it has been shown to have rapid and long-lasting effects on aspects of visual-spatial neglect.[82–84] Yoked prism with the base directed to the left or right (depending on the affected side) is used during therapy to alter the perception of space. Large amounts of yoked prism (approximately 20 prism diopters) are applied over the patient's habitual glasses with the bases directed into the neglected space. Then the patient performs a ballistic pointing motion toward one of at least two targets placed on the table in front of them either on the right or the left, always returning the hand to a center position between pointing. When prism adaptation is complete, the pointing will be accurate without corrections during the movement. The movement should be alternated toward rightward and leftward targets.

b. The patient should be instructed to stand at the entrance of a doorway and to identify the margins, such as the perimeter walls and furniture obstacles in the room. The patient should then practice going to places in the room with his eyes closed, using memory and visualization to navigate. The ultimate goal is for the patient to be able to use a combination of memory, sight, visualization, spatial orientation skill, and visual closure to allow him to accurately navigate through the room.

c. Another approach the author has developed and used successfully is to establish colors that are used as scan indicators. The color green is usually placed in the right field using colored tape or any green object. This colored object serves as the trigger that indicates to the patient that he should begin his scan to the left. The leftward scan is only completed once he can see the red marker, which signals him to stop. The red marker, which can also be colored tape or any red object, is placed on the left side. This trigger and extinguisher set may be used to define the scan required for a search, for example, scanning the width of a drawer, a cupboard, or a place setting at the table.

d. Place objects that create visual clutter on the left side of the patients' visual space and leave the right side of the space uncluttered. This serves to help bias visual attention to the left side.

e. Have the patient walk down a hallway with pictures on the right side. Have the patient note the location of these pictures. Have the patient locate them again on the return walk when they are on the left side.

f. Computerized visual search activities on wide diameter electronic boards such as Acuvision,[§§] Vision Coach,[***] Wayne saccadic fixator,[†††] or Dynavision,[‡‡‡] as well as computer games that provide surprise stimuli across the screen are good activities. It is important that the speed of the presentation and the level of challenge can be modified.

g. Place a vertical row of letters on either side of the doorframe. The patient should be encouraged to call out the letters top to bottom going left to right as he walks slowly toward the door.

h. Another activity that the author has developed to improve spatial relations in physical space is called "Hollywood Squares." Draw two squares, each 2 feet by 2 feet, and side by side on the floor. The therapist chooses a position in the first square. The patient has to stand in the corresponding position and direction in his square to that of the therapist. The next level on this activity is for the therapist to replace his square on the floor with a square drawn on a piece of paper. The therapist marks a position in the form of a directional arrow on the paper square. This arrow indicates to the patient the position and direction he should adopt in his square on the floor.

i. Draw a floor plan outline of the room in which the therapist and the patient are located. Draw landmarks on the outline such as a door or window. Ask the patient to indicate the position of the other objects in the room relative to the landmarks. The next level of this activity involves the patient locating objects

---

[§§] Acuvision: no longer commercially available.
[***] Vision Coach: available from info@visioncoachtrainer.com, Perceptual Testing, Inc., 6380 Rancho Park Drive, San Diego, CA, 92120.
[†††] Wayne saccadic fixator available from www.bernell.com, Bernell Corporation, 4016 N. Home Street, Mishawaka, IN, 46545.
[‡‡‡] Dynavision available from www.dynavision2000.com, 76 Major Buttons Drive, Markham, Ontario, Canada, L3P3G7.

in the floor plan outline of a familiar room, even though he may not be in the room

j. Encourage the patient to relate concrete positions in their physical surroundings to representative space on map drawings of the same area.

k. Arrange for the patient to hang a tennis ball loosely by a string from his shirt button. Have the patient walk forward with his feet on either side of a line guide. Allow the hanging ball to act as a plumb bob, deviating as the patient shifts his center of balance. The patient has to keep his weight balanced equally on his right and left side to keep the ball hanging in a centered position and dragging on the line. This helps reinforce midline awareness and bilaterality.

CASE EXAMPLE

A 65-year-old female, 8 months poststroke (right posterior parietal lesion) was referred for a vision consultation by a physiatrist.

Case history included complaints of bumping into objects on the left side, incomplete reading of sentences, and constantly losing personal items. Her daughter also described problems such as veering to the left as she walked, and sometimes leaving food on the left side of her plate.

Visual field testing: visual field analysis using automated perimetry revealed left homonymous hemianopia with macula splitting.

Neglect testing: line-bisection testing: she bisected 20% of the lines significantly to the right of center.

Visual midline projection: she projected her visual midline from the front of her right eye, rather than from the center of her nose.

Letter cancellation: she missed 30% of the letters that she was asked to mark.

On the 28 number cross: she reported that the scale extended 16 to the left and 24 to the right.

Wide layout pencil scan: she started her scan from about the middle of the row and only counted five of the total eight pencils.

Dynamic: she was observed to veer to the left when walking and was unable to center herself consistently in the passage or doorway. Testing, case history, and observation indicated hemianopic field loss and functional neglect.

Goals were established:

To develop her ability to orient herself accurately with respect to her surroundings
To develop her ability to walk without bumping into objects
To develop her ability to find the items she used everyday independently
To develop her ability to read fluently

Intervention was initiated with activities designed to improve body image awareness and visual-spatial orientation skills. Angels in the snow, mannequin projections, central passage, and obstacle course walking were practiced in the office and at home. As responses became more consistent, therapy was expanded to Acuvision search, balloon bunting, interactive computer programs that required searching for nonpredictive stimuli, and doorjamb saccades. She was also taught the color trigger method for scanning her closet, and was given a left side red margin for reading. The Margolis eye throwing technique was taught as follows: she was seated in the middle of a rectangular table with a therapist opposite her. She was instructed to close her eyes and to look as far to the left as possible, still with her lids closed. She was then asked to open her eyes and report what she saw. She responded by describing a picture that was to the far left of her body. She was then asked to throw her eyes to the left as far as they would go, now with them open, and then to scan to the right. Immediately on following this instruction, she accurately counted all the pencils laid out in front of her, in sequence from left to right. She was encouraged to practice this initially while sitting, then while standing, and eventually while walking. She was asked to practice the technique in her home setting, and was to wear the vibrating pager for several hours a day. In addition to learning the eye throwing technique, bright orange fluorescent strips were placed on the corners of the walls or furniture into which she frequently bumped. To assist her with finding items that she routinely used, I recommended that all toiletries and kitchen utensils be placed in the same designated place. After 8 weeks of the body image and general orientation training, the activities more appropriate for reading improvement were introduced. These included the red Velcro, T square, letter and word find, trail reading, and tape recorder reading. Worksheets were given for completion at home. To help her memorize where an object was, she was instructed to close her eyes and to visualize the object relative to its surroundings. She had great difficulty remembering and localizing the position of an object relative to her current position. We drew maps of her house and the office so that she could practice indicating her position on the map as she moved around. She was given visualization exercise to practice at home, using verbalization to generate visual images.

The patient was in a vision rehabilitation program, which included both office and home-based activities for about 10 months. She reached a point in her rehabilitation program that she could be left safely alone in her house during the day, and was also able to carry out primary ADLs in the house. She was able to read her mail accurately and independently without cueing. She still needed some support when in faster moving, busy environments such as in the supermarket.

SUMMARY

While visual field loss presents in a number of ways, a visual field loss is a relatively orderly deficit, as compared to visual-spatial neglect. Patients with visual field loss learn much more quickly where their blind areas are, and frequently are relatively quick at learning to compensate, once given the required skills, strategies, and tools, although in application of peripheral prism, for instance, there is a considerable amount of training and practice required. Visual field loss should prompt the rehabilitation team to think about the possibility of visual acuity loss, contrast sensitivity deficits, diplopia, perceptual speed, scanning, organization, and safety issues.

Visual-spatial neglect is more heterogenous and multidimensional than visual field loss, and brings a whole host of new concerns regarding safety and ability to carry out ADLs. Visual-spatial neglect is quite common following stroke and TBI. It is common for patients with visual-spatial neglect, without associated motor deficits, to leave the hospital undiagnosed and untreated. They may be misdiagnosed as having dementia, as family and caretakers are unable to understand why a person might end up with their pants on backward (when they put them on, they only acknowledged one leg, so there was no frontward or backward choice), or why they forget to finish a task or put away tools. It is not always as easy as noticing that they do not finish the food on one side of their plate. Patients with visual-spatial neglect are frequently misdiagnosed as having visual field deficits by vision care practitioners who are unaware of the possible diagnosis of visual-spatial neglect. Given the high incidence of visual-spatial neglect following stroke, every patient suffering CVA should be examined by an eye doctor with special expertise in post-brain injury rehabilitation. Appropriate diagnosis and treatment of visual-spatial neglect can make an enormous difference in the safety and quality of life for patients and the families who care for them.

REFERENCES

1. Stone, S. P., Halligan, P. W., & Greenwood, R. J. (1993). The incidence of neglect phenomena and related disorders in patients with an acute right or left hemisphere stroke. *Age and Ageing, 22*(1), 46–52.
2. Doricchi, F., Onida, A., & Guariglia, P. (2002). Horizontal space misrepresentation in unilateral brain damage. II. Eye-head centered modulation of visual misrepresentation in hemianopia without neglect. *Neuropsychologia, 40*(8), 1118–1128.
3. Rondot P., Odier F., & Valade, D. (1992). Postural disturbances due to homonymous hemianopic visual ataxia. *Brain, 115*(Pt. 1), 179–188.
4. Romano, P. E. (2003). A case of acute loss of binocular vision and stereoscopic depth perception. (The misery of acute monovision, having been binocular for 68 years). *Binocular Vision & Strabismus Quarterly, 18*(2), 101–103.
5. Zhang, X., Kedar, S., Lynn, M. J., Newman, N. J., & Biousse, V. (2006a). Natural history of homonymous hemianopia. *Neurology, 66*(6), 901–905.
6. Leo, F., Bolognini, N., Passamonti, C., Stein, B. E., & Ládavas, E. (2008). Cross-modal localization in hemianopia; new insights on multisensory integration. *Brain, 131*(Pt. 3), 855–865.
7. Paramei, G. V., & Sabel, B. A. (2008). Contour-integration deficits on the intact side of the visual field in hemianopia patients. *Behavioral Brain Research, 188*(1), 109–124.
8. Suchoff, I.B., Kapoor, N., Ciuffreda, K., Rutner, D., Han, E., & Craig, S. (2008). The frequency of occurrence, types and characteristics of visual field defects in acquired brain injury: a retrospective analysis. *Optometry, 79*(5), 259–265.
9. Townend, B. S., Sturm, J. W., Petsoglou, C., O'Leary, B., Whyte, S., & Crimmins, D. (2007). Perimetric homonymous visual field loss post-stroke. *Journal of Clinical Neuroscience, 14*(8), 754–756.
10. Schwab, K., Grafman, J., Salazar, A. M., & Kraft, J., (1993). Residual impairments and work status 15 years after penetrating head injury: Report from the Vietnam head injury study. *Neurology, 43*(1), 95–103.
11. Uzzell, B. P., Dolinskas, C. A., & Langfitt, T. W. (1988). Visual field defects in relation to head injury severity; a neuropsychological study. *Archives of Neurology, 45*(4), 420–424.
12. Wood, J. M., McGwin, G. Jr., Elgin, J., Vaphiades, M. S., Braswell, R. A., DeCarlo, D. K., Kline, L. B., Meek, G. C., Searcey, K., & Owsley, C. (2009). On-road driving performance by persons with hemianopia and quadrantanopia. *Investigative Ophthalmology and Visual Science, 50*(2), 577–585.

13. Racette, L., & Casson, E. J. (2005). The impact of visual field loss on driving performance: evidence from on-road driving assessments. *Optometry and Vision Science, 82*(8), 668–674.

14. Zhang, X., Kedar, S., Lynn, M. J., Newman, N. J., & Biousse, V. (2006b). Homonymous hemianopias; clinical-anatomic correlations in 904 cases. *Neurology, 66*(6), 906–910.

15. Shahinfar, S., Johnson, L. N., & Madsen, R. W. (1995). Confrontation visual field loss as a function of decibel sensitivity loss on automated static perimetry. Implications on the accuracy of confrontation visual field testing. *Ophthalmology, 102*(6), 872–877.

16. Johnson, L. H., & Baloh, F. G. (1991). The accuracy of confrontation visual field test in comparison with automated perimetry. *Journal of the National Medical Association, 83*(10), 895–898.

17. Fong, K. C., Byles, D. B., & Constable, P. H. (2003). Does frequency doubling technology perimetry reliably detect neurological visual field defects? *Eye, 17*(3), 330–333.

18. Wall, M., Neahring, R. K., & Woodward, K. R. (2002). Sensitivity and specificity of frequency doubling perimetry in neuro-ophthalmic disorders: a comparison with conventional automated perimetry. *Investigative Ophthalmology and Visual Science, 43*(4), 1277–1283.

19. Giunutsos, R., & Suchoff, I. B. (2001). An expanded visual field assessment for brain-injured patients. In I. B. Suchoff, J. K. Cuiffreda, & N. Kapoor (Eds.), *Visual and vestibular consequences of acquired brain injury* (pp. 114–130). Santa Ana, CA: OEP Foundation.

20. Silverstone, B., Lang, M. A., Rosenthal, B., & Faye, E. E., (2000). *The lighthouse handbook on vision impairment and vision rehabilitation.* New York: Oxford University Press.

21. Weiskrantz, L. (1986). *Blindsight; A case study and implications.* Oxford: Oxford University Press.

22. Danckert, J., & Rossetti, Y. (2005). Blindsight in action: what can the different sub-types of blindsight tell us about the control of visually guided actions? *Neuroscience and Biobehavioral Reviews, 29*(7), 1035–1046.

23. Leh, S. E., Johansen-Berg, H., & Ptito, A. (2006). Unconscious vision: new insights into the neuronal correlate of blindsight using diffusion tractography. *Brain, 129*(Pt. 7), 1822–1832.

24. Huxlin, K. R., Martin, T., Kelly, K., Riley, M., Friedman, D. I., Burgin, W. S., & Hayhoe, M. (2009). Perceptual relearning of complex visual motion after V1 damage in humans. *Journal of Neuroscience, 29*(13), 3981–3991.

25. Chokron, S., Perez, C., Obadia, M., Gaudry, I., Laloum, L., & Gout, O. (2008). From blindsight to sight: cognitive rehabilitation of visual field defects. *Restorative Neurology and Neuroscience, 26*(4–5), 305–320.

26. Boyle, N. J., Jones, D. H., Hamilton, R., Spowart, K. M., & Dutton, G. N. (2005). Blindsight in children: does it exist and can it be used to help the child? Observations on a case series. *Developmental Medicine and Child Neurology, 47*(10), 699–702.

27. Ishiai, S., Furukawa, T., & Tsukagoshi, H. (1987). Eye-fixation patterns in homonymous hemianopia and unilateral spatial neglect. *Neuropsychologia, 25*(4), 675–679.

28. Zihl, J. (1995). Visual scanning behavior in patients with homonymous hemianopia. *Neuropsychologia, 33*(3), 287–303.

29. Nelles, G., de Greiff, A., Pscherer, A., Stude, P., Forsting, M., Hugnagel, A., Gerhard, H. Esser, J., & Diener, H. C. (2007). Saccade induced cortical activation in patients with post-stroke visual field defects. *Journal of Neurology, 254*(9), 1244–1252.

30. Kerkhoff, G., Münβinger, U., & Meier, E. K. (1994). Neurovisual rehabilitation in cerebral blindness. *Archives of Neurology, 51*(5), 474–481.

31. Pambakian, A. L. M., Mannan, S. K., Hodgson, T. L., & Kennard, C. (2004). Saccadic visual search training: a treatment for patients with homonymous hemianopia. *Journal of Neurology, Neurosurgery, and Psychiatry, 75*(10), 1443–1448.
32. Zihl, J., & von Cramon, D. (1985). Visual field recovery from scotoma in patients with postgeniculate damage. A review of 55 cases. *Brain, 108*(Pt. 2), 335–365.
33. Nelles, G., Pscherer, A., de Greiff, A., Forsting, M., Gerhard, H. Esser, J., & Diener, H. C. (2009). Eye-movement training-induced plasticity in patients with post-stroke hemianopia. *Journal of Neurology, 256*(5), 726–733.
34. McFadzean, R. M. (2006). NovaVision: vision restoration therapy. *Current Opinions in Ophthalmology, 17*(6), 498–503.
35. Kasten, E., Müller-Oehring, E., & Sabel, B. A. (2001). Stability of visual field enlargements following computer-based restitution training – results of a follow-up. *Journal of Clinical and Experimental Neuropsychology, 23*(3), 297–305.
36. Gottlieb, D., Freeman, P., & Williams. (1992). Clinical research and statistical analysis of a visual field awareness system. *Journal of the American Optometric Association, 63*(8), 581–588.
37. Lee, A.G., & Perez, A. M., (1999). Improving awareness of peripheral visual field using sectorial prism. *Journal of the American Optometric Association, 70*(10), 624–628.
38. Gottlieb, D., Fuhr, A., Hatch, W. V., & Wright, K. (1998). Neuro-optometric facilitation of vision recovery after acquired brain injury. *NeuroRehabilitation, 11,* 175–199.
39. Peli, E. (2000). Field expansion for homonymous hemianopia by optically induced peripheral exotropia. *Optometry and Vision Science, 77*(9), 453–464.
40. Bowers, A. R., Keeney, K., & Peli, E. (2008). Community-based trial of a peripheral prism visual field expansion device for hemianopia. *Archives of Ophthalmology, 126*(5), 657–664.
41. Denes, G., Semenza, C., Stoppa, E., & Lis, A. (1982). Unilateral spatial neglect and recovery from hemiplegia: a follow up study. *Brain, 105,* 453–552.
42. Wilson, B. A., Cockburn, J., & Halligan, P. W. (1987). *Behavioral inattention test.* London, UK: Pearson Assessment.
43. Becker, E., & Karnath, H. O. (2007). Incidence of visual extinction after left versus right hemisphere stroke. *Stroke, 38*(12), 3172–3174.
44. Halligan, P. W., Marshall, J. C., & Wade, D. T. (1989). Visuospatial neglect: underlying factors and test sensitivity. *Lancet, 2*(8668), 908–911.
45. Halligan, P. W., & Marshall, J. C. (1991). Left neglect for near but not far space in man. *Nature, 350*(6318), 498–500.
46. Medina, J., Kannan, V., Pawlak, M. A., Kleinman, J. T., Newhart, M., Davis, C., Hillis, A. E. (2009). Neural substrates of visuospatial processing in distinct reference frames evidence from unilateral spatial neglect. *Journal of Cognitive Neuroscience, 21*(11), 2073–2084.
47. Gambarini, L., Seraglia, B., & Priftis, K. (2008). Processing of peripersonal and extrapersonal space using tools: evidence from visual line bisection in real and virtual environments. *Neuropsychologia, 46*(5), 1298–1304.
48. Tegnér, R., & Levander, M. (1991). Through a looking glass. A new technique to demonstrate directional hypokinesia in unilateral neglect. *Brain, 114*(4), 1943–1951.
49. Saj, A., Honoré, J., Richard, C., Bernati, T., & Rousseaux, M. (2008). Reducing rightward bias of subjective straight ahead in neglect patients by changes in body orientation. *Journal of Neurology, Neurosurgery and Psychiatry, 79*(9), 991–996.
50. Schindler, I., & Kerkhoff, G. (1997). Head and trunk orientation modulate visual neglect. *Neuroreport, 8*(12), 2681–2685.

51. Vuilleumier, P., Valenza, N., Mayer, E., Perrig, S., & Landis, T. (1999). To see better to the left when looking more to the right: effects of gaze direction and frames of spatial coordinates in unilateral neglect. *Journal of the International Neuropsychological Society, 5*(1), 75–82.

52. Halligan, P. W., & Marshall, J. C. (1989). Is neglect (only) lateral? A quadrant analysis of line cancellation. *Journal of Clinical and Experimental Neuropsychology, 11*(6). 793–798.

53. Mesulam, M.-M. (1981). A cortical network for directed attention and unilateral neglect. *Annals of Neurology, 10*(4), 309–325.

54. Valler, G., & Perani D. (1986). The anatomy of unilateral neglect after right hemisphere stroke lesions: a clinical CT scan correlations study in man. *Neuropsychologia, 24*(5), 609–622.

55. Smith, S. E., & Chatterjee, A. (2008). Visuospatial attention in children. *Archives of Neurology, 65*(10), 1284–1288.

56. Rorden, C., Fruhmann-Berger, M., & Karnath, H-O. (2006). Disturbed line bisection is associated with posterior brain lesions. *Brain Research, 1080*(1), 17–25.

57. Binder, J., Marshall, R., Lazar, R., Benjamin, J., & Mohr, J. P. (1992). Distinct syndromes of hemineglect. *Archives of Neurology, 49*(11), 1187–1194.

58. Husain, M., & Kennard, C. (1996). Visual neglect associated with frontal lobe infarction. *Journal of Neurology, 243*(9), 652–657.

59. Bartolomeo, P. (2006). A parietofrontal network for spatial awareness in the right hemisphere of the human brain. *Archives of Neurology, 63*, 1238–1241.

60. Doricci, F., Thiebaut de Schotten, M., Tomaiuolo, F., & Bartolomeo, P. (2008). White matter (dis)connections and gray matter (dys)functions in visual neglect; gaining insights into the brain networks of spatial awareness. *Cortex, 44*(8), 983–995.

61. Karnath, H.-O., Himmelbach, M., & Rorden, C. (2002). The subcortical anatomy of human spatial neglect; putamen, caudate nucleus and pulvinar. *Brain, 125*(Pt. 2), 350–360.

62. Sapir, A., Kaplan, J. B., He, B. J., & Corbetta, M. (2007). Anatomical correlates of directional hypokinesia in patients with hemispatial neglect. *Journal of Neuroscience, 27*(15), 4045–4051.

63. Bellgrove, M. A., Chambers, C. D., Johnson, K. A., Daibhis, A., Daly, M., Hawi, Z., & Robertson, I. H. (2007). Dopaminergic genotype biases spatial attention in healthy children. *Molecular Psychiatry, 12*(8), 786–792.

64. Buxbaum, L. J., Ferraro, M., Whyte, J., Gershkoff, A., & Coslett, H. B. (2007). Amantadine treatment of hemispatial neglect: a double-blind, placebo-controlled study. *American Journal of Physical Medicine and Rehabilitation, 86*(7), 527–537.

65. Azouvi, P., Bartolomeo, P., Beis, J. M., Perennou, D., Pradat-Diehl, P., & Rousseaux, M. (2006). A battery of tests for the quantitative assessment of unilateral neglect. *Restorative Neurology and Neuroscience, 24*(4–6), 273–285.

66. Albert M. L. (1973). A simple test of visual neglect. *Neurology, 23*(6), 658–664.

67. Suter, P. S. (2007). Peripheral visual field loss and visual neglect: diagnosis and treatment. *Journal of Behavioral Optometry, 18*(3), 78–83.

68. Kerkhoff, G., & Bucher, L. (2008). Line bisection as an early method to assess homonymous hemianopia. *Cortex, 44*(2), 200–205.

69. Nielsen, K. E., Intriligator, J., & Barton, J. J. S. (1998). Spatial representation in the normal visual field: a study of hemifield line bisection. *Neuropsychologia, 37*(3), 267–277.

70. Padula, W. V., & Argyris, S. (1996). Post trauma vision syndrome and visual midline shift syndrome. *Neuro Rehabilitation Journal, 6*(3), 165–171.

71. Warrington, E. K., & James, M. (1991). *Visual object and space perception battery (VOSP)*. London, UK: Pearson Assessment.

72. Lindell, A. B., Maarit, J. J., Tenovuo, O., Brunila, T., Marinus, J. M. V., & Hämäläinen, H. (2006). Clinical assessment of hemispatial neglect: evaluation of different measures and dimensions. *The Clinical Neuropsychologist, 21*(3), 479–497.

73. Antonucci, G., Guariglia, C., Judica, A., Magnotti, L., Paolucci, S., Pizzamiglio, L., & Zocolotti, P. (1995). Effectiveness of neglect rehabilitation in a randomized group study. *Journal of Clinical and Experimental Neuropsychology, 17*(3), 383–389.

74. Luauté, J., Halligan, P., Rode, G., Jacquin-Courtois, S., & Boisson, D. (2006). Prism adaptation first among equals in alleviating left neglect: a review. *Restorative Neurology and Neuroscience, 24*, 409–418.

75. Gordon, W. A., Hibbard, M. R., Egelko, S., Diller, L., Shaver, M. S., Lieberman, A., & Ragnarsson, K. (1985). Perceptual remediation in patients with right brain damage: a comprehensive program. *Archives of Physical Medicine and Rehabilitation, 66*(6), 353–359.

76. Pantano, P., Di Piero, V., Fieschi, C., Judica, A, Guariglia, C., & Pizzamiglio, L. (1992). Pattern of CBF in the rehabilitation of visuospatial neglect. *The International Journal of Neuroscience, 66*(3–4), 153–161.

77. Paolucci, S., Antonucci, G., Guariglia, C., Magnotti, L., Pizzamiglio, L., & Zoccolotti, P. (1996). Facilitatory effect of neglect rehabilitation on the recovery of left hemiplegic stroke patients: a cross-over study. *Journal of Neurology, 243*(4), 308–314.

78. Webster, J. S., McFarland, P. T., Rapport, L. J., Morrill, B., Roades, L. A., & Abadee, P. S. (2001). Computer-assisted training for improving wheelchair mobility in unilateral neglect patients. *Archives of Physical Medicine and Rehabilitation, 82*(6), 769–775.

79. Margolis N. W. (1996, May). Post stroke vision neglect and vision loss. Presented at the meetings of the NeuroOptometric Rehabilitation Association, Chicago, IL.

80. Margolis, N. W., & Suter, P. S. (2006). Visual field defects & unilateral spatial inattention: diagnosis and treatment. *Journal of Behavioral Optometry, 17*(2), 1–7.

81. Eglin, M., Robertson L. C., & Knight R. T. (1991). Cortical substrates supporting visual search in humans. *Cerebral Cortex, 1*(3), 262–272.

82. Rossetti, Y., Rode, G., Pisella, L., Farné, A., Li, L., Boission, D., & Perenin, M.-T. (1998). Prism adaptation to a rightward optical deviation rehabilitates left hemispatial neglect. *Nature, 395*(6698), 166–169.

83. Hatada, Y., Rossetti, Y., & Miall, C. (2006). Long-lasting aftereffect of a single prism adaptation: shifts in vision and proprioception are independent. *Experimental Brain Research, 173*(3), 415–424.

84. Jacquin-Courtois, S., Rode, G., Pisella, L., Boisson, D., & Rossetti, Y. (2008). Wheelchair driving improvement following visuo-manual prism adaptation. *Cortex, 44*(1), 90–96.

6 Egocentric Localization
Normal and Abnormal Aspects

Kenneth J. Ciuffreda and Diana P. Ludlam

CONTENTS

"Language should not obscure the concept."

– K. J. Ciuffreda

DEFINITIONS AND BASIC CONCEPTS

Interaction with the environment in an efficient and complete manner is critical to one's well-being. Hence, any factor that may impede this interaction adversely impacts on quality of life (QOL), which includes both one's vocational and avocational goals.

Related to the above in both visually normal individuals and in those with acquired brain injury (ABI) is the global concept of "spatial sense." This can be defined as "the means by which an organism establishes a stable, constant relationship with its surroundings"[1] (p. 4): that is, the relationship of objects in the world to the individual, and the relationship of the individual to the objects in the world.

We thank Dr. Irwin B. Suchoff for his numerous insightful discussions and comments on various drafts of the manuscript; Dr. William V. Padula for his helpful discussions on portions of the manuscript; Naveen Yadav, B.S. Optom., M.S., for his helpful discussions on egocentric localization and related prism adaptation/after effect aspects, Dr. N. Kapoor and Preethi Thiagarajan for help with the figures; and Drs. Penelope S. Suter and Lisa H. Harvey, the book coeditors, for their careful editing and queries related to the text.

This "spatial sense" has two components.[1] The first is "orientation," which provides information to know where we are with respect to objects in our environment. This involves factors such as static and dynamic equilibrium mechanisms, which primarily incorporates the vestibular and proprioceptive systems. With this information, in conjunction with the visual system, an individual can establish and maintain body orientation in the context of their everyday dynamic environment (see Chapter 9).

The second component of the spatial sense is "localization," which provides information to know where objects are with respect to the individual. This localization component has two aspects: "oculocentric" and "egocentric."

Oculocentric localization refers to a foveally based localization of objects in the environment. Thus, here the fovea of the eye is the center of the spatial coordinate system. In the visual field, objects are referenced with respect to the fovea. It is a monocularly based system only.[2] It is used, for example, during rifle practice or when aiming a camera through the viewfinder, with the fellow eye closed. It is also important for the understanding of some vision anomalies, such as eccentric fixation in amblyopic eyes and eccentric viewing in macular degeneration.[1,3]

However, of critical importance in the context of the present chapter is egocentric localization; that is, the localization of objects in the environment with respect to one's "self," or "egocenter." In contrast to oculocentric localization, egocentric localization refers to a body-based localization of objects in the environment. The center of the trunk along the body midline is the reference point for this spatial coordinate system.[4–6] It is a binocularly based system,[2] and as such would be used in nearly all of one's daily activities, such as ambulation and when reaching for objects. It too is important in the understanding of many binocular vision disorders, such as anomalous retinal correspondence. However, in the context of the present chapter focused on ABI, egocentric localization is *the* critical concept.

Three parameters are necessary to specify precisely the egocentric localization of an object in the environment: the meridian, eccentricity, and absolute distance, all with respect to this body-centric, *polar* coordinate system. However, sometimes only the first two parameters are sufficient, if one is simply concerned with an object's relative position and not distance per se, for example, "the object is over there a bit to my left."

The basic concept of egocentric localization is essential in understanding what occurs when its function goes awry, for example, in ABI. This occurs in many patients having traumatic brain injury (TBI), and even more dramatically in cerebrovascular accident (i.e., "stroke"; CVA). In such cases, there is an alteration in egocentric localization for the special case of one's "sense of straight ahead."[4–6] That is, under either a full cue or reduced cue environment, for example, in the clinic or laboratory setting, respectively, the individual's sense of straight ahead is altered from the veridical or "objective" straight ahead. In other words, in a visually normal person, the objective straight-ahead direction, per their normal body-based midline spatial coordinate system, is in agreement and consistent with their "subjective" sense of what appears to be straight ahead in both the horizontal and vertical directions: their subjective and objective perceptions of "straight ahead" are in basic agreement.

Thus, an object that is physically (i.e., objectively) centered on the person's body midline would also be perceived subjectively to be in the same two-dimensional direction from the self, or egocenter. In contrast, in individuals with an altered sense of straight ahead, that same object placed along their objective midline would be perceived elsewhere subjectively (e.g., to the left). This directional bias in egocentric localization likely extends across the whole (or most) of the visual field, but probably varies in a nonlinear manner.

An example is presented schematically in Figure 6.1. This hypothetical person has stroke and hemianopia with visual neglect (to be described later). Their subjective and objective directions of straight ahead do not match; in this case, the subjective sense of straight ahead is displaced laterally several degrees into the "seeing" hemifield,[4–7] presumably in an attempt "center" or bisect their effective visual world. In contrast, in visually normal individuals, the subjective and objective directions are in close agreement (<±2 degrees).[4,6]

This special case of egocentrically based, sense of straight ahead currently has several different terminologies. Perhaps the most common in the optometric, and legal, literatures is "visual midline shift syndrome" (VMSS), apparently coined and popularized by Padula.[8] However, this concept of a "shift" can be misleading. In the medical and dental literatures, "midline shift" suggests a lateral anatomical displacement of the brain or teeth, respectively.[9,10] In the case of VMSS, this is incorrect, as it suggests a lateral shift (rather than an angular deviation) of the perceived midline, for example, toward one's shoulder. Rather, there is a body-based, polar coordinate change as described earlier, similar to what one does when pointing with their arm to an object, for example, "up and to the right." Furthermore, Padula does not appear to differentiate between a "neuroperceptually based" alteration in this sense of straight ahead, as used

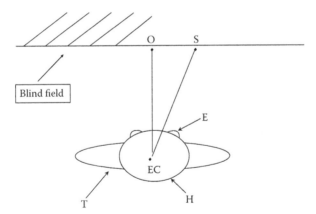

FIGURE 6.1 Schematic representation of anomalous egocentric localization in a patient with hemianopia and visual neglect. Symbols: E = eyes, EC = egocenter, H = head, T = torso, 0 = normal objective straight ahead, and S = anomalous subjective straight ahead. (From Suchoff, I. B. Ciuffreda, K. J. and Kapoor, N. (Eds.)., *Visual & Vestibular Consequences of Acquired Brain Injury*, Optometric Extension Program Foundation, Santa Ana, CA, 2001, p. 132. Reprinted with permission from the Optometric Extension Program Foundation [www.oepf.org].)

exclusively in this chapter and by many neurorehabilitative optometrists, and that which is primarily "mechanically based." This latter mechanical alteration is found in stroke patients without hemianopia and visual neglect but manifesting a shift, or bias, in body posture due to hemisided body motor weakness,[8,11] that is, of a mechanical nature.

Other terms have also been used to describe this phenomenon. These include "disturbed egocentric space representation," "perception of straight-ahead orientation," "egocentric spatial frame of reference," "perceived midline," "body midline perception," and "visual subjective body midline," to name a few. These terminologies have been used in a variety of nonoptometric disciplines: neurology, neuropsychology, and anesthesiology.[4,12–15] This concept of anomalous midline perception has also been described in the field of occupational therapy with respect to the use of yoked prisms (i.e., prisms having their bases in the same direction; to be described in detail later) as a compensatory optical approach in ABI vision rehabilitation.[16,17] Thus, while there have been, and continue to be, a range of terminologies to describe this phenomenon in the medical, legal, and optometric literatures, the basic neuroperceptually based concept remains the same. We prefer to use the term "abnormal egocentric localization" (AEL).

ASSOCIATED SIGNS, SYMPTOMS, AND CONDITIONS

Patients having this abnormal sense of straight ahead manifest a constellation of general symptoms, especially in the stroke population. These may include poor balance and posture, bumping into objects, spatial disorientation, lateralward bias in walking, dizziness, and a sense of being "out of synch" with their environment.[5,18] This last symptom is particularly insightful in the context of AEL. Whenever there is mismatch, or discrepancy, in the incoming perceptual information, such as in one's subjective versus objective sense of straight ahead, an individual exhibits difficulty interacting in their environment due to this spatial, and perhaps related temporal, perceptual "cue conflict."[19] This conflict produces visuomotor problems associated with walking and eye-hand coordination, as well as misperception of the apparent distances of objects in the environment.[1,20] However, this special type of cue conflict can be reduced with yoked prisms (Figure 6.2) and/or visuomotor adaptive training, as described later in this chapter.

There are three conditions that are strongly associated with this abnormal sense of straight ahead. The first is "hemianopia." This refers to the physiological loss of ability to see objects on one side of the visual field.[18] Second, and frequently related to the above, is "visual neglect" (e.g., "hemispatial neglect" or "hemi-inattention")[18] (see Chapter 5). This refers to the perceptual/cognitive loss of awareness of objects, even parts of one's own body, on one side of the visual field. Hemianopia and visual neglect can be independent entities; however, many stroke patients with hemianopia also have visual neglect, in conjunction with their abnormal sense of straight ahead. Visual neglect may extend to their personal (i.e., their own body awareness), peripersonal (i.e., their world within arm's reach), and extrapersonal (i.e., their world beyond arm's reach) spaces (reviewed by Suchoff and Ciuffreda).[18]

The third associated condition is "post trauma vision syndrome" (PTVS).[8,11] PTVS is the most common visual sequelae of TBI.[21] This refers to a constellation of ocular motor, attentional, and cognitive problems following a brain insult. Signs and

A   B

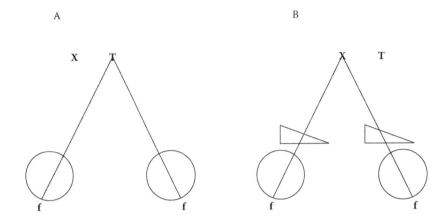

FIGURE 6.2 Schematic representation of yoked prism effect on spatial localization with subject instructed to gaze straight ahead. A: Without the yoked prism, where T = a midline object, X = an object to the left of midline. B: With the yoked prisms, where objects T and X are now optically displaced laterally to the right by the prisms *without* any change in eye position. (From Suchoff, I. B. Ciuffreda, K. J. and Kapoor, N. (Eds.)., *Visual & Vestibular Consequences of Acquired Brain Injury,* Optometric Extension Program Foundation, Santa Ana, CA, 2001, p. 132. Reprinted with permission from the Optometric Extension Program Foundation [www.oepf.org].)

symptoms may include exophoria, convergence insufficiency, diplopia, blur, light sensitivity, visual field loss, concentration difficulties, reading problems, visual memory lapses, and poor spatial judgment/depth perception and AEL. Presence of PTVS symptoms may adversely affect one's egocentric localization, for example dizziness and diplopia may bias its direction and/or increase its variability. Fortunately, most of the above symptoms can be remediated, at least to some extent, with the application of lenses, prisms, filters, occluders, and/or conventional optometric vision therapy.[22–24]

NEURAL SUBSTRATES

The neural substrates underlying computation of the egocentric spatial frame of reference, and its related adaptive aspects, remain an evolving area in light of advancing brain-imaging technology. The primary neural region involved in egocentric localization is the right posterior parietal cortex.[4,7] However, more recently, both the intraparietal sulcus and the lateral/right premotor frontal areas have been implicated.[25] Related to the above, regions of the brain involved in prism adaptation based therapeutic paradigms were the right cerebellum, left temporal-occipital cortex, left thalamus, left medial temporal lobe, and right posterior parietal cortex.[26] When there is damage to the right parietal cortex area, residual neuroplasticity makes possible recruitment of the left cortex to assume right cortex function.[26,27] Lastly, a recent fMRI study revealed interesting insights into the neural mechanisms involved in prism adaptation.[28] During the early phases, the anterior intraparietal sulcus was involved in positional error detection, while the parieto-occipital sulcus was involved in positional error correction. Moreover, during the latter phases of the prism exposure, the cerebellum and superior temporal cortex were activated and were believed to be involved in spatial realignment and higher-order spatial representations.

CRITICAL LABORATORY DEVELOPMENTS

There have been several critical laboratory developments in the area of human egocentric localization, both in normal and in brain-injured populations.

1. Werner et al. [29]: This group of research psychologists was one of the first to employ systematically a proprioceptively based, straight-ahead pointing task with the arm to assess what they referred to as the "apparent median plane" in young, visually normal adults. This approach has a long history in the perceptual adaptation literature, [30] and it is employed clinically with the VTE spatial localization board, [31] as discussed in the clinical section of this chapter.

2. Karnath[4]: This clinical neurologist was the first to test egocentric localization in brain-injured patients having right parietal lesions and left neglect (without hemianopia) using a remote laser pointing approach in an otherwise totally darkened enclosure (discussed later). He found a 15 degree, lateral, upsilesional displacement in their sense of straight ahead, with a normal vertical component. This abnormal lateral displacement could be influenced (usually reduced) by addition of either proprioceptive input (i.e., neck muscle vibration) and/or vestibular stimulation (i.e., caloric activation), both applied to the left side. The results suggested that the damaged cortical areas, which function to transform the incoming sensory information into an egocentric body-based coordinate frame of reference, produced a systematic directional error. Hence, aberrant subcortical sensory information can also adversely influence a patient's egocentric localization.

3. Rossetti et al. [32]: These psychologists extended Karnath's findings to the next level. They developed a prismatic, visuomotor-based therapeutic intervention. Patients with visual neglect and abnormal rightward biased egocentric localization performed a 2-hour manual-pointing task (without visual feedback) while wearing 10 degree bases-left (17.5 prism diopters [pd] rightward displacement) yoked prisms. Following the training and the removal of the adapting prisms, the patients exhibited a near normalization of their egocentric localization; that is, it was now more centrally positioned close to veridical zero. This centralward shift persisted throughout the 2-hour, posttask period. Alteration in the patient's egocentric localization reflected a prism adaptation after effect, as commonly found in prism-based perceptual experiments. [30] Of particular interest in this and related experiments in the ABI population (see Massucci for a review)[27] was the extended duration of this after effect (i.e., up to several months). Hence, prism adaptation training should be used in conjunction with yoked prism spectacles in this population to provide the most efficacious therapeutic approach.

4. Ciuffreda research group (2001)[6]: This optometric clinical research team developed a small and portable device to assess egocentric localization and related yoked prism application in the clinic setting. It produced reliable

and valid estimates of egocentric localization in both the normal and ABI population. This device can serve as an adjunct to the VTE spatial localization board (discussed later in this chapter) in the ABI population for the clinical assessment of egocentric localization,[31] as well as in its alteration by yoked prism spectacles and/or yoked prism treatment.

The explanation provided by Karnath,[4] and many others across disciplines, is simple, direct, comprehensive, and neurologically based: Damage to the posterior parietal cortex and related brain structures produces a systematic error in the body's spatial frame of reference. This involves visual, vestibular, and proprioceptive inputs. Furthermore, the prism adaptation experiments of Rossetti and colleagues,[32] with their therapeutically based prism after effect that acts to transiently counteract, and hence nearly normalize the AEL, is consistent with the Karnath hypothesis, both behaviorally and neurologically. Lastly, the unusually long duration of the prism after effect found in the ABI population can be accounted for by its effective reduction (i.e., near normalization) in the mismatch between their subjective and objective sense of straight ahead, just as it occurs with yoked prism spectacles, as described later. We subscribe to the above scenario.

However, a different possible scenario has been proposed.[11,8] Here the brain insult is speculated to have produced an "imbalance" between the "ambient" and the "focal" systems. The former system is believed to be involved in spatial aspects such as orientation and motion. It can be conceptualized as nonfoveal, peripheral, and magnocellular-like in its basic attributes. In contrast, the latter system is believed to be involved in fine detail vision. It can be conceptualized as foveal, central, and parvocellular-like in its basic attributes. However, the onus is on its ambient counterpart with regard to being the primary source of the overall dysfunction, as fine detailed vision is normal or nearby normal in this population.[5]

ASSESSING EGOCENTRIC LOCALIZATION IN ACQUIRED BRAIN INJURY

There are several clinical and laboratory approaches to the assessment of egocentric localization in patients with ABI, such as TBI and CVA. They range from simple gross observation to more formal quantification. The end result is the prescription of yoked prisms, either alone or in conjunction with vision rehabilitation therapy, plus lens spectacles for near work, vestibular therapy, and at times, occupational therapy.[22]

These procedures can also be applied to other populations, in our own experience and that of others,[33] such as autism and learning disability, where a small amount (e.g., 2 pd) of either horizontal or vertical yoked prism can result in considerable immediate benefit to visual performance, comfort, and posture. However, the underlying mechanisms (e.g., produce a shift in attentional space) are likely to be different in these other groups than in ABI; these applications are beyond the scope of this chapter.

CLINICAL APPROACHES

One of the simplest ways to evaluate egocentric localization at a gross level is to observe patient behavior in the reception area and as they walk to the examination room. Noting how the patient sits in the chair, and observing whether there is a marked head turn/tilt, or if the individual is leaning to one side, can yield valuable information regarding the presence of an abnormal egocentrically based directional bias. Observing them either from the side or behind as they walk to the examination room yields information as to any tendency to "drift" or bias toward one side of the hallway, presence of any unsteadiness, or use of their hand to "feel" the wall as they walk. Leaning/walking biased toward one side may suggest an alteration in their visual-perceptual sense of "straight ahead" and/or an undetected visual field deficit. Presence of gait unsteadiness might further suggest a slight motor weakness as a result of a CVA, a vestibular problem, or several other neurological possibilities. All of these observations must be taken into consideration with the findings revealed during the comprehensive vision examination. For instance, if a patient has a large anisometropia, an intermittent strabismus with or without attendant diplopia, or reduced visual acuity not correctable in one or both eyes (i.e., has low vision), these must be taken into consideration in developing a treatment plan.

Another simple technique developed by the authors is the "face-to-face" procedure. The patient is seated comfortably at a narrow table directly facing the examiner. The patient's chair or stool height is adjusted so that they are at the examiner's eye level. The patient is asked to "point" his/her nose directly at the examiner's nose, so that if both leaned forward, the tips of the noses would touch. Any turning, tilting, or misalignment of the head is noted as the individual attempts to follow these instructions. Another tactic is to ask the patient to "point" with their nose to objects held in different positions. Any horizontal or vertical directional error is again noted. However, such eccentric pointing may be confounded by parallax in the examiner's estimation of the patient's direction. This technique serves as a form of screening for any gross abnormal egocentric shift before more formal and quantitative testing.

One procedure developed by Dr. William V. Padula, which is easy to use to estimate and quantify any abnormality in the patient's subjective sense of "straight ahead," involves using a wand as a target with eye tracking, but without head movement.[8,11] The examiner is positioned to one side, so that the patient does not potentially cue off the examiner's own midline. As the target is tracked against a blank wall, the patient indicates when it appears to be straight ahead along their midline. To minimize any parallax error, the examiner moves back to the center of the field with the arm fixed, to assess the magnitude of offset. The test should be repeated twice, first with the target moving left-to-right and vice versa to prevent a directional bias, and the mean estimated. It should be performed both horizontally and vertically (see Chapter 5 for details). A modification of this procedure is used routinely by the authors (Figure 6.3). As the patient is comfortably seated directly in front of the examiner, they are told to follow the wand held vertically at about a 16-inch distance. They are further instructed to follow the target with only their eyes, with the head stationary. The wand is slowly displaced laterally, and the patient is asked to indicate verbally when it appears to be directly in front of their nose. This is repeated several times, and the misalignment/offset magnitude estimated, as well as its direction. This can be denoted in the clinic record by including a schematic of a simple face on the recording form and drawing lines representing the patient's response (Figure 6.4).[8] The procedure should be repeated, but this time with the target oriented horizontally and moved vertically.

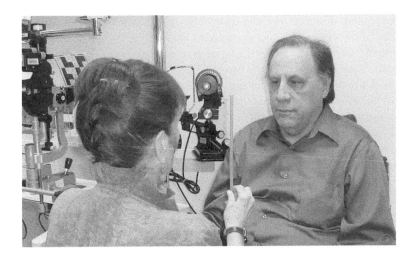

FIGURE 6.3 Examiner and patient performing test of egocentric localization using the modified "wand" procedure.

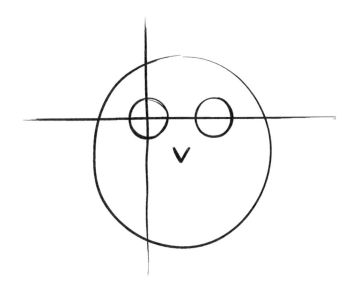

FIGURE 6.4 Schematic face representation of the wand test findings for egocentric localization in the horizontal and vertical directions.

The patient is asked to indicate verbally when the wand is directly in front of their eyes, so that if it were to be moved closer to them, it would be at eye level. This finding is added to the face schematic in the clinic record. If there is a marked directional shift in either or both of these tests, yoked prisms are added, until the target is perceived to be on or close to the true objective midline or eye level, respectively. This amount is usually between 2 and 6 pd,[22] but has been reported to be as high as 15 pd.[8]

The test procedure can be repeated without any eye tracking to remove the possible influence of the eye movements per se (e.g., extraocular muscle proprioception) on the sense of "straight ahead," per the findings of Karnath.[4] If there is a marked difference (more than 2 pd) between the two techniques, the authors use the prism amount found with eye tracking. The thinking is that much of daily life is spent in activities in which the eyes are actively engaged in tracking throughout the visual field. Lastly, while it is possible that the patient may cue off the examiner's midline, as mentioned earlier, this does not appear to be a major confound in our experience.

In the above case, the yoked prisms optically displace an object from the individual's anomalous subjective zero localization direction to their objective physical midline. However, this creates a perceptual mismatch between their abnormal subjective and veridical objective localization directions, and hence sensorimotor training may be required by the patient to adapt and optimize their visuomotor performance (as described later). In addition, in some patients, another mechanism has been speculated to be involved.[8] In those patients exhibiting "distortion" of visual space, that is, relative compression in one hemifield and expansion in the other, such neurologically based, nonuniform magnification is nulled optically by the yoked prisms, which themselves produce nonuniform magnification across the visual field (Figure 6.5).[20] As a by-product of this nulling effect, the patient's abnormal egocentric sense of "straight ahead" becomes veridical.

Another approach has been developed by Dr. Irwin B. Suchoff in patients with hemianopia, *with or without* either hemi-inattention (i.e., visual neglect) or AEL. The basics of this approach have been previously described by Suchoff and Ciuffreda,[18] and are more fully detailed here. The patient is directed to stand in the center of a long hallway that is deplete of objects, pictures, and so on, so that visual cues related to direction and distance are minimal. About 10–15 feet away, a person is positioned into the near edge of the hemianopic field, such that they are just *not* visible to the patient who is gazing straight ahead in primary position. The direction of the yoked prism bases is always the same as the visual field defect: that is, with left hemianopia, the bases are placed to the left. Small amounts of yoked prisms are introduced, until the patient is first visually aware of the formerly "hidden" person's shoulder and arm.

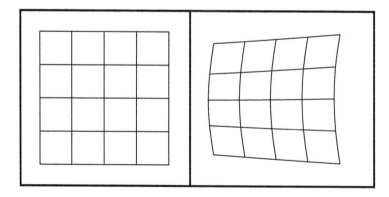

FIGURE 6.5   Illustration of nonuniform magnification distortion. Object is left, and image is right.

The next highest prism power is introduced, and this should make the patient visually aware of slightly more of the person's body. This is the indicated yoked prism prescription. Typical values are 2–6 pd, with a maximum of 10 pd at far, and up to 15 pd at near. The minimum amount of prism that accomplishes this goal should be used, as larger amounts may cause spatial distortion due to the nonuniform magnification properties of prisms[20] and/or substantial sensorimotor adaptation problems.[30] The patient is then instructed to ambulate down the same hallway, both with and without the yoked prisms, and to describe their overall perception. If it is substantially better with the yoked prisms, the walking process is repeated in a crowded environment. Lastly, they are asked to rate the improvement with the yoked prisms into one of three response categories: "Wow," "Very good," and "So what." If the response is "So what," they are discouraged from further pursuing this treatment plan. However, if it is positive, then at a subsequent visit the patient returns to confirm their initial perceptions. If it remains positive, the yoked prisms are prescribed for their intended application. For example, they might be used for ambulation and visual scanning, in which case 6 pd may be prescribed. However, if only for reading, larger amounts are typically prescribed (e.g., 12–15 pd) to shift more of the text that is physically positioned in the "blind" hemifield into the "seeing" hemifield.

The logic for the above procedure is as follows. In the case of hemianopia only and in the case that the patient's egocentric localization is veridical (i.e., objective and subjective "straight ahead" are coincident), the prisms optically displace objects throughout the entire visual field in the direction of the prism apex. In doing so, objects that were positioned into and near the edge of the "blind" hemifield, as well as any visible objects positioned along the patient's objective midline, are displaced laterally into the "seeing" hemifield. This introduces a directional mismatch between objective and subjective zero localization. Hence, the patient may require a period of sensorimotor training to use the prisms successfully and effortlessly, especially in dynamic situations such as walking or in grasping for an object. In contrast, in the case of hemianopia with visual neglect, in which their egocenter is shifted into the "seeing" hemifield,[4,5,18] the prisms also act to reduce the habitual perceptual mismatch between the veridical objective and the erroneous subjective egocentric localization. These patients are typically immediately happy with their yoked prisms, and usually do not require any subsequent sensorimotor training, that is, recalibration between their visual and kinesthetic directional information. Hence, in this case, the yoked prisms not only increase the effective and usable visual field, but also reduce the related perceptual directional mismatch. This is consistent with the results of Rossetti and colleagues with respect to the yoked prism's additional therapeutic effect.[32]

A novel technique to assess egocentric localization in combination with gross dynamic posturography was developed by Dr. Don Fong (Figure 6.6). His simple method incorporating weight bearing uses two bathroom scales, side by side, separated by approximately 6 inches, with each set to "0" lbs. The patient is asked to stand with one foot on each scale. A dowel is suspended from a ceiling mounted slide (such as a curtain rod), and a ruler is placed behind the sliding dowel on the ceiling, so that the examiner can read the numbers as the dowel is displaced laterally. The patient indicates when the dowel, which the patient tracks with their eyes, is perceived to be "straight ahead" on their midline. The magnitude and direction of

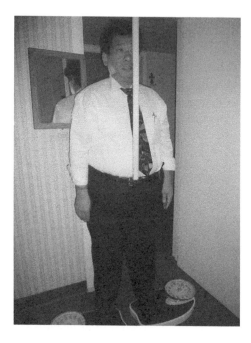

FIGURE 6.6 (See color insert following page 270.) Patient performing the combined weight bearing and visual egocentric localization tests.

any horizontal offset is noted. The examiner also denotes any changes in the readout of the scales as the above procedure is performed. Individuals with postural imbalances due to AEL may bear weight more on the side of the shift.[34] Application of yoked prisms is used to achieve equal weight bearing as measured on the scales, as well as more veridical direction sense. If there is a difference in yoked prism value between the weight bearing and rod settings, the latter is typically used in the spectacle prescription.

The last technique to be described is the newest in the clinical armamentarium. It was originally developed by experimental psychologists to assess visual adaptive processes[30] and incorporates the concept of arm pointing in the absence of visual feedback.[29] The VTE spatial localization board consists of a large translucent plastic platform.[31] One side rests with foam supports on the patient's shoulders, while the opposite side rests on some object or table that maintains the platform parallel to the ground, or it can be held by the clinician, while the patient either sits or stands. A large sheet of calibrated white paper is adhered to the bottom of the platform onto which the patient indicates their response. The patient faces a large, uncluttered wall to minimize visual cues to direction, with the dominant arm beneath the platform and with a pen marker held in the hand. The patient is instructed to move the unseen arm so that it "feels" to be "straight ahead," with the eyes gazing steadily in primary position. When the arm is believed to be pointing appropriately, the patient is asked to place a mark on the calibrated sheet. This represents their subjective egocentric sense of straight ahead. If there is a shift from objective zero, yoked prisms are

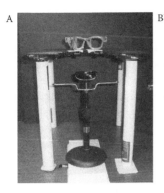
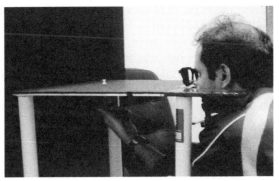

FIGURE 6.7 A: Modified VTE device. B: Patient performing test of egocentric localization using the modified VTE board.

added, until the offset is nulled. This is the starting point for prescribing the yoked prisms. Furthermore, by adding several of the small VTE targets to the top of the board, the general case of egocentric localization can be assessed collectively for a range of directions in near visual space.[31] Examples of measurements and cases using this device are presented in Chapter 7. In our own trials with the device, we have found it to be unstable physically. Hence, we have added considerable modifications, including table mounting, for use in both the laboratory and clinical settings (Figure 6.7A and 6.7B).

VISUOMOTOR TRAINING ASPECTS

We recommend visuomotor training in many of these patients. It may be required for the patient to feel that the now visually altered midline to be his/her perceived midline.[35] Furthermore, although the patient may be quite enthusiastic about the tentative amount of yoked prism, it may require recalibration of the previously learned sensorimotor programming for accurate grasping of a small object, as well as other general visuomotor tasks.

Training first takes place without ambulation. The training procedures include a variety of active sensorimotor tasks. A simple procedure is to ask the patient to touch the examiner's finger placed in different regions of the visual field. One can also use a large chalkboard with the numbers 1–10 marked on it in random positions. The individual is first asked to fixate, and then touch, the numbers to reestablish a match between perceived and physical space. Verbal feedback by the doctor or therapist is provided regarding the direction and magnitude of the initial error, and the task is repeated until accurate. If magnetic numbers are used, the patient also receives tactile feedback regarding their performance. A more demanding activity is "pointer in the straw," in which the examiner holds a drinking straw and asks the patient to insert a pointer into the straw rapidly without making any corrective movements, for example, by getting an error cue from first touching the end of the straw. The straw should be oriented horizontally, and then vertically and obliquely. One can customize this procedure to allow for such medical conditions as low vision, extension tremor, and so on, by using a larger diameter target and pointer, for example, a small mailing tube and pencil.

The training then takes place with ambulation. The patient is asked to walk through the reception area and pick up a magazine, touch the edge of a painting, sit in a specific chair, and so forth. The prism amount can be adjusted, and the procedure repeated depending on the response of the patient. Repeating these tasks, and having the patient match visual cues with motor activities, is crucial for establishing accurate perception of objects in physical space. In this way, the patient will develop a new and stable perceptual-motor map of visual space with the yoked prisms in place.

Continuation of this therapy should be reinforced at home and/or the rehabilitation facility, as well as in everyday work, play, and social settings, such as reaching for and grasping a water glass without mishap. Each successful experience builds the patient's confidence in relying on their sensorimotor perception of objects in their visual environment.

CLINICAL RESEARCH ASPECTS

There have been two primary groups who have assessed egocentric localization in patients having ABI in the clinical research laboratory, namely Karnath,[4] and Kapoor and Ciuffreda along with their clinical colleagues.[5,6] The intention in both groups was to obtain a "pure" measure of the brain's spatial map of one's "straight-ahead" egocentric direction sense.

The first attempts were by Karnath,[4] as mentioned earlier in this chapter. He used a laboratory room setting in which stroke patients with hemi-inattention (i.e., visual neglect) were assessed in total darkness to obtain a measure of their "straight-ahead" direction sense. With the patient gazing into primary position, an isolated small target in the visual field was laterally and vertically displaced, until it was perceived to be straight ahead by the subject. Other types of sensory stimuli could be introduced, such as proprioception, to assess their influence on egocentric perception. Karnath's work has provided considerable insights into the field of brain injury, in particular, stroke.

Several years later, the Kapoor and Ciuffreda group[5,6] developed a small (13-inch cube), portable device to more readily assess egocentric localization in the clinic and clinic research environment. Conceptually, it was a miniature version of Karnath's laboratory test environment (Figure 6.8). Essentially, the patient (or subject) was instructed to "gaze straight ahead into the device box, as if you are looking into a mirror shaving or applying eye make-up" in total darkness. The experimenter then introduced and slowly optically displaced a small laser-light target either horizontally or vertically, until it was perceived to be "straight ahead" by the test subject. This target was also visible to the experimenter through the back of the device, which contained a calibrated grid. The setting was read directly by the experimenter on the grid. The task was repeated several times, and the horizontal and vertical mean values, and their variabilities, were calculated. These values can be used in conjunction with other measures and correlates of egocentric direction sense for yoked prism applications.

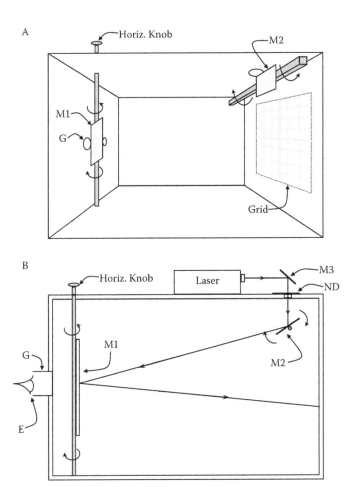

FIGURE 6.8 Egocentric localization device. A: Internal perspective view showing the viewing goggles (G), horizontally (M1) and vertically (M2) deflecting mirrors, as well as the calibrated grid (Grid), which is visible only to the experimenters and not to the subject. B: Internal side view showing subject's eye (E), viewing goggles (G), horizontally deflecting mirror (M1), laser (top of enclosure), mirror deflecting laser target into the enclosure (M3), neutral density filter (ND), and the vertically deflecting mirror (M2). (From Suchoff, I. B. Ciuffreda, K. J., and Kapoor, N. (Eds.)., *Visual & Vestibular Consequences of Acquired Brain Injury,* Optometric Extension Program Foundation, Santa Ana, CA, 2001, p. 140. Reprinted with permission from the Optometric Extension Program Foundation [www. oepf.org].)

This device has been tested in both visually normal subjects, as well as in stroke patients having hemianopia and hemi-inattention.[5,6] As found by Karnath,[4] normal subject's sense of straight ahead was quite accurate, with it being ±1 to 2 degrees horizontally and vertically of "objective" zero along the body midline. In contrast, the patients typically manifested an anomalous egocentric straight-ahead direction sense of several degrees and/or considerable directional variability. However, the AEL values were smaller than found by Karnath.[4] Additional experiments are needed in the area to develop the clinical correlates of this measure, as well as to develop more accurate prescription protocols for yoked prisms in this population in conjunction with active yoked prism visuomotor therapeutic applications.

CONCLUSIONS

There are several points that are critical to understanding the "spatial sense" in ABI patients having hemianopia, visual neglect, and an abnormal sense of "straight ahead" (Figure 6.9).

1. The main component of the spatial sense that is responsible for the problem is "abnormal egocentric localization" (AEL).
2. This lateralward bias, or error, in perceived midline is directed into the "seeing" hemifield. It is typically "perceptually based" and is attributed primarily to damage of the posterior parietal cortex. In a smaller percentage of ABI cases, however, it may be "mechanically based" due to neuromotor hemiparesis alone.
3. Specific visuomotor activities conducted with high-powered, bases-left yoked prisms promote prism adaptation. Upon their removal, the resultant prism after effect acts to reduce the error between the subjective, or perceived midline, and the objective, or veridical, sense of straight ahead in the ABI patient. In contrast, in visually normal individuals, the prism after effect acts to introduce a new and undesirable oppositely directed spatial error.
4. Since the error, or directional mismatch, is reduced in the ABI patient, it is beneficial.
5. Hence, it persists for an extended period of time.

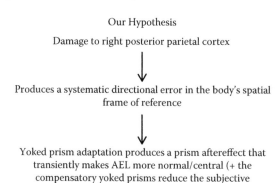

Our Hypothesis

Damage to right posterior parietal cortex

↓

Produces a systematic directional error in the body's spatial frame of reference

↓

Yoked prism adaptation produces a prism aftereffect that transiently makes AEL more normal/central (+ the compensatory yoked prisms reduce the subjective versus objective directional mismatch)

↓

The aftereffect persists as it is beneficial, that is, it reduces the subjective versus objective directional mismatch

FIGURE 6.9 A possible scenario to explain the effects of compensatory and therapeutic yoked prisms in patients with AEL.

6. The slow, and likely variable, dissipation of the prism after effect found in the ABI population may be the primary factor in, and a reflection of, their changing level of satisfaction with yoked prism spectacles. When the yoked prisms are initially dispensed, they immediately optically reduce the mismatch in the subjective versus objective sense of straight ahead. However, with continued wear and while performing various visuomotor activities in the home and work environments, prism adaptation will occur to some extent. Thus, upon removal of the prisms, the perceived midline error will be reduced per Rossetti et al.'s (1998) findings. The patient may now desire to abandon the yoked prism spectacles, and rightly so, as they are no longer beneficial. However, as the prism after effect slowly dissipates over the subsequent weeks or months, the patient's original problem reemerges. Thus, the yoked prism spectacles will once again be desirable. Of interest, the magnitude of the required prism is now typically less than originally prescribed. Presumably, this reflects incomplete dissipation of the original prism after effect.

7. As conventionally applied clinically, the typical yoked prism spectacles (e.g., 6 pd bases left) are immediately beneficial, as they reduce the subjective versus objective directional mismatch. Hence, they function in a "compensatory" manner. However, the newer notion of Rossetti et al. (1998) is to use larger magnitudes of yoked prisms (e.g., 20 pd bases left) in an adaptive approach. Here they function in a "therapeutic" manner to accomplish the same task.

8. The application of yoked prisms in both their compensatory and therapeutic modes is suggested. The appropriate power of the yoked prism spectacles required during the course of treatment and follow-up will be contingent upon the variable adaptive state of the ABI patient at that particular moment.

REFERENCES

1. Reading, R. W. (1983). *Binocular vision: Foundation and applications.* Boston, MA: Butterworths.
2. Solomons, H. (1978). *Binocular vision: A programmed text.* London, UK: William Heinemann Medical Books.
3. Von Noorden, G. K. (1969). The etiology and pathogenesis of fixation anomalies in the strabismus. *Transactions of the American Ophthalmological Society, 67,* 698–711.
4. Karnath, H. O. (1994). Subjective orientation in neglect and the interactive contribution of neck proprioception and vestibular stimulation. *Brain, 117,* 1001–1012.
5. Kapoor, N., Ciuffreda, K. J., & Suchoff, I. B. (2001). Egocentric localization in patients with visual neglect. In I. B. Suchoff, K. J. Ciuffreda, & N. Kapoor (Eds.), *Visual & vestibular consequences of acquired brain injury* (pp. 131–144). Santa Ana, CA: Optometric Extension Program Foundation.
6. Kapoor, N., Ciuffreda, K. J., Harris, G., Suchoff, I. B., Kim, J., Huang, M., & Bae, P. (2001). A new portable clinical device for measuring egocentric localization. *Journal of Behavioral Optometry, 12,* 115–119.
7. Stein, J. F. (1989). Representation of egocentric space in the posterior parietal cortex. *Quarterly Journal of Experimental Physiology, 74,* 583–606.
8. Padula, W. V. (1988). *Neuro-optometric rehabilitation.* Santa Ana, CA: Optometric Extension Program Foundation.

9. Weerakkody, Y. D., Feltman, R. L., & Leigh, A. J. (2009). Midline shift, seizures, and deterioration due to cranial vault metastases from prostatic carcinoma. *Journal of Clinical Neuroscience, 16,* 1506–1507.

10. Alcan, T., & Ceylanoglu, C. (2006). Upper midline correction in conjunction with rapid maxillary expansion. *American Journal of Orthodontics and Dentofacial Orthopedics, 130,* 671–675.

11. Padula, W. V., Nelson, C. A., Padula, W. V. III., Benabib, R., Yilmaz, T., & Krevisky, S. (2009). Modifying postural adaptation following CVA through prismatic shift of visuo-spatial egocenter. *Brain Injury, 23,* 566–576.

12. Bartolomeo, P., & Chokron, S. (1999). Egocentric frame of reference: its role in spatial bias after right hemisphere lesions. *Neuropsychologia, 37,* 881–894.

13. Ferber, S., & Karnath, H. O. (1999). Parietal and occipital lobe contributions to perception of straight ahead orientation. *Journal of Neurology, Neurosurgery, & Psychiatry, 67,* 572–578.

14. Sumitani, M., Schibata, M., Iwakura, T., Matsuda, Y., Inoue, T., Mashimo, T., & Miyauchi, S. (2007). Pathologic pain distorts visuospatial perception. *Neurology, 68,* 152–154.

15. Vallar, G., Lobel, E., Galati, G., Berthoz, A., Pizzamiglio, L., & Biham, D. L. (1999). A fronto-parietal system for computing the egocentric spatial frame of reference in humans. *Experimental Brain Research, 124,* 281–286.

16. Gianutos, R., & Suchoff, I. B. (1997). Visual fields after brain injury: management issues for the occupational therapist. In A. Scheiman (Ed.), *Understanding and managing vision deficits: A guide for occupational therapists* (pp. 333–358). Thorofare, NJ: Slack.

17. Zoltan, B. (2007). *Vision, perception, and cognition.* Thorofare, NJ: Slack.

18. Suchoff, I. B., & Ciuffreda, K. J. (2004). A primer for the optometric management of unilateral spatial inattention. *Optometry, 75,* 305–318.

19. Redding, G. M., & Wallace, B. (2006). Prism adaptation and unilateral neglect: review and analysis. *Neuropsychologia, 44,* 1–20.

20. Ogle, K. N. (1950). *Researches in binocular vision.* Philadelphia, PA: W. B. Saunders Company.

21. O'Dell, M. W., Bell, K. R., & Sandel, M. E. (1998). 1998 study guide: brain injury rehabilitation. Medical rehabilitation of brain injury. *Archives of Physical Medicine and Rehabilitation, 79* (Suppl. 1), 510–515.

22. Ciuffreda, K. J., Ludlam, D. P., & Kapoor, N. (2009). Clinical oculomotor training in traumatic brain injury. *Optometry & Vision Development, 40,* 16–23.

23. Ciuffreda, K. J., Rutner, D., Kapoor, N., Suchoff, I. B., Craig, S., & Han, M. E. (2008). Vision therapy for oculomotor dysfunctions in acquired brain injury. *Optometry, 79,* 18–22.

24. Kapoor, N., & Ciuffreda, K. J. (2002). Vision disturbances following traumatic brain injury. *Current Treatment Options in Neurology, 4,* 271–280.

25. Bremmer, B., Schlack, A., Duhamel, J. R., Graf, W., & Fink, G. R. (2001). Space coding in primate posterior parietal cortex. *Neuroimage, 14,* S46–S51.

26. Luaute, J., Michel, C., Rode, G., Pisella, L., Jacquin-Courtois, S., Costes, N., Rossetti, Y. (2006). Functional anatomy of the therapeutic effects of prism adaptation of left neglect. *Neurology, 66,* 1859–1867.

27. Massucci, M. E. (2009). Prism adaptation in the rehabilitation of patients with unilateral spatial inattention. *Journal of Behavioral Optometry, 20,* 101–105.

28. Luaute J., Schwartz, S., Rossetti, Y., Spiridon, M., Rode, G., Boisson, D., & Vuilleumier, P. (2009). Dynamic changes in brain activity during prism adaptation. *Journal of Neuroscience, 29,* 169–178.

29. Werner, H., Wapner, S., & Bruell, J. H. (1953). Experiments on sensory-tonic field theory of perception: effect of position of head, eyes, and of object on position of the apparent median plane. *Journal of Experimental Psychology, 46,* 293–299.

30. Welch, R. B. (1978). *Perceptual modification: Adapting to altered sensory environments*. New York, NY: Academic Press.
31. Valenti, C. A. (1996). Exploring a new technique to assess spatial localization. In A. Barber (Ed.), *Tools of behavioral vision care: Prisms* (pp. 52–73). Santa Ana, CA: Optometric Extension Program Foundation.
32. Rossetti, Y., Rode, G., Pisella, L., Farne, A., Li, L., Boisson, D., & Perenin, M. T. (1998). Prism adaptation to a rightward optical deviation rehabilitates left hemispatial neglect. *Nature, 395,* 166–169.
33. Keith, P. S. (1996). Prism lenses: an interview with an optometrist and a physical therapist. In A. Barber (Ed.), *Tools of behavioral vision care: Prisms* (pp. 33–49). Santa Ana, CA: Optometric Extension Program Foundation.
34. Gizzi, M., Khattar, V., & Eckert, A. (1997). A quantitative study of postural shifts induced by yoked prisms. *Optometry & Vision Development, 28,* 200–203.
35. Weiss, N. J., & Brown, W. L. (1995). Uses of prism in low vision. In S. A. Cotter (Ed.), *Clinical uses of prism—a spectrum of applications* (pp. 279–299). St. Louis, MO: Mosby.

7 The Use of Lenses to Improve Quality of Life Following Brain Injury

Paul A. Harris

CONTENTS

It's not what a lens does to a person but what a person does with a lens.

(Kraskin 2002, p. 83)[1]

INTRODUCTION

Lenses are one of the many tools that may be used in helping a person with traumatic (TBI) or other acquired brain injury (ABI). Lenses can be used in many different ways such as to compensate for a loss, to treat a problem, to reduce effort, or to improve the efficiency of the visual interactions the person has with the things they choose to involve themselves in. Examples of conditions that often benefit from or require lenses are neglect, hemianopsia, and posttraumatic strabismus. "Lenses" in this context is being used as a general term inclusive of concave and convex spheres, astigmatic, prisms, filters, diffusers, and those lenses fit to address aniseikonia. This chapter will concentrate on the use of prisms in its many forms for aiding patients who have had brain injury as (1) the subject of prisms itself is rather large, (2) there are many other sources of information on how to prescribe standard ophthalmic lenses clinically, and (3) the majority of special modifications of lens application in the cases of brain injury involve ocular motor issues, which require the use of prisms in ways that generally do not arise in the neurotypical population. It is important to note, however, that many of the principles that are discussed in the context of prescribing prisms may be applied to prescribing all lenses for all members of the human race.

    Prisms may be used monocularly or binocularly. Prisms may be used pointing in various directions; *yoked*, with both bases in the same direction; *nonyoked complementary*, which encompasses the standard base in and base out pairs or with a base up in front of one eye and a base down in front of the other; or *nonyoked irregular,* where the bases may point in directions that are not complementary to each other nor are they the same. An example of this might be where a prism is applied with the base pointed at one angle relative to the horizon in front of one eye and at some different angle in front of the other eye. Prisms may be used over the entire field of view in front of one or both eyes and they may be used only over a sector or portion of one or both eyes. Prisms may be incorporated into the design of the fabricated lens by being ground in or achieved by lens decentration. Prisms may be applied to one of the surfaces of the spectacles in Fresnel form or in the application of a piece of prism that is glued or fused with the carrier lenses. Knowing which cases may benefit from prism and which application of prism to probe with and ultimately which to prescribe in both amount and duration is the goal of this chapter.

TRADITIONAL VIEW OF PRISMS

From classical optics courses one learns that a prism is a wedge of refractive material that shifts the primary or chief ray of light that traverses the prism 1 cm/prism diopter for every meter traveled away from the prism. This chief ray is shifted toward the base (see Figure 7.1). The greater the power of the prism, the more the chief ray is shifted. This is accomplished by either increasing the apex angle of the prism or by making the prism of a medium that has a higher index of refraction.

A person viewing an object through a prism will notice a displacement of the object toward the apex of the prism. The greater the power of the prism the greater the displacement of the chief ray when looking at the pathways of light and greater the displacement of the apparent position of the object when looking at an object through the prism in reference to where it would be seen without the prism in the line of sight.

If this were all that prisms did, both, to the light rays that traverse them and to the perception of the people that look through them, then the application of prisms in clinical practice would certainly be much simpler than it has proven to be.

CHROMATIC ABERRATION

When white light passes through a prism the light is broken down into the color spectrum because different wavelengths of light are slowed down different amounts in the medium (see Figures 7.2A and 7.2B). The greater the amount of prism, the greater the chromatic aberration produced. Some people are very demanding in

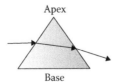

Apex

Base

FIGURE 7.1 A typical wedge prism showing one possible pathway for the light that is deviated toward the base.

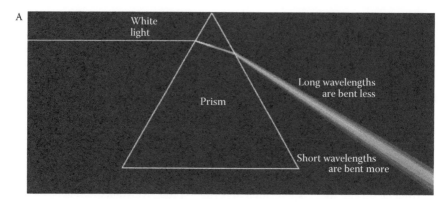

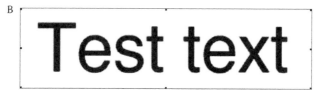

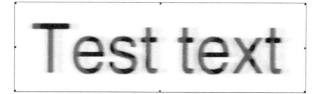

FIGURE 7.2   (See color insert following page 270.) A: This figure shows white light being broken down into the spectrum by a prism. B: This is a demonstration of how high-contrast, square-wave, black on white text looks after passing through a prism. There is an apparent doubling with a ghost yellow image to the right and a "blurring" effect, which is produced by a blue color fringe to the left of the core of the letter and with a red fringe to the right of the black letter.

terms of clarity, contrast, and detail, and if this chromatic aberration becomes significant, they will choose diplopia or a patch over the use of the prisms.

The Abbe number is used to describe the dispersion properties of a lens. It is the ratio of the angle of deflection to the mean dispersion angle. A low Abbe number indicates a high level of dispersion. The Abbe number should not be lower than 30 to ensure that color fringes do not impair peripheral vision.

Figure 7.3 shows the relationship between the Abbe number on the left-hand side of the graph and the index of refraction along the bottom of the graph.

Lower index of refraction media has a higher Abbe number and therefore creates less color fringes than high index of refraction media. However, it takes much more of the lower index of refraction media to bend the light to the same degree and

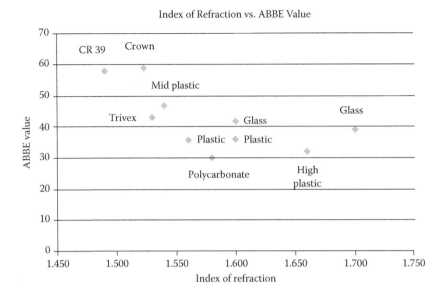

FIGURE 7.3 This figure shows a plot of the Abbe number on the vertical axis and the index of refraction of a number of currently available and in-use materials along the horizontal axis. The higher the Abbe number, the lower the chromatic aberration present.

therefore to produce the same power prism. In general, a thicker lens is heavier. One consideration in prescribing prisms is to keep in mind the trade off between weight, color dispersion, and image quality. A thin pair of lenses made from a high index of refraction material is generally going to have more color fringes.

ARE PRISMS MORE THAN CHIEF RAY SHIFTERS?

So far only the chief ray has been given consideration. Once we begin to look beyond the chief ray we get to see more of the complex modifications or transformations that prisms produce. One of the most difficult things in working with prisms and people who have ABI is in identifying which of these many different transformations will be the ones that the patient before you will react to. In addition, they may react differently to the same lens in different lighting conditions or in different postures. To understand the clinical responses people make to these lenses, on both a conscious and subconscious basis, it is important to have as much knowledge as possible about both the transformations that prisms make to the light and the varied way our brain and mind interpret these changes. Then and only then will we have an understanding of how to use this powerful clinical tool to the maximum benefit of our patients.

DISTORTION

Prisms cause a distortion of the light. The word "distortion" takes on several meanings in clinical practice. One meaning of *distortion* might be the nonlinear transformations introduced into the image as it passes through a nonuniform medium. This

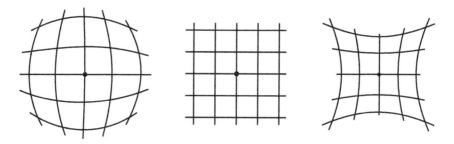

FIGURE 7.4   Compared to the reference pattern in the center, the right pattern shows the type of distortion one would see from a minus sphere lens, and the left pattern shows the type of distortion one would see from a plus sphere lens.

would be similar to the changes seen when polycarbonate lenses are made slightly too large and inserted into a heavy gauge metal frame and the lens wire is overtightened. Nonlinear transformations take place that are seen as waviness similar to the metamorphopsia seen in some early forms of macular degeneration. This is *not* the type of distortion typical of prisms, though prisms made of nonuniform media could certainly produce these types of nonlinear transformations.

Rather "distortion" when used in reference to a prism is used in a manner consistent within the field of geometric optics. The Seidel Sums relate to the five monochromatic aberrations of optical systems. Jenkins and White (1976) state, "No optical system can be made to satisfy all these conditions at once. Therefore it is customary to treat each sum separately, and the vanishing of certain ones corresponds to the absence of certain aberrations" (p. 151).[2] If a lens is manufactured so that the first Seidel Sum is equal to zero, then the lens has no spherical aberration. If both Seidel Sum's one and two are both zero then the lens has no spherical aberration and it has no coma. In the case where the first four Seidel Sums are all zero then the lens would be free of astigmatism and curvature of field. Finally, it takes a lens where all five of the Seidel Sums are zero to eliminate distortion. "To be free of distortion a system must have uniform lateral magnification over its entire field" (p. 318).[3] The types of distortion are the familiar barrel and pincushion distortions as shown in Figure 7.4. These diagrams are the type seen with spherical lenses.

PRISMS BEND SPACE

"A wedge prism has the effect of curving the retinal image of all straight lines that are parallel to the base of the prism. The reason for this is that the angle of incidence of the rays of light from the ends of the line to the prism is greater than the angle of incidence of the rays of light from the center of the line. The greater the angle of incidence, the greater is the refractory displacement effect of the prism" (p. 318).[3] When one looks through a prism held with its base to the right or to the left and looks at a vertical line on the other side of the prism, the vertical line appears curved. This apparent bending of space is a result of the distortion (see Figure 7.5).

Figure 7.6, from Kaufman,[4] helps to give some insight into how a regular grid that is perpendicular to the line of sight of the observer looking either through one eye

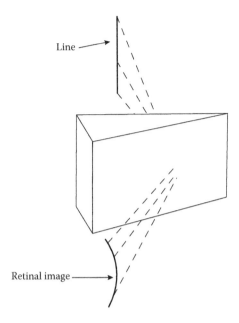

Line

Retinal image

FIGURE 7.5 The vertical line at the top of the picture is in object space. The curved line results from the distortion of the prism and sends a curved line into the eye rather than a straight line. (From Rock, I., *An Introduction to Perception*, Macmillan Publishing, New York, 1975, p. 320. Reproduced by permission of Pearson Education, Inc.)

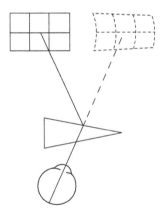

FIGURE 7.6 This figure requires some visualization to understand. The lower section of the diagram is to be seen from above or in aerial view. However, from that view the pattern and its projection would appear as only a line. The reference pattern at the top of the picture is a frontal view with the figure at the left being the actual "test pattern" or grid that is viewed by the person and the dashed line from the prism goes to a projection of the reference pattern that the person would project out into space. This shows the curvature of each of the vertical lines that result from distortion plus the compressions and expansions through the base and apices. (From Kaufman, L., *Sight and Mind, An Introduction to Visual Perception,* Oxford University Press, New York, 1974, p. 414. By permission of Oxford University Press.)

with a base left prism or looking through yoked prisms with bases both pointing left and with equal amounts of prism would be perceived.

Notice in Figure 7.6 that in the image on the right there is an additional transformation that has yet to be discussed. Each of the four vertical lines has been curved, convex side pointing to the right. However, each of the newly produced arcs is not of the same height. The right most arc, the one closest to the apex, is slightly shorter vertically than the one to the left, and as you proceed to the left each of the arcs is slightly bigger vertically.

Under some conditions of observation, people will report seeing the transformed image this way but still in the frontal plane, meaning they see it with the right and left edges the same distance away from them. However, others interpret this image rather as a version of the left hand original object but now rotated in space about a vertical axis through the center of the object. The right side of the transformed image is vertically shorter than the left side. By using size constancy and by seeing the object as the same size as it was before the transformation, the object is now seen as rotated with the right side further away from the observer and the left side brought closer to the observer by a complementary amount. It helps to see this spatial rotation if the grid that is observed is truly a separate object in front of the background. Simply viewing a grid that is tacked to a wall or viewing a grid-like pattern that is part of the wallpaper causes most people to see the curves of the vertical lines and the spatial variations in the heights of the vertical crosspieces. Move an object with the same pattern off the wall, and often now what is perceived is the rotation of the object in space with the portion toward the apex shifted away from the observer and the section through the base being seen as shifted closer to the observer.

Earlier in his book, Rock deals with our ability to adapt to the primary shift in location in space induced by prisms. He wondered if people would easily adapt to this curvature. Do people straighten out the curved appearance of things that we knew were straight, such as doorframes on the same time scale as we adapt to the past pointing that occurs with prisms? There is some adaptation but it is very small and it does not last very long. The differential adaptations to curvature versus displacement most likely demonstrate that different brain centers are involved with each and that there may be different underlying perceptual mechanisms that rely on or use these observations. If indeed the processing of this information is done in different areas of the brain, this may serve as the basis for why some patients react one way to a lens and other patients react in an opposite way to the same lens.

DUAL STREAMS AN EXPLANATION?

Goodale and Milner[5] discuss the separation of the visual pathways for functional reasons:

> Visual perception is there to let us make sense of the outside world and to create representations of it in a form that can be filed away for future reference. In contrast, the control of a motor act requires accurate information about the actual size, location, and motion of the target object. This information has to be coded in the absolute metrics of the real world. The dorsal stream works in real time and stores the required visuomotor coordinates only

for a very brief period—at most for a few hundred milliseconds. The ventral stream, on the other hand, is designed to operate over a much longer time scale. The use of scene-based metrics means that the brain can construct this representation in great detail without having to compute the absolute size, distance and geometry of each object in the scene. (p. 73)

They make a compelling case for two separate but dependent parts of the visual process. The one we are aware of and the one that we respond to consciously when describing visual events or putting into words how it feels to look at this or that does not use absolute metrics but only computes spatial relationships in a relational way. This object is closer than that but the absolute amount is not easily available to our conscious processes. To calculate all spatial relationships on an absolute basis would take so much computation power that we might not make the decision to avoid the oncoming car fast enough. Since the visual perception system, the part of our visual process we are conscious of, is used primarily to identify goals for the movement and manipulation systems to act on, we leave it to the action system to work out the metrics for those movements. In this way, the absolute metrics only need to be calculated for a few objects at any one time. "The visuomotor system is largely isolated from perception. Its modus operandi seems to be to disregard information from much of the scene when guiding goal-directed movements like grasping, restricting itself to the critical visual information that is required for that movement" (p. 88).[5]

This isolation of the visuomotor system from visual perception may be the basis for why there is selective adaptation to various aspects of the spatial transformations created by prisms. It will be for future research to help us more fully understand this phenomenon.

NOT ALL CURVATURES OF SPACE ARE THE SAME

A real curved rod in space will be projected differently on our retinas as we move through space (Figure 7.7A).

A straight line viewed through a prism is different. Rock states, "When a straight line is seen through a prism, its retinal image is curved, but the curvature of this image never changes as we change our position in relation to the line...So the fact that the image does not transform as we move around a rod is potential information that the rod is a straight one. We do not know if the perceptual system makes use of such information" (p. 318).[4]

A result of these effects that many of us see regularly in the vision therapy room is the curvature of the walking rail with lateral yoked prisms (Figure 7.7B). Here the bases are both base left. Generally, one needs the power to be 5 diopters or more to see this effect. Some people can see it at lower powers than this. At 10 diopters nearly everyone will see the curvature of the walking rail or a straight line on the floor in front of them.

One reason that there is less adaptation to the curvature may be that this is critical information for us in deciding if the object being viewed is indeed straight or curved. Rock speculates that it may be the flow of the images over the retina through time as we move relative to the object that gives us the ability to differentiate straight from curved. Figure 7.7C shows these movements attribute as it would overlay the image of the object. Movement and object recognition are processed in different parts of the brain.

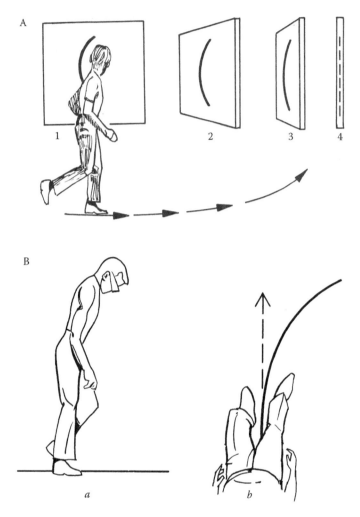

FIGURE 7.7　A: Projection of a curved rod onto the retina from four perspectives as a person moves around it. In this case, moving counterclockwise around the rod, at 90 degrees from the starting point the rod appears to open up and to have less and less curvature until it is viewed on edge and appears to be just a straight line. (From Rock, I., *An Introduction to Perception*, Macmillan Publishing, New York, 1975, p. 321. Reproduced by permission of Pearson Education, Inc.) B: The subject here is wearing base left yoked prisms. The line that is a straight line on the floor appears to be curved toward the subject's right. (From Rock, I., *An Introduction to Perception*, Macmillan Publishing, New York, 1975, p. 322. Reproduced by permission of Pearson Education, Inc.) C: Here Rock shows how a real curved line and a straight line that has a curved retinal projection are differentiated. In the case of the truly curved line, each part will move parallel to each other part of the line as an observer moves relative to that line. In the case of the straight line with the curved retinal projection, the movements will be along the length of the line. (From Rock, I., *An Introduction to Perception*, Macmillan Publishing, New York, 1975, p. 323. Reproduced by permission of Pearson Education, Inc.)

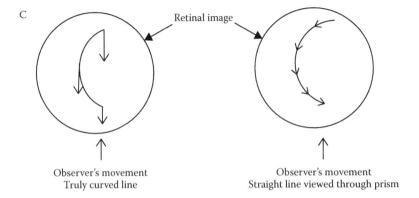

FIGURE 7.7   Continued.

THE SPACE BOARD TO THE RESCUE

It was left to the profession of optometry to find ways to understand the true nature of how prisms act as spatial transformers. In the late 1980s, Claude Valenti, an optometrist from La Jolla, CA, demonstrated a simple device used to demonstrate the manner and degree that people misperceive the location of objects in space. C. A. Valenti (personal communication, January 1986) stated that the inspiration for developing his method came from another optometrist, John Streff, who had demonstrated a procedure he called "touch points." In the touch point procedure, the practitioner holds a finger vertically in front of the patient from above with the finger pointed down at the floor. The finger is normally placed at eye level although this can be varied. The patient is told to look directly at the finger and then, in a single, fast, ballistic type of movement, move one hand upward to allow the index finger on that hand to attempt to touch the finger of the examiner. It is important that the patient not slow down and adjust after beginning the movement, as the examiner is looking for slight misalignments as the finger approaches the stationary target finger. The misalignments were read as misjudgments of space.

Valenti's original procedure was modified extensively by Paul Harris. An early version of the space board was a thin board mounted on a structure that allows the height of the instrument to be shifted up and down to match the height of the patient. The board projects horizontally from the wall. There is a small cutout on one side for the patient to put their nose into, assuring that the patient remains properly aligned during testing. The patient looks across the board and out into open space rather than at the wall (Figure 7.8). Seven small-headed pushpins are placed on the top of the board. The numbers next to the "•'s," which show the relative position of the pins, show the recommended order of testing.

A piece of paper is attached to the underside of the board, premarked with the actual pin placements. When the paper is properly attached underneath the board, the markings are directly below the pins that are on the top of the board. The patient is then given a marker to hold in both hands (Figure 7.9). She cannot see the marker. She stands on both feet, with equal weight on each foot, and with her knees slightly

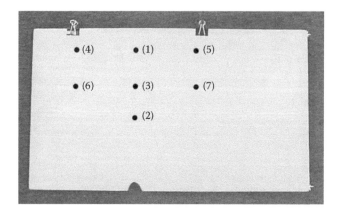

FIGURE 7.8 This shows the pattern of the pins on the top of the actual space board. The patients stand with their nose in the small cutout at the bottom of the picture. The single pin is closest to the nose and is directly in front of the patient. The pins all fit within the boundary of an 11" × 17" piece of paper. The right side of the board is attached to the wall so that the patient is looking out into the room rather than into the wall. The numbers next to each pin show the order of testing. The first points are all on the midline. Then the points alternate sides. This is done to reduce the influence that one sideways movement might shift all subsequent marks to one side.

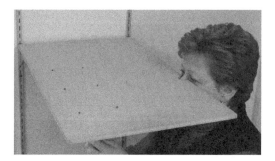

FIGURE 7.9 This shows the space board in use. The patient's nose is in a small cutout that is directly lined up with the centerline of pins. The recording paper is held onto the bottom of the board such that the marks on the paper line up directly with the pins. The patient performs the marking bilaterally with both hands clasped together around the marking pen.

bent. She looks first at the pin on the midline furthest away from her. She is asked to bring the marker up from below and touch where she sees the pin to be. She is directing action in space to where she is looking. This is a very basic request of the person and their visual process. The sequence of how the pins are looked at and marked can be seen in Figure 7.8.

Figures 7.10, 7.11, 7.12, and 7.13 are a series of drawings by actual patients; the legends describe each type of topological transformation seen in each situation. Because the paper is on the bottom and is turned over to read the results,

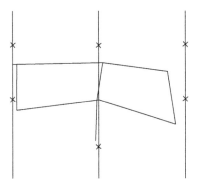

FIGURE 7.10 Note with this patient that the middle point is almost exactly on target. If this happened to correspond to the point where a phoria measure was taken it would show very good alignment. However, note how the other points are shifted in different directions, with some closer and some farther away.

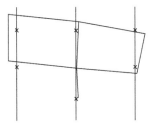

FIGURE 7.11 Once again this patient has the middle point almost exactly on target. However, notice how the markings on one side are shifted inward, toward the person, and on the opposite site the pins are shifted outward, away from the patient. This patient happened to be a competitive equestrian rider. She complained about her horse having difficulties with the turns, turning too sharply one way and too wide the other. How surprised she was to find that the problem was hers and not that of the horse!

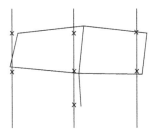

FIGURE 7.12 This patient shows six of the seven marks being displaced to one side. In cases like this, one often sees an asymmetry in movement and in motor performances such as those involved in sports. Yoked prisms are often investigated as a possible treatment option when this kind of shift is demonstrated.

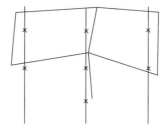

FIGURE 7.13 In this final example, the patient lost her left eye in a riding accident while on a horse. This drawing was done by her, using light input from her intact right eye. The space board can help give insights into a person's spatial perception when a standard phoria type of measure cannot be taken, since phorias require two eyes.

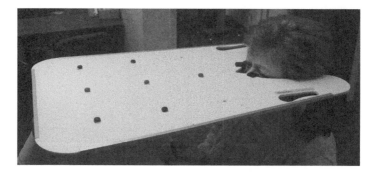

FIGURE 7.14 The VTE space board.

right and left are reversed. The diagrams here have been flipped over for ease in explanation and interpretation. To help the reader see the patterns on each of the figures, lines have been drawn to connect the actual data points of the patient. If the patient touched exactly at each of the pin points, the lines drawn would connect each of the Xs. When the line does not touch the corresponding X, there was a mismatch between the actual position of the object in space and the perceived position of the object.

Figure 7.14 is the Space Board made by VTE (the Italian vision therapy equipment manufacturer) that is distributed in the United States by Bernell Corporation. This device has greatly simplified space board measurements.

To this point, the figures shown on the space board have all been done with the person's habitual prescription on. Figure 7.15 shows the spatial transformation that occurs when yoked prisms are used. The test was done three times: the first with habitual lenses on and then the next two with 5-diopter yoked prisms on, one set bases right and the other set bases left. The first few times this was done, it helped to fully dispel the simple view of a prism as a chief ray deflector and helped the author fully understand prisms as space transformers.

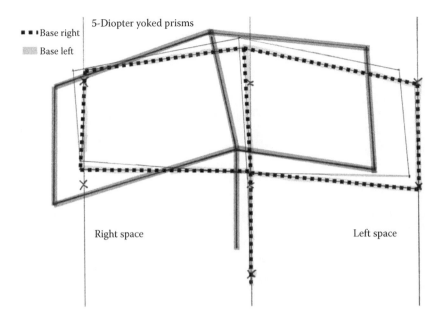

FIGURE 7.15   Here is a recording of data points done with the same person wearing at first only their habitual glasses followed by trials with 5-diopter yoked prism sets with bases right (dashed line) and bases left (thick gray bar). Remember that this is the recording paper from the underside of the space board, and thus the directions are reversed.

What can be seen here is that there is a shift to the left or right of the points on the midline but there is also a forward and backward shift of the points on either side resulting in a spatial rotation as well as a shift. The side with the base is shifted outward away from the person, while the side toward the apices is shifted inward.

To imagine how vertical yoked prisms work, one has to do some visualization or use visual imagery as to date no such recording device has been made. However, if such a device did exist, the following would be the results. Yoked prism base up and base down pairs of glasses alter the space board results in similar ways. For example; yoked prism base up shifts each point on the space board results downward. However, the lower portion of the recordings would be shifted inward toward the person and the upper points would be shifted outward away from the person. Space in the lower section that is brought toward the person are also relatively more compressed than the upper portion that is shifted outward; however, since the further away parts shift outward faster than the closer areas of space, there is a relative spatial expansion along the Z axis in upper space. With base down yoked prisms, the exact opposite occurs.

CHIEF RAY SHIFTER VERSUS SPACE TRANSFORMER

The information on prisms presented above should help the reader begin to understand that there is more to understanding the response patients make to prisms in clinical settings. In clinical practice, prisms have almost always been viewed as chief ray shifters and have been prescribed to shift images from one place in space to another. Many of those patients who got prisms prescribed on this basis were able to use the lenses successfully. However, some had varying degrees of difficulty in learning to use the prisms. Some of those patients returned to complain and some simply went on to another eye care professional or chose to live with their visual problem and to stop seeking visual care.

The chief ray shifting effect of the prisms cannot be separated from the spatial transformations of the prisms. In many instances, the benefits of the prescribed prisms may result more from the spatial transformation than from the image shift. A number of clinicians over the years have advocated an approach to using very small amounts of prism to affect significant change in how a person uses their visual process to interact with the world. Some of the performance differences in patients aided by these small amounts of prisms have been out of proportion to the small amount of image shifting. Without a way to explain the large changes in behavior secondary to the small amount of prism used, some have resorted to explanations that border on mysticism or magic to explain their results. Once one shifts away from thinking exclusively of the prism as a chief ray shifter and begins to include the notion of a prism as a spatial transformer, then the potentials of even small amounts of prisms to greatly alter human behavior shifts from the unexplainable to something with a solid basis for understanding.

The implications are that our probes of human behavior as well as clinical thinking will need to go beyond chief ray shifting. These new insights point out that those tests such as phorias, associated phorias, and fixation disparities, which concentrate so heavily on deriving the exact amount of chief ray shifting needed to bring about alignment, may be far less relevant in many patients as sound ways from which to derive treatment options than is thought by some. A new series of probes will need to enter the clinical domain to help gain insight into those with unmet needs who may require the spatial transformation effects of prisms.

NOMENCLATURE

One thing that is certain is that as a clinical profession, optometry will need to develop a standard nomenclature that goes with a standardized series of tests that can encapsulate these spatial shifts, both those made by the lenses to the light and those perceived by subjects, for easy recording of our observations and for communicating with our colleagues and other professions. At this point in time we are reduced to relatively long narratives to describe what we observe. For the newly initiated into the field, many of these observations go unseen secondary to a lack of knowledge that such transformations may be present.

LENS AND PRISM CLASSIFICATION

Over the years the profession of optometry has evolved its use of terms to help communications. Terms such as *compensatory, treatment, directive, disruptive,* and others have been used to describe various uses of prisms. One difficulty in working with these terms is that at some level we would like the categories denoted by these modifiers to be discrete entities with little overlap from category to category. When taught or discussed in various forums, each is taken in turn as if they are mutually exclusive methodologies with little or no overlap in use, purpose, or operational changes. In truth, each category may overlap to a high degree with the others and there may be very little that allows an objective categorization of specific treatment options with specific patients and specific times in their clinical care.

For the purpose of our discussion, we might use the following definitions of *compensatory* and *treatment* as modifiers for prisms or lenses:

1. *Compensatory*—the lens that allows the person to function better with their asymmetry.
2. *Treatment*—any lens other than the compensatory lens, usually prescribed on a basis other than clarity, or in the case of prisms, a lens other than that which matches exactly the misalignment measured.

As with many other aspects of the recovery from an ABI, often a treatment modality may be hard to classify, and over time the manner in which such a treatment may be useful to a person may evolve from one type to another. As an example, a compensatory lens may be used early on during the early phases of a sixth nerve palsy. The patient may present wearing a patch, with a face turn, covering or closing their eye or with complaints of double vision that they are simply choosing to ignore. A Fresnel prism may be applied to allow for use of the flow through both channels simultaneously.

In one instance, the clinician may choose to fully compensate for the entire amount of turn measured. This would allow the minimum of effort on the part of the patient and may allow a more normal use of the binocular flow. This might be the treatment option of choice and might be considered purely *compensatory*. However, it might be precisely what is wanted and needed at a particular point in a person's recovery. For example, a person might have multiple other issues going on concurrently, and the choice is to aid binocular flow as much as possible and to allow the person to address other health/life concerns before working to reduce dependency on the prism. On the surface, this use of the prism might be thought of as being purely compensatory in nature, almost by definition. However, even in this instance one could say that some portion of this lens is certainly helping to treat the underlying problem, making the future treatment of the problem easier by allowing for the continued use of the binocular flow without the need for extended occlusion of the flow from one of the eyes. For a turn that measures 35 prism diopters in primary gaze, a 35-diopter Fresnel may allow for fusion in primary gaze without the need for a face turn to achieve this fusion.

In this same patient, the clinical decision might be to provide the minimum prism necessary to establish binocular flow, allowing for some conscious effort and some face turn to be used by the person to maintain use of the binocular flow. The actual amount of prism may be only slightly less than the amount that would fully compensate for the palsy. As little as 3–5 prism diopters less than full compensatory power could be thought of now as a treatment lens, since it is setting the stage for a potential resolution of the problem by leading the system toward a new posture at some time in the future. In the above patient, a 30-diopter Fresnel prism could be used initially to restore the use of the binocular flow with some face turn and some effort.

Thus, initially one might classify the 35-diopter prism as "compensatory" and the 30-diopter prism as a "treatment" lens. It should be recognized that some portion of both of those lenses is aiding in reestablishing the use of the flow through both channels and that there is more a difference in degree than there is a substantial difference in type. Interestingly, over time the expectation is for the person wearing the 30-diopter prism to adapt to this prism amount so that at a future date this level of prism may be just right for primary gaze and if left on too long may actually cause problems. So, over time a prism fit with guidance, development, or adaptation in mind may take on a different role, and to remain effective as a stimulus for change may need to be changed. In fact, for this patient there is a high expectation that the prism will need to be changed; failure of the patient to adapt and need such a reduction would be more cause for concern.

LENS TYPES: STABILIZATION—GUIDANCE

Thus, it may be easier to classify prism types by what they are designed to do rather than how the measurements relate. We may think of lenses that are prescribed to stabilize a patients' condition. Such a *stabilization* lens would be prescribed in light of a long-term view that sees the patient remaining with the same degree of physical or neurological deficit in both the short and long term. The *stabilization* lens would have the goal of allowing the person to use their binocular system as it is today with maximum effectiveness and efficiency and to reinforce the current patterns of use to embed this posture.

A *guidance* lens would be one prescribed with the desire of shifting the posture* to some different status in the future. The shift may be accomplished with varying amounts of prism and in some cases even with prisms with their bases in the exact opposite directions to each other. To clarify: in one instance a set of three prisms all in the same direction but of different amounts may relate to a particular person such that one might stabilize the posture over time, another might help guide the posture toward less dependence on the use of the prism, while the third may build in a greater dependence on prisms in the future. In this instance all prism bases could be in the same direction.

However, in some situations the key factor might be the direction of the base of the prism. Here, a prism in one direction of a certain power might be the stabilization lens. A prism with the base in the opposite direction may cause some people to alter their use of the binocular flow in such a way that after a given period of time their need for the prism in any form is reduced or eliminated. Such an opposite-direction-base prism may not be useable by some people. However, in others this approach to the use of prism may be exactly what they will benefit from most. This option is most likely not available for everyone at all points in time. Often this type of lens will increase the visual stress a person is under and concurrently their overall stress levels would be increased by such a treatment modality. In most instances of patients recovering from an ABI their energy reserves are needed to recover essential functions (e.g., consciousness, speech, attention, swallowing, etc.), and this idea of increasing local and general stress using an opposite-direction-base prism is not recommended. However, as the patient recovers

---

* Note: *posture* here is being used intentionally in at least two ways. One way refers to the posture of the eyes relative to one another and the second is the posture of the person's body as they engage in performing various tasks.

essential functions and rises up through the various levels of recovery, such a lens at a critical point in time may be just what is needed to help the person let go of a particular compensatory strategy and to find a new way of using their visual process. A prism used in this way might be compared to processes that set the stage for an "Aa-ha" effect or a paradigm shift; the emergence of a new organization, new posture, or new use of self, which is different in type and not just a shifted form of a prior mode.

Figure 7.16 shows how relative eye alignment is radically altered following a stroke. The diagram is intentionally ambiguous in that the misalignment could be in any direction away from a prior frame of reference. Once at the new position, three possible future paths showing different eye alignments over time are shown moving to the right. Figure 7.17 shows a close up of the small point from which the

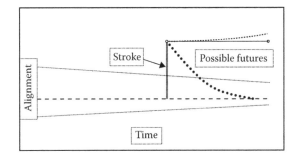

FIGURE 7.16 This figure shows the alignment of the eyes over time. The center dashed line would be absolute alignment with the flanking dotted lines showing tolerance ranges throughout which actual alignment can take place. The vertical double line represents the time when an event takes place, in this example a stroke, which shifts the actual alignment of the eyes. Three lines of possible futures are shown emerging from this new point. The dotted line slopes down during the patient's recovery and alignment returns to its prior condition over time. The upper most dashed line shows degradation over time beginning rather slowly and increasing over time. The thin line that goes horizontally to the right from the new post-stroke position shows absolute stabilization from this point in time.

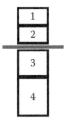

FIGURE 7.17 This is a highly magnified view of the point in Figure 7.16 at the top part of the double vertical line, which depicts the stroke event. This new position is outside of the person's ability to align their binocular system without assistance. The boxes were drawn in different sizes to remind the reader of the nonlinearity we are dealing with in the visual process. Options 1 and 2 represent prism in excess of the measured deviation and options 3 and 4 are options with less prism use than the exact measurement of the new deviation, which is represented by the center line.

new futures emerge. The horizontal line between areas 2 and 3 shows the new measured misalignment, which is well outside of the range within which the person can compensate for. This figure shows four regions about the new alignment position that vary in size. Zones 1 and 2 are on the side of the new alignment area that lies on the side away from the prestroke condition. Zones 3 and 4 are on the side toward the former prestroke alignment. In zone 1 the patient would have prism in place that is more than the measured amount of the red line deviation and would require some degree of face turn to compensate for this excessive amount of prism. However, as long as the amount of prism is in zone 1, the person can compensate for it with a face turn and without suppression or having to block or cover one eye. In zone 2 the person would be wearing more prism than is measured but no face turn is noted. In zone 3 the person would be wearing less prism than is measured and no face turn is noted. In zone 4 the person would be wearing less prism than is measured but some face turn is required to compensate and allow for fusion. Any prism amount that puts the patient above zone 1 or below zone 4 results in no establishment of binocular flow.

ABSOLUTES AND UNIVERSALS

A word about the use of universals or absolute statements is in order. In much of the literature that addresses the use of prisms there exist statements such as, "In condition X the prism must be placed in direction Y." The exact form of the statement may be different but the message is that there is but one way to apply the prism for this condition. Some authors have had different clinical experiences with certain conditions and have come to different conclusions that one type of lens is right, while another method or application of a prism is wrong. It is important for the reader to recognize these absolute directives and take them as a genuine observation of the writer that may, under certain conditions of observation, be different and therefore not hold as an absolute. The visual process is an extremely complex process. The underlying control mechanisms for ocular motor control are also extremely complex. There are multiple different types of neurological insult that can lead to similar looking clinical entities. Until one tries an actual potential treatment on an individual, one cannot know what will work best for that person. In many instances studies that average the results over a large number of subjects may lose the variations that are present in such populations. Not all brain injuries are the same; in fact one could say that this might be the best universal: No two brain injuries are exactly the same. Therefore, we need to probe each patient as an individual and evaluate what we see anew each time.

SPATIAL MAPS—MULTIPLE REPRESENTATIONS

When working with patients who have sustained head trauma it is important to have an understanding of the complexity and diversity of spatial maps that can be found in the brain that are used in various situations by the person to solve real-world problems. The idea of there being a homunculus and there being a single site in the brain where a three-dimensional holographic type of map with the person at the origin pervades much of the early thought on the visual process. From that point of view the primary purpose of the visual process is to help assemble this view of the world, and impairments could be seen as blockages that would lead to incomplete assembly or distortions, which lead to inaccurate representations of reality. The basis of this type of thinking was that there was a single view of reality that was represented within the person that matched in some way consciousness.

As mentioned above, Milner and Goodale found that there are at least two different metrics used by the dorsal and ventral streams with the latter being only relative in nature and the former being absolute for just the few objects that are about to be acted upon. Even this, however, is a great simplification. The implication of the Milner and Goodale work is that both systems are egocentric and refer to the person at the origin. In addition to these egocentric maps there are many additional spatial maps with different origins or reference points that are used by the person for an array of different purposes that we are just beginning to learn about. A few will be highlighted here simply to form the basis of understanding why, on occasion, very different prisms may be needed to help people with very similar conditions or why the same prism on the same person may have very different effects at different times or under different situations.

Graziano and Gross[6] give us a sense of the different types of spatial maps and spatial encoding used in different parts of the brain. "Space is encoded in different brain structures for different behavioral functions, e.g., premotor cortex (PMv) and the putamen for visuo-motor space; frontal eye fields (FEF), lateral intraparietal sulcus (LIP) and the colliculus for oculomotor space; and the lateral prefrontal cortex for short-term mnemonic space" (p. 126).

Graziano and Gross[6] then discusses the findings of bimodal cells in the putamen. These cells respond maximally when two different types of stimulation are present. A number of such cells that combine visual and tactile responses have been identified and had their visual and tactile receptive fields mapped. What emerged is a sort of linking of the two maps, the area on the skin of the body part being mapped and the area of space around or near to that body part. These shifted dynamically as the body parts were shifted in space and in particular when that body part was about to be used to manipulate something in the environment and during the actual manipulation. The premotor cortex contains many of these visual-tactile bimodal cells.

In an experiment mapping the linkage between the visual and tactile receptive fields in monkeys Graziano and Gross[6] found that as the arm moved, the areas of the visual field that were associated with the arm moved with the arm (Figure 7.18). "When the arm was placed in different locations, the visual receptive fields also changed location, remaining in rough register with the arm. Clearly, this visual receptive field was not fixed to one site on the retina; that is, it was not retinocentric. It was arm-centered, encoding the locations of visual stimuli with respect to the arm. Most bimodal PMv cells with tactile responses on the arm (88% of 42 cells tested) had similar, arm-centered visual receptive fields" (p. 123).[6]

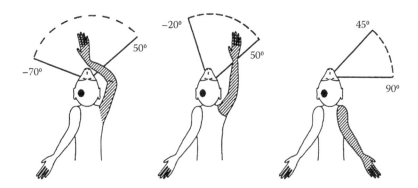

FIGURE 7.18   Bimodal cells were mapped from the left premotor cortex (PMv), designated by the black circle. The tactile receptor fields of the cells are marked by the shaded area on the monkey's right arm. As the arm moves so does the part of the visual field that the PMv cell responds to. The eyes were fixed in the head in a straight-ahead gaze. (From Graziano, M., and Gross, C., *From Eye to Hand*, 3rd Appalachian Conference on Behavioral Neurodynamics, 1995, p. 124, ISBN 0-8058-2178-3 Reprinted with permission.)

What purpose might these cells and the maps they make serve and why is this relevant to our discussion of prisms for head injured patients? "Arm-centered neurons would be useful for hand-eye coordination, guiding the arm toward or away from visual targets. Indeed, a high proportion of neurons in the putamen and PMv are active during reaching. In PMv, the cells are spatially tuned, responding best when the arm reaches into a particular region of space" (p. 124).[6] In a healthy individual, these maps and all the flow of the information needed to keep these maps coordinated and adaptable is intact. In the head injured patient transformations, distortions, loss of information, corrupting of information, and other problems can be introduced by damage at any point in this complex system. Even in cases of similar looking brain scans from similar types of damage, there is still likely to be variations from patient to patient.

SPRAGUE EFFECT

One more very confounding problem when dealing with head injured patients is something called the Sprague effect named after Dr. James Sprague who discovered this in his lab in 1966. He was working with cats with surgically induced lesions of their right visual cortices. He was doing pioneer work on what would later be called *blindsight* though it took Weiskrantz until 1989 to build on this work. Sprague found that the cats at this stage showed no interest in objects in their left visual fields. This is consistent with the condition seen in right side strokes in humans called *neglect*, or *hemi-inattention*. Sprague subsequently lesioned the left superior colliculus (SC) in a few of these cats. After recovery from the procedure the cats now showed interest in objects in their blind field. Thus, the paradoxical observation that a lesion on the opposite side of the brain could cause a function that appeared to be gone to reappear was made. Sprague's explanation for this is that the SC is dependent on excitation from the cortex of the same hemisphere. So in the first condition after the lesion to the right visual cortex, the right SC was not getting excitatory stimulation. Input to the SC is balanced by inhibitory input from the contralateral substantia nigra. When the left SC was surgically destroyed its inhibitory effects were removed from the right SC.[7] The key point here is that many types of head injury include a primary assault with many other secondary effects that occur remote to the primary site, and many of these areas of secondary affect may be below the threshold of today's scanning technology to identify the areas of injury. Thus, until one probes a patient's behavior with lenses, one will not know for certainty how that patient will react. This is very strong support for the statement by Robert A. Kraskin, OD, "It's not what a lens does to a person but what a person does with a lens" (p. 83).[1] As clinicians we must be prepared to look at our patients from different viewpoints and be prepared that in some cases the exact opposite lens will bring about the desired changes.

TYPICAL SPATIAL SHIFTS

Table 7.1 gives the expected canonic responses of healthy subjects either to yoked prisms or to prisms in the same direction when experienced under conditions of monocular viewing. Kraskin[41] states that there is no difference between how a person reacts to a yoked prism versus a prism in front of one eye with the other eye patched. Table 7.1 assumes in all circumstances that both before and after prism application, the person looks at the same object before them.

TABLE 7.1
Canonic Responses to Prisms

Prism Effects	Base Right	Base Left	Base Up	Base Down
Space shift	Right side further away and expanded on the z-axis but compressed on the x-axis Left side closer and compressed on the z-axis but expanded on the x-axis	Right side closer and compressed on the z-axis but expanded on the x-axis Left side further away and expanded on the z-axis but compressed on the x-axis	Above the line of sight shifted further away and expanded Below the line of sight shifted in and compressed	Above the line of sight shifted in and compressed Below the line of sight shifted further away and expanded
Eye movement	Left	Right	Down	Up
Center of gravity shift/ postural change	Shifts right	Shifts left	Shifts back	Shifts forward
Pelvis shift	Rotation right	Rotation left	Upward (front)	Downward (front)

TESTING

ALIGNMENT PROBES

One of the consequences of many ABIs is a change in the balance within the elements of the ocular motor control system, which often lead to various forms of strabismus. We have six ocular motor muscles that move each eye, innervated by a total of three pairs of cranial nerves. Recently, each of the muscles has been found to have two divisions, an ocular portion of the muscle that does the actual work of moving the eye and an orbital part that seems mostly involved with redirecting the force vectors of the ocular portion of the muscle. At first it was thought by Demer[8] that the orbital portion moved actual pulleys to redirect the force of the ocular portion of the muscle. Work by Ruskell and others[9] have shown that Demer's original theory is incomplete at the anatomic level. Rather, Ruskell et al. histologically identified a series of connective tissue and muscle bands that can contract at different places along the axis of the ocular portion of the muscle acting like a pulley system, without there being a single pulley that is shifted forward and backward in the orbit.

The significance of this complexity is that there are many different places for problems to occur from the brain centers involved with planning an eye movement, to the brain centers involved in mapping the movements to be made, to the brain centers responsible for taking the mapped instructions and turning them into specific commands to the individual muscles, to the nerves anywhere along their pathway from the back of the brain to their insertion into the muscles, to problems in the orbit secondary to facial injuries or frank injuries to the muscles themselves.

Thus, there are a myriad of potential causes that could lead to the development of a change in the habitual posture of the two eyes, one relative to each other; strabismus. The clinician needs a battery of probes that can be used to assess the relative positions and paint a clinical picture without which the potential benefits of prisms can be determined. There are many such probes that the clinician may use. The few selected examples presented here are

- Observation
- Cover test: objective and subjective
- Maddox rod testing
- Cheiroscopic tracing
- Fixation disparity (FD) or associate phoria testing

Each will be taken in turn.

Observation

As ocular alignment is so important to understanding the nature of the ABI the clinician is observing eye alignment informally during most of the time they are engaged with the patient. Observation of the eye alignment is often one of the first things that make an impression on the optometrist along with, certainly, mobility issues and any gross asymmetries in posture. When ocular alignment issues are revealed early in the testing, observation would include a number of different qualities and quantities that are summed over the encounter with the patient. It is as if the recognition by the clinician that there is a problem here opens the door to them spending time evaluating ocular alignment before any formal testing begins. These include but are not limited to the following:

- Degree of time the patient makes eye contact.
- Is eye contact made with a face turn, head tilt, or with the chin up or down relative to what in the judgment of the optometrist would be their natural line of sight?
- Do the relative positions of the eyes stay the same during movement and change of posture?
- Do the relative positions of the eyes stay the same or change as the person answers questions or thinks of things to say during the case history?
- Does the person change fixation pattern during this early period looking at the examiner directly with one eye, both eyes, or do they alternate?
- If they alternate, what percentage of time is the person spending with one side as the leader versus the other side?
- If binocular fixation is intermittent, what percentage of the time does the person seem to be aligned versus turned?
- If binocular fixation is intermittent, what kinds of events seem to trigger suspension of binocular alignment and what kinds of events seem to trigger a reestablishment of binocular alignment?

These are just some of the aspects of an ocular motor alignment that can be evaluated informally, but which may yield most of the information needed to know how to proceed probing for treatment alternatives. In many instances the formal probes are only done to confirm or deny the observations made during this informal period of getting to know the patient. It is recognized that the ability to make these informal observations while engaged in what appears to be casual conversation is the mark of an experienced clinician. New practitioners to this field may find that until they have done many hundreds of formal evaluations of ocular motor alignment, gaining insights into the above aspects of binocularity may not come as easily.

Cover Test

It is beyond the scope of this chapter to go into full detail of how to perform a cover test and all of its variations. Suffice it to say that the cover test may be of paramount importance in cases where the patient's language, speech, and motor functions may impair their ability to respond to other probes of ocular alignment that require a response by the patient other than simply looking at a specific location in space.

In working with ABI in cases where prism may be needed as a part of the treatment program, there are several clinical guides that may help gain insight more easily into the patient's condition. The baseline against which to measure the effects of the cover test are the cumulative observations made as indicated above in the section: observation. This is the baseline for all of the factors to be looked at.

It is highly recommended that you use a translucent occluder (Figures 7.19 and 7.20) to give you the best opportunity to see what the patient does with the eye that you cover. Set up whatever target you feel will be the best target to help you gain insight into your patient and begin at whatever testing distance you feel will give

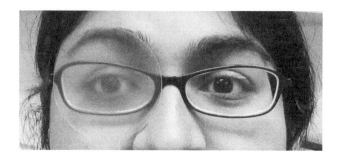

FIGURE 7.19 This shows how easy it is to see the patient's eye behind the translucent occluder.

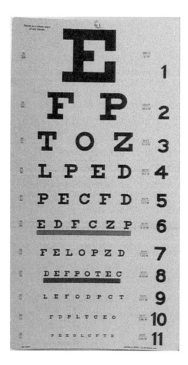

FIGURE 7.20 This shows two views of the same Snellen chart with the one on the right being what is seen through the same translucent occluder used in Figure 7.19. Note how much the image is degraded by the occluder, but how well the clinician can see the eye through it when held close to the patient.

you the greatest insights. In some instances where the visual acuity through one or both channels is 20/80 or worse, the translucent occluder may not be enough of a disturbance to the patients' habitual condition to make the observation meaningful. In these instances you may need to change over to a more conventional opaque occluder.

In most instances cover-uncover should be done first to give you insight into the degree the patient is aligned or how fragile their alignment is. Before introducing the cover the first time, get in position to observe your patient and just watch how they look at the target for a few seconds. Watch to see if they change the way they look or if it stays the same. As you bring in the cover from the side watch to see if there is any change in body posture, facial expression, head position, and of course in the positions of the eyes both relative to each other and relative to the target.

In general, with patients with ABI, it is best to slow down your rhythm of testing and to give the patient time to equilibrate with the new condition before moving to the next step in the testing situation. Thus, you should keep the cover in the covered position for as long as it takes for the person to stabilize in a new posture or to see if in this new condition (with a cover over one side) they continue to alter their posture(s) (body, head, and eyes). It is as if you run through the entire gamut of questions in your mind that are listed in the "observe" section above; maybe not all of the questions but any of the ones that you had made significant notations on. Here is a chance to see if the unilateral cover alters the patterns at all. Equally important would be to get a sense of whether similar changes occur when the cover is over the right eye and when it is over the left eye or if some of the changes only occur when one side is covered. These observations may be more important in the end than the actual measure of the angle of eye turn.

Once you feel that you have received as many insights as the cover-uncover will give you, move on to sustained alternate cover. In the cover-uncover test you give the patient a chance to restore their habitual pattern of looking in between disruptions. In the alternate cover, you continue your disruption unabated and new qualities may emerge that were not revealed until this point. Again it is important to take your time with this portion of the evaluation, remaining with the cover over each eye for significantly longer than you normally would to give yourself time to watch what the patient explores during this extended time without the chance to return to their habitual pattern. NOTE: When you shift the cover from eye to eye, this should still be done quickly. The extra time recommended should be spent with the cover stationary over an eye, while you observe what the patient is doing. It is recommended to continue the alternate cover until such time as new behavior patterns stop emerging.

Then prepare yourself to observe all the steps the person goes through immediately after you perform the uncover. It might help to give you a framework to place your observations in if you are familiar with the concept of the binocular continuum as presented by Paul Harris[10] (Figure 7.21).

Rather than thinking of a person having a single relative position of their eyes that is maintained all the time, the concept here is of a dynamic system. Throughout the day, based on many factors, including the fatigue level of the patient, their level of attention devoted to the topic of interest, their motivation involved in the task

The Binocular Continuum

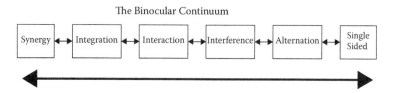

FIGURE 7.21   The binocular continuum showing the six different ways that a person can use their visual process. Although each type has solid boxes around it, this is only for descriptive purposes. In reality each type dissolves seamlessly into the next to the right and left.

at hand, as well as the nature of the demand of the task in addition to many other factors, they may shift up and down the continuum. Instead of characterizing a person by a specific number it would be desirable to establish a binocular profile. This would be a graph overlaid onto the binocular continuum with a frequency distribution of the time and conditions during which the person is at each of the conditions. During the observation phase until the very point that you remove the cover, a judgment is made as to where the person is on the binocular continuum. As the cover comes off they may travel along the continuum and if you watch carefully you may be able to judge where they are at any point based on an overall evaluation of their postures (head, body, and eyes) as well as their facial expression, breathing rates, and so on. The binocular continuum may be helpful in organizing your observations.

Estimation versus Prism Neutralization

When classifying the relative positions of the two eyes to each other in response to a request to look at an object there are times when all that matters is a gross classification into rather broad categories and there are times when measuring the angles requires more precision.

When gross classification will do one might choose to use the three categories of small, medium, and large. In this scheme small might refer to anything up to about 10 prism diopters of turn. Medium would then be used for from 10 to 25 prism diopters of turn. Large would be anything over 25 prism diopters.

In general, when the case calls for some prescribing of prism these general categories are not going to be sensitive enough to manage the needs of the patient. Prism neutralization combined with the alternate cover may be an excellent way to gain insights into the ranges of potential lenses available for use with a particular patient here. Depending on the individual and their specific needs, you may choose a variety of different targets, lighting conditions, and postures for the patient to be in and redo this test several times to get a sense of the relative stability/variability of the postures. The more variability is found, the further one might delve into additional variations to discover the factors that influence how the person alters the relative posture of the eyes in space in response to differing demands. The finding(s) that you get with prism neutralization will be a data point(s) from which your consideration of the benefit of prisms will begin.

One strong case for beginning with estimation and then moving to prism neutralization is that once prisms are introduced into the line of sight of the patient they may alter very significantly their manner of looking in such a way that the system is now functioning in a different manner than before the introduction of the prisms. For example, what might look on gross observation and be estimated to be a small turn might get much larger once even a small amount of prism is introduced. In this case, the patient might be working very hard to hold their visual world together as it is at that moment. Once the prism is introduced, rather than allowing for a reduction of tension in the system and moving to a more stable alignment, they might shift to a new pattern of organization that includes a discontinuity. A discontinuity would imply rather than a smooth transition along a continuum of responses similar in kind but different in degree, it would imply that at some point along the continuum there is a transition state that occurs and on the other side of that the person is now using their visual system in a very different manner. Part of the reason for doing the prism neutralization is to identify when a system seems to be a continuum within a similar state all along its range as opposed to those where these discontinuities may exist. All of these observations should be made note of and will factor in to the clinical decision to prescribe prism.

Range of Lenses

An operational concept here is the concept of deriving a range of lenses that may be available for use with this patient. Rather than looking for a single measure that is *the* prism or sphere power amount to be prescribed, it is generally more productive to look at a series of probes as yielding a range of lenses that under different circumstances may be useful to accomplish different objectives.

In one condition in Figure 7.22, there is a rather narrow range of probe lenses that the patient finds useable to achieve binocular flow. In the second condition the range of lenses is much wider. This patient might be considered to be more flexible and the optometrist has more choices in terms of the prisms available. When a high degree of flexibility exists, even when the condition of no prism would yield diplopia, the

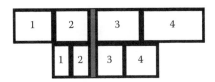

FIGURE 7.22 The lower portion of this diagram is similar to Figure 7.17, which has now been turned on its side. This diagrammatically shows patients with two different results from the test probes. The line between zones 2 and 3 is the same measurement for each patient and represents only the central tendency of the testing. The patient at the top has a much wider range of acceptable lenses, while the patient on the bottom has each zone being smaller showing tighter ranges of acceptable lens powers. Zones 2 and 3 could be thought of as being an area within which the person is in integration on the binocular continuum. In zones 1 and 4 they are shifting more to interaction or interference on the binocular continuum. To the right of zone 4 or to the left of zone 1 for either patient causes massive disturbance to their binocularity.

patient may not actually need prism to be prescribed, particularly if some postural factors can be manipulated to achieve alignment for periods of time. These might include a face turn, a head tilt to one side, or a tipping of the head chin up or chin down. The range of lenses found for any one patient will include elements from each of the probes done, and variability between the responses to these probes is expected rather than having the expectation that they should all come up with the same exact measure of the relative positions of the eyes in space.

Maddox Rod Testing

In some cases, the optometrist might suspect that a factor making it difficult for the patient to achieve binocular flow is that a relative rotation in the perception of verticality between the two channels has become significant. When present, this might explain why in the cases of even small eye turns, the person is complaining of symptomology and finds it impossible to reconcile the flows through each channel with each other. A simple way to identify any cyclorotation is to perform a double Maddox rod probe (Figures 7.23 and 7.24).

One red and one white (unless other colors are available) Maddox rods are used, one before each eye. One side will become the reference and the other will be the measuring side. You can set the reference Maddox rod to any orientation but for practical purposes setting them so that the patient sees them at or near vertical is preferred. If they were set horizontal, the lines would overlap at some point and if the measuring Maddox rod were rotated slowly at some point the person might make a compensatory cyclorotation and bring about a premature alignment, which could give a reading that was not a central tendency measure. If done this way one might have to do a series of measures from both directions of rotation to get a

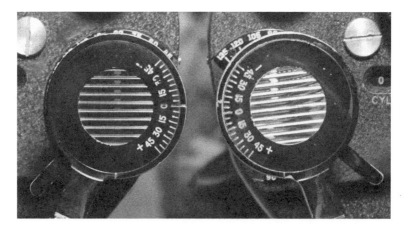

FIGURE 7.23 (**See color insert following page 270.**) This shows the setup for doing the double Maddox test for cyclo rotations. Shown is the Bausch and Lomb phoropter, which allows for both Maddox rods to be rotated through 360 degrees. Here the red Maddox rod, which is before the patient's right eye is set to "0" and is the vertical reference line. The white Maddox rod, which is before the patient's left eye is close to 10 degrees of excyclorotation.

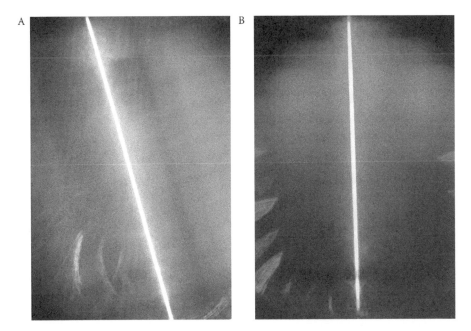

FIGURE 7.24 **(See color insert following page 270.)** This gives a patient's view of the double Maddox rod test. A: The right eye sees the vertical red line, which can easily be seen to be perpendicular to the horizontal segments of the lens. B: The left eye sees the white line. Here the white Maddox rod is shown rotated, with the top to the left. The white Maddox rod is rotated until the patient subjectively reports the two lines to be parallel to each other.

sense of the degree of compensatory cyclorotation that might go on. It is assumed that there is less of this when the two vertical, or near vertical lines, are separated horizontally by some space. It is possible that the same type of compensatory cyclorotation might go on with the vertical samples. Thus, it is recommended to do multiple measures, even with the vertical arrangement and to alternate which side you come from; one time from the ex-cyclo side and the next time from the in-cyclo side.

Note that the patient will see the line perpendicular to the ribs seen on the front surface of the Maddox rod. Thus, the Maddox rod is set so that the ribs are seen to be horizontal. Then rotate the second Maddox rod a good 15–20 degrees away from the vertical setting. Instruct the patient to attend to both images of the Maddox rods simultaneously and to tell you when they are parallel to each other. The goal is not fusion of the two rods but the achievement of parallelism. Record the degree of in- or ex-cyclorotation. The amount of cyclorotation may change from distance to near and therefore should be checked at both distances. The presence of a cyclo-rotation between the two channels is generally a contraindication for prism applica-tion. The prisms may bring the perceived images into overlap but may not result in perceived fusion due to the twisting of one flow relative to the other. In these cases other solutions may need to be looked for, including the use of blur in one image or degrading the image using occlusion foils or "cling patches"; Bangerter Foils[†] being one type of such occlusion foil.

Cheiroscopic Tracing

One very helpful way to gain insight into spatial perception shifts a patient has made is to perform a cheiroscopic tracing. This uses a stereoscope into which a simple line drawing is placed. This line drawing is placed before one eye and the person is asked to trace over the figure with a pencil. By virtue of the way a stereoscope works, only one eye can see the actual line drawing and only the other eye is able to view the tracing as it is being made. Once the first tracing is done, the figure is shifted in front of the other eye and the pencil shifts hands so that the other eye can view the tracing. This results in two tracings, one on either side of the line drawing, which can be compared. The main comparisons would be relative position (inward indicating an eso shift, outward indicating and exo shift, or with figures shifted up or down, indicating vertical misalignments of the eyes), size (larger or smaller from right to left or in different parts of the tracings), and rotations (if both tracings are rotated relative to each other in similar amounts then a true cyclorotation of the eyes, one relative to the other may be diagnosed—see crossed Maddox rod procedure above for an explanation of this).

If a patient is able to perform a cheiroscopic tracing you may get strong indications either for or against the use of prism as a treatment option following an ABI. If the patient can stand, it is best to use a stand-up cheiroscope such as the unit shown below (Figure 7.25) that is distributed by Bernell. If the patient cannot stand up then an attempt should be made to get a cheiroscopic tracing with a desktop stereoscope. The following is an example of the suggested target to use along with tracings from a patient without brain injury.

Figure 7.26 provides an excellent opportunity for the examiner to see if either a cyclorotation of one image as compared to the other exists. It also provides an excellent opportunity to see if a significant size perception difference exists between the two sides. This is called an *aniseikonia*. Significant and consistent size perception differences between the two sides are also contraindications for early use of prisms if the angle of strabismic deviation is large. If prisms are used to overlap two significantly different perceptual sized images the person may have more difficulty in moving through space and in understanding of what they see than if the two images were left further apart. When left further apart they may actually be able to learn to alternate and use both channels, with one leading for some activities and the other leading for other activities more easily than if they are directly superimposed over another.

Figures 7.27A and 7.28 show renderings of what the tracings would look like in an idealized fashion for both the cyclorotation example and the aniseikonia example. Some patients may display symptoms of both. Note the difference between the

---

[†] Bangerter occlusion foils are available from Fresnel Prism & Lens Co., 6824 Washington Ave. S, Eden Prairie, MN, 55344, Phone: 1–800–544–4760, www.fresnel-prism.com; as well as from Bernell, 4016 N Home St., Mishawaka, IN, 46545, Phone: 1–800–348–2225, www.bernell.com

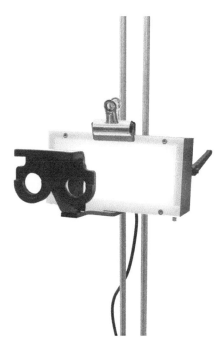

FIGURE 7.25   Wolff Stand-Up Cheiroscope available from Bernell Corporation. The heavy metal base stabilizes the unit well and the light box and prism head can be slid up and down through a large range of heights.

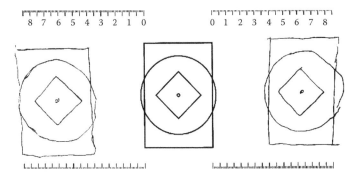

FIGURE 7.26   This is a cheiroscopic tracing of a patient that is not suffering from double vision. Asymmetries can be seen in this drawing but this patient does not require prisms to use her visual process in a balanced manner and very efficiently nearly all of the time.

apparent rotations of the drawings in Figure 7.27A versus 7.27B. The former indicates cyclorotation, while the latter demonstrates a different type of distortion in spatial perception. Also note that under different testing conditions and different real-life conditions that the patient may demonstrate significant variations on all of these asymmetries. In general, the greater the asymmetry and the more robust that

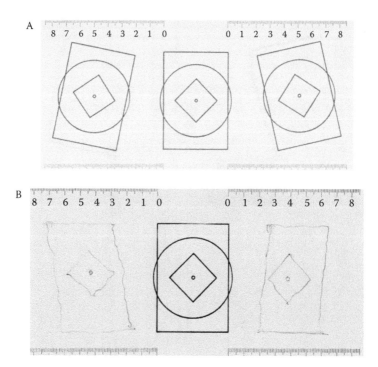

FIGURE 7.27 A: This figure shows an idealized cheiroscopic tracing with a cyclorotation of the perceived images between the two eyes. A key aspect that characterizes the cyclorotation is that all lines are rotated from one image relative to the other. B: This figure was made by a patient who has tremendous difficulty with his binocularity. At times tracings like these have been interpreted to demonstrate a cyclorotation due to the diagonal sloping of the sides. However, notice that the upper and lower parts of the tracings are not rotated. This type of pattern indicates that in downward gaze spatial computing is centripetally shifted toward the individual, while in upper gaze it is centrifugally shifted outward toward the person. Notice that although both images are the same size in the vertical dimension, in the horizontal dimension is the left drawing significantly wider than the right most drawing. This patient does not have any anisometropia or astigmatism but does require 7 diopters of vertical prism to achieve fusion. This drawing was done with his glasses on, which do incorporate his prism.

asymmetry is the more it may act as a bar to the simple application of prism as a way to relieve the symptoms associated with induced misalignments between the two channels.

Fixation Disparity—Associated Phoria

Under conditions of the use the binocular flows in what has been called *fusion*; it has been recognized that some degree of slippage in the alignment of the two channels can occur that does not grossly disrupt the use of the binocular flow. Mental constructs that have most people maintaining exact levels of *fusion* throughout extended periods of their waking hours are most likely incorrect. To do so would

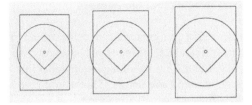

FIGURE 7.28 This is an idealized cheiroscopic tracing pattern showing approximately a 10% size difference between the two channels with the size distortion occurring equally in all meridians. It is important to see a similar amount of enlargement on one side as there is shrinkage on the other side and that the size change is similar in amount in all dimensions. NOTE: Clinically we may see variations on this theme with the size variations occurring in only one dimension. In some cases the size discrepancy might appear to be only on one side. In this instance one must suspect either a motor problem on one side of the body or that the person may have significantly altered posture between the two tracings. Rotations of the body around the "Y" axis, where one side of the body might be shifted closer to the instrument with the other rotated away from the instrument can cause just such a tracing. Therefore, attention to posture is very important throughout the task.

require a great expenditure of effort and energy at very little potential gain for the person. There are some life experiences that may require such exactitude, and during those times, if the person deems the end result to be of the level of import to require such an investment, then and only then is the system kicked into aligning to a finer degree. This state would generally only be maintained as long as it is necessary to perform the task at hand. One can imagine athletes who have periods where bursts of such a high degree of alignment may assist them in their tasks. A baseball player who might get up to bat four to five times a game comes to mind. They may see only four to six pitches on average at bat having to use their binocular system at peak levels for a total of 8–10 min game as a batter. So much of their preparation during the off season, in spring training, in the batting cage before the game, in visualization and visual imagery practice during the day and just before each at bat, and finally in the on-deck circle, all to be ready to raise the probability that they get one to two more hits per week, which is the difference between the average baseball player and the superstar. Simply reading most efficiently would be another such example.

While using the binocular flows in either integration or interaction and in particular in interference, it is expected that for ever-increasing amounts of time, as one moves from Integration to Interaction to Interference, precise alignment time decreases and the degree of variability in alignment increases. Both the amount of time out of highly precise alignment and the amount of motion through that less precise zone would tend to vary over the same set of states along the binocular continuum. Tests of FD, and *associated phoria*, are probes of this slippage. The FD being the amount of slippage, and for a test of FD to be of any meaning, one must first be able to achieve fusion of some sort. In those cases, where some of the above probes of alignment have resulted in periods of fusion, testing of FD may provide additional insights into the range of prisms that may be useable by the patient.

It is important to clear up a common misconception about FD testing that seems to have entered into the clinical use of many of these tests. As first conceived and used in clinical practice, FD testing was done in a manner that gave a plot of alignment over a wide range of challenge lenses. This would give a graph that showed both the range of lenses through which alignment was, practically speaking, exact, and the ranges just at the edges of this "fused" area, where fusion was still within Panum's areas but a measurable degree of slippage—not enough for the patient to notice frank double vision—had occured. Clinicians now seem to do the testing much more quickly, and rather than looking at a range of lenses, they seem to be content with the central tendency only, which they do by finding *the* prism amount that brings exact alignment. This is correctly called the *associated phoria*. They view this as another measure to be "thrown in the hat" with all other central tendency measures, such as phorias or the angle as measured by prism neutralization on the cover test, and miss a great opportunity to explore the width or depth of the range of potential lenses.

Some Tests of Fixation Disparity

There are many tests of FD and associated phoria. It is beyond the scope of this chapter to discuss all such tests. A few will be presented to give the reader a sense of what to look for in these probes that may help in evaluating the usefulness of other such probes. Figure 7.29 is a picture of the Wesson card produced by Dr. Michael Wesson.

This card can be used either directly in the phoropter, clipped to the near point rod and illuminated with the normal near point light, or put on a stand, such as a Vectogram stand or cook book stand, and used in more of a free space environment. Polaroid filters are used over the patient's eyes. This limits the view through each channel to seeing either the lower half of the gray area in the figure above through one channel and the indicator lines in the upper gray area through the other channel. By design, the gray areas covered by the Polaroid filters are very small and the arrows and indicator lines are very fine. The purpose of everything in black on the front surface of the card is to give the visual process ample amount of stimuli to "act normally" and to posture the binocular system as it usually does when looking at high-contrast high-spatial frequency targets. This is a test designed to be used at near only.

When used with patients with ABI, for whom the clinician is thinking that prism use may be warranted, it is preferred to do this test in free space, out from behind the phoropter. This allows the clinician the opportunity to observe the patient, as well as allowing the patient ample opportunity to alter their posture. It also removes the potential difficulties of field limitations induced by the phoropter, which act as very significant field stops. For many people the contribution to binocularity that is derived from the mid periphery and the wider periphery is very important and phoropters block this out. Thus, for more clinically relevant findings, it is recommended to use the Wesson card on a Vectogram or cook bookstand with extra illumination directly onto the card. The purpose of the extra illumination is to reduce the amount of suppression that may make the test difficult to run and frustrating for the patient.

If the patient has frank diplopia without any compensatory prism in place, begin the testing with the minimum amount of compensatory prism that allows for the patient to report a single view of the Wesson card with both the arrow and the measuring lines being visible. Record this amount of prism. Hand-held or prisms mounted on a holder are then introduced before one eye.

NOTE: Not all prisms are created equal. Some lesser quality prism sets have enough surface irregularities that they destroy the polarization, and the patient will report that the arrow is aligned with ALL prism powers. They are not aligned, rather they see both the arrow and the indicator lines through both eyes and may only be reporting seeing a single set that is lined up. Test all prisms that you will use before testing with some commercial polarized product to be sure that the polarization is maintained after the light has traveled through the prisms.

Proper measuring technique involves probing over as wide a range as the person is able to keep the main card single and through which they can see both the arrow and the indicator lines. It is important to look at the full range in both directions, not just the side toward less dependence on prism. In general, over some portion of the range, however small in some people, there will be a lens and posture that brings about some degree of alignment where the arrow points directly up to the center red line. From this point in 1-diopter steps, base in and base out for probing a horizontal

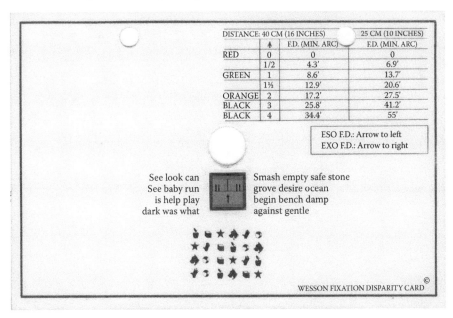

		DISTANCE: 40 CM (16 INCHES)		25 CM (10 INCHES)
		♠	F.D. (MIN. ARC)	F.D. (MIN. ARC)
RED	0		0	0
	1/2		4.3'	6.9'
GREEN	1		8.6'	13.7'
	1½		12.9'	20.6'
ORANGE	2		17.2'	27.5'
BLACK	3		25.8'	41.2'
BLACK	4		34.4'	55'

ESO F.D.: Arrow to left
EXO F.D.: Arrow to right

See look can
See baby run
is help play
dark was what

Smash empty safe stone
grove desire ocean
begin bench damp
against gentle

WESSON FIXATION DISPARITY CARD ©

FIGURE 7.29 (See color insert following page 270.) This is the Wesson fixation disparity card. The only portion with Polaroid filters is the very center portion. The small lower arrow is seen through one channel and the colored lines above are seen through the other channel. Everything else on the card is seen by both eyes and is to act as a form of fusion lock, fusion hold or stimulus to fusion, depending on the model used by the clinician.

FD and base up and base down for probing a vertical FD, the clinician should introduce lenses and record the patient's observation.

It is important when introducing the probe lenses to let the patient know that
they may see an initial jump of things and then there is some movement that slows
down and then stabilizes. Some patients want to give a narrative of the entire experience. After a while most will get the idea to wait an appropriate period, which
may be very different for different patients, and once the movement settles down
to report at which indicator line the arrow points. This should be recorded for plotting onto the recording chart. Figure 7.30 shows the data for a patient with a very
steep FD curve.

In the instance of the above patient there is only exactly one amount of prism,
6 diopters of base in prism that gave him perfect alignment of the arrow on the red
indicator line. One diopter either way and alignment was off by half the distance
to the green indicator line on either side of the red center line. This represents a
degree of slippage. It was not enough for him to see double, but was recorded as a
misalignment. The above patient has Duane's retraction syndrome and was capable
of compensating for this with a slight face turn and did not require prism lenses to
eliminate his diplopia. This was taken in primary gaze and was before any vision

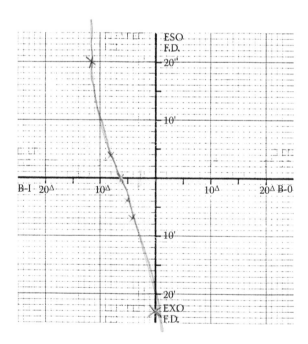

FIGURE 7.30 This fixation disparity plot is of a patient with unilateral Duane's retraction
syndrome. This graph is before vision therapy and shows an intersection point with the zero
fixation disparity line at a single point at 6 diopters of base in prism. With 5 diopters of base
in prism he showed alignment half way in between the red center line and the neighboring
green line on the exoside. With 8 diopters of base in prism he was off the same amount but
this time on the esoside.

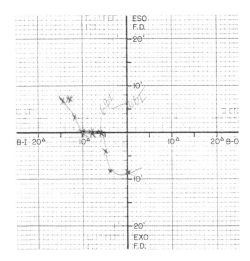

FIGURE 7.31 This is the same patient after a few months of vision therapy. Notice now the range of four diopter from six base in to ten base in through which no fixation disparity is measured. Also notice that the lines on either side of the flat zone are not as steep (close to vertical) as in the previous figure. This indicates a wider spatial area of slippage through which this patient can maintain a higher degree of binocular flow.

therapy. The FD curve in Figure 7.31 is from the same person a few months into a program of vision therapy.

A few months later, this patient now has a 4-diopter flat zone from 6 diopters base in to 10 diopters base in through which he reports alignment of the arrow on the red indicator line. Also the "slippage" zones on either side of the "flat zone" are wider. This means that over a greater variation of prismatic demands he is able to continue using the flow through both channels. Since he is a person with unilateral Duane's retraction syndrome, he is able to compensate by turning his face just a small amount. He now turns less than before as he only needs to get into the slippage area to experience perceptually better visual comfort. If this were an ABI patient, at this point less prism may be needed to achieve resolution of symptoms.

It can easily be seen in this case that 8 diopters of base in prism is the center of the range. Other prism measures might tend toward this amount. The use of the FD makes sense in terms of viewing this range clinically. Here it indicates that in spite of many other tests lining up saying that 8 diopters are needed, this shows that 6 diopters still do the job and don't even enter into the slippage area. In this case, prism powers from 6 to 8 might be considered stabilization lenses, the result of which might be to keep the deviation at about this level. There is no reward for the person to alter the position of the flat zone.

Lenses prescribed in the slippage area closer toward the no prism condition would be considered to be guidance lenses as they are setting the stage to attempt to trigger a recalibration or a normalization of the system. If the person finds a way to shift slightly toward the slippage area and now flattens the curve, even momentarily into this area, then there is a reward and this is a shift up the binocular continuum, with more information available for deriving meaning and directing action with less effort and energy. If the person is capable of making this change, either on their own through the lens treatment program or through the more concentrated effort of an in-office with home practice vision therapy program, then new lenses may need to be made with the power constantly being shift downward in prism power to remain in the slippage area. Vygotsky in reference to language development called this the *zone of proximal development* (as cited in Sacks).[11] In successful prism therapy, where the goal is working toward less dependence on the prisms, the FD test shines in helping identify the slippage area and thus the optimal guidance lens values.

Figure 7.32 shows the FD curve for the same patient at the conclusion of his vision therapy. The range of lenses through which the arrow is aligned with the red indicator line is now from 4 diopters of base in prism to 15 diopters of base in prism. With no prism at all, still in primary gaze with no face turn, he now shows a slippage of the arrow to half way between the red line and the green line. He does not appreciate diplopia between the ranges of 25 diopters base in to 10 diopters base out.

Mallett Test   Another excellent test for FD was produced by Bernell and designed by Mallett and is shown in Figure 7.33.

Figure 7.33 shows only the central portion of the Mallett card as produced by Bernell. There is additional text above and below the section shown, and the entire card is framed in a black border all of which is seen by both eyes. Only the small green arrows, which do not show up well in the figure, are polarized, with one arrow on the vertical and the lateral boxes being seen with one eye and

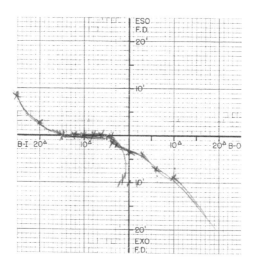

FIGURE 7.32   This is the final fixation disparity curve with the same Duane's retraction patient described above after completion of vision therapy. This shows a tremendous change in the range of challenge lenses through which he reports seeing the arrow pointing right at the center red indicator line.

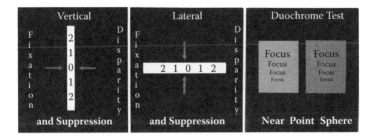

FIGURE 7.33   (See color insert following page 270.) This is the center portion of the Mallett fixation disparity card as produced by Bernell. It is meant to be used in the back holder part of the Macular integrity tester. It can also be used on a Vectogram stand.

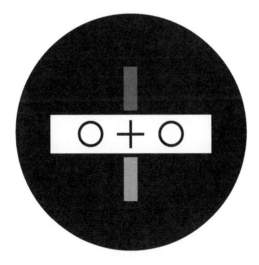

FIGURE 7.34   (See color insert following page 270.) This simple demonstration of a Mallett target for fixation disparity uses glasses with one lens red and one lens blue. The black and white areas are seen by both eyes and the red and blue lines become the indicators. In general, this type of measure yields much cruder information that the Wesson card and it becomes difficult to do much more than find the central tendency.

the other arrow in each box being seen by the other eye. Quantification with this is a bit more difficult than with the Wesson card as the indicator markers are much further apart than on the Wesson card. For the same distance between the "0" and the "1" on the Mallett card, one would have moved through multiple indicator lines on the Wesson card. Figure 7.34 is a picture of a Mallett test done anaglyphically.

The Saladin Nearpoint Balance Card   One final card of note is the Saladin near-point balance card (Figure 7.35). Here multiple vertical and horizontal arrangements

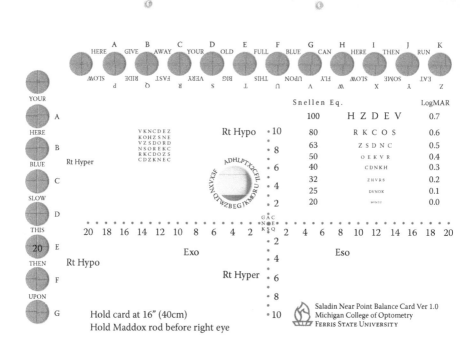

FIGURE 7.35 The Saladin card. This is made to be attached to the near point rod on most phoropters. The hole in the center allows for retinoscopy to be performed while the chart is in use.

of the indicator lines appear on the card. The patient again looks at the target through a pair of polaroid filters. The patient here, once they have attained fusion, need only look across the upper row of circles to find the one or ones that have the two vertical lines in alignment. When looking at the vertical FD, they would look up and down along the column of circles on the left side of the card. In practice, this has been quite easy to administer but the data obtained is more difficult to interpret than the graphs obtained by use of the Wesson card.

Other Probes   There are many other probes of alignment of the visual axes that clinicians may find helpful. Some of these may include

- Brock posture board
- Worth 4 Dot
- Phoria testing: various methods
- Vectograms
- Hess Lancaster Screens
- Computerized testing

Each of these under the right set of circumstances may yield significant insights into understanding how the patient is using their visual process and may impact on the treatment decisions derived. A general principle that can be used in the selection of which tests may be the most helpful is the following:

> **Principle:** Tests that are more similar to the way that particular patient uses their visual process in life, are more apt to give clinical insights, which have a higher chance of success when turned into a treatment plan.

TREATMENT

PRISM APPLICATION FOR ALIGNMENT

It would be desirable to now present a formal decision tree that could be followed, which would help guide the clinician through the process of using the data collected to derive a lens or range of lenses to help the patient meet their unmet needs. Any attempt at such a decision tree is fraught with danger as it would imply that all the steps in such a process are known and verifiable and have been found to be correct. This is not the case. However, an attempt will be made to give the clinician a decision tree that could be used to act as a guide to clinical thinking. This is written more in the language of principles and guidelines rather than in specific directives.

The decision tree flow chart presented in Figure 7.36 provides a conceptual framework for coming to a decision on how to deal with alignment issues with your patients. In the first bubble the patient presents with a binocular problem. The first decision point hinges on the answer to the question of whether the patient's unmet needs can be met with nonprism methods. If so, then try these methods first. If in the course of monitoring the effects of these treatments, the patient still has unmet binocular vision needs, then you may face having to answer this question again in the future.

Assuming that you feel you cannot meet their needs with nonprism methods or visual therapy, then we move to the second decision point, which asks if there is any place in space that binocular interaction can be achieved. If it is reasonably possible to achieve binocular interaction this should be attempted. If there is no place in space where binocular interaction can be achieved then an additional question needs to be answered. If the flow through both channels is causing interference to the point that the person is experiencing diplopia or confusion to a level that they find disturbing, then you should consider some form of occlusion. This is beyond the scope of this chapter on prisms. However, there are many forms of occlusion short of full field patching. It is a general principle that the larger the amount of the visual field that can be allowed to be visible, the better it is for the person's function. Thus, when looking at patching options the goal would be to disrupt the least volume of the visual field to the least degree possible. Thus, options such as a Bangerter occlusion foil is more desirable than an opaque spot patch, and a small spot patch would be more desirable over a patch that takes up a much larger area of the visual field.

Once you find a place in space where with prism you can achieve some degree of binocular interaction then it becomes important, as mentioned earlier in the text, to perform a series of tests to find the ranges of prisms through which the person can achieve different degrees of binocularity. In most instances you will find that there

Alignment Prism Prescribing Decision Tree

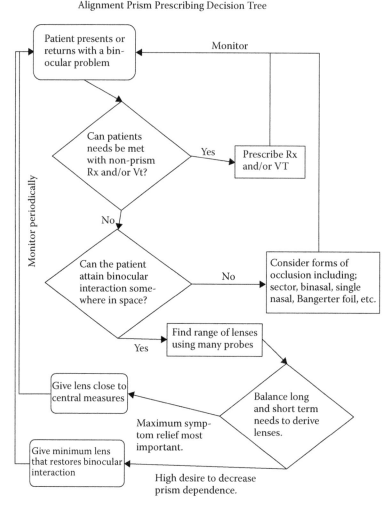

FIGURE 7.36 This is a flow chart to help you make decisions when prescribing prism for helping a patient with alignment issues.

is a range of lenses from which you can select. Once you have this range of lenses then you will need to factor in the patient's visual needs into their overall current life needs. If, for instance, the person has been seen in the hospital and their immediate medical needs are very significant, you may choose to give a bit more prism to minimize the amount of extra work they need to do to attain binocular interaction. If, however, most of the person's other needs have been met and they express a strong desire to work toward less dependence on prism, then you may choose to shift as far into binocular interaction away from binocular integration as possible, while requiring the patient to actively work to achieve this with some degree of face turn, head tilt, and/or conscious attention.

Naturally, all choices will require monitoring at various intervals. General guidelines would be the following. Shorten the monitoring time interval in cases

- That present narrower ranges of lenses to choose from
- When you prescribe toward the interface between binocular interaction and binocular interference
- Where the person's health/life condition is more labile

PROVIDING THE PRISM

Once all the data has been collected and the clinician has worked through the decision tree for giving prism and all signs point to providing the prism to the patient, the following should help make sure that the prism is delivered in the most efficacious manner possible. The first step should be to try the prism in the office. Depending on the power of the prism, this may be done with a Halberg clip and a prism from a trial case or it may require the use of a Fresnel prism.[‡] Fresnel prisms come in two forms (Figures 7.37 and 7.38). One is the large flexible plastic disk that can be cut and applied to an ophthalmic lens and be used in the office on a trial basis or for vision

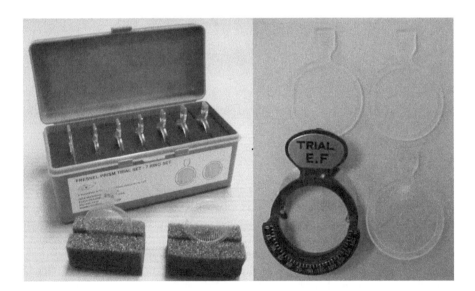

FIGURE 7.37 The Fresnel prism trial set is an excellent way to test the use of prisms in the power range of from 12 diopters and higher in the office. They are made to fit into most trial frames and Halberg clips. Unlike single cut wedge prisms, which may have too much thickness to fit into a trial frame with other lenses, the Fresnel lenses are relatively thin, even in the 40-diopter prism power.

[‡] Both the trial lens set and the ones for application on ophthalmic lenses are available from Fresnel Prism & Lens Co., 6824 Washington Ave. S, Eden Prairie, MN, 55344, Phone: 1–800–544–4760, www.fresnel-prism.com.

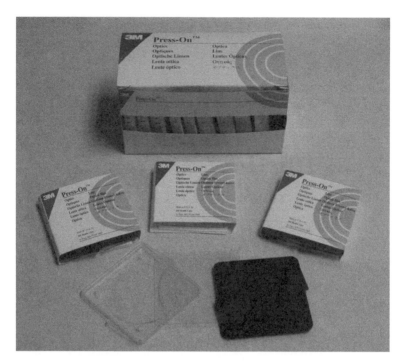

FIGURE 7.38 The Press-On optics are Fresnel prisms and are available in 1-diopter steps in the low powers up to 40 diopters when lots of power is needed.

therapy or it can be dispensed. Then there are rigid trial Fresnel prisms that are sized to fit trial frames or Halberg clips.

TRIAL PERIOD WITH PRISMS IN OFFICE

In some instances a patient's initial reaction to any lens may change over time and in this regard prisms are no exception. If scheduling permits, it may be best to have the patient you are preparing to dispense prisms to have an extended in-office experience with the lenses. If you can have them engage in some movement activity or an activity where they must use their visual process to interact with real objects in the physical world this is best, rather than sitting and reading, taking a nap, or playing on a small computer console or laptop. The ideal situation is where you can have them get involved in an activity like this for 20–30 minutes and then check in and see if the prism amount and direction seems to be useable by the patient and is beginning to help them achieve the goals you both have agreed on. If the alignment measures seem to be changing and the prism amount and direction you chose seem now to not be addressing the patient's unmet needs, then you may consider altering the prism amount and/or direction and then have the patient engage in similar movement experiences in or around the office and continue the sequence until you are both confident that you have found the right starting amount and direction of prism.

TABLE 7.2
Fresnel versus Ophthalmic Prism Decision Matrix

Action: Stay with the Fresnel	Action: Shift to Ground in Prism
You anticipate making changes in weeks or months	You anticipate few if any changes over time
The prism amount is greater than 12–14 diopters	The prism amount is below 12 diopters
Weight is a factor	The patient can tolerate the weight
Clarity through the one side is not a high priority	Clarity through both channels is very important
Appearance is not as important	Best appearance needed (actor, TV personality, etc.)
Cost is a factor	The higher cost is not a concern
Changes are needed right away	Time lag when changes are made
Prism only needed in parts of the visual field	Prism will be used full field

TEMPORARY PRISM ON THE RX

Before having the prism ground into the patient's glasses, it is usually best to extend the trial period of the lenses by affixing a Fresnel prism and having the patient return a few days to a week or so later. Once the response to the prism has stabilized and you have made any adjustments to the Fresnel to balance the needs of the patient, you will have to make the judgment of whether or not it is in the patient's best interest to shift to a ground in prism.

General guidelines for when to shift to a ground in prism versus a Fresnel prism are shown in Table 7.2.

YOKED PRISMS

Prisms are said to be yoked when the bases in front of both eyes point in the same direction and when the prism amounts are the same. For example, 10 base-out in front of the left eye and 10 base-in in front of the right eye could be said to be 10 diopter base left yoked prisms. Yoked prisms have a long heritage in the profession of optometry as a clinical tool used in many visual therapy protocols, as well as being prescribed to provide various benefits to patients who either have significant asymmetries or who work in asymmetric postures for whom the use of yoked prisms may help them deal with the asymmetric demand better. In addition, the fields of psychology, cognitive psychology, neuroscience, and others have used yoked prisms to investigate the spatial transformation effects on adaptation and visual perception. It is beyond the scope of this chapter to recount the entire theoretical basis of yoked prisms. However, yoked prisms have become an integral part of the treatment of patients with head injury, particularly those with visual field loss and with the subsequent shifts or rotations of egocentric location. The use of the prisms has been associated with the conditions of homonymous hemianopsia (HH), and neglect or unilateral spatial inattention (USI), which are discussed in detail in Chapter 5.

Homonymous Hemianopsia

One of the frequent sequelae of stroke is a HH. When the stroke affects the right visual cortex (V1) or the pathways into the right V1 after they leave the right side lateral geniculate, the neural substrates for sight in the left visual field are lost. When the stroke affects the left visual cortex or the pathways into the left V1 after they leave the left side lateral geniculate, the substrates for sight in the right visual field are lost. "As many as one third of stroke survivors in rehabilitation have either homonymous hemianopsia or hemineglect. In the United Kingdom, 50% of neurological admissions are attributable to strokes and 30% of these cases have hemianopsia" (p. 453).[12] In some instances of HH there may also be the confounding symptom of neglect.

A number of approaches to help patients with HH fall squarely within the scope of practice of optometry and involve the use of prisms. Peli states, "Rehabilitative approaches to homonymous hemianopsia typically fall under three categories: (1) Training patients to make better compensatory scanning eye movements; (2) restoring a portion of the blind hemifield through training, and; (3) the use of optical devices, most commonly prisms"(p. 492).[13] Margolis and Suter state, "The purpose of using optical prism systems in glasses for homonymous hemianopsia compensation is to shorten the time required to access information from the affected field, and to decrease the time that attention is being diverted from the functional side" (p. 34).[14] As will be discussed later, there are several different methods of using prisms to attempt to achieve this goal, and the clinician needs to know and understand each of these methods, as the many variations of presentation from patient to patient may necessitate using one approach with one patient and a different approach with another despite both having HH.

Neglect

One of the most striking disorders of cognition is unilateral neglect, also known as hemi-inattention. Patients with this syndrome act as though whole regions of space contralateral to their lesions do not exist. In early stages, patients may deny ownership of their contralateral limb and also neglect parts of their own body. When dressing, they might not clothe the contralateral side and may fail to groom their hair or shave parts of their faces on that side. Right hemisphere damage is a more common and is the more severe cause of unilateral neglect than left hemisphere damage.[15] Damage causing left-sided neglect is usually centered on the inferior parietal lobule or superior temporal lobe of the right hemisphere. Patients with such damage ignore events occurring on the left side of space.[16] Patients may even fail to eat the food on the left side of their plate or bump into obstacles on their left side. "The various manifestations of unilateral neglect share one major feature—patients remain unaware of the deficits they exhibit or at least fail to fully consciously attend to these deficits" (p. 534).[17]

When neglect was first encountered many explanations that were rather simplistic in nature were offered leading to the oversimplified concepts that a patient was felt to either have it or not. "Neglect is a heterogeneous disorder whose different symptoms can be explained in terms of damage to (at least) one of three different cognitive mechanisms mediating attention, intention, and/or space representation. Recent evidence has begun to challenge the traditional distinction in the standard clinical definition between low level sensori-motor deficits and those assumed to involve higher level/cognitive systems" (p. 25).[18]

Each of these mechanisms, attention, intention, and space representation, do not reside in single locations in the brain but rather are distributed through large areas around the brain and are each dependent on multiple subareas working together in complex networks. Neglect can result from damage to each of these main systems or in combination, and at a lower level each of the systems can become faulty through various constellations of damage. Thus, no single lesion site will most likely even be found to explain all forms of neglect. However, "The frequent parietal locus of the lesion producing neglect reflects the impairment of coordinate transformation used by the nervous system to represent extra-personal space" (p. 166).[19] This shows that in the area of the parietal cortex many of these spatial maps come together or are related to each other and damage here often results in odd behaviors, some of which are classified as neglect.

Symptoms of neglect also may appear on a continuum from being present for all instances of objects in a field be they personal or extrapersonal. However, in some instances the lack of attention, intention, or spatial awareness may involve only some objects and only in some situations. It is beyond the scope of this chapter to fully explain neglect. The critical point here is that since neglect is not caused by lesions to one specific area of the brain or through one specific mechanism, that any systematic approach to using yoked prisms or visual field expanding prisms, such as the Peli prisms, will not be able to address all patients with neglect. The clinician should have an open mind and be prepared to probe similar clinical entities with various approaches to using prism, including trying for a period of time bases in directions opposite to those one might anticipate to be helpful. The complexity of the neurological causes of the condition of neglect requires flexibility of approach by the clinician in its treatment.

It is also important to keep in mind that with many patients, the longer in time they are removed from the event that led to their neglect, the less likely they are to show neglect in all forms of clinical probes. Many patients show deep neglect on all probes within days of their stroke but over a period of months they may lose the neglect-like characteristic responses in many of the clinical probes, while retaining them in others. Because of the variability of expression of the condition, this also follows an unpredictable time course and clinical course. Some patients may seem to retain the full expression of neglect for very long periods of time, though this is the exception rather than the rule.

For a long time, patients with neglect had the additional stigma of family and others believing that they were confabulating or were simply playing a game with those around them. As stated by Suchoff and Ciuffreda, "...*neglect* carries the connotation of a willful act on the part of the individual, while *inattention* more accurately describes the individual's unawareness of, and lack of attentional control over, the condition" (p. 305).[20] Thus, inattention became the key concept to build many of the observed behaviors around. The modifiers, unilateral and spatial, are descriptive; *unilateral* because the problem is one-sided, and *spatial* because the problems involve mapping or representation problems.

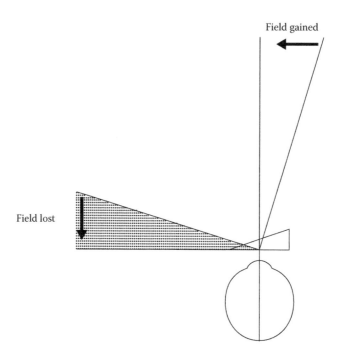

FIGURE 7.39 This shows monocularly how the visual field is altered as a result of the yoked prism applied this way. The patient here has a right visual field problem. Two right triangles are formed with their apices at the prism. The one labeled "Field Gain" shows some of the right visual field that was not being seen by the patient to be shifted leftward into the person's seeing area. The triangle to the left labeled "Field Lost" shows a portion of the formerly seen field that is shifted now into nonseeing area. The main idea here is to trade some less relevant visual field for more important field. The area just to the right of the physical midline or projected saggital plane is more critical more of the time in avoiding obstacles when moving.

Suchoff and Ciuffreda have used yoked prisms with patients with USI (Figure 7.39).

Our greatest successes with USI patients have been with full-field ground in yoked prisms. This has the effect of shifting the patient's locus of true, or objective, "straight ahead" toward the apices. This results in a reorganization of the wearer's visual space. The patient now becomes somewhat more aware of people and objects in the compromised field. This does not ameliorate the total effect of USI, but rather provides an "early warning system" in that an approaching person, vehicle, or an object in that field comes into the patient's visual awareness perhaps several seconds before it did without the yoked prisms. (p. 314)[20]

They are recommending a specific orientation of the prism and this may have worked well with the clinic population that they saw. However, as was noted above and as will be explained a bit more differently below, a uniform approach where prisms in a single direction are expected to work on all such patients is most likely not going to stand the test of time. Suchoff and Ciuffreda add the following caveat,

"The power of the prisms should be the least at which the patient reports a visual awareness of objects or people in the compromised field that was not present without the yoked prisms" (p. 314) [20] In the end, the criteria of altering patients' awareness may be the key to their success. It is assumed that a number of patients did not have their awareness altered and therefore they were not represented in their work. In other words, to be successful the person wearing the prisms had to be aware of the shift. To be aware of the shift, symptoms of neglect or USI had to be below a certain level, low enough to allow for the awareness.

ABNORMAL EGOCENTRIC LOCALIZATION

One of the very interesting observations made with people with acquired visual field problems are a series of shifts in several aspects of how that person perceives or functions in space (further discussed in Chapter 6). These shifts may include a shift in the persons' perceived egocentric locus, a shift in their perception of what straight ahead is when directing actions in space, or redistributions of weight, which may alter their canonic postures in fundamental ways. Unfortunately, we find too often that all of these shifts are all referred under a single umbrella term of *midline shift*. This term is too general in light of the many different observations that have been grouped under it.

In addition, the word *shift* is not well defined and seems to imply in some writings a right or leftward shift of the point from which a person looks from, while others talk of an angular rotation of the perceived straight-ahead point. Some of these definitions of *shift* use the person as the reference point and the others use where they point in space in an open loop (they can't see where they are pointing) pointing activity as the reference point. For example, Margolis and Suter state, "Persons with one eye enucleated have been shown to undergo a significant shift of their egocenter" (p. 33).[14] Here they are clearly talking about the person's perception of where they look at the world from. In an intact binocular individual this is generally from inside the middle of the head directly between the two eyes. In the person who only has one eye, there is a shift to looking at the world from directly behind the intact eye. This shift often takes the person who loses an eye a considerable amount of time to adapt to.

It is possible to see combinations of all of these factors. A person may have a shift of their egocentric locus, while not having an angular rotation in their perception of straight ahead and vice versa. With each of these combinations, a person may or may not have alterations of weight bearing; when the weight bearing shifts occur they may occur to varying degrees in different situations in the same patient depending on the activity and on where the person's attention is directed (e.g., Where they are directed to put their attention, how they feel [both muscle tone as well as emotionally], where the object is that they are looking at, etc.). Thus, it is easy to find rather conflicting statements about these shifts when the definitions of what is observed are so general and incompletely specified or they only refer to one of the types of shifts/rotations that could be observed.

Few speak of the actual amount of shift or rotation. An exception is Kapoor et al., where they note, "In some patients, their subjective egocentric localization does not coincide with their objective midline representation, and thus there is a spatial mismatch between their subjective and objective visual spaces. This anomalous shift in their spatial egocenter can be 15 degrees or more with respect to the normal objective straight ahead along the body midline" (p. 132).[21]

Pisella et al. help delineate the problem well, "Orienting in space requires an integration of retinal, eye-position and head-position signals, together with vestibular information. These signals are classically considered to be further transformed to build a unitary egocentric reference, aligned with the saggital body axis. A reference-shift hypothesis of neglect has been proposed, according to which all the orienting biases observed in neglect patients are due to an "illusory rotation of the egocentric reference, somewhat as if the subject felt being constantly rotated toward the lesion side" (p. 327).[22] As has been noted above in the work by Graziano and Gross, there is no one place in the brain where the master maps are kept. For many different kinds of activities and for different relationships to those objects or movements, different maps exist and they are not all affected the same in each person with similar looking visual field problems.

These shifts are far from universal characteristics of visual-spatial neglect. In three studies recently published, where 2, 23, and 18 neglect patients were studied, the researchers "…challenged this reference shift theory of hemispatial neglect by showing that not all patients exhibited a rightward shift of the egocentric reference. In those three studies, a total of 43 patients were examined, and only 27 of them exhibited a deviation of the manual straight-ahead to the right. In addition, Farné et al showed that the same proportion of right brain-damaged patients without neglect exhibited a similar trend" (p. 328).[22]

Padula and Argyris state, "A high correlation has been found with a shift in midline away from the neurologically affected side" (p.168).[23] It is of interest that this was in a work published in 1996. Since that time the field has matured a great deal. In 2006, a full 10 years later, Margolis and Suter state, "The egocentric visual midline shift, or perception of 'straight ahead', tends to be in the opposite direction for patient with unilateral spatial inattention, vs. those with homonymous hemianopsia. That is, the perceived visual midline is shifted toward the defect for patients with 'pure' hemianopsia, and away from the defect for patients with 'pure' unilateral spatial inattention. Interestingly, patients with both homonymous hemianopsia and unilateral spatial inattention have no shift in their perception of straight ahead" (p. 35).[14] This shows how quickly the field is maturing and how quickly new insights are helping to reorganize our observations, resulting in different and evolving clinical approaches.

The primary reason for spending so much time on this topic is that, "Application of yoked prism spectacles reduces the mismatch between their subjective and objective visual space, as the prisms optically shift the visual world in the direction of their anomalous egocentric projection with the eyes maintaining straight ahead gaze. We have observed that some of these patients immediately experience greater perceptual and motor stability upon application of the yoked prisms, especially during ambulation" (p. 133).[21] In those patients who experience such major benefits from the yoked prisms in the office, a trial period should be considered following the suggestions in the prescribing prism for alignment section. It was recommended that you try the prism for an extended period of time in the office before prescribing it on a temporary basis with Fresnel prisms and then moving to having the prisms ground

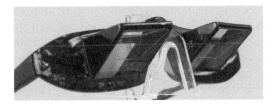

FIGURE 7.40 "Bed" or "Postural" glasses.

into their prescription if the benefits continue on for an extended period of time. Many clinicians have had positive experience with this.

However, as will be seen just a bit further on in the text it may be that the benefits of wearing the prisms on a long-term basis are actually coming from another phenomena that has been described and researched extensively outside of the eye care professions may be the primary reason why yoked prisms are having the positive effects they are.

"Bed" or "Postural" Glasses

Nonprescription high-powered direction shifting glasses (Figure 7.40) that allow a 90-degree shift in viewing direction are marketed for laying flat in bed and watching television. These glasses, though they look like prisms and are indeed made in a wedge form do not function like the rest of the prisms discussed in this chapter. One side of the prism has an inward facing mirrored surface. Light enters the wedge and is bounced off the mirror and then bounced again off the first surface that is functioning as a beam splitter, sending light back through the third surface, through which the person looks. This results in a full 90-degree shift in the direction of light that enters through these glasses. These glasses may be very helpful for patients who have supranuclear palsies that prevent them from moving their eyes into downgaze, allowing them to reconnect visually with their hands to fixate them during therapy or specific tasks. Similar, but much lower powered (25^Δ) "postural" prism spectacles are also available in both directions in clip-on form so that the patient can use their habitual glasses for clarity.[§] These clip-ons have been made in two forms that allow them to be used for seeing either upward or downward in reference to the person's body orientation and are useful for patients who need less prismatic help getting into downgaze (base down), as well as those who have postural difficulties in raising their heads (base up).

Top-Down/Bottom-Up

It was mentioned earlier that some approaches to working with patients with visual field defects or visual-spatial neglect involve top-down or high-level cognitive approaches. This requires that the person have an awareness of their problem for these approaches to be effective. The patient is given strategies or activities to do to

---

[§] Available through: Chadwick Optical, Inc., 1763 Old River Road, White River Junction, VT, 05001, Phone: 1–800–410–1618, www.chadwickoptical.com

help them overcome the problems they know they have. Because they know they have the losses they can cognitively associate the new learned strategy with the problem and see the relevance of the potential work around as being helpful. These patients generally do well because there is a match between their loss, their awareness of the loss, and high-level or cognitive strategies that can be of assistance. However, where there is no such awareness of the problem, these types of techniques or counseling do not work well, if at all.

In some neglect research there is recognition that prisms can be used in a way that alters visual perception, below the threshold for conscious awareness, that is capable of bringing about significant and lasting change.[6,17–19,22,24–27] This change may be immediate but the exciting part of the treatment is the long-term aftereffects that occur after the prisms are removed. These interventions, which do not rely on any strategy changes or conscious awareness of the problem, are of special importance to understand. These effects of prisms applied below a level of conscious awareness in this patient population are considered to be a bottom-up approach. By altering the sensory data as it comes in, in a subtle way, the stage is set for recalibrations of some of the mapping areas in the brain in such a way that having had the prism experience may help to realign the system on a long-term to permanent basis. In fact, it may be that it is this effect, when the prisms are removed, which actually accounts for the majority of the changes that occur when yoked prisms are prescribed for this population. It will await further research to help us understand precisely what is going on. The next section presents the data from this body of work, which may become the staple for optometric treatment of midline shifts/rotations and weight distribution changes.

PRISM ADAPTATION AFFECTS ABNORMAL EGOCENTRIC LOCALIZATION

A large body of literature, outside of the optometric field, exists where yoked prisms have been used in conjunction with prism adaptation work with subjects with HH with various degrees of neglect or USI.[17–19,22,24–27] These researchers have paid more attention to what happens directly after relatively brief exposure to the yoked prisms. Their subjects were given various activities that involved pointing to objects in space or navigating themselves through space with the prisms on.

To get baseline measures of misalignments and for measurements after adaptation, this group of experimenters used open-loop measures. In the open-looped condition the person does not see the consequences of their actions, but the experimenters can see where the person is pointing relative to the real object's location in space. The subjects were blindfolded and they were asked to point straight ahead while their head was kept aligned with the body's sagittal plane. They were asked to move their hand forward from their midline to a wall that was at their full arms' length. Ten trials were done to get a baseline measure of their straight-ahead position and to get an idea of the degree of variability in the subjects' pointing. This is very much like the space board where the person cannot see directly where they make the mark until after the paper is removed for inspection.

At this point the subjects engaged in active pointing tasks for adaptation. This body of researchers used 10 degree prisms or about 17.5 prism diopters with the bases left. During most of the active adaptation, the person is involved in closed-loop tasks. Here they can see the results of any mismatches or misalignments that result from the prisms. The subjects looked directly ahead at a target that is on their midline. A small shelf is set up under their chin below which their hand is hidden when in the starting position. The subject looks at the target and then ballistically thrust their hand forward toward the target making whatever adjustments they need to get their index finger directly on the target. They repeat this motion over and over until they are consistently hitting the target. Adaptation times may be from 5 to 10 minutes total.

The subjects then return to the blindfolded situation and another 10 trials are taken in the open-loop (no visual feedback) situation. What emerged was the exciting observation that, "The perceived midline of neglect patients can be shifted to the left following adaptation to prisms" (p. 26).[28]We are all quite aware of the aftereffects when working with prisms. When the prisms are on, if a person engages in active closed-loop activities where they are generating the movements, rather than being passively moved by someone else, they adapt to the prism. Over time their movements now properly guide the hand to the correct location in space. If a person does this long enough, when the prisms are removed there is an opposite shift effect. So the above statement does not seem that exciting. The startling thing is that rather than simply seeing a short-lived opposite shift of similar magnitude to what we see in people without visual field loss that dissipates over a few minutes, they saw several very significant things.

Michel et al.[25] note that, "Neglect patients show an extraordinary level of adaptation to prisms, while also exhibiting a lack of awareness of the optical deviation" (p. 348). The amount of adaptation is far in excess of what we see with normal controls. "Neuronormals" show an aftereffect of about 4 degrees of shift to the left that dissipates rather quickly over time. Patients with neglect, with a right-side lesion, begin the open loop showing a shift to the right of the target of about 9 degrees. Their aftereffect shifts them to the left, from this position to just about 2 degrees to the right of the target, a full 7 degrees of shift, nearly twice the shift found in the "neuronormals." A key thing is that this "aftereffect" in the neglect patients did not seem to be a typical aftereffect in that it had effects in many profound areas that lasted not just for minutes but in many cases for hours, days, and longer.

Once this observation was made, many experimenters delved into the entire body of knowledge of prism adaptation and looked into what other aspects of prism adaptation were different between neuronormals and patients with visual field disturbances and neglect, particularly those with neglect. Some found a lack of body part specificity of the adaptation and aftereffect that occurs in neuronormals. Others found very abnormal time courses, where the aftereffects seemed to last an extraordinary period of time in the neglect patients. This triggered other investigators to look at the actual measures of neglect and what they found sets the stage for some different views of the use of prisms in optometric care.

Rossetti et al. state, "Unlike other physiological manipulations used to improve neglect, patients demonstrating the classical features of severe visual neglect after right-brain damage showed a strong and reliable improvement after a short adaptation period to a prismatic shift of the visual field to the right. This finding also stands in contrast with the usual specificity of wedge prisms aftereffects in normal subjects, found to be arm-specific or even task-specific under several experimental conditions" (p. 166).[19] Luauté et al. state, "A brief period of right prism adaptation with left-ward compensatory aftereffects has been repeatedly shown to improve left neglect across a variety of different standard tests. Short-term exposure to visuomotor adaptation is sufficient to stimulate a long-term reorganization of the neural representation of space that develops autonomously after removal of the prisms" (p. 1859).[26]

In the classic types of probes of the depth of the neglect where patients are given a picture to copy, Pisella[17] showed very significant changes that lasted 8–10 hours and in some cases got better over time. The classic representation is that the subject only copies a few parts of the picture from the extreme right most part of the picture. After prism adaptation they begin copying more of the picture, in many instances crossing the center line of the picture, paper, or target being viewed and these changes lasted for hours, in some cases actually getting better over time.

Michel who collaborated with Pisella on several research protocols states, "Simple prism adaptation modulated visuo-spatial neglect performance in a directionally specific way on many of the established clinical tests thought to assess the effect of damage to high-level spatial cognition. Collectively, these findings question the assumption that only higher level cognitive disorders (e.g., attention, intention and/or representational) are involved in producing the characteristic clinical picture of unilateral neglect" (p. 27).[28] Thus, something more may be occurring in these patients. This work opens up new avenues of treatment and gives potential alternate explanations as to why earlier methods of prescribing yoked prisms may have been beneficial.

WHAT PARTS OF THE BRAIN MIGHT BE INVOLVED?

Some of the workers have used brain scanning technology to help identify which parts of the brain may be affected by the prism work. Luauté et al. state, "The network of significant brain regions associated with improvement of left neglect performance produced by prism adaptation involved the right cerebellum, the left thalamus, the left temporo-occipital cortex, the left medial temporal cortex, and the right posterior parietal cortex" (p. 1859).[26] The neurology involved is complex and involves interaction between both halves of the brain. If the right cerebellum has also been affected these changes may be markedly less.

YOKED PRISM AS ACTIVE TREATMENT NOT SPACE SHIFTER

What this body of literature is pointing to is the role that yoked prisms and their aftereffects play in the neurological reorganization of the affected person's neurology to allow for a recalibration in many patients. Pisella et al. state, "The neural mechanisms underpinning visuo-manual plasticity can be viewed as a powerful rehabilitation tool that produces straightforward effects not only on visual and motor parameters, but on visuo-spatial, attentional and higher cognitive neurological functions. The use of prism adaptation therapy in neglect and other visuo-spatial disorders has just started to reveal its potential, both at a practical and theoretical level" (p. 534).[17] They go on to discuss how many other areas the prisms and the aftereffects have been shown to affect. "The fact that different tasks based upon other sensory modalities can be improved (haptic circle centering) and that several nonmanual tasks (postural control, wheelchair driving, imagery, verbal reports) were also improved, demonstrates that the effects of prism adaptation on visuo-spatial defective abilities go well beyond the visuo-manual parameters usually affected in normal subjects" (p. 537).[17]

One of the most startling areas affected will be described. Before the prism training experience, participants with neglect were asked to visualize a map of France, the country in which the people lived and where the work was done; they were asked to call out the names of all the cities they could see on the map. The list of cities given by each participant was then plotted on a map of France. For each participant, the geometric center of this cluster of cities was well to the right of the map of France, with no cities called out being past the actual geometric center of France. After the prism adaptation work, the list of cities given by the subject now ranged throughout all of France with the center coinciding rather closely to the actual geometric center of the country. This shows linkages to how these internal mapping systems are kept that goes well beyond real-time processing of current visual input.

Pisella et al. state, "Prism adaptation can be considered the most-promising rehabilitation method for unilateral neglect to date, especially in light of the fact that spontaneous recovery from neglect is very limited" (p. 540).[17] This leads to the strong recommendation that before looking to prescribe yoked prisms for long-term wear on a compensatory basis that one should go through a rather intensive period of active-closed-loop prism adaptation work in a myriad of settings involving as much movement as possible. These sessions should allow for periods of time with no yoked prism use between the active works to allow a chance for the emergence of the beneficial aftereffects of the prism. Rossetti states

> Our results contrast with those obtained when Fresnel prisms were used to shift the left visual field toward the central retina, rather than to study the effect of adaptation. Under these later conditions, no significant improvement of neuropsychological testing was observed after the patients kept using the goggles daily during four weeks. A permanent exposure to a shift of the visual field in a direction compensating for the left hemispatial neglect is thus less effective on neglect than the adaptation to this optical deviation, because it produces mainly a sensory, peripheral effect rather than a central effect on space representation. (p. 167)[19]

Clinical Pearl

With all patients with neglect and/or unilateral spatial inattention, try active-closed-loop prism adaptation activities before prescribing of yoked prisms on a long-term basis.

Clinical Technique

The procedure involves the patient wearing base left yoked prisms; generally 10 diopters should be just about right. Several points or targets should be marked on a vertical surface that is within arm's reach in front of the patient, but not too close to them. They should not have to lean forward to touch the vertical surface but should extend their arm to near full length. A card board, about the size of a sheet of standard 8.5 × 11" or A4 size is held under the patient's chin so that they cannot see their hand when the hand is held close to the body. The patient then looks at one of the points on the vertical surface and ballistically (very quickly in one movement, not slowly and certainly, not with any adjustments being made as the arm is moved) thrusts their index finger toward the target. They are to attempt to hit the target directly, in one swift movement, without any corrections made during the movement. This is very important. This should be done over and over to different points with each hand for 5–10 minutes. It can be done several times per day as well, but is better done in multiple short sessions rather than in one continuous long session. This should be repeated daily for 7–10 days and then discontinued, with observations related to the neglect and unilateral spatial inattention being made over time.

PRESCRIBING FULL FIELD YOKED PRISMS

The preceding section has documented both the complexity of the visual process, as well as the many ways patients with brain injury may react in both the short term and long term to yoked prisms. One should have yoked prisms on hand for testing. Nearly all of the work done outside of optometry has been done with "wedge" or flat prisms rather than prisms with a positive front base curve. The clinician should have both sets on hand for testing purposes. In particular, if you get to the stage that you are considering prescribing yoked prism by having the prism ground into the final eyeglass prescription for the patient, then you should have some curved prisms to assess your patient's behavior with.

Prisms can be obtained in several forms for trial purposes. Bernell Corporation[**] and VTE Stress Point Test from Italy[††] produce holders that allow the prisms to be rotated independently of each other (Figure 7.41). To make the prisms into yoked prisms, one need only rotate both prisms so that the bases are pointing in the same direction. One benefit to these prisms is that you can invest in just a few pairs and that will allow you to cover a wide range of powers and all possible directions of prism.

It is recommended to have several powers of prisms for both testing and training. Most optometric testing begins with 5-diopter prisms. However, greater powers are often used when probing visual field conditions. It is recommended to have 10-, 15-, 20-, and 25-diopter prisms in addition to the standard 5-diopter prisms. One may find situations where less power is also helpful. Some practitioners find having sets with 1 and 3 diopters of prism are helpful as well. Pairs of Fresnel trial prisms (Figure 7.37) can be used in a trial frame, but the image quality isn't as good as with full field prisms and when assessing behavioral changes to prism it is best to have prisms like that pictures above. Of course, there are situations where you may decide to try very high-powered prisms and these may only be available in Fresnel form.

[**] Bernell, 4016 N Home St., Mishawaka, IN, 46545, Phone: 1–800–348–2225, www.bernell.com.
[††] VTE equipment can be obtained through Bernell Corporation.

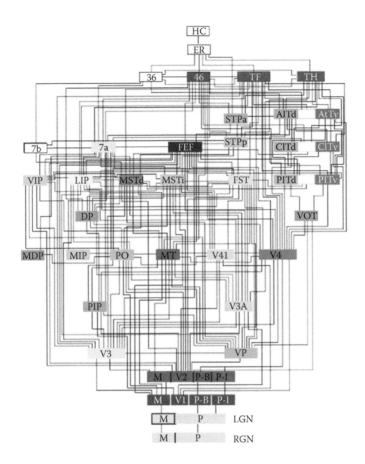

FIGURE 4.1 Hierarchy of visual areas. This hierarchy shows 32 visual areas. These areas are connected by linkages, most of which have been demonstrated to be reciprocal pathways. (From Felleman, D. J. and Van Essen, D. C., *Cerebral cortex*, 1991, 1, 1. Reprinted with permission.)

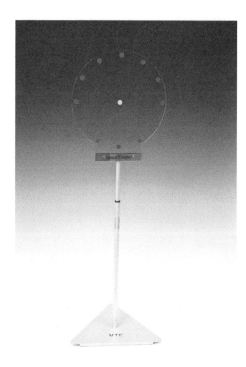

FIGURE 4.7 Space fixator. The transparent background and swiveling head allows for excellent feedback regarding localization in three-dimentional space when the patient attempts to touch each of the dots in a programmed therapy regimen.

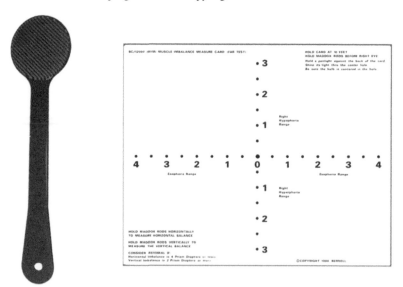

FIGURE 4.12 Maddox rod and phoria card (modified Thorington method) for assessing phoria in a two-dimensional plane. (Reprinted with permission from Bernell, V. T. P. www. bernell.com, 4016 N. Home St. Mishawaka, IN. 46545.)

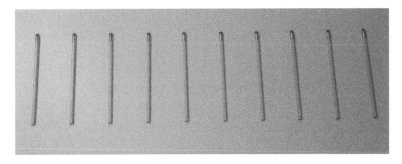

FIGURE 5.7   Pencil layout test for visual-spatial neglect.

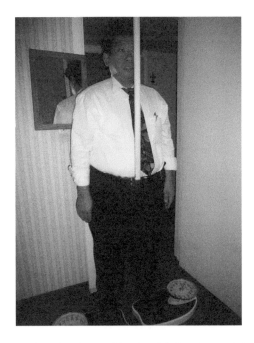

FIGURE 6.6   Patient performing the combined weight bearing and visual egocentric localization tests.

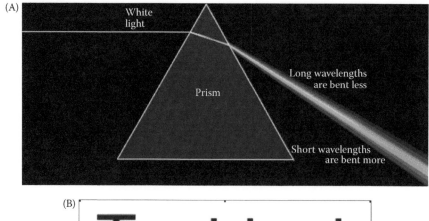

FIGURE 7.2 (A) This figure shows white light being broken down into the spectrum by a prism. (B) This is a demonstration of how high-contrast, square-wave, black on white text looks after passing through a prism. There is an apparent doubling with a ghost yellow image to the right and a "blurring" effect, which is produced by a blue color fringe to the left of the core of the letter and with a red fringe to the right of the black letter.

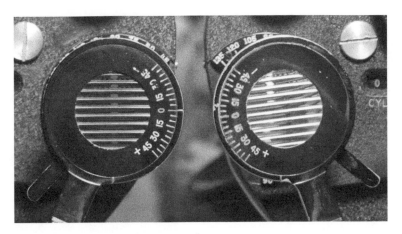

FIGURE 7.23 This shows the setup for doing the double Maddox test for cyclo rotations. Shown is the Bausch and Lomb phoropter, which allows for both Maddox rods to be rotated through 360 degrees. Here the red Maddox rod, which is before the patient's right eye is set to "0" and is the vertical reference line. The white Maddox rod, which is before the patient's left eye is close to 10 degrees of excyclorotation.

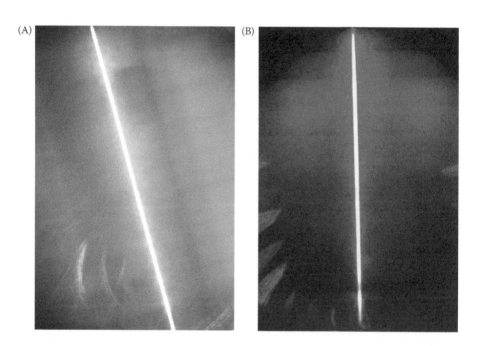

FIGURE 7.24 A: This gives a patient's view of the double Maddox rod test. A The right eye sees the vertical red line, which can easily be seen to be perpendicular to the horizontal segments of the lens. B: The left eye sees the white line. Here the white Maddox rod is shown rotated, with the top to the left. The white Maddox rod is rotated until the patient subjectively reports the two lines to be parallel to each other.

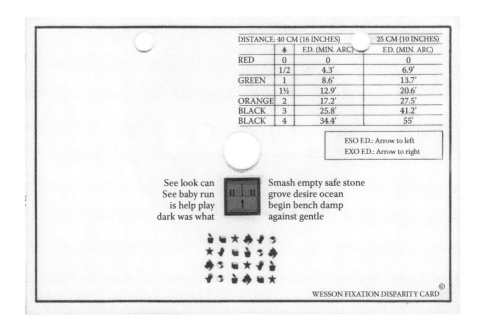

DISTANCE: 40 CM (16 INCHES)			25 CM (10 INCHES)
	⬆	F.D. (MIN. ARC)	F.D. (MIN. ARC)
RED	0	0	0
	1/2	4.3'	6.9'
GREEN	1	8.6'	13.7'
	1½	12.9'	20.6'
ORANGE	2	17.2'	27.5'
BLACK	3	25.8'	41.2'
BLACK	4	34.4'	55'

ESO F.D.: Arrow to left
EXO F.D.: Arrow to right

See look can
See baby run
is help play
dark was what

Smash empty safe stone
grove desire ocean
begin bench damp
against gentle

WESSON FIXATION DISPARITY CARD ©

FIGURE 7.29 This is the Wesson fixation disparity card. The only portion with Polaroid filters is the very center portion. The small lower arrow is seen through one channel and the colored lines above are seen through the other channel. Everything else on the card is seen by both eyes and is to act as a form of fusion lock, fusion hold or stimulus to fusion, depending on the model used by the clinician.

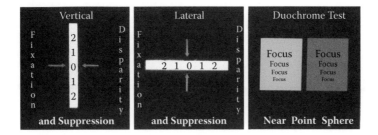

FIGURE 7.33 This is the center portion of the Mallett fixation disparity card as produced by Bernell. It is meant to be used in the back holder part of the Macular integrity tester. It can also be used on a Vectogram stand.

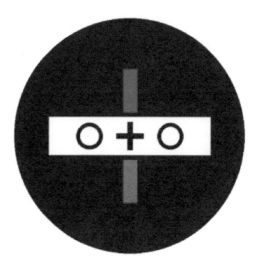

FIGURE 7.34 This simple demonstration of a Mallett target for fixation disparity uses glasses with one lens red and one lens blue. The black and white areas are seen by both eyes and the red and blue lines become the indicators. In general, this type of measure yields much cruder information that the Wesson card and it becomes difficult to do much more than find the central tendency.

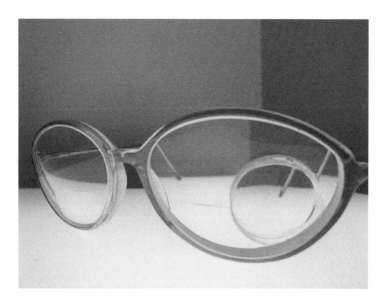

FIGURE 7.42 This figure shows a Gottlieb Visual Field Awareness System™ lens mounted in the temporal field of the left eye. (Courtesy of Dr. Daniel Gottlieb, www.gottliebvision-group.com)

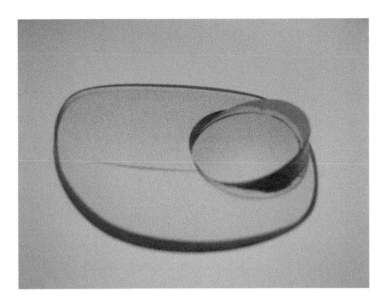

FIGURE 7.43 This figure shows the inside surface view of the Gottlieb Visual Awareness System™ lens. The lens was tinted for the patient's comfort. (Courtesy of Dr. Daniel Gottlieb, www.gottliebvisiongroup.com)

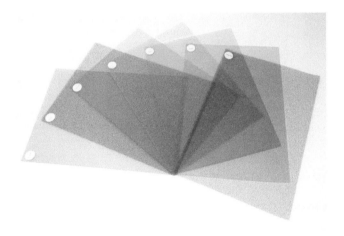

FIGURE 8.1 Colored overlays.

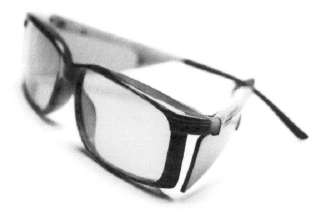

FIGURE 8.2 Wellness Protect Eyewear. (Courtesy of Eschenbach Optik of America, www.eschenbach.com)

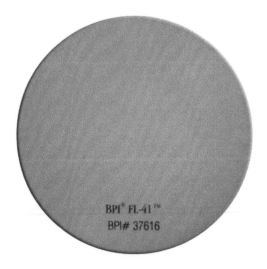

FIGURE 8.3 FL-41 lens. (Courtesy of Brain Power Incorporated, www.callbpi.com)

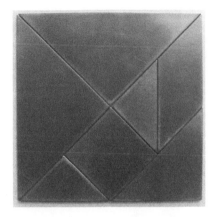

FIGURE 11.1 On the left, is a Tangram puzzle to be solved by placing the Tangram pieces, shown on the right, to create the puzzle figure.

<pre>
Perceptual Speed   00.33
           Choose 1 that is like: 7 Q U X N

   7 X N U Q   7 U N X Q   7 U Q X N   7 Q U X N
   A X 6 H 3   H X 6 A 3   H 6 X A 3   H 6 3 A X
   N M P I 9   I M P N 9   I 9 P N M   I 9 M N P
   T Z B E R   T R B E Z   T R B Z E   B R T Z E
   N 9 5 P V   N P 5 9 V   N P V 9 5   N V P 9 5
   N K Z 2 G   N K Z G 2   G K Z 2 N   G K Z N 2
   P R 3 4 X   X R 3 4 P   X R P 4 3   4 R P X 3
   1 U I 9 K   1 I U 9 K   I U 1 9 K   K U 1 9 I
   Q Y 0 5 S   Y Q O 5 S   Y 5 0 Q S   Y 5 Q 0 S
   J R K Y C   R J K Y C   R Y K J C   R K Y J C
   9 E V D M   W E V D 9   W D V E 9   E W V D 9
   M 3 B T 1   B 3 M T 1   3 B M T 1   3 1 M T B
   L A N 4 V   L A V 4 N   V A L 4 N   A L V 4 N
   4 W K 9 Y   4 Y K 9 W   W Y K 9 4   W Y 9 K 4
   8 M J X C   8 X J M C   8 X J C M   X 8 J C M
                        1 of 5
</pre>

FIGURE 11.2 Perceptual speed module from *Computerized Perceptual Therapy.* (Home Therapy, Inc.)

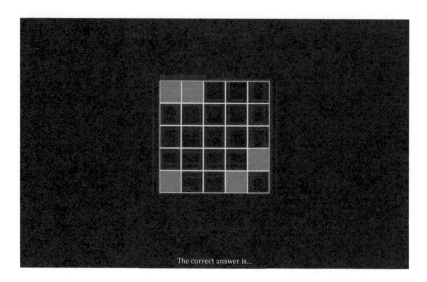

FIGURE 11.3 Visual memory module from *Computerized Perceptual Therapy*. (Home Therapy, Inc.)

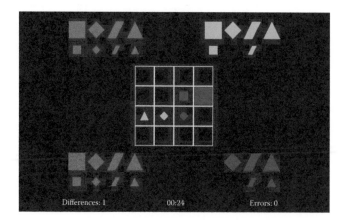

FIGURE 11.4 Visual thinking module from *Computerized Perceptual Therapy*. (Home Therapy, Inc.)

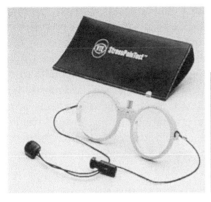
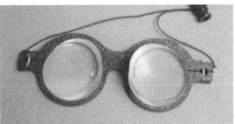

FIGURE 7.41   Commercially available prisms that can be rotated to be yoked prisms are shown above. The prisms shown at the left are available from VTE StressPoinTest, an Italian company. The prisms shown on the right are available from Bernell Corporation in the United States. Bernell also distributes the VTE prisms in the United States. (Photo from www.bernell. com. Reprinted with permission.)

In those circumstances, the use of the Fresnel prisms is desirable as a probe. The expense and time lag of getting prisms made by a lab simply to test a new condition is generally not practical.

It is important to keep in mind that due to the complexity of the conditions as noted earlier in the text that the patient may best be served by trying several varied sets of prisms, including different powers and base directions. If a particular set of prisms seems to bring about positive changes then the use of these should be pursued. It is important to be certain that the changes seen are repeatable. Therefore, with whatever types of activities you prefer to engage the patient in while observing them you should cycle through pairs of opposite bases in addition to frames or holders without any prism. As is seen sometimes in visual therapy and, in particular, with some intermittent exotropes, simply having a frame on the face may be enough to facilitate the person to change the way they look at the world.

Once a helpful direction and the amount of prism has been identified and once you have exhausted the prism aftereffects training benefits as mentioned above, then it is suggested to go through the same basic steps as outlined above in the alignment prism section. After in-office probes some in-office extended wear should take place. You might schedule the patient back for the duration of an hour or two and have them wear the proposed prisms while they are involved in various tasks that involve visually guided movements. At this stage it would be best to have curved yoked prisms near the amount you will be prescribing to get the most out of your observations.

When prescribing full field yoked prisms for visual field problems you may also have to consider at what distances you would like to have the prisms worn for. If you feel the benefit is primarily for gross motor movement tasks and not for activities that will be done while the person is at rest, then you might consider two pairs of glasses. One would be set up primarily for distance tasks and would include the yoked prisms, while the second pair would be set up primarily for near tasks and would not include the yoked prisms. NOTE: This type of prescribing has been done traditionally, and over time many patients have found that they use the yoked prism glasses less and less. This has sometimes been taken as a sign that the yoked prisms are not effective. The contrary may be what is actually true. The on and off of the yoked prisms, with the yoked prisms being used mostly for visually guided movements may have facilitated, through the aftereffects produced upon their removal, a form of vision rehabilitation therapy, the end results of which are more awareness of the full visual field and less need for the field shifting, resulting in a decreased need for the lenses and decreased benefit from wearing them.

> **Clinical Pearl**: Patients with yoked prisms should be monitored more frequently over the first few months of wear and decreases in wearing times should be noted. The clinician will have to sort out compliance problems from those instances where the use of the prisms is causing a measurable change in the patient's condition.

MIRRORS

Though this chapter is about the use of prisms in the care of patients with brain injury, it should be noted that some clinicians have used mirrors, both monocularly and binocularly in lieu of prisms to attempt similar spatial transformations. In general, these approaches have not yielded significant clinical success. Suchoff and Ciuffreda state, "Mirrors are either mounted of clipped to the nasal side of the spectacle lens that is on the same side as the affected field (i.e., left spectacle lens for a left field defect). The mirror is tilted to reflect the compromised field into the patient's left eye. The patient is then required to actively look into the mirror to obtain a view of that field. There are some difficulties with this device: the patient sees a reversed image of that field and must resolve the superimposition of the mirror's image of the other eye. Further the cosmetic appearance of the device is not acceptable to many patients" (p. 312).[20] Gottlieb, Freeman, and Williams report that, "Clinical experience has proven that mirrors used to expand the patient's visual field awareness can cause significant disorientation and perceptual confusion due to image reversal" (p. 581).[29]

SPOTTING/SECTOR PRISMS

Two additional methods for using prisms in cases of acquired visual field problems and visual-spatial neglect have been to use small sections of prisms mounted either on or through a portion of the lens on one side of the patient's glasses. The two basic applications of these prisms, the Gottlieb Visual Field Awareness System™ and the Peli Lens™ are based on different principles. Margolis and Suter refer to the use of sector prisms in the case of the Gottlieb System, as a spotting or alerting system; "With peripheral prism systems, the patient is also taught how to fixate quickly into the prism to gain awareness of objects in the hemianopic field, ignoring the double vision that this creates. If something of interest is viewed in the prism, the patient must then turn her head toward the target to view it outside of the prism" (p. 5).[14]

As has been stated before, this type of system requires awareness on the part of the person of their field defect as the effective use of the system is a cognitively top-down type of system.

An alternate approach to the use of monocular sector prisms was developed by Eli Peli. The Peli Lens™‡‡ prism system is not based on a top-down approach to the use of the prisms, but on a bottom-up development of a wider field of view. Peli states, "The effects of these devices may be classified as providing either field-of-view relocation (shifting) or field-of-view expansion. Field-of-view expansion is the preferred effect, because the simultaneously seen field-of-view is wider with the device than without it. A wider field-of-view enables the patients to monitor more of the environment at any instant and thus offers safer mobility. Field-of-view relocation only exchanges the position of the field loss relative to the environment or relative to the body's midline" (p. 454).[12]

Both prism systems have effects on the visual system. The reader should be familiar with both methods as additional tools for assisting patients with acquired visual field problems. The Gottlieb system has been demonstrated to be associated with actual recovery of visual field along the border zone in many patients, perhaps due to the necessity of scanning into the blind field on a consistent basis. Because the Peli prism is a "bottom-up" system that does not require scanning into, it may be quite useful for patients with visual-spatial neglect who will not scan, will not necessarily recognize the effect, but will functionally benefit from it, as well as other patients with visual field deficits, as it provides immediate optical expansion of the visual field. Each system will now be discussed individually.

Gottlieb Visual Field Awareness System™

The Gottlieb Visual Field Awareness System™§§ uses a single round prism button that is mounted through a hole that is cut through the carrier lens (Figures 7.42 and 7.43). The carrier lens holds the standard prescription and can be any plastic lens that will allow the hole to be drilled in it without cracking.

Prism diameters of 7/8 inches, 1inch, and 1–1/4 inches are available, along with a trial lens kit and fitting guide from Rekindle. A prism of 18.5 prism diopters is typically used.[30] The prism is mounted within a spectacle-borne single vision or multifocal prescription near the edge of the individual's perceived visual field, within the area of the visual field loss. Thus, the prism is unseen until the patient scans into it. The patient's spectacle prescription is ground into the prism button so that the view when scanning into the button is relatively clear, as there are the typical distortions one would expect from an 18.5-diopter prism. According to Gottlieb and Suter,[30] the prism works by superimposing images from the unseen field over those from the seen field, when the prism is scanned into. Gottlieb and Suter further state that the system allows patients with field loss to better fill in the gaps and understand the missing area, which is invaluable for both function and safety.

---

‡‡ Available through Chadwick Optical, Inc., 1763 Old River Road, White River Junction, VT, 05001, Phone: 1–800–410–1618, www.chadwickoptical.com
§§ Rekindle™, Gottlieb Vision Group, 10700 Medlock Bridge Rd., Suite 103, John Creek, GA, 30097, USA, 1–678–417–9778, www.rekindlevision.com

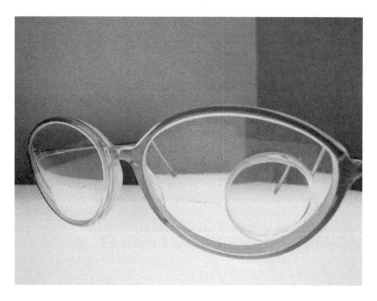

FIGURE 7.42 **(See color insert following page 270.)** This figure shows a Gottlieb Visual Field Awareness System™ lens mounted in the temporal field of the left eye. (Courtesy of Dr. Daniel Gottlieb, www.gottliebvisiongroup.com)

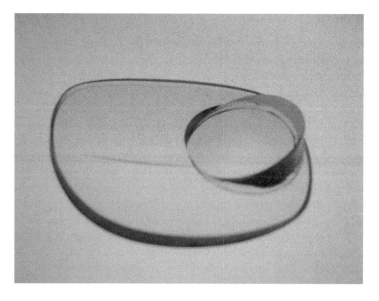

FIGURE 7.43 **(See color insert following page 270.)** This figure shows the inside surface view of the Gottlieb Visual Awareness System™ lens. The lens was tinted for the patient's comfort. (Courtesy of Dr. Daniel Gottlieb, www.gottliebvisiongroup.com)

Gottlieb et al.[29] conducted a study, which was later replicated. "Of the 16 subjects in the replication phase of the research protocol, eight chose to utilize the system full-time and three chose the system for selective part-time use. This represents a 69 percent (11 of 16) acceptance" (p. 587).[29] It would be helpful to see long-term follow up with these patients, including probes into other symptomology of neglect and homonymous hemianopia. Gottlieb does not discuss the use of his system for providing just the right type of life experience that might trigger some degree of field recalibration as mentioned earlier. However, the fact that this might be in play is evidenced by the following statement. "A review of the general statistics from all of the subjects ($N = 34$), documents increased visual field awareness of 6°–19°, with a mean of 13.25°" (p. 587).[29] These increases in sighted visual field were documented with Humphrey visual fields testing paying particular attention to fixation, and blindspot location, using the Humphrey comparison measures.

Peli Lens™ Prism System

Eli Peli conceived the idea of placing high power prisms (base toward the direction of the field loss) across the top and bottom of a spectacle carrier lens with a prism-free central area in between. This allowed objects on the blind side to be viewed on the seeing side without interfering with central vision. Peli[12] ran a study of 12 hemianopic patients, 9 of whom reported increased mobility and quality of life. For this study, Peli initially used a 40-diopter prism, the highest power available in a Fresnel Press-On, which shifted the image about 22 degrees. He stated that because the prism affected only peripheral vision, a higher power prism could be used despite the degradation of optics through the higher power prism.

Great emphasis is made when these prisms are prescribed to have the patient learn to look straight ahead through the portion of the lens where the carrier is and where the prism is not. The prism images are automatically picked up in the patient's superior and inferior periphery without interfering with central vision. Some patients describe these as "ghost images" that act as an early warning system for obstacle avoidance and provide true field expansion. The person automatically becomes aware of what is on the blind side and can then use head and eye movement to view the object through the central prism-free portion of the lens. The narrower strip prisms that have been developed leave room for the patient to look below the prism—either below the glasses if it is a narrow frame or in the bottom portion of the lens—to assist with placing feet without confusion at curbs and steps.

The following is from his fitting guide:

> The overall goal of the prism fitting is to determine the lowest position at which the upper prism can be worn and the highest position at which the lower prism can be worn i.e., to fit the prisms as close together as possible while still allowing comfortable central vision and a natural head posture when walking. In order to achieve this goal, the protocol lays out a standardized procedure for fitting, adjusting and evaluating the position of the upper prism segment and then the lower prism segment. (p. 2)[31]

Later refinement of this protocol in clinical practice showed that the two prisms should be at least 12 mm apart in the vertical dimension and that beginning with the prisms at this separation is recommended and widened as necessary.[32] In collaboration with Peli in 2003, Chadwick Optical, Inc., a specialty ophthalmic lens laboratory, developed permanent 40$^\Delta$ Peli Lens™ glasses (Figure 7.44). A 74% patient acceptance rate was reported at 6 weeks, with 47% continuing to wear the lenses after 12 months, in a recent multisite trial on the Peli Lens™.[33] A point of interest in this study was that clinicians who fit more of these prisms had a much higher success rate than those clinicians who fit very few. Careful adherence to the fitting guide developed and provided by Chadwick Optical appears to enhance success rates. Chadwick has continued this line of development on the Peli prism concept, including a 57$^\Delta$ Peli Lens™ in both horizontal (Figure 7.45) and oblique (Figure 7.46) configurations. These lenses were introduced in 2009, and provided 30 degrees of field expansion

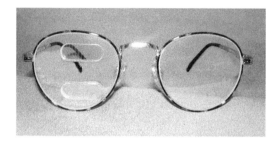

FIGURE 7.44 Photograph of 40$^\Delta$ horizontal Peli Lens™ glasses. The permanent Fresnel-type lenses are fused into the lens. (Courtesy of Chadwick Optical, Inc.)

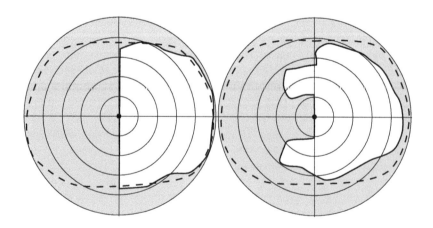

FIGURE 7.45 A comparison of hemianopic visual fields tested binocularly without (on the left) and with (on the right) the patient wearing 57$^\Delta$ Peli Lens™ glasses. It is easy to see the optical expansion into the blind visual field. (Courtesy of Chadwick Optical, Inc.)

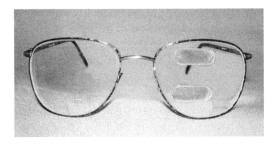

FIGURE 7.46 Photograph of 57$^\Delta$ oblique Peli Lens™ glasses. (Courtesy of Chadwick Optical, Inc.)

as opposed to the 22 degrees of the 40-diopter lenses. The oblique design uses tilted prisms to bring objects from upper and lower fields into midline view.

YOKED PRISM AND SECONDARY CONTRACTURE

Some conditions lead to an asymmetric shift in the posture of one eye relative to the other, such as that which occur in a lateral rectus paresis or paralysis. A mild paresis may result in a head turn that allows the person to restore the use of the binocular flow without the need for prism. A more pronounced paresis may be beyond the ability of the person to compensate for with a face turn, and, therefore, they may slip into diplopia and confusion causing them to begin developing alternate strategies for use of the flows from both channels.

One concern when there is an introduction of a sudden imbalance in the ocular motor system is a contraction or shortening of the unaffected muscle over time. In general, there is a minimum of two muscles acting as an agonist-antagonist pair. This muscle pair lives in a dynamic balance with a degree of dynamic tension between them. A certain amount of background contraction of healthy muscle tissue is present all the time and may be called the tone of that muscle. The sum of the background tones in the muscle pair is thought to be a factor in determining the balance point between the muscle pair. When there is a removal or reduction in the tone to one side the balance point shifts away from the affected side. The unaffected side then is more contracted.

Several options are available to the person to attempt to normalize the use of the affected system. One of these would be to decrease neurological output in the unaffected side to decrease background tonus to reduce the pull on the eye toward the unaffected side, allowing a shift back toward the habitual balance point. This does not seem to happen in most cases, leading to the conclusion that background tonus to single muscles may have rather narrow limits through which they can be modified in the short term.

There is evidence that if a muscle that was a certain length for a long period of time is functionally shortened by reduced opposition from its paired muscle or muscle groups then the length of the contractile sarcomeres shortens over time. This contracture can lead to problems should the originally affected neurological muscle unit recover. Once its strength returns to normal, if the problem was severe enough for a long enough period of time, the opposing muscle now may function as though it were shorter; even in the case of a full recovery, the baseline balance in the agonist-antagonist pair or group may not be restored.

To avoid this situation, London[34] recommends using yoked prism to shift the center point over into the affected side. He suggests a 15-diopter yoked prism with the base in the direction that would shift the eyes toward the affected side. A simpler clinical method to achieve this might be to give the patient stretching activities to get them to move their eyes to extreme positions of gaze for short periods of time throughout the day. If this is done, it is important to move in both directions, not just in the direction that would pull against the muscle that is at risk to shorten.

In this same vein of the discussion and for completeness, the condition progressive supranuclear palsy merits mention. A presenting symptom of this condition, which may mimic certain characteristics of Parkinson's disease, is a restricted movement of the eyes in downward gaze. Although there is a loss of neurological signal to move the eyes downward, the lack of movement into that field can lead to a secondary contracture that would further restrict movement. Thus, the first recommendation in these conditions is to have the patient move their eyes regularly to the extremes of gaze in all directions to avoid the embedding of these further restrictions. In addition, some have found clinically that some of these patients may benefit, not only from "bed" glasses discussed above, but also from vertical yoked prisms, and exploring their use in these conditions may be beneficial.

GENERAL LENS DESIGN CONSIDERATIONS

In providing patients with prisms, certain principles should help guide the eye care professional to choices that minimize distortions and maximize the patient's ability to benefit from the lenses. The first is the principle of minimum deviation. Figure 7.47 shows that there is an angle of incidence to a prism, at which the deviation of the light is at a minimum. This coincides to the path through a wedge prism where the chief ray passes through the lens parallel to the base of the prism.

The key point is that the prism power rating is based upon the minimum deviation pathway. It is important to note that rays of light that enter at angles steeper or flatter

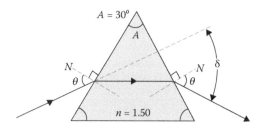

FIGURE 7.47   This figure shows the minimum deviation path of light through a prism.

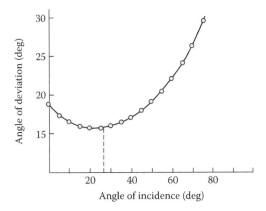

FIGURE 7.48 This figure shows how the effective power of a prism varies as a result of the angle of incidence of the light on the surfaces of the prism.

than the minimum deviation angle will cause the prism to act as a more powerful prism. Figure 7.48 shows how the angle of deviation varies as a factor of the angle of incidence of the light.

The practical point to consider when using prisms is to attempt to fabricate the lenses in a form that will deliver the desired effects and minimize the negative effects. One can easily see that this consideration led Gottlieb to mount his 18.5-diopter prism through the carrier lens so that a portion of the prism projects out in front of the lens and a portion projects behind the carrier lens to be closer to the patients' eye. In this manner he helps to bring the power of the lens as close to its rated power as possible. Of course, this is a more expensive way to mount such a prism.

CONCLUSION

Prisms are powerful tools that can be used to help patients who have suffered loss as a result of brain injury. Because the brain is so complex, and injuries vary from person to person, as well as having varied expression in the same person in different life situations, the good clinician needs to have a wide array of tools at his disposal to aid in recovery from brain damage. Prisms can be used in many different ways to help the patient recovering from ABI/TBI. The astute clinician will need to use his power of observation as different alternatives are tried to detect which may be the best for the particular person in front of him and to take the time to see both the immediate effects of the lenses and the rebound effects if any are present. Clinicians are routinely well out in front of the research in finding ways to utilize the tools at our disposal to help our patients. It remains for additional research guided by these insightful clinical minds to help elucidate the underlying mechanisms whereby prisms have the effects that they do. Invariably, as both clinicians gain insights by working with their patients and more research is done, we will identify and use prisms in more and varied ways to help the public.

REFERENCES

1. Kraskin, R. J. (2002). *Lens power in action*. Santa Ana, CA: Optometric Extension Program Foundation.
2. Jenkins, F. A., & White, H. E. (1976). *Fundamentals of optics* (4th ed.). New York: McGraw-Hill.
3. Rock, I. (1975). *An introduction to perception*. New York: Macmillan.
4. Kaufman, L. (1974). *Sight and mind, an introduction to visual perception*. New York: Oxford University Press.
5. Goodale, M., & Milner, D. (2004). *Sight unseen*. New York: Oxford University Press.
6. Graziano, M., & Gross, C. (1995). From Eye to Hand. In J. King, & K. Pribram (Eds.), *Scale in conscious experience: is the brain too important to be left to the specialists to study?* (pp. 117–132). Hillsdale, NJ: Lawrence Erlbaum.
7. Schwartz, E. L. (1993). *Computational Neuroscience*. Cambridge, MA: MIT Press.
8. Demer, J. L. (2004). Pivotal role of orbital connective tissues in binocular alignment and strabismus. *Investigative Ophthalmology and Visual Science, 45*(3), 729–738.
9. Ruskell, G. L., Kjellevold Haugen, I., Bruenech, J. R., & van der Werf, F. (2005). Double insertion of extraocular rectus muscles in humans and the pulley theory. *Journal of Anatomy, 206*(3), 295–306. doi: 10.1111/j.1469–7580.2005.00383.x.
10. Harris, P. (2002). The binocular continuum. *Journal of Behavioral Optometry, 13*(4), 99–103.
11. Sacks, O. W. (1989). *Seeing voices: A journey into the world of the deaf*. Berkley, CA: University of California Press.
12. Peli, E. (2000). Field expansion for homonymous hemianopia by optically induced peripheral exotropia. *Optometry and Vision Science, 77*(9), 453–464.
13. Giorgi, R., Woods, R., & Peli, E. (2009). Clinical and laboratory evaluation of peripheral prism glasses for hemianopia. *Optometry and Vision Sciences, 86*(5), 492–502.
14. Margolis, N. W., & Suter, P. S. (2006). Visual field defects & unilateral spatial inattention: diagnosis and treatment. *Journal of Behavioral Optometry, 17*(2), 31–37.
15. Chatterjee, A. (1998). Motor minds and mental models in neglect. *Brain and Cognition, 37*(3), 339–349.
16. Bartolomeo, P., & Chokron, S. (2002). Orienting of attention in left unilateral neglect. *Neuroscience and Biobehavioral Reviews, 26*(2), 217–234.
17. Pisella, L., Rode, G., Farné, A., Tilikete, C., & Rossetti, Y. (2006). Prism adaptation in the rehabilitation of patients with visuo-spatial cognitive disorders. *Current Opinion in Neurology, 19*(6), 534–542.
18. Michel, C., Pisella, L., Halligan, P., Luauté, J., Rode, G., Boisson, D., & Rossetti, Y. (2003). Simulating unilateral neglect in normals using prism adaptation: implication for theory. *Neuropsychologia, 41*(1), 25–39.
19. Rossetti, Y., Rode, G., Pisella, L., Farné, A., Li, L., Boisson, D., & Perenin, M.-T. (1998). Prism adaptation to a rightward optical deviation rehabilitates left hemispatial neglect. *Nature, 395*(Sept. 10), 166–169. doi:10.1038/25988.
20. Suchoff, I. B., & Ciuffreda, K. J. (2004). A primer for the optometric management of unilateral spatial inattention. *Optometry, 75*(5), 305–318.
21. Kapoor, N., Ciuffreda, K. J., & Suchoff, I. B. (2001). Egocentric localization in patients with visual neglect. In Ciuffreda, K., Suchoff, I., & Kapoor, N. (Eds.). *Visual & vestibular consequences of acquired brain injury*. Santa Ana, CA: Optometric Extension Program Foundation.
22. Pisella, L., Rode, G., Farné, A., Boisson, D., & Rossetti, Y. (2002). Dissociated long lasting improvements of straight-ahead pointing and line bisection tasks in two hemineglect patients. *Neuropsychologia, 40*(3), 327–334.

23. Padula, W., & Argyris, S. (1996). Post trauma vision syndrome and visual midline shift syndrome. *NeuroRehabilitation, 6,* 165–171.

24. Pisella, L., Michel, C., Gréa, H., Tilikete, C., Vighetto, A., & Rossetti, Y. (2004). Preserved prism adaptation in bilateral optic ataxia: strategic versus adaptive reaction to prisms. *Experimental Brain Research, 156*(4), 399–408.

25. Michel, C., Pisella, L., Prablanc, C., Rode, G., & Rossetti, Y. (2007). Enhancing visuomotor adaptation by reducing error signals: single-step (aware) versus multiple-step (unaware) exposure to wedge prisms. *Journal of Cognitive Neuroscience, 19*(2), 341–350.

26. Luauté, J., Michel, C., Rode, G., Pisella, L., Jacquin-Courtois, S., Costes, N., Rossetti, Y. (2006). Functional anatomy of the therapeutic effects of prism adaptation on left neglect. *Neurology, 66,* 1859–1867.

27. Luauté, J., Halligan, P., Rode, G., Jacquin-Courtois, S., & Boisson, D. (2006). Prism adaptation first among equals in alleviating left neglect: a review. *Restorative Neurology and Neuroscience, 24*(4–6), 409–418.

28. Michel, C., Pisella, L., Halligan, P., Luauté, J., Rode, G., Boisson, D., & Rossetti, Y. (2003). Simulating unilateral neglect in normals using prism adaptation: implication for theory. *Neuropsychologia, 41*(1), 25–39.

29. Gottlieb, D. D., Freeman, P., & Williams, M. (1992). Clinical research and statistical analysis of a visual field awareness system. *Journal of the American Optometric Association, 63*(8), 581–588.

30. Gottlieb, D. D., & Suter, P. S. (2001). Visual field loss (homonymous hemianopsia) and visuospatial neglect. Retrieved from http://www.gottliebvisiongroup.com/Suter_Gottlieb_paper.htm (Accessed February 25, 2010).

31. Bowers, A., Keeney, K., & Peli, E. (2004). Community-based trial of peripheral prism visual field expansion device of hemianopia – fitting and training protocol. Retrieved from http://www.eri.harvard.edu/faculty/peli/shared/Fit_n_train_protocol_web.pdf

32. Chadwick Optical, Inc. (2008). *EP-horizontal fresnel press-on expansion prism system fitting guide.* White River Junction, VT: Author.

33. Bowers, A. R., Keeney, K., & Peli, E. (2008). Community-Based trial of a peripheral prism visual field expansion device for hemianopia. *Archives of Ophthalmology, 126*(5), 657–664.

34. London, R. (2005, August). Review of management strategies for the diplopic patient. Pacific University online course documentation. Retrieved from http://www.pacificu.edu/optometry/ce/list/14717.cfm (Accessed February 26, 2010).

8 Photophobia, Light, and Color in Acquired Brain Injury

Cathy D. Stern

CONTENTS

INTRODUCTION

Light, in the visible spectrum, is processed both for vision, and for nonvision modulation of human function. A critical part of light for vision is spectral sensitivity, which allows us to perceive an almost limitless array of colors from the combined input of less than a half dozen different types of light receptors. Nonvision responses to light resulting from eye-brain connections include regulation of circadian rhythms through the action spectrum for melatonin regulation and neuroendocrine modulation.[1]

Deficits in the processing of light and color are common following acquired brain injury (ABI). Deficits in the processing of light often lead to photophobia, dark adaptation deficits, or hypersensitivity to strong patterns, resulting in migraine, reading difficulty, or even seizure activity. Deficits in color perception can occur due to damage to the eye, optic nerve, and chiasm, interrupting the reception of color, or due to cortical damage interfering with the perception of color. Congenital color deficits are not considered in this chapter.

Deficits in processing light and color can have a significant impact on overall rehabilitation of the patient following brain injury. Careful diagnosis is critical for determining the best treatment as these deficits have multiple etiologies. Current treatments for these deficits include multiple modalities, from tinted lenses, tinted overlays, and light exposure therapy sessions, to addressing the underlying causal defect through vision rehabilitation therapy.

PHOTOPHOBIA

Photophobia, or extreme light sensitivity, is characterized by intolerance to light. It is a common symptom following ABI that frequently persists after other symptoms have resolved.[2] While all of us encounter circumstances where the amount or quality of light is bothersome, many ABI patients have a lower threshold for light tolerance. They demonstrate not only increased sensitivity to bright illumination but impaired performance in dim illumination.[3] They are often affected indoors as well as outdoors and their condition is different from the photosensitivity of ocular disease.

Causes for photophobia include cortical changes in light sensitivity, binocular vision disorders, post trauma vision syndrome (PTVS), and ocular damage. Photophobia has a significant impact for activities of daily living including work, school, and recreation. Therefore, comprehensive patient history and vision evaluation is critical for proper diagnosis and treatment.

Photosensitivity following ABI has been called *functional photophobia* by Lane.[4] The source of the photosensitivity is nonocular, rarely accompanied by pain and often seen along with headache, nausea, and dizziness. Some patients also report a perception of waviness or shimmering of their surround that is greater in bright light.[5] This is different from glare hypersensitivity experienced by the person with a traumatized eye or when photopigments are depleted as in malnourished individuals or those with ocular albinism.

Patients with photosensitivity following ABI were found to have an objective increase in sensitivity to light, both within 3 weeks of minor head injury[6] and 6 months following mild head injury for those with persistent postconcussion symptoms.[7] While patients often report sensitivity to normal or bright light, they are often less likely to report reduced visual performance in the dark and a thorough history should include questions about visual ability in the dark.

Photophobia may be associated with reading difficulty despite normal binocular vision and is found to be closely related to visual stress.[8] Wilkins[9] uses the term visual stress to describe symptoms of eyestrain, headaches, and even seizures provoked by reading. Patients may report movement or blurring of print, letters changing size or doubling, patterns or illusions of color appearing on the page, nausea, dizziness, and discomfort.[8] Photophobia and accompanying symptoms such as eyestrain, nausea, or dizziness can have a significant effect not only while reading, but for general mobility, driving, work, and other activities of daily living.

Treatment may include remediation of binocular vision disorders, colored filters or overlays, prism lenses, binasal or other selective occlusion, tinted contact lenses, or syntonic phototherapy. Other neurologic disorders may present with symptoms similar to those accompanying photophobia.[9] These include migraine headache, computer vision syndrome, dyslexia, epilepsy, and multiple sclerosis. Patients with these conditions may respond to similar methods of treatment.

CAUSES OF LIGHT SENSITIVITY

Photosensitivity following ABI has been attributed to a variety of causes, including magnocellular damage, cortical hyperexcitability, binocular vision disorders, and PTVS.

Magnocellular Damage

Dark adaptation is the process by which the visual system maintains a constant level of light sensitivity regardless of the level of ambient illumination. Elevated dark adaptation thresholds mean the patient demonstrates decreased photosensitivity in the dark. Jackowski[10] assessed dark adaptation in patients with ABI reporting varied levels of light sensitivity. All patients were found to have elevated dark adaptation thresholds. Those patients experiencing the most pronounced photophobia had the most elevated thresholds. Rod-mediated visual sensitivity was significantly impaired. Cone-mediated visual sensitivity was also deficient but only mildly impaired in comparison to the rod-mediated visual loss. The rods and cones, respectively, feed into the magnocellular and parvocellular visual pathways. Jackowski hypothesized that as these pathways are mutually antagonistic the reduction in rod-mediated response may allow for an exaggerated cone pathway response to light leading to hypersensitivity to light in typical room illumination. Zihl and Kerkhoff[3] assessed dark adaptation in ABI patients with varied sensitivity to light as well as with patients reporting difficulty functioning in dim illumination. Forty percent of the patients reported experiencing both symptoms, while 22% were asymptomatic. More than 50% of the patients who reported visual light adaptation problems demonstrated reduced light sensitivity or elevated dark adaptation thresholds.

Du, Ciuffreda, and Kapoor also found that more than 50% of patients with ABI who reported photosensitivity exhibited elevated dark adaptation thresholds.[11] They propose that two separate mechanisms exist and both are damaged during

ABI. There is an abnormality in cortical gain control for photopic light stimulation resulting in hypersensitivity while those with elevated dark adaptation threshold develop an anomalous cortical adaptive response as an attempt to attenuate light at all levels that leads to excessive attenuation and therefore elevated dark adaptation thresholds.

Visual field study utilizing frequency doubling technology (FDT) was carried out by Jackowski to further investigate magnocellular deficits in acquired ABI. Jackowski utilized FDT, which is particularly sensitive to magnocellular loss, to measure visual field sensitivity throughout the central 30-degree field.[10] This was in response to the degree of rod-mediated sensitivity losses and the common complaint of loss of peripheral visual field awareness. All of the patients complaining of light sensitivity demonstrated visual field sensitivity losses throughout the central 30 degrees. The most affected patients exhibited a constriction of the visual field for each eye with preservation of sensitivity within the central 10 degrees. All the patients with loss of sensitivity also reported episodes of "collapsing" of the visual field and dimming of field brightness during the testing. These symptoms increased with time and were alleviated with eye closure.

Visual field study is important in identifying the generalized visual field constriction seen in patients reporting photophobia. Langerhorst and Safran[12] attribute this to an organic disturbance in attentional mechanisms, revealed when executing dual task demands. Jackowski attributes it to a common postretinal mechanism given the high degree of correlation between visual field sensitivity losses and the losses found in rod-mediated activity upon dark adaptation.[10]

Cortical Hyperexcitability

Wilkins proposes a theory of cortical hyperexcitability. He hypothesizes that black and white stripes or other strong geometric patterns cause a nonuniform spread of excitation among neighboring pyramidal neurons with resulting perceptual distortion, and normal cortical inhibition may be insufficient to stop the spread of excitation.[9,8] This cortical hyperexcitability or under-inhibition may be caused by lack of uptake of the excitatory amino acid glutamate causing glutamate overactivity.[13] It may also be caused by an imbalance of the inhibitory neurotransmitter gamma aminobutyric acid or GABA.[14] An individual's degree of susceptibility to the visual distortion increases with, and reflects, the degree of cortical hyperexcitability.[15,13] The visual patterns that provoke sensations of visual distortion in patients with photophobia are similar to those that trigger seizures in patients with photosensitive epilepsy.[9] Photosensitivity has even been described as a form of reflex partial epilepsy and can be suppressed with drugs that promote GABAergic transmission.[16]

Noseda et al. found that blind individuals experience exacerbation of migraine headache by light even in the face of massive rod/cone degeneration.[17] They propose that the non-image-forming retinal pathway, involving ganglion cells known as melanopsin containing intrinsically photosensitive retinal ganglion cells or ipRGCs, modulates the activity of dura-sensitive thalamocortical neurons. ipRGC axons converge on dura-sensitive neurons in posterior thalamus.

Binocular Vision Disorders

Binocular vision and accommodative disorders are common vision disturbances following ABI.[18] The symptoms of binocular and accommodative dysfunction may be difficult to distinguish from the symptoms of visual stress, as described by Wilkins.[8] He emphasizes the importance of optometric testing to sort out the cause of the photophobia.[19] Ample evidence exists demonstrating the effectiveness of optometric vision therapy for binocular and accommodative dysfunction (reviewed by Scheiman and Galloway).[20]

Lane found that students with functional photophobia demonstrate an accommodative fatigue syndrome and variability of binocular convergence.[21] The symptoms of photophobia were dramatically relieved by having the student cover one eye. Treatment to reverse the accommodative and binocular dysfunction included low power plus lenses and optometric vision therapy.

Wilkins found that children in his study who benefited from colored lens therapy demonstrated slightly poorer performance for near point of convergence and prism vergence but it was rarely clinically abnormal and many of the children had normal binocular function.[22] He relates the symptoms to visual stress, but, again, he does emphasize the importance of optometric testing to sort out the cause of the photophobia.[19] Wilkins does report that epileptic visual sensitivity as well as pattern sensitivity is greater under binocular stimulation and covering one eye attenuated the photoconvulsive response to flicker,[23] which might be expected from reducing the photic input by half. However, pattern sensitivity was also reduced by covering one eye.[24]

Monocular eye closure in sunlight is often seen in patients with strabismus or intermittent exotropia. During testing with high intensity light, subjects were found to have a mean monocular photophobia threshold significantly higher than the binocular threshold (i.e., monocularly, subjects tolerated higher intensity light before reporting photophobia) and binocular photophobia thresholds were significantly lower in those reporting eye closure. None of the subjects reported diplopia so the conclusion is that monocular eye closure in sunlight is a mechanism used to reduce photophobia.[25]

Post Trauma Vision Syndrome

Post trauma vision syndrome has been described as the most common visual sequela following traumatic brain injury (TBI).[26] Signs and symptoms may include high exophoria or exotropia, convergence insufficiency, ocular motor dysfunction, accommodative dysfunction, low blink rate, spatial disorientation, diplopia, headaches, and photophobia. These signs and symptoms are hypothesized to result from an imbalance in central (focal) versus peripheral (ambient) processing.[27] Padula et al.[28] reported reductions in N1–P1 amplitudes of visual evoked cortical potentials (VECP) in patients diagnosed with PTVS; VECP amplitudes increased immediately with application of binasal patches or bases-in prism in these patients. Full-field electroretinography (ERG) and VECP were used by Freed and Hellerstein to assess patients with mild TBI.[29] Full-field ERG results were unremarkable in patients with mild TBI. VECP studies revealed waveform abnormalities in a large percentage of the mild TBI subjects indicating probable primary visual pathway deficit.

Mydriasis

Pupil dilation of one or both eyes can lead to a complaint of photophobia. This may be a result of trauma to the iris sphincter, CN III damage, or a reaction to medications such as amphetamines or antihistamines. Many widely prescribed antidepressants may also cause mydriasis. Tinted lenses, tinted contact lenses, or, in extreme cases, artificial pupil contact lenses may be beneficial for reducing excessive light.

Dry Eye Syndrome/Lagophthalmos

Dry eye is extremely common after ABI and may contribute to photophobia. Lagophthalmos, incomplete closure of the eye, is also very common following TBI and leads to exposure keratitis, causing photophobia. In both cases, ocular lubricants and/or therapeutic contact lenses can be beneficial.

IMPACT ON DAILY LIFE

Following TBI, patients frequently present with complaints of visual dysfunction.[2,18] The impact on everyday tasks can be significant. Activities of daily living as well as academic, occupational, and recreational activities may be a challenge. Patients frequently report light sensitivity and reading discomfort. They are less likely to be aware of difficulty in dim illumination or of the effects of visual field constriction while driving. Careful questioning of patients will help the clinician match symptoms to diagnostic testing and allow for appropriate application of treatment alternatives. Hellerstein et al.[2] report significantly more visual symptoms in TBI patients compared to controls. Light sensitivity and reading problems were prominent. Jackowski notes that patients with photosensitivity may also report reading discomfort, loss of visual function in the dark, peripheral visual field reduction, visual distortion, and asthenopia.[10]

Wilkins discusses how reading can provoke "pattern glare" resulting in eyestrain, headaches, and visual distortion.[9] He proposes that successive lines of text resemble a pattern of stripes. Pattern from text is known to induce perceptual distortions leading to headaches and eyestrain in susceptible individuals. Wilkins found that symptoms are reduced if change is made to spacing between the lines of print or if a reading mask similar to a typoscope is introduced that covers all but the text being read.[9,30] In general, reading comfort is increased when the spacing between the lines of print is about 1.5 times the font point size (e.g., if point size is 12, the line spacing should be about 16–18 point spacing). This appears to have a similar effect to a reading mask or typoscope.

Knowledge of the patient's symptoms and the possible effects on performance is critical to helping the patient function on a daily basis. Even when treatment will not fully alleviate the symptoms or will take time, patients are appreciative of the recognition that their symptoms are real and related to their injury. Often, simple adaptations such as change in classroom placement or modifications to positioning of reading material are very effective in helping the patient function in everyday life.

COLOR VISION DEFICITS FOLLOWING ACQUIRED BRAIN INJURY

Color perception refers to our ability to see color and is commonly tested with Ishihara color plates or Waggoner's *Color Vision Testing Made Easy*™ (CVTME). Passing of Ishihara or CVTME requires both normal color perception as well as adequate figure-ground ability. Further testing with the Farnsworth D-15 color vision test should be considered for patients who fail Ishihara or CVTME to confirm that failure does indeed indicate loss of color perception.

Optic Nerve and Chiasm Color Deficits

Damage to the optic nerve and chiasm, may occur in TBI. The Farnsworth D-15 or desaturated D-15 or the Lanthony 15 can be helpful in detecting subtle optic neuropathy. Acquired color vision loss usually does not respect the color visual axes (as indicated on these tests). A differential color vision deficit between the two eyes implies an acquired deficit, as congenital color vision defects are symmetrical between the two eyes. A comparison of saturation of colors between the two eyes and monocularly across the vertical midline (as in the red cap test) can provide a quick screening for optic neuropathy.[31]

Cortical Color Deficits

As reviewed by Tranel, central color vision deficits fall into four categories: color naming, color imagery, color recognition, and color perception.[32] Color naming deficits (color anomia) are those not caused by aphasia or defective color vision, in which the patient is unable to name colors or point to objects of that color, given the color name. Loss of color imagery is determined by self-report. Loss of color recognition or color agnosia prevents a person from identifying the color of an object even though the eyes are capable of distinguishing color. Color naming should be tested as well as the standard "color vision" tests mentioned above. Cortical color vision deficits following ABI are rare and are typically treated with compensatory or cognitive therapies where they affect function during daily activities.

VISION EVALUATION

Vision evaluation for patients with brain injury is often overlooked because vision deficits are hidden, while other medical and behavioral considerations appear more prominent. Vision evaluation typically includes a detailed history, determination of refractive status, and assessment of ocular health. Primary care optometric evaluation also includes sensorimotor examination with assessment of ocular motor, accommodative, and binocular vision status.[2] The color testing described above should be included and several other tests, described below, may be added that are helpful in assessing the impact of photophobia and subsequent treatment.

Pupillary Responses

Pupil responses should be carefully evaluated. Third nerve damage may lead to the presence of mydriasis, asymmetric or fluctuating pupil diameter. Less obvious is careful observation of response time and pupillary release. When a penlight is beamed into one eye, pupillary constriction is expected. The constriction should hold for at least 10 sec. When pupillary release takes place, this is called *pupillary escape*. If the pupil dilates within a few seconds, this is known as an alpha–omega pupil.[33] According to Gottlieb and Wallace,[34] the faster the pupillary escape, the smaller the functional visual field. Any sluggish pupillary response most likely indicates autonomic system imbalance.

CONTRAST SENSITIVITY

Contrast sensitivity measurement can be useful in understanding complaints of blurry or foggy vision in the presence of normal visual acuity. Loss of contrast sensitivity for middle to low spatial frequency results from damage to the magnocellular system and may help to explain the frequently reported foggy vision and difficulty with daily activities.

VISUAL FIELD

Visual field study is important not only for identifying characteristic visual field deficits related to primary visual pathway lesions (retina-LGN-V1) but also for identifying the generalized visual field constriction that is common in patients reporting photophobia. This is best done with either FDT[10] or kinetic functional visual field evaluation.[33] The degree of visual field constriction often correlates to the severity of symptoms. Wallace has demonstrated good correlation between kinetic perimetry obtained by use of a moving stimulus from a nonseeing area toward the fixation point until it is seen and FDT visual fields.[35]

PHOTOPHOBIA VERSUS GLARE SENSITIVITY

Photophobia is an abnormal sensitivity or intolerance to light, while glare sensitivity is discomfort or reduced visual performance from a strong or dazzling light source. Glare testing measures the effect of a glare source on visual acuity or contrast sensitivity. Common glare testers include the Marco brightness acuity tester (BAT), Stereo Optical Optec Rehab Vision Tester, VectorVision CSV-1000HGT (Halogen Glare Test), and Miller-Nadler Glare Tester.

FUNCTIONAL PHOTOPHOBIA GRADING SYSTEM

One may want to better quantify the level of photophobia. While no formal scales have been proposed, Lane has defined five behavioral stages of functional photophobia.[21]

- Stage PP-Zero—no apparent hypersensitivity
- Stage PP-1—newly experienced, usually short-lived hypersensitivity to extremely bright outdoor sun illuminating a large, bright peripheral field, walls, pavement, or other surfaces
- Stage PP-2—chronic hypersensitivity especially to hazy-bright skies

- Stage PP-3—usually many years of hypersensitivity resulting in great discomfort in supermarkets where the whole ceiling is brightly illuminated
- Stage PP-4—the final stage of a long chain of decreasing binocular vision skills or a degenerative chain instituted by trauma, characterized by intolerance even to usual relatively low levels of illumination used in home lighting

Others make note of the degree of subjective symptoms, whether they are present some or all of the time and whether patients present wearing dark glasses indoors or ask that room lighting be kept to a dim level.

PHOTOPHOBIA TREATMENT ALTERNATIVES

For most patients with photophobia following ABI, due to cortical changes, colored filters will be the treatment of choice. However, photophobia must be treated based on the diagnosis. Photophobia caused by binocular dysfunction or PTVS is treatable with lenses and/or vision rehabilitation therapy that decreases associated symptoms along with the photophobia. Patients with dry eye or lagophthalmos will be treated by keeping the eye moist, using ophthalmic lubricants, contact lenses, or in the most difficult cases, perhaps surgical intervention that will relieve the causal exposure keratitis.

LIGHT AND COLOR THERAPIES

The scientific bases for phototherapy are emerging from research in a number of different fields. For instance, light therapy for seasonal affective disorder is now commonplace, based on non-image-forming light pathways, and has been found to be safe and effective.[36] Non-image-forming light pathways involve ganglion cells known as melanopsin containing ipRGCs. They are most sensitive to short wavelength blue light and project to nonvisual areas of the brain including the suprachiasmatic nuclei (SCN) of the hypothalamus (the circadian pacemaker of the brain) and to the olivary pretectal nucleus for pupillary regulation. Further neural pathways to the pituitary and pineal glands allow for photic entrainment or synchronization of circadian rhythm via melatonin suppression and contribute to pupillary constriction. Light exposure via the non-image-forming light pathways is also involved in neuroendocrine modulation for mood and immune regulation.

Research in dyslexia has demonstrated an imbalance between the magnocellular and parvocellular visual subsystems.[37] As the magnocellular and parvocellular systems respond to different wavelengths of light, it has been suggested that specific wavelength filters help to balance the interaction between these visual subsystems.[38] Indeed, Solan et al.[39] and Ray et al.[40] demonstrated improved reading through colored filters, as has Wilkins, as discussed above. Jackowski also hypothesized a similar magno-parvo imbalance in her work with patients with ABI, as discussed above.

Colored Filters

It is well established in the literature, that while for the healthy neurologically normal visual system, gray filters provide relief from discomfort glare such as excessive

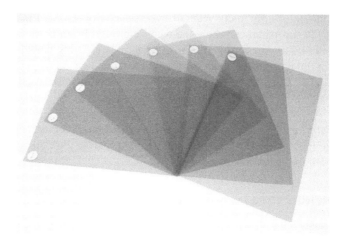

FIGURE 8.1   **(See color insert following page 270.)** Colored overlays.

sunlight, ABI patients respond to colored filters, known as wavelength specific treatment, for relief from photosensitivity. Colored filters can be tinted lenses worn as eyeglasses or may be colored overlays (Figure 8.1) placed on top of a page of print while reading. Some patients may be uncomfortable with the look of tinted lenses, and, if most bothered while reading, will choose the colored overlays. Since most patients experience photophobia during tasks other than reading, colored filters worn as eyeglasses may be a more effective treatment.

Determining the best choice of color has been carried out with methods that require only subjective responses as well as with more objective testing. Blue, yellow, and rose have all been documented as having reduced photophobia and improved reading *performance.*[10,41,42]

The Intuitive Colorimeter is a device developed by Arnold Wilkins that illuminates a page of text and allows the hue and saturation of the color to be varied independently at constant brightness.[43] The color is then presented in tinted trial lenses under more natural viewing conditions.[8] The device is used to obtain a color that reduces perceptual distortion or provides the greatest increase in reading speed. The lenses are designed to provide the appropriate color under white fluorescent lighting. While some patients may require refinement of the color if they spend most of their time under another type of visible light, fluorescent lighting is prevalent in schools, offices, and shops. In fact, it is often true that patients report the most discomfort where there is both fluorescent lighting and a busy visual environment such as in a grocery store.

The Intuitive Colorimeter is a relatively quick and precise way of determining the specific wavelength filter that provides the greatest subjective relief and greatest improvement in reading rate. However, many extremely photophobic patients will then request additional attenuation (neutral gray filters that are added to the wavelength filter). This may make them feel more comfortable for a few minutes, but it may ultimately be too dark for indoor wear. The patient must also be advised whether the lenses may be worn for driving, as particular filters will decrease ability to see stoplights. This information is provided from the Cerium tinting lab where the specific wavelength filter match is obtained.

Intuitive colorimeter testing is frequently useful for patients who not only have photophobia, but also for patients with dyslexia or those with neurological conditions, other than reading difficulty, associated with an increased risk of seizures such as migraine, and photosensitive epilepsy.[44]

Richman, Baglieri, and Cho evaluated a 47-year-old female who presented with photophobia, blurry vision, movement of print, nausea, and dizziness while reading.[41] She was 5 years post-brain injury after being trapped in a falling elevator. Colored Intuitive Overlays™ were tried based on the screening protocol of Wilkins.[45] This involves placing colored overlays on top of selected text to determine which, if any, color minimizes the patient's symptoms. In this case, the patient selected a specific blue overlay and when tried with print and lighting that typically maximized her symptoms, she reported less motion of the print, loss of place, and vertigo. Tinted lenses matching the luminance characteristics of the blue overlay were mounted in a clip-on frame. The patient used them over her bifocal eyeglasses for reading. One month later she reported significant improvement in reading comfort and significant reduction in reading fatigue, headaches, vertigo, and photophobia. It was not reported if she continued with the clip-on lenses or considered tinting of her own eyeglasses.

While Richman et al.[41] tinted the lenses to match the overlay; Wilkins[8] frequently finds that the chosen color of the overlay is different than the chosen color of the tinted lenses. He attributes this to the overlays providing a surface color in the presence of white light adaptation while the tinted lenses have an effect similar to changing the color of the lighting.

Jackowski reported decreased reading rates and normal contrast sensitivity for patients with photophobia.[10] These patients experienced increased reading rates and marked enhancement of contrast sensitivity (in spite of their initially normal contrast sensitivity) when tested while wearing light filtering lenses. She tested subjects with Corning Photochromic Filters: CPF 450-S (yellow), CPF 527-S (orange-amber), and CPF 550-S (orange-red). In five out of six cases, the CPF 450-S provided the greatest improvement in contrast sensitivity so it was used to test reading rate. All of the mild brain injury patients tested demonstrated significant improvement in reading rate. Two patients out of seven did as well with a neutral density (gray) filter that was luminance matched to the CPF 450-S and they preferred it as cosmetically more acceptable. The Corning CPF lenses were dispensed and used for reading, driving, and some outdoor activities. At a 1-year progress evaluation, the lenses continued to provide faster reading speed, control of light sensitivity, and reduced headache.

Eschenbach Optik recently released Wellness Protect Eyewear (Figure 8.2). It features yellow lenses similar to the Corning 450-S lens. It protects the eyes by blocking light 470 nm in wavelength and less thereby cutting out most blue light. The eyeglasses can be ordered in any prescription and with other standard filtering tints, including orange (525 nm), amber (511 nm), plum (400 nm), or deep red (550 nm).

Photophobia, blepharospasm, and headaches have been treated by Kathleen Digre, MD, of the University of Utah, utilizing lenses tinted a rose color called *FL-41*. She had patients compare FL-41 lenses to gray tinted lenses, and while gray lenses

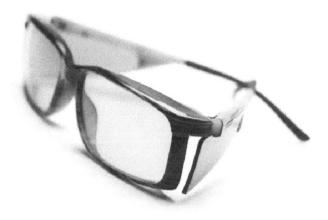

FIGURE 8.2   (See color insert following page 270.) Wellness Protect Eyewear. (Courtesy of Eschenbach optik of America, www.eschenbach.com)

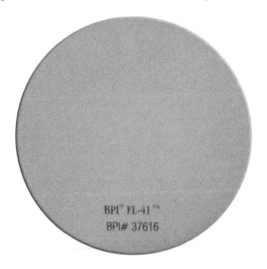

FIGURE 8.3   (See color insert following page 270.) FL-41 lens. (Courtesy of Brain Power Incorporated, www.callbpi.com)

also reduced symptoms for patients with blepharospasm, they preferred the FL-41 lenses (Figure 8.3).[42] The lenses are generally effective when tinted to a darkness of 50% and therefore allow for better cosmesis and eye contact than very darkly tinted lenses.

While there are many positives to colored overlays and tinted lenses, there are some special considerations. Children and adults are often concerned about cosmesis and fitting in and will be less likely to wear tinted lenses even when they are helpful. Contact lenses prescribed along with lightly tinted spectacles that mask the contact lens color may be more acceptable. Tinted lenses may adversely affect perception of objects such as traffic signals. In addition, color reduces the amount of light entering the eyes and therefore can create concerns similar to those expressed by early cataract patients. There is also some question whether wearing lenses that block wavelengths to which ipRGCs are sensitive could cause, exacerbate, or improve sleep disorders. Safety must be considered and patient education is of prime importance.

Syntonic Phototherapy

Syntonic phototherapy describes the application of colored light delivered through the eyes by way of specialized instrumentation rather than being worn as spectacles or used as a transparency. Constriction of functional visual fields, as described above, is a common phenomenon following ABI. The goal of syntonic phototherapy is expansion of constricted visual fields and reduction or elimination of visual symptoms. Syntonic phototherapy treatment as prescribed by the College of Syntonic Optometry curriculum consists of a 20-minute light treatment 3–5 days/week. Twenty to forty sessions of treatment are generally necessary to reduce symptoms and expand the visual field. Progress evaluation is recommended every eight to ten sessions with reevaluation of visual field. If the visual field is not expanding, reassessment of the colored light filter(s) is recommended. Treatment is discontinued when the visual field is normal or a recovery plateau is reached with the understanding that recovery may vary depending on the severity and type of brain injury.

For mild TBI, blue, blue-green, or green light treatments are prescribed if symptoms are present and the injury occurred less than 3 years before the treatment. Very deep blue or indigo may be added for headache or pain. Yellow-green light is used for more chronic conditions. Syntonic phototherapy treatment is a noninvasive, safe, and effective treatment for many patients.

POST TRAUMA VISION SYNDROME TREATMENT

Padula et al. demonstrate the value of bases-in prism and binasal occlusion in treating PTVS, which frequently includes the symptom of photophobia. [28] Both, bases-in prism and binasal occlusion resulted in increased visual evoked potential amplitudes in the PTVS group, but not in a control group.

BINOCULAR VISION DYSFUNCTION TREATMENT

Lane in writing about functional photophobia notes the reversal of symptoms after treating the underlying accommodative and binocular dysfunction with low power plus lenses and optometric vision therapy.[21] Tinted lenses enable performance in persons with otherwise fragile binocular fusion, especially intermittent exotropia, but may not be treating the underlying accommodative fatigue syndrome.

If the binocular dysfunction is consistent with PTVS, then bases-in prism and/or binasal occlusion should be attempted. If positive results are not achieved in this manner, then vision rehabilitation therapy may be necessary to remediate the underlying accommodative and/or binocular dysfunction.

Contact Lenses

Tinted contact lenses have been used cosmetically and therapeutically. Tinted contact lenses may be preferred to tinted spectacle lenses as they are often more cosmetically acceptable. Tints can be translucent or opaque over the entire lens or even opaque over a portion of the lens. Custom tinted lenses can help decrease photophobia and glare and may be used for monocular occlusion if necessary. Lenses with an artificial pupil can be helpful for patients with mydriasis. Several specialty labs are available to make these prescription contact lenses.

APPROACHES TO TREATING PHOTOPHOBIA

For many patients, lightly tinted lenses for indoor use along with more darkly tinted lenses or polarizing lenses for outdoor use are a simple first step for treating photophobia. Patients should also be checked for the appropriate refractive correction.

Suchoff and colleagues found that 50% of TBI patients required a prescription for spectacles. Patients may require different lenses for long distance, intermediate, and near working distances and may also require different lenses for indoor versus outdoor activities.[46] It is a challenge reducing the number and types of glasses to the minimum possible for good comfort and efficiency so that the patient with brain injury can keep track. Progressive lenses have distortion in the periphery that may contribute to symptoms and patients often find relief when switched to flat top or round segment bifocal lenses for distance/near sight along with single vision lenses for intermediate tasks such as computer or piano playing. Low power plus lenses, bases-in prism, and binasal occlusion alone or in combination frequently provide relief from photosensitivity. Padula hypothesizes that they do so by restoring balance between the focal and ambient visual systems.[28]

Patients with normal pupillary responses demonstrated increased contrast sensitivity and reading rate while using CPF 450-S (yellow) lenses.[10] These lenses also enhanced contrast sensitivity for light sensitive individuals. Yellow lenses are also known to increase convergence and accommodation.[40] Patients with abnormal pupillary responses preferred neutral gray filters for overall light reduction.[10]

While blue tinted lenses have been advocated for glare control (e.g., the Harley-Davidson® Viva® Eyewear Riding Glasses with blue tinted lenses), blue blocking lenses such as the rose color FL-41 lens have been shown to reduce light sensitivity and the perceived flicker of fluorescent lighting. A study of children with migraine revealed no improvement for those wearing blue tinted lenses but significant reduction of headache frequency in the children who wore rose colored tinted lenses.[47]

Outdoor tints are most effective when the tint is 85%–90% attenuation (10%–15% light transmission). Patients who preferred the CPF 450-S lens indoors preferred neutral gray lenses outdoors. Gray lenses produce the most natural color vision but some patients prefer brown lenses because they enhance contrast by blocking a larger percentage of blue light.

Polarizing sunglasses decrease the effect of reflective glare and are optimal when light is reflected off water, snow, or wet roadways. They are less effective in icy conditions, if a car windshield is already polarized or while viewing liquid crystal displays (LCD) such as TVs, clocks, or computer monitors.

With such a dizzying array of choices, how do the doctor and the patient work together so neither is overwhelmed in the process? If an intuitive colorimeter is available, it makes finding the specific wavelength filter for indoor wear easier. In my office, we keep a "trial set" of lenses for quickly working with patients. We have single vision lenses of low power plus (+0.25, +0.50, +0.75) without and with 1–2 prism diopters of bases-in prism. We have them in spectacle form but you can easily use lens holders and place them together to create the combinations. We also have both lens holders and clip-on frames with the most frequently used color tints (neutral gray, light blue, yellow, and rose). We trial these lenses and tints while the patient is viewing the distance letter chart and with reading material. For outdoor use, those patients who prefer yellow tinted lenses are prescribed SolarShield® lenses in yellow, while those who respond well to the FL-41 lenses can wear their lenses for indoor and outdoor activities. We generally prescribe gray or brown lenses and frequently polarizing lenses for general light attenuation. Today polarizing lenses are available in a range of colors so you have greater flexibility to combine glare control with lenses that enhance contrast. If possible, you may want to go outdoors with patients to gauge their response to these lenses but more often our recommendation is based on the patient's report of symptoms, level of discomfort, and daily activities.

It is not uncommon to prescribe several pairs of eyeglasses. For example, one patient may require polarized prescription sunglasses for outdoors, single vision distance lenses with a 30% gray tint for indoor use, and bifocal lenses with a computer lens on the top, reading lens on the bottom, and a 15% tint in whatever tint makes the patient the most comfortable for indoor nearpoint work. We like to tell patients that they own several pairs of sneakers to maximize sports performance (running shoes, walking shoes, and tennis or basketball sneakers) and it will take several pairs of eyeglasses to maximize visual performance. Sometimes a clip-on sunglass over the indoor distance prescription and tint can further decrease the number of glasses required. Compliance is sometimes an issue, so it is best to provide patients with a written summary of when and how to use their eyewear as memory function is frequently impaired after brain injury. Most patients will do whatever it takes to relieve their discomfort so by prioritizing the patient's needs, it is possible to recommend all the potentially helpful options without overwhelming the patient or their families.

SUMMARY

Photophobia following brain injury is common, and it differs from that associated with ocular disease. It frequently persists after other symptoms have resolved. Discomfort with normal illumination includes sensitivity to indoor as well as outdoor lighting, enhanced sensitivity to fluorescent lighting, reduced vision in dim lighting, reduced visual field sensitivity, and loss of contrast sensitivity.

The initial treatment for photosensitivity, after a proper refractive analysis, is most often tinted lenses for indoor use along with sunglasses for outdoor activities. Specific wavelength filters, either prescribed as tinted lenses or applied as overlays improve post-brain injury symptoms in many patients, including those with photo-sensitivity, migraine, seizure disorder, and feelings of confusion and disorientation in visually busy spaces. While these may provide immediate reduction of symp-toms, the use of low power plus lenses, bases-in prisms, and binasal occlusion should also be explored, as they have been demonstrated to be effective in treating PTVS. Progressive lenses should not be used for sensitive patients. Multiple pairs of eye-glasses may be needed for enhancing a patient's ability to perform the tasks of daily living that are important to them. Photosensitive patients frequently require lenses for activities at varied working distances as well as for both indoor and outdoor activities. Syntonic phototherapy is another treatment option that can be offered either in-office or as a home-based therapy.

Traumatic damage to the optic nerve or chiasm can result in a desaturated percep-tion of red. Central color vision deficits following ABI, including color perception, color imagery, color recognition, and color naming, are somewhat rare and typically treated with compensatory or cognitive therapies where they affect function during daily activities.

The neuro-optometrist has special training to assess, diagnose, and treat the func-tional visual deficits that frequently accompany brain injury. Patients need treatment that not only brings immediate relief but also remediates any underlying visual condi-tions such as binocular or accommodative dysfunction. Patients treated for photophobia, PTVS, and binocular dysfunction frequently report not only decreased light sensitivity but enhanced visual performance including improved visual acuity, reading speed, and contrast sensitivity along with reduction or elimination of asthenopia and headaches.

REFERENCES

1. Roberts, J. E. (2000). Light and immunomodulation. *Annals of the New York Academy of Sciences, 917,* 435–445.
2. Hellerstein, L. F., Freed, S., & Maples, W. C. (1995). Vision profile of patients with mild brain injury. *Journal of the American Optometric Association, 66,* 634–639.
3. Zihl, J., & Kerkhoff, G. (1990). Foveal photopic and scotopic adaptation in patients with brain damage. *Clinical Vision Science, 5,* 185–195.
4. Lane, B.C. (1963). Functional photophobia: preliminary observations from optometric analysis of 100 cases. *Eastern Seaboard Conference on Visual Training, 8,* 32–51.
5. Jackowski, M. M., Sturr, J. F., Taub, H. A., & Turk, M. A. (1996). Photophobia in patients with traumatic brain injury: uses of light filtering lenses to enhance contrast sensitivity and reading rate. *Neurorehabilitation, 6,* 193–201.
6. Waddell, P. A., & Gronwall, D. M. (1984). Sensitivity to light and sound following minor head injury. *Acta Neurologica Scandinavica, 69*(5), 270–276.
7. Bohnen, N., Twijnstra, A.,Wijnen, G., & Jolles, J. (1991). Tolerance for light and sound of patients with persistent post-concussional symptoms 6 months after mild head injury. *Journal of Neurology, 238*(8), 443–446.
8. Wilkins, A. J. (2003). *Reading through color.* West Sussex, UK: John Wiley & Sons.
9. Wilkins, A. J. (1995). *Visual stress.* New York: Oxford University Press.

10. Jackowski, M. (2001). Altered visual adaptation in patients with traumatic brain injury. In I. B. Suchoff, N. Kapoor, & K. J. Ciuffreda (Eds.), *Visual and vestibular consequences of acquired brain injuries* (pp. 145–173). Santa Ana, CA: Optometric Extension Program.

11. Du, T., Ciuffreda, K.J., & Kapoor, N., (2005). Elevated dark adaptation in traumatic brain injury. *Brain Injury. 19*(13), 1125–1138. doi:10.1080/02699050500149817

12. Langerhorst, C.T., & Safran, A. B. (1998). Progressive shrinkage of the visual field during automated perimetry following traumatic brain injury Patients' experience. *Neuro-Ophthalmology, 20*(4), 177–185.

13. Wilkins, A. J., Huang, J., & Cao, Y. (2007). Prevention of visual stress and migraine with precision spectral filters. *Drug Development Research, 68*(7), 469–475.

14. Palmer, J. E., Chronicle, E. P., Rolan, P., & Mulleners, W. M. (2000). Cortical hyperexcitability is cortical under-inhibition: evidence from a novel functional test of migraine patients. *Cephalalgia, 20*(6), 525–532.

15. Huang, J., Cooper, T. G., Santana, B., Kaufman, D. I., & Cao, Y. (2003). Visual distortion provoked by a stimulus in migraine associated with hyperneuronal activity. *Headache: The Journal of Head and Face Pain, 43,* 664–671.

16. Carolis, P., Tinuper, P., & Sacquegna, T. (1991) Migraine with aura and photosensitive epileptic seizures: a case report. *Cephalalgia, 11*(3), 151–153.

17. Noseda, R., Kainz, V., Jakubowski, M., Gooley, J. J., Saper, C. B., Digre, K., Burstein, R. (2010). A neural mechanism for exacerbation of headache by light. *Nature Neuroscience, 13*(2), 239–245.

18. Kapoor, N., & Ciuffreda, K. J. (2002) Vision disturbances following traumatic brain injury. *Current Treatment Options in Neurology, 4*(4), 271–280.

19. Wilkins, A. J. (2005). Visual stress in neurological disease. *Advances in Clinical Neuroscience & Rehabilitation, 4*(6), 22–23.

20. Scheiman, M., & Galloway, M. (2001). Vision therapy to treat binocular vision disorders after acquired brain injury: factors affecting prognosis. In I. B. Suchoff, N. Kapoor, & K. J. Ciuffreda (Eds.), *Visual and vestibular consequences of acquired brain injuries* (pp. 89–113). Santa Ana, CA: Optometric Extension Program.

21. Lane, B. C. (2001, March). *The functional photophobia syndrome and binocular fusion in neuro-rehabilitation.* Neuro-Optometric Rehabilitation Association Conference. New York.

22. Scott, L., McWhinnie, H., Taylor, L., Stevenson, N., Irons, P., Lewis, E., Wilkins, A. (2002) Coloured overlays in schools: orthoptic and optometric findings. *Ophthalmic & Physiological Optics, 22*(2), 156–165.

23. Jeavons, P. M., & Harding, G. F. (1975). *Photosensitive epilepsy.* London, UK: Heinemann.

24. Wilkins, A. J., Darby, C. E., & Binnie, C. D. (1979). Neurophysiological aspects of pattern-sensitive epilepsy. *Brain, 102,* 1–25.

25. Wiggins, R. E., & von Noorden, G. K. (1990). Monocular eye closure in sunlight. *Journal of Pediatric Ophthalmology & Strabismus, 27*(1), 16–20.

26. O'Dell, M. W., Bell, K. R., & Sandel, M. E., (1998). 1998 Study guide; brain injury rehabilitation; pain rehabilitation. *Supplement to Archives of Physical Medicine and Rehabilitation, 79*(3, Suppl. 1), S1–S92.

27. Padula, W. V., Argyris, S., & Ray, J. (1994). Visual evoked potentials (VEP) evaluating treatment for post-trauma vision syndrome (PTVS) in patients with traumatic brain injuries (TBI). *Brain Injury, 8*(2), 125–133.

28. Padula, W. V., & Argyris, S. (1996). Posttrauma vision syndrome and visual midline shift syndrome. *NeuroRehabilitation, 6*(3), 165–171.

29. Freed, S., & Hellerstein, L. F. (1997). Visual electrodiagnostic findings in mild traumatic brain injury. *Brain Injury, 11*(10), 25–36.

30. Wilkins, A. J., & Nimmo-Smith, I. (1987). The clarity and comfort of printed text. *Ergonomics 30*(12), 1705–1720.

31. Miller, N. R., Newman, N. J., Biousse, V., & Kerrison, J. B. (Eds.), (2008). *Walsh and Hoyt's clinical neuro-opthalmology: The essentials.* Philadelphia, PA: Lippincott Williams and Wilkins.
32. Tranel, D. (2001). Central color processing and its disorders. In M. Behrmann (Ed.), *Handbook of neuropsychology* (2nd ed., Vol. 4, pp. 1–14). Amsterdam, Netherlands: Elsevier Science.
33. Fast, D. A., Shayler, G., & Pharr, W. (2000). Functional visual fields and dural torque. *Journal of Optometric Phototherapy, April,* 5–10.
34. Gottlieb, R., & Wallace, L. (2001). Syntonic phototherapy. *Journal of Behavioral Optometry, 12*(2), 31–38.
35. Wallace, L. (May, 1999). *Functional field-new data, new equipment.* Conference on Light and Vision. Washington, D.C.
36. Gallin, P. F., Terman, M., Remé, C. E., Rafferty, B., Terman, J. S., & Burde, R. M. (1995). Ophthalmologic examination of patients with seasonal affective disoreder, before and after bright light therapy. *American Journal of Ophthalmology, 119*(2), 202–210.
37. Lehmkuhle, S., Garzia, R. P., Turner, L., Hash, T., & Baro, J. A. (1993). A defective visual pathway in children with reading disability. *New England Journal of Medicine, Aug, 19, 329*(8), 579.
38. Dain, S. J., Floyd, R. A., & Elliot, R. T. (2008). Color and luminance increment thresholds in poor readers. *Visual Neuroscience, May–June, 25*(3), 481–486.
39. Solan, H.A., Ficarra, A., Brannan, J.R., & Rucker, F. (1998). Eye movement efficiency in normal and reading disabled elementary school children: effects of varying luminance and wavelength. *Journal of the American Optometric Association, July, 69*(7), 455–464.
40. Ray, N. J., Fowler, S., & Stein, J. F. (2005). Yellow filters can improve magnocellular function: motion sensitivity, convergence, accommodation, and reading. *Annals of the New York Academy of Science, 1039,* 283–293.
41. Richman, J. E., Baglieri, A. M., & Cho, O. (2007). Tinted lenses in the treatment of visual stress in a patient with a traumatic brain injury: a case report. *Journal of Behavioral Optometry, 18*(6), 149–153.
42. Adams, W. H., Digre, K. B., Patel, B. C. K., Anderson, R. L., Warner, J. E. A., & Katz, B. J. (2006). The evaluation of light sensitivity in benign essential blepharospasm. *American Journal of Ophthalmology, 142*(1), 82–87.
43. Wilkins, A. J., Nimmo-Smith, M. I., & Jansons, J. (1992). A colorimeter for the intuitive manipulation of hue and saturation and its application in the study of perceptual distortion. *Ophthalmic and Physiological Optics, 12,* 381–385.
44. Wilkins, A. J., & Evans, B. J. (2009). Visual stress, its treatment with spectral filters, and its relationship to visually induced motion sickness. *Applied Ergonomics,* doi:10:1016/j.apergo.2009.01.011
45. Wilkins, A. J. (2002). Coloured overlays and their effects on reading speed: a review. *Ophthalmic and Physiological Optics, 22,* 448–454.
46. Suchoff, I.B., Kapoor, N., Waxman, R., & Ference, W. (1999). The occurrence of ocular and visual dysfunctions in an acquired brain-injured patient sample. *Journal of the American Optometry Association, 70*(5), 301–309.
47. Good, P. A., Taylor, R. H., & Mortimer, M. J. (1991). The use of tinted glasses in childhood migraine. *Headache: The Journal of Head and Face Pain, 31*(8), 533–536.

9 The Vestibular System
Anatomy, Function, Dysfunction, Assessment, and Rehabilitation

Velda L. Bryan

CONTENTS

INTRODUCTION

The human vestibular system develops early in the womb and is doing its job long before we are born. At birth, a highly developed vestibular system is the reason babies love movement. The structure and chemistry of the vestibular system alone is interesting, but its intricate interaction with the visual system and the somatosensory system is even more fascinating. When each system is functioning and interacting normally, we are able to maintain uprightness in relation to gravity whether standing still or moving. However, when disease or trauma impairs any portion of these interactions, disability can be severe.

PURPOSE

There is an abundance of literature about the vestibular system. That bank of knowledge will continue to grow as ongoing research provides greater insight into the workings of this system. For this reason, the purpose of this chapter is to provide basic rather than detailed information in an effort to understand (1) the anatomy and functions of the peripheral and central vestibular systems; (2) the vestibular system's interactive functions with the visual and somatosensory systems; (3) the causes and symptoms of dysfunction; (4) the methods of diagnostic evaluation; and (5) the various rehabilitative approaches.

EPIDEMIOLOGY

Head and/or brain trauma is a frequent cause of vestibular pathology. In the United States, the annual occurrence of traumatic brain injuries (TBIs) seen in emergency departments (EDs) is approximately 1.4 million. Approximately 1.1 million of those patients are diagnosed with mild TBI (mTBI) or concussion and are released.[1] However, the true number of patients with mTBI is unknown in that many concussed patients are never seen in an ED and, therefore, are never captured in any database. Another category of unrecognized concussion patients are those admitted through an ED with major injuries, such as fractures, spinal cord injury, and/or internal injuries, but no obvious neurological signs of significant brain injury. Evidence of concussion goes unnoticed until symptoms are manifested as the patient is activated in the later stages of recovery. Among the cluster of symptoms of postconcussion syndrome are dizziness and disturbances in vision and spatial orientation.

Of the overall known annual TBI population, approximately 80% complain of dizziness and balance problems. In 1982, Healy[2] reported approximately 2 million clinic visits involving complaints of dizziness from traumatic or nontraumatic causes. In 2008, a study reported that as many as 5.6 million clinic visits involved complaints of dizziness.[3] On occasion, a differential diagnosis to rule out a possible evolving stroke will be imperative. Included in our concern are the approximately 1 million children and adolescents who are hospitalized annually from TBI. Approximately 17,000 are left with permanent disabilities including disturbances in vision and vestibular function.[4]

It must be said that any clinician assessing post-TBI patients who present with dizziness, imbalance, and/or visual dysfunction must have some understanding of the importance of the interactive processes of the three sensory systems. In many cases, a dysfunction is unrecognized and the patient needlessly suffers. For example, post-TBI visual dysfunction is often overlooked only to be discovered later and be treated by vision specialists. This underscores the importance of listening to the patient and taking proper diagnostic action. When all dysfunctional components are in view, a multidisciplinary treatment process can begin to reduce further disability and enhance the patient's highest potential for independence.

ROLE OF THE VESTIBULAR SYSTEM

The vestibular system is responsible for (1) detecting linear and angular head movement and head position in space; (2) assisting gaze stabilization of the visual field; (3) maintaining balance and postural control; and (4) providing spatial orientation or perception of body movement. The vestibular system continually makes adjustments with the cooperation of interacting systems in response to movements. The primary role of the vestibular system is to provide the central nervous system (CNS) with information to regulate posture and to coordinate eye and head movements.[5] The system represents our sense of balance or equilibrium and is often referred to as the "sixth sense."[6,7]

PRIMORDIAL DEVELOPMENT OF THE PERIPHERAL VESTIBULAR SYSTEM

Before 5 weeks gestation, the embryonic beginnings of the human peripheral vestibular and auditory structures emerge as one unit called the *otocyst*. At 5 weeks gestation, differentiation of the two structures occurs with the vestibular organ developing more rapidly than the hearing (cochlea) organ. This may be an indication of the vestibular system's important role in the development of other portions of the nervous system. Between 7 and 14 weeks gestation, the *semicircular canals* (SCC or canals) and *receptor hair cells* form and begin to attract neurons of the vestibular nerve to synapse (connect) with them. The tiny *receptor hair cells* are the common sensory receptors in the vestibular and cochlear organs. Some vestibular neurons will grow toward the brainstem. By 12 weeks gestation, reflexive eye movements respond to changes in head position.[5,6,8]

By the last week of the first trimester, the vestibular nerve has become the first fiber tract in the brain to begin myelination. Myelin is a white lipid substance that insulates axons to promote rapid transmission of electrical signals throughout the entire nervous system. By 5 months gestation, the vestibular organ has reached full size with ongoing myelination of pathways to the eyes and the spinal cord. Myelination of other vestibular pathways occurs but at slower paces well into puberty. The fetus is able to sense an orientation to gravity through this early maturation of the vestibular system. As the time for birth approaches, the head begins to turn downward. It has been suggested that presence of vestibular dysfunction in the fetus could be the cause for a breech presentation.[6]

Development of the newborn's vestibular function can be tracked by observing the *oculocephalic reflex* (OCR) also known as "doll's head eye movements."[5] When the head is rapidly turned approximately 15°–20°, the reflex causes conjugate eye deviation to the opposite side. Maturation of the vestibular system promotes development of postural abilities for the exploring baby. They love movement and respond to rocking and bouncing, which is also beneficial for activation of other sensory systems in the developing infant brain.

ANATOMY AND FUNCTION OF THE PERIPHERAL END-ORGANS

THE MIDDLE EAR: ANATOMY AND FUNCTION OF AUDITORY OSSICLES

The external auditory canal takes us toward the air-filled middle ear. The auditory canal, middle ear, and inner ear are enclosed within the hardest bone of the human skull: the *petrous* (rock) portion of the temporal bone. The cavern within this space is called the *bony labyrinth* or *osseous labyrinth*. The external auditory canal stops at the *tympanic membrane* (ear drum), which covers and protects the entrance of the middle ear. The air-filled chamber of the middle ear houses three tiny odd-shaped bones or *auditory ossicles*: *malleus*, *incus*, and *stapes*. Attached to the inner surface of the tympanic membrane is the malleus which attaches to the incus which attaches to the stapes. The footplate of the stapes connects with a barrier between the middle and inner ear. These auditory ossicles form a bony chain called the *ossicular chain*. Bony conduction of sound is transmitted through the ossicular chain and collected by receptor hair cells in the cochlea (peripheral auditory end-organ) inside the inner ear.[5] The auditory signal is transferred to the cochlear portion of cranial nerve (CN) VIII (vestibulocochlear nerve), which then transmits the signal into appropriate nuclei in the brainstem. From the brainstem the signal is transmitted upward into the auditory cortex located in the superior temporal lobe.

When sound is prevented from reaching the bony labyrinth or if there is a disarticulation in the ossicular chain, hearing loss will occur. Neurosensory hearing loss can occur from disease or TBI when hair cell receptors, cochlear nerve fibers, or cochlear nuclei are damaged.[5,9,10] Hair cell receptors may also deteriorate in the aging process.

INNER EAR: ANATOMY AND LABYRINTHINE FLUIDS

In the air-filled middle ear, the footplate of the stapes bone sits in a recess or *oval window* on the lateral wall of the *vestibule* located in the fluid-filled inner ear. A secondary tympanic membrane forms the *round window* on the cochlear structure in the inner ear. These windows (membranes) form a barrier between the middle ear and inner ear. The bony labyrinth of the inner ear is filled with *perilymph fluid*. Trauma to the head may cause a rupture or *fistula* in a window, allowing perilymph to leak into the middle ear. While the amount of perilymph fluid is minute, loss of fluid through a perilymphatic fistula (PLF) will cause inner ear dysfunction.

Suspended within the bony labyrinth is the *membranous labyrinth*, a continuous, closed system. The membranous labyrinth is filled with *endolymph fluid*, which is produced by special cells located in multiple areas throughout the membranous labyrinth. The fluid is continually produced and circulated through the ducts of the inner ear. Endolymph eventually flows into an endolymphatic duct and out of the labyrinth. As it reaches the endolymphatic sac, found in the dura covering the inner wall of the temporal bone, the endolymph is reabsorbed. If circulation of endolymph is obstructed or in some way defective, the membranous labyrinth will swell leading to symptoms of *Ménière's disease* or *endolymphatic hydrops*.[5]

The chemical make up of each fluid also plays an important role. Perilymph has a fluid concentration low in potassium and high in sodium. In contrast, endolymph has a high potassium concentration and low sodium concentration. The resting electrical potential needed for normal receptor hair cell function is dependent upon the sustained stability of the differences in chemical composition.[5,9,11,12] Separation of perilymph and endolymph is maintained by a barrier made up of "tight junctions" at the top of the hair cells. If the chemical composition of one fluid is changed, both the vestibular and auditory end-organs could be incapacitated.

INNER EAR: ANATOMY AND FUNCTION OF THE
PERIPHERAL VESTIBULAR END-ORGAN

The peripheral vestibular end-organ and the auditory end-organ (cochlea) are housed in the inner ear (Figure 9.1). Structures include the three bony SCC, the bony

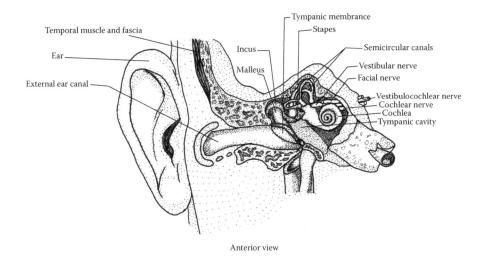

Temporal muscle and fascia

Ear

External ear canal

Tympanic membrane

Stapes

Incus

Malleus

Semicircular canals

Vestibular nerve

Facial nerve

Vestibulocochlear nerve

Cochlear nerve

Cochlea

Tympanic cavity

Anterior view

FIGURE 9.1　Coronal view of three sections of the ear. External ear with auditory canal and tympanic membrane. Air-filled middle ear: auditory ossicles (malleus, incus, stapes). Fluid-filled inner ear: semicircular canals, vestibule, cochlea. Vestibular nerve, cochlear nerve, facial nerve, and vestibulocochlear nerve (CN VIII). (Adapted from Moore, K. L., and Dalley, A. F., *Clinically Oriented Anatomy*, 5th ed., Lippincott Williams & Wilkins, Philadelphia, PA, 2006, p. 1023.)

cochlea, and the bony vestibule. The cochlea is actually an extension of the vestibule. Remember, the tiny sensory hair cells are the common sensory receptors of the inner ear. As the head moves, hair cells interpret the motion of endolymphatic fluid and translate that motion into a neuronal electrical discharge that is forwarded through the vestibular nerve to the brainstem, brain, spinal cord, and cerebellum.

The Vestibule

The endolymph-filled membranous labyrinth is a closed system suspended within the perilymph-filled bony labyrinth. The vestibule (Latin: room) contains two enlargements of the membranous labyrinth called the *utricle* and the *saccule*. They are *otolithic* end-organs. The function of the otolithic organs is to detect linear acceleration and position of head tilt from the force of gravity, while moving in a horizontal or vertical plane. In the lining of the utricle and saccule are supporting cells or *kinocilia* and sensory receptor hair cells or *stereocilia* all of which are referred to as the *macula*. The macula is covered by a gelatinous matrix within which tiny crystals of calcium carbonate called *otoconia*, from the Greek term for "ear dust." In some literature, the term "otoconia" is used interchangeably with the term "*otolith*," which comes from the Greek term for "ear stones."[5] In this chapter, the more commonly used term "otoconia" will be used.

As head position changes, the force of gravity and linear acceleration change the direction of *otoconia* movement which then bends the stereocilia of the macular hair cells in the same direction. The plane of the utricle's macula is nearly horizontal and, therefore, detects head position changes while moving on a horizontal plane, as turning the head while walking. The nearly vertical plane of the saccule detects movement in an up/down plane, as riding in an elevator.[5,9,11,12]

The Semicircular Canals

In each inner ear are three bony SCC within which a semicircular duct, a part of the membranous labyrinth, is suspended. Each end of a canal is connected to the utricle. Each canal is oriented in a different plane from the others. The horizontal (lateral canal) is tilted slightly backward to about 30°. The posterior canal (inferior canal) and the anterior canal (superior canal) are somewhat oriented in vertical positions but at approximately 45° to the saggital plane, which divides the cerebral hemispheres. Each SCC represents one of the three planes of space. The function of each canal is to detect a specific movement of the head in one of those planes. For example, detection of head movement in bending forward, looking upward, or head turning. The SCC detect angular acceleration and changes in velocity but will not detect constant velocity. For example, as the head is accelerated through a plane of movement, any change in the velocity of that movement is detected in that direction. However, once constant velocity is reached, the sense of motion disappears.[12]

At one end of each canal is a bulge or *ampulla*, where the canal attaches to the utricle (Figure 9.2). Each ampulla contains a *crista*, a rise of tissue covered by stereocilia, which protrude into the ampulla and endolymph in the membranous labyrinth. These stereocilia of the *crista ampullaris* are the sensory receptor organs that bend in response to head acceleration in the plane of an individual canal. The hair cells are imbedded in a gelatinous matrix called the *cupula*, which covers the crista and extends over the ampulla forming a partition. At the opposite end of the crista, the

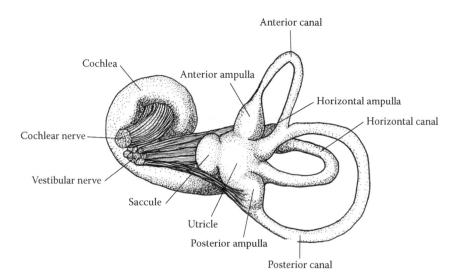

FIGURE 9.2 Vestibular labyrinth: three semicircular canals (posterior, anterior, horizontal), ampulla, saccule, and utricle. (Adapted from Baloh, R. W., and Halmagyi, G. M. (Eds.), *Disorders of the Vestibular System*, Oxford University Press, New York, 1996, p. 4.)

hair cells synapse with vestibular nerve fibers and afferent signals are sent to the CNS. It has been suggested that the top of the cupula may function as a "relief valve" during the extreme angular acceleration forces, such as those caused by head trauma.[12,13]

The Vestibulocochlear Nerve (CN VIII)

The superior section of the vestibular nerve transfers information from the anterior canal and horizontal canal, utricle, and a little from the saccule. The inferior section of the vestibular nerve transfers information from the posterior canal and from most of the saccule. The inferior portion of CN VIII transmits signals from the cochlear (auditory) end-organ. The transmitted peripheral signals synapse with brainstem nuclei specific to vestibular or cochlear input signals.

The facial nerve (CN VII) winds through the temporal bone within the internal auditory canal in close proximity to CN VIII. Thus, paralysis of facial muscles may occur from temporal bone fracture, disease, or compression from a tumor in the auditory space.[5,9]

Under normal circumstances, misinformation coming into the brain is avoided because the afferent signal moving along the vestibular nerve on one side is inhibited while the afferent signal on the opposite side is excited. Nolte coined the term "functional pairs" to describe how head movements that "affect one [canal] will affect the other" canal on the opposite side[5] (p. 358). For example, the posterior canal of one side is parallel to the anterior canal on the opposite side. They form a "functional pair." The horizontal canals of both sides form a "functional pair." How vestibular signals are processed through central regions of the brainstem, subcortex, cerebral cortex, spinal cord, and cerebellum is discussed later in this chapter.

INTERACTIVE ROLES OF VESTIBULAR, SOMATOSENSORY, AND VISUAL SYSTEMS

The business of maintaining stable head and body positions in relation to gravity cannot be done by the vestibular system alone. This requires cooperative interaction between three systems. Sensory receptors or *hair cells* in the peripheral vestibular end-organ collect and transfer information regarding head position and head movement to the brain. However, the peripheral vestibular receptors do not provide information about body position. That information is collected by somatosensory receptors in body joints, ligaments, muscles, and skin and are transferred as *proprioceptive* information to the brain. When the somatosensory system senses a need for postural control it stimulates automatic postural responses or *protective reactions* through the spinal cord to maintain balance. If the body extends beyond its base of support or *center of gravity* a fall may occur unless a *protective reaction* causes an automatic step or a hand reaching out to a wall or object to prevent the fall. If balance cannot be maintained while standing with a narrow base of support (feet close to or touching each other) a disturbance somewhere in the coordinated systems is indicated.[5,8]

Sensory receptors in the eyes provide important feedback regarding orientation of the body in space. In other words, where is the head in relation to the horizon?

As discussed in Chapters 5 through 7, dysfunction in the visual perception of "straight ahead," common following brain injury, can cause dizziness, disorientation, and imbalance. In the process of orientation, visual input also provides information regarding possible environmental hazards, barriers or avenues of escape. In the presence of impaired inputs from either the somatosensory or vestibular or both systems there is a strong dependence upon visual input. Defective input from one of the three systems may be compensated for by the remaining intact systems such that the patient is able to function, albeit with some discomfort and loss of efficiency. However, dysfunction in two of the three systems will result in significant disability.

INTERACTIONS BETWEEN VESTIBULAR AND VISUAL (OCULAR MOTOR) SYSTEMS

The vestibular system plays an important role in the generation of eye movements that compensate for head movements. Through vestibular nuclei in brainstem, each SCC is able to communicate with motor neurons of extraocular muscles to cause eye deviation in the each canal's own plane. This interaction is the basis of the *vestibulo-ocular reflex* (VOR), which stabilizes gaze upon an image or the visual world during head movement.[9,14] If the VOR is impaired, loss of gaze stabilization is the result. For example, as the patient turns the head while walking an object in the visual field or the whole visual environment appears unsteady or "bouncing."

Demer[15] described the VOR as a "synergistic" interaction between the vestibular and ocular systems. Normal VOR stabilization is needed for "functional vision, and vision optimizes the performance of the VOR" (p. 73).[5,15] *Dynamic visual acuity* (DVA) plays a role in maintaining a sharper image on the retina, while the VOR steadies gaze during head movement. This interaction is called the *visual vestibulo-ocular reflex* (VVOR).[15] The DVA test (DVAT) is performed to assess the VVOR, discussed later in the chapter.

The VOR also plays a cooperative role with another reflex. The OCR (or "doll's eyes") is tested with a "head thrust" or "head impulse" by rapidly turning the head to 30° from midline. The eyes normally move to the opposite side to maintain focus on a fixed object. ED physicians use this test for a quick assessment of a possible location of brainstem damage in comatose individuals. If damage is present in the reticular core of the brainstem, the "head thrust" results in eyes moving to the opposite side but rapidly drifting back to midline because gaze maintenance is deficient. This was found to be true whether testing was performed in the supine position or in the sitting position. Leigh[16] suggested that when individuals with normal OCR function were tested in the supine position the response was essentially a VOR. Nolte[5] reported a similar suggestion. When the OCR is activated in conscious individuals the VOR is suppressed as the head and eyes move to one side spontaneously. Pathways from the brainstem's vestibular nuclei to the lateral gaze centers, near the sixth motor nucleus on the same side, are intact with normal functioning.[15–17]

A rarely mentioned reflex is the *cervico-ocular reflex* (COR). Not to be confused with the OCR, which involves ocular (eye) and cephalic or brain (visual) mechanisms, the COR involves somatosensory inputs from cervical (neck) muscles and joint facets and ocular mechanisms. The COR complements the VOR. When gaze stability is deficient in patients with bilateral vestibular dysfunction, exercises to enhance the COR may increase VOR function in short low frequency head movements. However, compensation will not occur when head movements are rapid in the presence of VOR loss.[15]

VESTIBULAR AND SPINAL INTERACTIONS

While the VOR is involved in coordination of eye and head movements, the *vestibulospinal* reflex (VSR) is involved in controlling movement and stabilization of the body to maintain balance. The two reflexes help to orient the eyes, head, and body regarding the self and the environment. Gravitational forces on the head and body during linear acceleration stimulate the otolithic receptors and angular movement stimulates the SCC. Receptors from the SCC and the otoliths transmit their signals through the vestibular nerve and synapse with spinal nuclei in the brainstem. The response is the VSR, which serves to stabilize the head and control upright balance by involving antigravity (extensor) muscles of the neck, trunk, and extremities.[14,18] A response occurs whether in a static or dynamic state.

Control of muscle tone in the antigravity muscles is the function of *deep tendon reflexes (DTRs)*. The DTRs are, in turn, influenced by combined inhibitory and excitatory neuronal centers located above the spinal cord in the brainstem, basal ganglia, and cerebellum. If brain trauma impairs the inhibitory influence of the frontal cortex and basal ganglia, the antigravity muscles go into a state of contraction known as *decerebrate* rigidity. The DTRs are hyperreflexive. The vestibular system is likely a significant contributor to the increased muscle tone since a marked increase in tone occurs when destruction of the labyrinths is bilateral.[9,14,18]

NYSTAGMUS

As an indicator of normal peripheral vestibular system function, nystagmus is not a voluntary movement of the eyes but a physiological response to stimulation of the vestibular or ocular motor systems. The reflex may be physiological (normal) or pathological (abnormal). Normal nystagmus is characterized by a rhythmic conjugate oscillation or beating of the eyes with a slow component and a fast component (saccade). The slow component moves in the opposite direction away from the direction of head movement. The saccade phase occurs as the eyes return and fixate gaze at the original position. Control of eye movements involves both peripheral and central components through the medial longitudinal fasciculus (MLF) of the brainstem. On occasion, speed of eye movement during nystagmus may be the same in both directions and may be horizontal, vertical, or torsional. If head rotations are too rapid to allow the VOR to compensate, very rapid eye movement may be seen in the opposite direction.[5,9,19,20]

Visually mediated or *optokinetic* (OKN) eye movements supplement the VOR if SCC function is normal during sustained slow head rotation. This prevents continual and annoying "jumping" of the visual field while walking.[19] Alterations of saccadic movements may be an indicator of central abnormality, especially within the brain-stem or frontal cortex.

CENTRAL VESTIBULAR PROCESSING

Within the brainstem's ponto-medullary juncture is an area referred to as the *vestibular area* because it is primarily made up of vestibular nuclei. Each SCC and otolithic organ makes a connection with its own vestibular nucleus. Also, the vestibular nuclei of one side communicate with the contralateral vestibular nuclei. Projections from the cerebellum and spinal cord are also received in various vestibular nuclei. Projections from the vestibular nuclei, in turn, connect with nuclei of the spinal cord, cerebellum and CN III, IV, and VI (ocular motor nuclei). The brainstem system that relays vestibular information to the brain is found in a central core of neurons called the *reticular formation* (RF). In the RF are converging and diverging sensory and motor pathways, which are integrated and organized before being sent on to specific targets. Tracts in the RF ascend and descend neuronal information to and from the brain. The *ascending reticular activating system* (ARAS) projects vestibular signals into subcortical structures before entering the cerebral cortex.[5,11]

Is there a "primary vestibular cortex"? The short answer is "no." There is, rather, a complex of cortical targets many of which remain difficult to understand. From the brainstem, vestibular signals reach a subcortical structure called the *diencephalon*. Tucked in between the cerebral hemispheres the diencephalon houses such important structures as the pineal gland, hypothalamus, and thalamus. Compared to the cerebral cortex, the diencephalon is small in size but is very rich in nuclei for sensory, motor, and limbic pathways. The thalamus is a central relay station for all incoming sensory signals excepting olfactory information.[5] Afferent vestibular signals connect with specific thalamic nuclei and are forwarded through the internal capsule to the cortex.

The confusion about cortical connections has been somewhat cleared in recent years with advanced neuroimaging technology. Functional neuroimaging (positron emission tomography [PET], functional magnetic resonance imaging [fMRI]) has allowed us to observe the metabolism of brain fuels (oxygen, glucose) as specific areas were activated. In 1994, Bottini et al.[21] used PET imaging to identify areas of central vestibular activation. After the left and right peripheral vestibular structures were stimulated with cold water injections, cortical activation was found in the right temporoparietal area, posterior insula, putamen, anterior cingulate cortex, and the right primary sensory cortex. Vestibular connections were also found in the hippocampus and frontal lobe. Studies have suggested that vestibular information may be projected to these areas via cerebellum and thalamus.[19,22]

Descending cortical projections influence multiple functional movements involving the vestibular, visual, and somatosensory systems. Regulation of posture and coordination of eye and head movements is a function of the vestibular system through its connections with the spinal cord, cerebellum, and motor nuclei. Cortical influences on eye-hand coordination are processed through vestibular nuclei and reticulo-spinal pathways. Smooth, coordinated head and body movements receive additional input through the thalamus from the cerebellum, basal ganglia, and limbic system.[5,9,11,14]

INDICATORS OF VESTIBULAR DYSFUNCTION

Vestibular pathology was little understood until the 1970s when many pioneering clinicians began to explore and establish a process of evaluation and treatment. Even throughout the 1980s and the early 1990s, outside of the world of specialization, recognition and understanding of vestibular pathology remained fuzzy. However, during the 1990s, sports media began to bring attention to problems related to repeated concussions suffered by notable athletes. Decreased ability in speed of processing and recall of information were acknowledged but a decline in high level motor speed and coordination were not recognized as a potential vestibular dysfunction until later.

Since 2003, military actions in Iraq and Afghanistan have produced their "signature injury," the "blast injury TBI" or "BITBI," as it is called in recent literature. In 2008, the Defense and Veterans Brain Injury Center published a consensus on "acute management of concussion/mTBI in the deployed setting."[23] In 2009, a study reported that the "top three" complaints from service members of a U.S. Army brigade combat team were headaches, dizziness, and balance problems.[24] In both civilian and military post-mTBI patients, headaches, vision changes, balance difficulties, and dizziness/vertigo, are being increasingly investigated for possible accompanying vestibular pathology.[25] As the media reports on this increased awareness of the disabling residuals of concussion, the general public is raising an eye to the reality of "mild" TBI as a "not so mild" condition. Neuroscientists and neurorehabilitation specialists are beginning to suggest that the label "mTBI" be changed to remove the illusion of a "benign" status.

Dizziness/Vertigo

Although the terms "dizziness" and "vertigo" are used interchangeably throughout the literature, there are clinical definitions for both. The patient may refer to "dizziness" in relation to feeling disoriented, especially in dark areas, or feeling spacey, floating, rocking, or lightheaded. When dizziness is mentioned in relation to balance difficulties, involvement of vestibular dysfunction must be considered. "Vertigo" is the illusion of movement, typically rotational, when no actual movement is observed. True vertigo refers to vestibular system involvement.

Dizziness is not always related to vestibular dysfunction but may indicate nonvestibular causes such as orthostatic hypotension, cervical injury, cardiac disease, medication side-effects, systemic diseases (diabetes), and visual disorders (discussed in Chapters 4, 6, and 7), or psycho-physiologic factors, including anxiety or phobic disorders. Alcoholism, either acute or chronic, alters inner ear chemistry. Following TBI, common causes include peripheral or central vestibular dysfunction, hypoglycemia, hyper- and hypotension, orthostatic hypotension from prolonged inactivity, and hyponatremia (low sodium levels in the blood caused by excessive sweating, persistent diarrhea, or overuse of diuretic drugs). The patient simply wants to know "what is happening?" and "what can be done for relief?" and "how soon." Seemungal and Bronstein suggest asking the patient if the problem is in "the legs or in the head" and if there is a feeling of faintness versus being on a merry-go-round or a boat.[26] The location of the lesion may be peripheral or central or both. Understanding the vestibular system is best done through exploration of its dysfunctional states, which are discussed below.

INAPPROPRIATE NYSTAGMUS

Spontaneous nystagmus, occurring when the head is static (still), is an indicator of acute peripheral vestibular loss. Nystagmus is often along the horizontal plane. Vertical or torsional spontaneous nystagmus usually indicates a direct injury to the brainstem. The cause of this inappropriate nystagmus is a direction-specific imbalance in the VOR as brainstem neuronal circuitry is activated. Inappropriate nystagmus may also be related to medication toxicity, such as some antiseizure medications.

In the presence of normal peripheral vestibular function, head shaking does not provoke nystagmus or may provoke 1–2 beats. However, nystagmus provoked with head shaking indicates an imbalance of dynamic vestibular function. The clinical assessment involves placing the patient's head in 30° of anterior flexion, which positions the horizontal (lateral) SCC toward the ground. The head is then vigorously shaken from side to side about 30 times and then stopped. If nystagmus occurs, it may be immediate or there may be a latent period of about 10 sec. Nystagmus normally extinguishes after about 20–30 sec. Inappropriate nystagmus may also originate from abnormalities in some brainstem or cerebellar structures.

Inappropriate nystagmus can persist for as long as 24 hours when a peripheral otolithic organ (vestibule) is damaged. This persistent nystagmus continues while the head is held in the position that provokes it. However, nystagmus of peripheral origin may be suppressed by visual fixation while in a lighted room. In a dark room, visual fixation is not possible and nystagmus intensity will increase with the slow phase becoming faster.[26–28]

Central vestibular dysfunction produces a nystagmus of longer duration than from peripheral origins. An indicator of inappropriate nystagmus of central origin is often the inability to inhibit nystagmus with visual fixation. The dysfunction could be at the brainstem level or in the cerebellum. Therefore, if spontaneous nystagmus can be suppressed in lighted conditions, the indication is for an intact central mechanism, especially the cerebellum. Impairment of eye movement coordination may arise from peripheral or central receptors if the MLF malfunctions. Frenzel goggles or an ophthalmoscope may assist in observing a subtle inability to inhibit visual fixation during inappropriate nystagmus. Beating can also be observed with the eyes closed.[26,27]

Gaze-provoked nystagmus is the inability to maintain a stable gaze position in an eccentric direction. It is characterized by the eyes drifting back toward the central position and then jerking back to the eccentric object of regard. This dysfunction is of central origin, probably not vestibular in nature, and is often seen in patients with brain injury or other central pathology.

Inappropriate Nystagmus and the Cupula

In the SCC, a gelatinous *cupula* sits on top of hair cells and attaches to the ampulla forming a diaphragm across the ampulla closing it off to the flow of fluid. Longer hair cells actually project into the cupula. The thickness of the top or center of the cupula is thinner than the rest and may be subject to detachment during the extreme angular acceleration forces caused by head trauma.[12] Hillman et al.[13] suggested that this detachment may function as a "relief valve" and serve "to prevent damage to receptor structures." If detached, it may reseal at a later time.

Nystagmus accompanied with vertigo may indicate involvement of the cupula in the peripheral end-organ. A normal cupula has the same density as the surrounding endolymph. Gravity does not cause movement of the cupulae relative to the crista and the SCC are insensitive to head position. If a situation changes the relative densities of cupulae and endolymph, the SCC would then be sensitive to gravity. This, in turn, causes an illusion of movement in response to certain orientations of the head. For example, vertigo and nystagmus typically occur when the density of the cupulae changes after excessive alcohol intake. High levels of blood alcohol result in alcohol leaving capillaries and infiltrating the cupulae making them less dense than the surrounding endolymph. Nystagmus continues until alcohol concentrations of the cupulae and endolymph become equal. The alcohol will leave the cupulae as blood alcohol concentrations drop leaving the cupulae more dense than endolymph. This results in several hours of head position-dependent nystagmus in the opposite direction.[5]

PERIPHERAL VESTIBULAR PATHOLOGY

Temporal Bone Fractures

Transverse basilar skull fractures of the temporal bone are often caused by traumatic blows to the occipital or frontal areas of the head. As a result, damage to the acoustic nerve, cochlea, or labyrinths may occur. Symptoms are manifested by sensorineural hearing loss, vertigo, and disequilibrium. A traumatic blow to the temporoparietal area of the head will likely cause longitudinal fractures of the temporal bone. Symptoms are manifested by conductive hearing loss from ossicular chain disarticulation.

Longitudinal fractures are more common but have a lower incidence of fracturing through the labyrinthine capsule. A transverse fracture is less common but has a higher incidence of fracture into the labyrinthine capsule. Locations of CN VII and CN VIII make them vulnerable to damage with transverse fractures. Hearing loss on the same side as the fracture is typically complete, and complete ablation of the vestibular function on that side is also common. If normal vestibular function remains intact on the opposite side, there will be several days of extreme rotational vertigo accompanied by nausea and vomiting. Normal functioning may then return. Age and presence of other related injuries may or may not be factors. In the patient age 60 or older, recovery is much slower and fine balance skills may never be regained.[5,10,29,30]

PERILYMPHATIC FISTULA

The protective membrane between the middle and inner ear prevents leakage of perilymphatic fluid into the middle ear. A fistula is an unnatural opening or hole in a pliable membrane. Causes for perilymphatic fistula (PLF) include trauma or barotrauma. A fistula usually occurs in the oval or round window. Symptoms are quite disabling with rapid onset of severe hearing loss, a loud roaring-type tinnitus, severe rotational vertigo with nystagmus, and severe disequilibrium accompanied by visceral autonomic symptoms of nausea and vomiting.[9]

BENIGN PAROXYSMAL POSITIONAL VERTIGO

This is an inner ear disorder involving a spinning sensation provoked by changes of head position relative to gravity. A common cause is head trauma but less common causes may include ear infections or Ménière's disease. True benign paroxysmal positional vertigo (BPPV) occurs when an otoconia is dislodged from its normal placement in the macula of the saccule or utricle in the inner ear and moves into a canal. Bhattacharyya et al. (2008) raised concern about the commonly used word "*benign*" in BPPV diagnosis. Again, as in "mild TBI," the implication was that the disorder was not serious.[3] However, if not diagnosed, the patient's quality of life could be seriously impaired and far from being "benign." The term *paroxysmal* refers to the rapid and sudden onset of the BPPV episode. BPPV has also been called *benign positional vertigo* (BPV), *paroxysmal positional vertigo* (PPV), *positional vertigo* (PV), *benign paroxysmal nystagmus* (BPN), and *paroxysmal positional nystagmus* (PPN).

There are two variants of BPPV: posterior canal BPPV and horizontal canal BPPV. Approximately 85%–95% of cases of BPPV involve the posterior canal. There are two theories used to describe how otoconia dislodgement occurs. The *cupulolithiasis* theory suggests that the loosened otoconia moves and attaches to the ampulla of a canal. The ampulla becomes sensitive to gravity due to the added otoconia mass. The cupula alone normally responds to angular acceleration. However, the dislodged otoconia causes deflection of the cupula during different movements of the head and not to angular acceleration alone.[9]

The second theory, *canalithiasis*, is considered, but debated, to be the most common cause of posterior canal BPPV. Otoconial debris is displaced from a normal state of floating freely in the vestibule's endolymphatic fluid and becomes trapped in the posterior canal. When the head moves in the same plane as the canal, labyrinthine fluid moves unilaterally deflecting the cupula resulting in inappropriate nystagmus and vertigo. In some cases, a combination of cupulolithiasis and canalithiasis may be present.[9,31,32]

Benign paroxysmal positional vertigo can occur at any age but is more prevalent in the aging population (5th to 7th decade). In the younger population, BPPV interferes with daily activities and loss of work days. However, the elderly have the added impact of other health issues that cause additional loss of quality of life. Oghalai et al.[33] estimated that 9% of older patients seen for comprehensive geriatric assessments for "non-balance-related complaints" are found to have undiagnosed BPPV. It is well known that falls secondary to a variety of causes or, more specifically, secondary to BPPV often result in serious injuries, including fractures and/or head trauma.

ACUTE PERIPHERAL VESTIBULOPATHY

An episode of vestibular neuritis has a rapid onset of vertigo, nausea/vomiting, nystagmus, unsteady gait, and intolerance of head movement. The visual environment appears to spin but when eyes are closed there is a sense of the self spinning. Symptoms intensify when the head is moved and are reduced by keeping the head motionless. An episode may persist for days or weeks. The etiology is typically a viral infection within the labyrinthine space known as "labyrinthitis." Vestibular neuronitis is a viral infection of the vestibular nerve.[34]

VESTIBULAR PSEUDONEURITIS

While acute peripheral vestibulopathy is a self-limited condition, a more threatening condition mimicking symptoms of peripheral origin is an acute vestibular syndrome of central origin. This central syndrome, known as "vestibular pseudoneuritis," may indicate a posterior circulation stroke involving an infarct in the brainstem or cerebellum. Small studies by Norrving et al.[35] and Lee et al.[36] found that 25% or more patients presenting with acute vestibular syndrome were experiencing posterior circulation strokes. The patient complains of dizziness but has no classic stroke symptoms or other neurological signs. Without further evaluation via MRI, the patient may be discharged with the assumption that symptoms are of benign origin. However, if a stroke is evolving, a precious window of time for an early diagnosis and implementation of a potentially beneficial treatment may be lost. Patients with a history or high risk for stroke should be evaluated.

In an effort to find a method of assessment to quickly differentiate between peripheral neuritis and central vestibular pseudoneuritis, Cnyrim et al.[37] and Newman-Toker et al.[38] conducted "proof of concept" studies with a goal of finding a cost effective method that would be as reliable as using an MRI and other neuro-otological equipment. A differentiation between posterior circulation stroke and benign peripheral vestibular neuritis was found to exist in alterations of eye movement. *Peripheral vestibular nystagmus is typically suppressed by visual fixation but vestibular nystagmus of central origin is not.* The method of quick assessment, found in the Newman-Toker et al.[38] study involved a penlight and the examiner's hand or other occlusive device. The penlight-cover test was more easily performed with actual acute pseudovestibular patients because their nystagmus was continuous rather than rapidly decaying over 30–60 sec as in a peripheral origin. While the study was acknowledged as needing further investigation, it did offer the possibility of a low-cost, rapid, and simple form of disrupting visual fixation and quickly indentifying brainstem or cerebellar stroke.[38]

OTHER ETIOLOGIES OF DIZZINESS/VERTIGO

CERVICOGENIC DIZZINESS/VERTIGO

Little thought is given to the possible relationship between complaints of dizziness, disturbed eye movement, and cervical (neck) muscle pain following a "whiplash" injury or "whiplash associated disorders" (WADs).[39] The most common mechanism of "whiplash" injury involves neck hyperextension and hyperflexion resulting from the forces of acceleration and deceleration during a rear-end collision. In recent decades, WAD injuries decreased when vehicles became equipped with seatbelts, air bags, and head restraints. However, lateral (T-bone) motor vehicle accidents or accidents causing spinning of the vehicle produce torsion of the neck and head. Mallinson et al.[40] reported that lateral impact accidents have "inflict[ed] more severe injury than rear-ending collisions."[40] Of course, motor vehicle accidents are not the only cause of WAD. Physical altercations or other mechanisms of injury causing severe shaking of an unprotected head or torso can produce the same effect.

Somatosensory postural control becomes impaired when the proprioceptive receptors in neck musculature are overexcited by excessive stretch. The receptors then misinform the brain about head position, which causes dizziness/vertigo. Children are particularly vulnerable due to less mature (weaker) neck musculature. Cervicogenic vertigo is accompanied by neck pain and headaches. Impairment of eye movement causes difficulties in reading. The sensation of dizziness is typically mild with a sense of movement of self or of the environment. Symptoms, including imbalance, worsen with head movement, significant movement in the visual environment, or holding the head in one position for a long period of time. Duration of symptoms may be minutes to hours.[3]

MÉNIÈRE'S SYNDROME AND POSTTRAUMATIC MÉNIÈRE'S SYNDROME

The etiology of Ménière's syndrome is not completely understood but is considered to be idiopathic endolymphatic hydrops. Symptoms occur when excessive amounts of endolymphatic fluid swell the endolymphatic space in the membranous labyrinth. Onset is typically spontaneous with symptoms of severe rotational vertigo, fluctuations in hearing, tinnitus, and aural fullness. Intervals between episodes are symptom-free and may be days, weeks, months, or years. Triggers may be stress, fatigue, changes in barometric pressure, some foods, excessive dietary salt, or by other illnesses. When the initial episode of Ménière's occurs following TBI, it is identified as posttraumatic Ménière's syndrome. It is uncommon and symptoms may not be manifested for weeks or months or years after the injury.

Hamid[41] reported that a diagnosis of Ménière's syndrome is "certain" in the presence of (1) two or more spontaneous episodes with rotational vertigo for 20 minutes or longer, (2) audiological assessment showing hearing loss (unilateral or bilateral), on at least one occasion, (3) tinnitus or aural fullness reported in the affected ear, (4) other etiologies were excluded (i.e., vestibular schwannoma), and (5) histopathological findings in the temporal bone.

Treatment begins with a trial of medical management with diuretic therapy and a restricted salt diet (2000 mg/day). During severe episodes of vertigo, diazepam (antianxietal), or meclizine (antihistaminic vestibular suppressant) may help. Abstinence from alcohol, nicotine, and/or caffeine can be beneficial. Studies involving intratympanic injections of gentamicin (an ototoxic antibiotic) are exploring other methods to relieve severe vertigo. However, vertigo may be relieved but some hearing loss could occur.[42–44] Vestibular rehabilitation can be beneficial for teaching the patient to use movement and balance strategies. Prognosis may be good with early identification and treatment. If aggressive medical management fails, a final resort involves surgery to destroy vestibular tissue or to prevent vestibular signals from going to the brain.[7,9,45]

LABYRINTHINE CONCUSSION

Pathophysiology of a labyrinthine concussion or "inner ear concussion syndrome" is not completely understood. Tangeman[46] defined the syndrome as a "descriptor for the spectrum of inner ear symptoms that may occur following many mild to severe head injuries." A clearer definition proposed by Luxon[29] noted that "microscopic hemorrhages" would be found in the cochlea and labyrinth from mechanical membrane disruption caused by acceleration/deceleration forces to the head. Symptoms include vertigo and disequilibrium, with or without hearing loss, and tinnitus or a sense of pressure in the ear.[47]

The most commonly used tool for diagnosis is electronystamography (ENG). On occasion, the platform posturography, is used for confirmation of diagnosis. Recovery depends upon the extent of injury and presence or absence of associated abnormalities. Recovery is often complete in a few weeks. If recovery is slow, the patient may benefit from vestibular rehabilitation. If unilateral weakness is confirmed and is significant, consideration of surgical ablation of the injured labyrinthine end-organ may be needed.[9]

GAIT ATAXIA

When a patient requires a broad base of support or widened center of gravity to stabilize balance during ambulation, it is named "gait ataxia." An ataxic gait is a residual of acquired cerebellar damage and/or of bilateral peripheral vestibular loss. Vestibular ataxia is caused by inappropriate or abnormal activation of vestibulospinal pathways.[28] When ambulating, the patient will be observed using a cane or touching walls or furniture to maintain steadiness. If visual cues are reduced in darkened areas, a functional somatosensory system could be inadequate to maintain spatial orientation. The ability to stand upright would then be impaired. This dysfunction influences gradual changes in the patient's daily habits such as avoidance of walking or driving at night in poorly lighted areas. The consequences of drug or alcohol intoxication also affect inner ear fluids leading to ataxia and balance difficulties.

OSCILLOPSIA

An illusory movement of stationary objects or of the general visual environment is oscillopsia. Presence of impaired bilateral peripheral vestibular and cerebellar function will produce a sense of visual unsteadiness and blurring of vision when the head is moved. Oscillopsia does not occur during slow head movement or at rest. Eye movement in oscillopsia is horizontal or vertical.[48] Residual deficits are frustrating and impact daily life. Imagine objects in your visual environment continually "jumping." You would have to stop and stand still to clearly see an object or read a street sign.

MIGRAINE VERTIGO

This type of vertigo is included in differential diagnostics for Ménière's syndrome or peripheral BPPV. Migraine symptoms include headache, sensitivity to light (photophobia), sensitivity to sound (phonophobia), and visual aura. Migraine-associated vertigo involves chronic nonparoxysmal (nonsudden) motion sensitivity, lightheadedness, or disequilibrium. The most prevalent origin of this type of vertigo appears to be central. A mild low frequency unilateral hearing loss or bilateral hearing loss may be present. Diagnostic criteria include episodic vestibular symptoms; migraine, as defined by the International Headache Society; and at least two migraine symptoms during at least two vertiginous episodes. Vertigo is not rotary as seen in Ménière's disease. In most cases, the patient has a family history of migraine with associated nausea, light and sound sensitivity, and changes in vision.[41,49]

ISOLATED EPISODES OF ACUTE VERTIGO

Seemungal and Bronstein[26] reported that acute isolated vertigo is "usually benign"; however, a differential diagnosis must be considered to rule out other causes. Vertigo that persists several hours should raise concern for possible cerebellar stroke, migrainous vertigo, labyrinthitis, and even a BPPV diagnosis that may have been missed. Other possible causes of dizziness/vertigo include low blood sugar (hypoglycemia), chemical intoxication, psychophysiological episodes, oculomotor paresis, or adjusting to a new pair of glasses.

CENTRAL VESTIBULAR PATHOLOGY

Dysfunction of central origin may be related to traumatic or nontraumatic causes involving brain tumors, vascular, cardiac, or other central neurological pathologies. Central vertigo indicates damage to areas responsible for integrating and processing balance information as in brainstem nuclei. While nystagmus of peripheral origin is provoked by head movement, nystagmus of central origin is spontaneous without provocation. Symptoms include dizziness, nausea, vomiting, imbalance, and/or gait problems. Neurologic symptoms accompanying central disorders may include confusion, headaches, extremity and facial weakness and/or numbness, poor coordination, visual deficits, and dysarthria. Episodes of central origin do not fatigue making duration longer than with peripheral origin. Gait is typically more unstable. On occasion, both central and peripheral origins are present. Age is also a factor.[50]

CEREBELLAR STROKE

Onset of cerebellar infarct or hematoma presents with an intensive acute onset of vertigo. Diagnosis may be difficult in that symptoms are similar to vestibular neuritis. However, if the "head thrust test" demonstrates an intact peripheral vestibular function, a cerebellar stroke may be present. An early computed tomography (CT) scan would reveal a large cerebellar hemispheric stroke. If the CT scan appears to be negative but cerebellar stroke remains suspect, an MRI could provide confirmation.[35–38]

Vertigo and balance difficulties related to cerebellar involvement are experienced only when standing or trying to ambulate. Nystagmus is very strong with eyes open or closed.

POSTTRAUMATIC VASCULAR LOOP

There are occasions when the anterior inferior cerebellar artery (AICA) is displaced as a result of trauma to the head. The displacement causes the artery to compress CN VIII in the cerebello-pontine angle at the brainstem. The patient is unable to function while suffering from a constant severe PV accompanied by nausea and vomiting. Any movement will increase symptoms. Infrequently, the patient will complain of unilateral tinnitus and hearing loss. An auditory brainstem response (ABR) may reveal evidence of CN VIII pathology. Once the diagnosis is confirmed, surgical decompression may be beneficial.[9]

THE PSYCHOLOGICAL IMPACT OF DIZZINESS AND IMBALANCE

There are a variety of reasons why patients suffering from episodes of vertigo develop anxiety, depression, poor self-esteem, and a growing sense of disability. The fear of falling or the fear of heights is common. Concern for a sudden onset of vertigo and the loss of control in public venues often leads to avoidance behaviors or "safety-seeking behaviors," as coined by Gurr and Moffat.[51] The appearance of staggering, falling, and confusion may lead observers to believe that the person is intoxicated. The patient soon finds him/herself avoiding social events and staying home to avoid embarrassment. Physical activity is avoided for fear of provoking an episode.

There is no doubt that many patients undergoing a vestibular rehabilitation program require a coupling of counseling sessions to address a variety of emotional symptoms stemming from the dysfunction. While most vestibular rehabilitation therapists are physical therapists with specialized training, the counseling aspect is typically addressed by a psychotherapist (clinical psychologist) or licensed marriage-family therapist. Many balance clinics include or refer to the services of psychotherapists who have knowledge of the vestibular components. However, it is often difficult to locate a psychotherapist with this knowledge. If the vestibular therapist and psychotherapist establish a team effort with regular intercommunication, the patient will benefit.

A key factor in achieving the best outcome will be patient compliance. Education is the greatest tool used by a good therapist to engage a patient's willing participation in what is usually a difficult treatment program. Between, both, the vestibular therapist and the psychotherapist the patient is assisted in understanding the basics of the dysfunction: Why symptoms occur; the emotional response; and how treatment should help. Initial treatment typically provokes unpleasant symptoms but feeling worse comes before feeling better. Another factor in achieving the best outcome involves adequate intensity and duration of the treatment program.

In cases where only partial symptom resolution is the best that can be obtained, the psychotherapist will play an even more important role. Adjustment to disability will require strong coping strategies to help the patient through anxiety, depression, and loss.

DIAGNOSTICS OF THE AUDITORY SYSTEM

Vestibular symptoms following TBI may or may not include hearing disturbance. If diagnosis of BPPV has been confirmed but hearing loss is not evident, an audiometric assessment may not be needed.[3] Testing is appropriate if conductive hearing loss is evident. This may occur in the presence of hemotympanum (blood in middle ear); foreign debris in the ear canal or middle ear; transverse fracture of the temporal bone; or auditory tumors. The patient's history may include exposure to ototoxic medications leading to hearing loss.

Acoustic immittance testing identifies disarticulation in the ossicular chain. After TBI, some patients are unable to complete standard audiometric evaluations due to cognitive or behavioral problems. An ABR may be helpful.[10]

NEUROSENSORY HEARING LOSS

Neurosensory hearing loss is related to loss of cochlear hair cells and/or damage to CN VIII due to trauma, aging, and/or chronic exposure to extremely loud noise without ear protection. Other causes include endolymphatic hydrops, PLF, autoimmune ear disease, virus in the cochlea, or metabolic disorders (hypothyroidism). A frequent complaint involves difficulty in distinguishing speech sounds while attempting to converse in environments with competing noises. Neurosensory hearing loss has no known medical treatment but may respond to hearing aids or the more recent cochlear and brainstem implants.[9,10]

TINNITUS

Complaints of noise in the ears (ringing, roaring, high-pitched whistling) is termed "tinnitus." It may be an indication of a physiological disturbance of CN VIII. There is no known medical treatment to reduce or stop tinnitus. Episodes may be intermittent, continuous, or may completely disappear after an episode or two. Tinnitus is aggravated by prolonged exposure to excessive noise levels and/or excessive use of aspirin. The patient may not be as aware of tinnitus during normal exposure to daily environment noise. However, awareness will arise significantly in quiet environments or if congestion from a cold or ear infection is present. The annoying sound can be quite disturbing to some patients when attempting to fall asleep or concentrate on work. A device that "masks" tinnitus has been helpful for some patients. The sound from an oscillating fan, or device making "white noise" or falling water are some examples.[5,10]

CENTRAL HEARING LOSS

Signals from the cochlea into the cochlear portion of CN VIII are normal. However, lesions impairing cortical or subcortical levels result in defective central auditory processing.

DIAGNOSTICS OF THE VESTIBULAR SYSTEM

Specialists in neurological disorders of the auditory and vestibular systems are neuro-otologists as well as some but not all audiologists and otorhinolaryngologists (ENT). The patient's general history is reviewed, including medications, over-the-counter supplements, dietary habits, and intake of caffeinated and/or alcoholic beverages. Symptoms are reviewed as well as what, if any, seems to provoke symptoms and what seems to relieve them. Also, nonvestibular causes for dizziness are ruled out. Specific assessments for possible vestibular causes are then initiated. Once a diagnosis is made, identification of a trained vestibular/balance therapist, usually a physical therapist, is the next step. Another referral to consider would be to a neuro-optometrist or rehabilitation-optometrist specializing in the evaluation and treatment of vision-related dysfunctions, which can cause dizziness and difficulties with balance. This is especially true for the patient after a TBI. It is unfortunate that many regions of the United States do not have these specializations and the cost of traveling significant distances for services is not always just monetary. Many individuals will not tolerate repetitive travel, which continually provokes symptoms and, therefore, have the benefit of a treatment session undone.

Vestibular function testing is warranted in the following situations: (1) atypical nystagmus; (2) suspected additional vestibular pathology; (3) failed or repeatedly failed response to otolith replacement; or (4) with frequent recurrences of BPPV.[3] Thabet's study[52] found that the majority of cases with acute vertigo syndrome were related to BPPV in the right posterior canal. Another point in evaluating patients was made by Shumway-Cook[53]: always consider the influences presented with accompanying disabilities, such as hemiplegia, or spinal pathologies.

Postural control is measured in static (stationary) and dynamic (moving) conditions. A *perturbation* is a disturbance in balance during static conditions. If the standing surface and the visual field are altered, sensory inputs in the CNS can be measured in terms of functional balance, mobility, and gait performances when the entire body is in motion. Some tests measure performances of functional balance and mobility during tasks requiring combined activity and divided attention. Even nonambulatory patients can be tested for sitting balance during various activities.[8]

Once a diagnosis is made, it is not the end but the beginning of treatment.

PERIPHERAL VERSUS CENTRAL

Remember that visual fixation can suppress nystagmus when dysfunction is in the peripheral system but fixation is more difficult when dysfunction is in the central system. Smooth ocular pursuit mechanisms must be intact for suppression of nystagmus of peripheral origin to occur. Nystagmus provoked by head positions presents with latency, adaptability, and fatigability. Latency refers to the time between the stimulus (provoking head position) and the beginning of the response (nystagmus). Adaptability refers to the peripheral system's ability to adapt to the stimulus through treatment. Fatigability refers to the cessation of the nystagmus after a period of time. For example, nystagmus that occurs after twirling around several times will normally fatigue within about 10–20 sec. Abnormal function typically results with a prolonged nystagmus (about 60 sec). If nystagmus is of central origin, it lacks latency, adaptability, or fatigability.[50]

Central vestibular lesions may be found in the brainstem, cerebellum, or vestibulocerebellar pathways but rarely from lesions in the thalamus or other of the multiple central vestibular regions. Central disorders of otolithic function often involve a history of hypertension, myocardial infarction, or stroke. Gait instability is more pronounced when a central lesion is present. For example, gait ataxia could signify a disorder of dynamic otolithic-spinal function or cerebellar involvement.[54,55]

THE DIZZINESS HANDICAP INVENTORY

This 25-item self-assessment scale is a commonly used tool to quantify the patient's perception of handicap as a result of dizziness. Influences of dizziness on daily life are explored in three spheres: physical, emotional, and functional. The highest score is 100 with physical 28, emotional 36, and functional 36. A high score indicates a greater level of handicap. The dizziness handicap inventory (DHI) is a reliable measure of outcome during treatment.[56–58]

PERILYMPHATIC FISTULA

Confirmation of PLF is difficult due to the inconsistent symptoms and acute onset is often masked by more serious injuries or delayed symptoms. For this reason, appropriate testing is required before decisions for treatment can be made. Rapid onset of symptoms occurring immediately after a trauma indicates necessity of an initial assessment by audiometry and dynamic platform posturography. Audiometrics find sensorineural hearing loss. Platform posturography involves applying pressure to the external auditory canal to measure increases or decreases at the tympanic membrane and middle ear. A fistula is present if postural sway is abnormal as pressure changes.[59]

Once PLF is identified, surgical repair involves placing a graft over the oval and/ or round window to stop leakage. It would seem simple to explore the middle ear for leaking fluid; however, perilymph fluid in the inner ear is miniscule (0.07 cc). Roland[9] indicated that even with magnification, leaks of 5%–10% of perilymph fluid are almost impossible to see "in an operative field flooding with local anesthetics, irrigating fluids, and even minimal bleeding." If fistula repair is successful vertigo will disappear. On occasion, there will be an improvement in hearing.

WHIPLASH-ASSOCIATED DISORDERS

Symptoms arising from WAD may involve pathology from peripheral vestibular end-organ, CNS, or proprioceptive receptors in the cervical column.[60] Consider also the neck pathology from other causes, including degenerative cervical spine disease or cervical spondylosis as often found in elderly patients. Complaints of lightheadedness or fainting may occur when extending the neck to look upward. Vertebrobasilar insufficiency can occur when neck pathology compresses the vertebrobasilar artery in the extended position. Peripheral vestibular testing includes the Dix-Hallpike and caloric testing. CNS causes are ruled out with normal findings from a visual evoked

potential (VEP), ABR, saccade test, and caloric suppression test. If no neuropathological signs were identified, the conclusion is that neck torsion caused the overexci-
tation of proprioceptive receptors in the cervical column.[60]

Most patients improve with conservative therapy involving gentle mobilization of
the cervical spine, muscle stretching, exercises, and instruction in proper posture as
well as vestibular therapy. If smooth pursuits and saccades are affected the patient
often complains of reading difficulties. Neuro-optometric evaluation and subsequent
vision therapy will improve the outcome.

TESTS OF STATIC STANDING BALANCE

ROMBERG AND SHARPENED ROMBERG

The standard Romberg tests the status of the vestibulospinal tracts along the posterior column during static standing.[61] Abnormal findings may indicate a dysfunction
in the vestibulospinal tracts along the posterior column or indicate dysfunction in the
processing of sensory organization in the CNS. The patient stands with feet together
(narrow base) with eyes closed for 20–30 sec. The Romberg is normal if the patient is
able to stand steadily without sway or loss of balance. However, the more challenging
"sharpened" or "extended" Romberg test requires the patient to stand with feet in a
heel-toe position and arms folded across the chest and eyes closed for 60 sec. After
four trials, a normal score would be 240 sec. To determine dependence on visual
input, have the patient perform trials with and without eyes open.

ONE-LEG STANDING TEST

The One-Leg Standing Test (OLST) is another test of static standing commonly used
by both physicians and therapists. The patient stands on both feet with arms folded
across the chest and eyes remain open. One leg is bent at the knee and not pressed
into the standing leg. Holding balance for 30 sec, each leg separately, is the normal
range for young adults. However, older adults may have a shorter range. Each leg is
tested over five trials. The normal total would be 150 sec.

TIMED STANCE BATTERY

This reliable and valid battery was developed by Bohannon and Leary[62] to assess
balance capabilities during variations in foot position. The battery is also sensitive to
changes through serial testing over time. The four stance positions have the patient
stand with feet apart (broad base), together (narrow base), tandem, and on single leg.
Each stance is performed with eyes open and eyes closed. The maximum duration
for normal is 30 sec with a possible total score of 240 sec.

MULTIDIRECTIONAL REACH TEST

Measurements of sway are made while reaching forward, backward, and to each
side. Observation can be made of any limitations on the control of the center of

gravity. Another reach test is the Limits of Stability Test, which requires a computerized forceplate to measure postural control sway from midline into eight different directions.[8]

OTHER STATIC TESTS

The Postural Sway Test and the Motor Control Test use computerized forceplates to measure postural responses. The equipment is more likely to be used in specialty balance clinics and not in acute or postacute rehabilitation settings. Allison and Fuller[8] noted that postural sway measurements "detect more subtle problems" with greater sensitivity to changes in performance following treatment than rating scales or timed measures. Postural sway is measured while the patient stands normally for about 30 sec. The forceplate measures the degree of sway required to maintain balance or center of gravity. The motor control test measures automatic postural responses when the forceplate becomes dynamic. A quick shift of the plate forward or backward causes a postural adjustment to bring the center of gravity over the base of support.

When computerized equipment is not available, the clinician can use the "nudge-push" test to get a sense of the patient's automatic postural responses. There is no need to warn the patient before this test but the therapist must be prepared to prevent a fall. This is not a quantifiable test nor are there reliable measures. As the patient stands, the clinician gives a moderate push backward at the sternum followed by a push forward between shoulder blades. Loss of balance and postural responses, such as bending from the hip or stepping, can be recorded as normal, fair, poor, or unable.[8]

TESTS OF DYNAMIC BALANCE

A test of dynamic balance requires input from the VOR to stabilize the visual field and an ability to make rapid adjustments in posture. Heel-toe ambulation and walking on a straight line on the floor or on a low balance beam forward and backward are performed to 50 feet with eyes open. An error is counted each time a step is taken outside of the straight line or off the balance beam. The following exercise may be too difficult for some patients but for those who are able, it will challenge higher level dynamic balance skills. Hop 10 times each with feet together, on the left foot, and on the right foot. Notice whether the patient maintains a consistently steady rhythm. Two more challenging tests involve jumping rope. The patient first jumps 10 times with the feet together with one rhythm. The second challenge is jumping rope, while alternating hops from the floor to an elevated level (step 10 inches high) with one rhythm up to 20 times.[9]

UNTERBERGER TEST

Another assessment of vestibulospinal function involves the patient standing with eyes closed and making 50 steps in place. Dysfunction is present if the patient rotates more than 45° to the right or left. Direction of rotation indicates the side of lesion.[63]

BABINSKI–WEIL TEST

While keeping the eyes closed, the patient imagines a straight line ahead and steps five steps forward and five steps backward. The side of lesion is indicated if the patient consistently drifts toward that side going forward and away from that side going backward.

MODIFIED UNTERBERGER AND BABINSKI–WEIL TESTS

Both tests are performed as described above but the patient wears headphones to eliminate environmental sounds that would otherwise provide spatial orientation.

SENSORY ORGANIZATION TEST

The Sensory Organization Test (SOT) requires computerized forceplate equipment (computerized dynamic posturography) to measure the sensory inputs while maintaining postural control. Both visual environment and standing surface components are changed in various patterns to measure how the patient utilizes visual, vestibular, and somatosensory inputs. The six assessment conditions include (1) a fixed surface position and fixed visual input; (2) eyes closed while surface fixed position; (3) visual environment moved while in surface fixed position; (4) surface moved with eyes open; (5) surface moved with eyes closed; and (6) both visual environment and surface moved. If the patient perceives movement of the body away from midline or center of gravity, a normal response would be to initiate protective or righting actions. If the perception is incorrect, the attempt to return to center of gravity would be inaccurate and loss of balance could occur.[64]

CLINICAL TEST FOR SENSORY INTERACTION ON BALANCE

The Clinical Test for Sensory Interaction on Balance (CTSIB) is a version of the SOT that does not require computerized equipment. Instead of moving forceplates to measure responses in the same six conditions, the CTSIB involves observation while the patient stands on a thick foam surface. A helmet (Japanese lantern) completely covering the head has been used to imitate the moving visual environment. However, most therapists have currently modified the CTSIB by eliminating the helmet and testing in four conditions: (1) eyes open and (2) closed while (3) standing on a firm surface and (4) repeated while standing on a foam surface. A stopwatch is used to measure how long the patient can balance without stepping, reaching, or falling. The normal range is 30 sec. Results of testing should provide the clinician with information to focus treatment. It is noted that patients who are able to compensate for vestibular system dysfunction while maintaining a fixed head position may demonstrate a dependence on visual input if head movement is added during tests.[65]

TINNETTI BALANCE ASSESSMENT

This is an easy clinical evaluation of balance and gait under varying challenges. Balance is assessed by quiet standing and then challenged with eyes closed. Gait balance is assessed for quality, speed, and symmetry.[66]

Fukuda Stepping Test

This assessment of labyrinth function can be used to determine if a patient is able to detect movement without benefit of visual input.[67] However, it is not used as a true diagnostic assessment due to a low degree of reliability. The patient stands with eyes closed and arms outstretched in horizontal position. Instruction is given to take 100 marching steps (knees raised high) in place. Observation notes the angle and distance of drift from center. A normal result demonstrates that the patient is able to complete 100 steps with forward progression of no longer than 3 feet and an angle of rotation of no larger than 45°. A normal performance rarely demonstrates the patient progressing backward. When the finding is abnormal, the drift away from center is toward the side of dysfunction. It is possible for persons with normal vestibular functioning to test positive on the Fukuda. For this reason, it is imperative to perform a battery of tests.

Dynamic Gait Index

Eight gait tasks including walking and walking at different speeds, walking moving the head in pitch (around the intra-aural axis) and yaw (movement on vertical axis) planes, pivoting, walking over objects, walking around objects, and going up and down stairs. The maximum score is 24. Scores of less than 19 typically identify patients with vestibular disorders who have falls. Age is of no concern.[68]

Timed Up and Go Test

Measure speed in standing up from a chair and walking 3 m (around 10 feet), turning around, walking back, and sitting down. Measurements of 13.5 sec or more, typically, identified individuals with increased risk of falls. This is particularly seen in the elderly.[69]

Five Times Sit-to-Stand Test

In this test, the patient is asked to come from sitting to standing with arms crossed as quickly as possible for five times. Height of the seat from the floor should be about 43 cm (16–17 inches). This test is considered to be a valid measurement of balance and lower extremity strength in the elderly. However, the test is applicable to younger patients with lower extremity weakness and possible vestibular dysfunction.[70]

ELECTRONYSTAGMOGRAPHY

This tool provides a clinical assessment of vestibular function. Recommendations from the Bhattacharyya et al. study[3] provided simple but clear diagnostic criteria for posterior canal BPPV. They are as follows:

1. The patient's history includes repeated episodes of vertigo with changes in head position.

2. The physical examination findings are the following:
   a. Vertigo associated with nystagmus provoked by the Dix-Hallpike test[71]
   b. Latency period between completion of the Dix-Hallpike test and onset of vertigo and nystagmus
   c. Provoked vertigo and nystagmus increase and then resolve within 60 sec

A patient complaining of dizziness may or may not have an obvious nystagmus by simple observation. Pathology may be missed unless an electronystagmography (ENG) battery is performed. The ENG records nystagmus by using electrooculography (EOG), which measures movement of the eye globe within the orbit. The two terms, ENG and EOG, have been used interchangeably in the literature; however, ENG is actually a battery of eye movement tests and is more commonly heard in balance/dizziness venues. The ENG is a noninvasive tool utilized by the neuro-otologist to detect abnormalities in each labyrinth separately or to indicate potential dysfunction at the brainstem level. Intact extraocular function is necessary for more accurate measurement of responses. ENG is also able to detect nystagmus with eyes closed. Electrodes are placed on the skin around the patient's orbits. The patient wears Frenzel goggles with 20-diopter lenses to magnify the eye globes for better detection of nystagmus on observation. Since nystagmus from peripheral dysfunction can be suppressed by visual fixation, the lenses magnify to the point that the patient sees nothing but light.

A disadvantage in using the ENG is that the stimulus is not physiologic and stimulus intensity is only partially under the examiner's control. In that regard, Roland[9] appropriately advised that the examiner must be "meticulous" with calibration of equipment before each examination and provide an agreeable environment for the patient. Measurements recorded during ENG assessments provide documentation for comparison on subsequent assessments.

COMPONENTS OF A COMPLETE ELECTRONYSTAGMOGRAPHY BATTERY

A complete ENG battery includes (1) the Dix-Hallpike maneuver, (2) bithermal caloric test, (3) optokinetic test, (4) visual tracking test, (5) gaze test, (6) saccade test, and (7) positional test.[9] If a diagnosis of BPPV is uncertain by positional testing or if other unrelated neurological symptoms are present, additional assessments may be required. However, unless a patient has an atypical clinical presentation, the Bhattacharyya et al. study demonstrated that neuroimaging or more extensive vestibular testing was seldom of diagnostic value.[3] Diagnostic neuroimaging would be important to rule out a possible lesion in the brainstem, cerebellum, thalamus, or cortex. It must be noted that CT or MRI techniques cannot detect BPPV alone due to the microscopic nature of pathology in the SCC.

Dix-Hallpike Maneuver

The Dix-Hallpike maneuver (Figure 9.3) is the standardized test used to determine presence of BPPV. Patients with significant vascular disease or physical limitations related to spinal pathologies, Down syndrome, severe rheumatoid arthritis, or morbid obesity should be excluded from testing. Also, before beginning the test, the examiner should explain the procedure in full and describe expected symptoms.

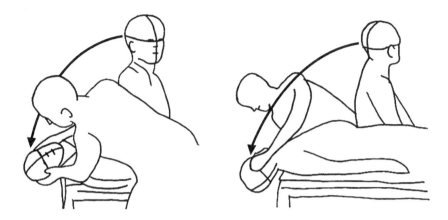

FIGURE 9.3 Dix-Hallpike maneuver test for benign positional nystagmus. (Adapted from Baloh, R. W., and Halmagyi, G. M., *Disorders of the Vestibular System*, Oxford University Press, New York, 1996, p. 331.)

From a sitting position, the examiner holds the patient's head at 45° to the right or left and 20° neck extension, while taking the patient to a supine position. The patient's head is hanging off the table maintaining neck extension at 20°. This position is held for about 30 sec. The eyes are observed for nystagmus, which may be present or absent. The direction of nystagmus is recorded for each side.[71]

Dix-Hallpike Test for Posterior Canal Benign Paroxysmal Positional Vertigo

The right posterior canal BPPV is the most common cause of peripheral vertigo. Therefore, it makes sense to begin the examination with the head turned to the right side. Diagnostic for posterior canal BPPV is positive if the Dix-Hallpike test causes vertigo with nystagmus. A latency period from the time the supine position is completed until onset of nystagmus ranges from 5 to 20 sec or, rarely, as long as 1 minute. The fast component of nystagmus is typically mixed torsional and vertical eye movement. Torsional movement is the upper pole of the eye beating toward the dependent ear (*geotropic*) and the vertical component beating toward the forehead. Inquire if the patient has subjective vertigo. Resolution of vertigo and nystagmus typically occurs within 60 sec. After nystagmus has ceased and the head has been returned to the upright position, nystagmus may be seen in the reverse direction. A patient with a history of TBI should have both ears tested since bilateral posterior canal BPPV is more likely to occur in those cases. A negative finding on an initial Dix-Hallpike test does not necessarily rule out posterior canal involvement. A repeat test should be performed at another time to avoid a false-negative result.[3,71,72]

Assessment for Horizontal (Lateral) Canal Benign Paroxysmal Positional Vertigo

Horizontal canal BPPV is the second most frequent BPPV diagnosis. If the Dix-Hallpike test was negative for posterior canal BPPV but the patient continues to have repeated episodes of vertigo provoked by changes in head position relative to gravity, another type of test should be performed. On occasion, a maneuver performed to reposition a displaced otoconia in the posterior canal may result in displacement of the otoconia into the horizontal canal. If symptoms persist, testing for horizontal canal BPPV should be conducted.

Although the supine roll test is used for preliminary testing for horizontal canal BPPV, it is not yet considered to be an absolute validation. Before testing, the examiner must warn the patient of the possibility of provoked symptoms. The patient lies in the supine position with the head in neutral position (nose up). The head is rapidly rotated 90° to one side. While holding that position the examiner observes for nystagmus. Once nystagmus subsides or if no nystagmus occurred, the head is returned to neutral position. If nystagmus recurs while the head is in the neutral position, wait for it to subside and then rapidly turn the head 90° in the opposition position. Following observation for and ceasing of nystagmus, the head is returned to neutral.[73]

Diagnosis of horizontal canal BPPV involves two possible conditions: *geotropic* type and *apogeotropic* type. The *geotropic* type involves an intense horizontal nystagmus when pathology is present. The fast component beats toward the ground (*geotropic*). When rotated to a healthy side, the horizontal nystagmus is also *geotropic* but is less intense. *Apogeotropic* type is less common. The supine roll test results in horizontal nystagmus with beats toward the upper most ear (*apogeotropic nystagmus*). When the patient rolls to the opposite side, nystagmus again changes directions with beats toward the upper ear. Diagnosis of horizontal canal BPPV typically indicates a lesion in the ear in which the direction producing the most intense nystagmus.[73]

Bithermal Caloric Test (Caloric Irrigation)

A portion of the horizontal canal protrudes into the middle ear thus making it available for thermal stimulation. This standardized test involves irrigation of warm and cool water into an ear. Water temperature warms or cools the tympanic membrane and changes the temperature in the middle ear. Each ear is tested separately. About 10 cc of warm water (~44°C) is injected into an ear. The moving endolymphatic fluid deflects the cupula, which stimulates the vestibular nerve. The provoked nystagmus is observed with EOG. The same is performed with an injection of cool water (~30°C). The resulting nystagmus is measured in terms of the fast phase. The pneumonic "COWS" refers to the expected response. Cold stimulus ("C") results in fast beating nystagmus toward the opposite ("O") side. Warm stimulus ("W") results in fast beating nystagmus toward the same ("S") side. Suppression of visual fixation may also be tested during caloric irrigation. While nystagmus is brisk, the patient is to keep eyes open, which may reduce the intensity of nystagmus.[9]

Calculations determine peak responses and assess the integrity of the labyrinth. The record may indicate a percentage of "weakness" of one side compared to the other and a threshold for abnormality may range from 35% to 30% difference from ear to ear. Responses to thermal testing are reliable and the test is relatively easy to perform at bedside. However, before testing, the examiner should rule out a possible perforated tympanic membrane or obstructions in the external auditory canal. The patient should be warned that nausea and vomiting could occur.

Optokinetic Testing

A rotating drum with alternating black and white stripes is placed at the center of the patient's visual field. The drum is rotated in each direction at 20° per second and at 40° per second. Nystagmus is the normal response. However, a normal OKN-provoked nystagmus in one direction but absent in the other direction is an abnormal response. A normal nystagmus may occur with slower rotations but be abnormal at higher rotations. Abnormalities point to central pathology at the brainstem level.

Visual Tracking Tests

While normal and abnormal visual tracking are discussed in greater detail elsewhere in the text, assessments of the vestibular system cannot ignore the importance of visual input. Visual tracking is assessed by observations of ocular motility and the VOR. If the peripheral vestibular end-organ is impaired, the VOR is impaired. As previously mentioned, during the acute phase of TBI, the "head thrust" test can provide a quick evaluation of the integrity of the VOR.

Following TBI, abnormal visual tracking should be suspected when the patient frequently complains of losing his/her place and/or headaches while reading. When lines are skipped the patient not only becomes increasingly frustrated by repeated searches for the starting point but concentration and comprehension are lost as well. The patient has poor eye-hand coordination, balance, and general clumsiness. Reading and other activities are then avoided or modified in some manner. Impairments in visual and vestibular components are, unfortunately, often overlooked. This underscores the necessity of comprehensive post-injury evaluations, which should include vestibular as well as ocular motor and vision testing by appropriate specialists.

Gaze Test

While sitting, the patient is instructed to look straight ahead, 30° each right and left, and 30° each up and down. At each point, gaze is sustained for 20–30 s with the eyes open and then closed. If gaze nystagmus occurs, pathology may be present in either peripheral or central vestibular systems. More definitively, pathology in the central system is indicated when nystagmus is present with eyes open but absent with eyes closed.

Saccade Test

This test may be used as a formal or informal assessment for brainstem dysfunction. The patient is instructed to keep the head in a static position while moving the eyes back and forth to specific points on a wall. A normal response is demonstrated when the eyes move from point to point and maintain focus on each point. An abnormal finding shows the eyes missing or overshooting/undershooting the targeted points.

While the ENG can be used to evaluate subtle dysfunctions in visual tracking another tool is the dynamic visual acuity test (DVAT). The DVAT is a computerized screening test of the visual-vestibular ocular reflex (VVOR). If visual acuity decreases during head turning, impairment of visual-vestibular interaction is the result of excessive retinal slip. DVAT results may correlate with the patient's symptoms of blurred vision while walking or inability to read road signs while driving.[74]

Positional Test

Electronystamography records nystagmus in four different positions: (1) sitting and looking straight ahead, (2) in supine position looking straight ahead (up), (3) in supine with the right ear down, and (4) in supine with left ear down. ENG recordings examine nystagmus provoked by one position or more of these positions. If a preexisting spontaneous nystagmus is known, recordings may show alterations in the underlying nystagmus pattern. Peripheral disorders show a direction-fixed nystagmus. Central disorders show a direction-changing pattern. However, determination of etiology is difficult due to various exceptions to these rules. An indicator of CNS pathology is related to changes in nystagmus patterns while the head is maintained in one position.[9]

Vestibular Autorotation Test

Decades ago, clinicians performing field evaluations tested the VOR by stimulating the SCC during spinning. The patient sat in a swivel chair and closed the eyes while being spun or rotated at a steady rate for about 30 sec. When stopped, observation was made for nystagmus. In a more sophisticated clinical setting, rotations were performed while the patient sat in a motorized rotational chair. When rotations were stopped, magnification through the Frenzel goggles allowed a better observation of post-rotatory nystagmus. The test was fairly helpful in detecting suspected bilateral vestibular function loss. To date, testing protocols and instruments have become increasingly sophisticated allowing for more quantitative and qualitative information.

The VAT[75] was designed to assess horizontal and vertical VOR gains (comparisons between magnitude of rotation and induced eye movement) and phases (latency). A sensor detecting rotations is placed on the patient's head and ENG electrodes are fixed to the patient's face. When ENG alone could not confirm that dizziness was of peripheral origin, the VAT provided more reliable information.

NEUROCHEMISTRY IN THE VESTIBULAR SYSTEM

A brief word about the world of neurochemistry involved in the peripheral and central vestibular systems is necessary to broaden our appreciation of how these systems function. The synaptic transfer of information from peripheral receptor hair cells to the vestibular nerve is in chemical form. Afferent neurotransmitters called "excitatory amino acids" (EAAs) include glutamate, kainite/AMPA, N-methyl-D-aspartate (NMDA), and metabotropic glutamate receptors (GluRs) with several subtypes. The central vestibular system uses EAAs for signal transmission between the vestibular nerve and the vestibular nuclei in the brainstem. Ocular motor function benefits from the actions of glutamate and ketamine hydrochloride (an NMDA receptor/channel antagonist), which play an important role assisting vestibular nuclei neurons in reaching "target motoneurones." Nitric oxide (free radial gas) works within the vestibular labyrinth in the transmission of EAAs. Nitric oxide appears to play an important role in ocular motor function.[76,77]

Excitatory amino acids are balanced or modulated by "inhibitory amino acids" (IAAs) such as y-aminobutyric acid (GABA). Inhibition between bilateral vestibular nuclei comes from GABA interaction. The specific function of glycine, an IAA in the central vestibular system, is not yet understood, but it is known to decrease with age. Another inhibitor, nociceptin, was found to decrease VOR gain and prolongation of post-rotatory nystagmus in a dark environment.[78,79] Spontaneous and evoked activity of vestibular nuclei neurons were found to be modulated by the amino acid, arginine vasopression. Although many other EAAs and IAAs have been identified, studies have yet to completely understand their role in peripheral or central vestibular functions.[76]

MOTION SICKNESS

What causes those "unpleasant vegetative effects" called *motion sickness*? Many healthy individuals have experienced motion sickness whether traveling by car, sea, air, or in space. Studies have indicated that the most susceptible individuals are children and adult women. The least susceptible tend to be toddlers under age 2 and adults 50 years and older.[80]

Vision, as proposed by Bronstein, had a dominant role or "hierarchical preference" over proprioceptive input in the process of maintaining upright posture and balance.[81] However, Mallinson et al.[40] suggested that a "visual preference strategy" would not apply to some individuals who have an intolerance for any disagreement between visual and vestibular signals. Paige[82] had previously called this disagreement between the two systems as a "visual vestibular mismatch" (VVM) and others referred to it as a "sensory conflict." By 1996, the "sensory conflict" theory for the development of motion sickness had been accepted within the scientific field studying this subject.[80]

The theory states that a "provocative motion stimulus" is detected by peripheral sensory receptors in the inner ear (otoliths and SCC), eyes, and somatosensory system. The collected sensory signals are forwarded to and integrated in the brainstem and then presented to a "neural store" in the brain, where previously established sensory patterns are stored. If the new incoming sensory pattern does not agree with or match previously stored sensory patterns, a "sensory conflict" occurs. The "sensory conflict" then activates a "neural process" responsible for mediating the emetic (vomiting) response.[80–83] This "neural process" involves three afferent pathways: the labyrinth, the chemoreceptor trigger zone (CTZ) in the floor of the fourth ventricle, and the visceral afferent of the gastrointestinal tract. Each afferent pathway sends its signal through a neuropharmacological mechanism, which is independent from the other two pathways. For example, input from the labyrinth to the emetic center is through histamine (H_1) receptors. A signal from the CTZ is relayed through dopamine (D_2) receptors and visceral afferents relay signals through serotonin ($5HT_3$) receptors. Neurotransmitters involved in the neural processes of motion sickness include H_1, acetylcholine, and norepinephrine. The initial symptom of the emetic response is nausea, which will evolve into vomiting if the stimulus is prolonged.

PHARMACOLOGICAL TREATMENT OF
VESTIBULAR-RELATED SYMPTOMS

The unpleasant symptoms related to vestibular dysfunction have driven many a person to search for a magic remedy. Some would chew on ginger root to soothe an upset stomach. Others resort to a dark, quiet room and avoid movement, especially of their heads and eyes. Physicians have prescribed such medications as amphetamines, benzodiazepines, anxiolytics, muscle relaxants and antiseizure medications. To date, the most commonly prescribed medication is an antihistamine: meclizine. Others are diphenhydramine, zolantidine, and betahistine. Antihistamines seem to "*suppress*" the central emetic center thus relieving vegetative symptoms of nausea and vomiting. It is thought that the histaminergic system in the hypothalamus could be involved in the vestibular-autonomic response to motion sickness.[80] Another *vestibular suppressant* is scopolamine, an anticholinergic, which reduces neural mismatching as it blocks the action of acetylcholine. Benzodiazepines (diazepam, clonazepam) are prescribed to reduce anxiety and relax muscles. The antiseizure properties of benzodiazepines involve the inhibitory effect of the GABA system. However, all of these *vestibular suppressants* have one undesired property: sedation.[3,76]

As a rule, patients with TBI are warned to avoid or at least minimize use of sedating medications, if possible. In the field of neurorehabilitation, it is recognized that sedation negatively impacts the patient's performance in tasks requiring attention, concentration, thought processing, problem solving, or initiation. A seizure-prone patient may find that these medications, as well as opioids and barbiturates, exacerbate encephalopathies.

Vestibular suppressant medications may relieve the vegetative symptoms; however, the "core cause," a dysfunction somewhere within the vestibular system, remains untreated. When medication is discontinued after a prolonged dependence, the rebound of symptoms is a reminder that the "core cause" is waiting to be treated. The result of multiple studies on this subject is that use of *vestibular suppressant* medications is not recommended.[3,84,85] This is especially true if medication is the only treatment offered to the patient. Patients and physicians should also be aware of a possible adverse interaction with other medications.[84]

On the positive side, studies have clearly demonstrated that vestibular exercises provide the most beneficial treatment and best outcomes. In cases of severe nausea and vomiting, short-term use of a suppressant will help the patient as vestibular rehabilitation is started. The patient may be requested to discontinue medication before Dix-Hallpike testing to assure test accuracy.

Studies continue to search for pharmacological agents to relieve symptoms related to peripheral or central vestibular disorders. Most have been unable to find effective agents. Interactions between the endocrine and vestibular systems are being researched for possible influences on vestibular function. While it is known that steroids, amines, and peptide hormones influence the peripheral vestibular system, a complete picture is yet to be known.[56,76,85,86]

VESTIBULAR REHABILITATION

Progression of function is the best gauge for the effectiveness of treatment. The rehabilitation discipline most involved in vestibular rehabilitation is physical therapy. The process of treatment involves strategies for adaptation and substitution by using other strategies, habituation (desensitization), and retraining of balance. As the patient is able, exercises are expanded to include cardiorespiratory conditioning. Goals of vestibular rehabilitation are to (1) optimize compensation in the balance system; (2) habituate abnormal vestibular responses to rapid movements; (3) reduce fall risks by improving balance and postural control; and (4) educate the patient.

Before treatment, many suffering patients succumb to subtle changes in posture and movement to avoid the triggering of symptoms. These changes impose dramatic alterations in a patient's once active lifestyle. There will be occasions when medication can be helpful for the short term. Surgery is the rare choice. Therapists take caution when a patient has other disabilities (brain trauma, stroke, peripheral neuropathy, spinal conditions, and/or vision disorders), which may limit choices of exercises.[87]

The effectiveness of rehabilitation will be enhanced if the patient is advised that symptoms will worsen before getting better as habituation is established. The therapist is the motivator giving encouragement to help the patient stay the course. Home programs are instructed to increase intensity of treatment; however, it is strongly suggested that patients begin the course of treatment with one-on-one sessions with a therapist. This approach will assure that the patient is compliant and consistent. Therapist involvement will be able to monitor the effectiveness of treatment and make modifications when needed. If symptoms remain severe or long-lasting, treatment may be discontinued and reevaluation made by the neuro-otologist.

Effective treatment starts with stabilization of static balance before moving on to the more challenging dynamic balance treatment.

TREATMENT FOR BALANCE AND GAIT IMPROVEMENT

In the 1940s, Cawthorne[88] first described vestibular rehabilitation habituation exercises. Although still an effective protocol, clinicians have modified the original protocol as education on this subject advanced. Herdman's[87] approach to address unilateral vestibular hypofunction provided a clear application of exercises for both the therapist and patient. The following adapts Herdman's protocol.[89]

The initial portion includes treatment for cases with severe vertigo, nausea, and vomiting. These patients prefer a dark and quiet room because any stimulus seems to trigger an episode. Habituation begins with graduated introduction of light into the room. Gentle head movement is next introduced. As habituation increases, the patient is advanced to assisted ambulation and graduated to more independent ambulation as fall risk decreases. At that point, the patient should be able to begin the next phase of treatment.

Exercises to Improve Static Balance

Try to achieve a successful performance for each step before advancing to the next step.

1. Stand with a wide base of support. Gradually narrow base of support a few inches. Hold each position 15 sec. Continue until balance is stable for 15 or more seconds with feet together.
2. Increase challenge by standing in heel-toe position for 15 sec. Switch position of feet and repeat stance for 15 sec.
3. Increase challenge of heel-toe position by holding arms close to body, outstretched, or folded across chest. Hold each position 15 sec (eyes open and closed).
4. Advance balance challenge by standing on thick foam pad or cushion. Tilt the head upward to 45° (eyes open and closed).
   a. Stand with feet as close together as possible to maintain balance for 15 sec. Wall touch may be used until balance is achieved without support.
   b. While standing, turn the head horizontally to right and left while holding visual fixation on a target ahead. Practice for 1 minute without interruption.
   c. As able, gradually bring feet closer together until wall touch is not needed.

Exercises to Improve Dynamic Postural Sway

Try to achieve a successful performance for each step before advancing to the next step:

1. In acute phase, start with walking, even if assistance is needed for safety.
2. Walk with as narrow base as possible for balance. Gradually narrow the base. (Wall touch is allowed until practice gradually eliminates that need.)
3. Walk while turning the head to the right and to the left. Try to visually focus on different objects during this exercise. As improvement occurs, attempt to increase speed of head turning.
4. Walk forward several feet and then return using a wide turning circle. Gradually make the turning circle smaller. Alternate turns to both directions.
5. Challenge balance by sitting and bouncing on a Swedish ball or trampoline.
6. Catch a ball by starting with small stepping movements. Then increase challenge with larger stepping movements needed to catch the ball.
7. Walk an obstacle course on varying surfaces (smooth, rocky, grass, hills) with turns. Use small and large steps. Practice on stairs and stepping on/off curbs.
8. Walk in a mall or other busy environment. Start by walking when the environment is quiet (stores closed). Then advance to walking when the environment is busy. Walk with the flow of traffic and then against the flow of traffic.

REHABILITATION FOR BILATERAL PERIPHERAL VESTIBULAR DYSFUNCTION

The patient with bilateral vestibular loss has difficulty with balance and seeing environmental objects clearly while the head is moving. These difficulties do not occur while the patient is still. Treatment for bilateral vestibular loss focuses on a "substitution" strategy instead of an "adaptation" strategy.

Substitution Exercises for Bilateral Vestibular Loss

Functional visual and somatosensory inputs are "substituted" to compensate for bilateral vestibular function loss. To determine if the somatosensory system is intact, assessment includes evaluation of the patient's ability to detect vibration, kinesthetic sense in the feet, and proprioception (sense of limb position without looking). If somatosensory deficits are present, the patient will have significant difficulty in achieving a functional recovery after bilateral vestibular loss. However, if the somatosensory system is intact but the patient has a progressive vision disorder (macular degeneration, cataracts), this poses a major problem for recovery. As previously discussed, there is a hierarchical preference to rely on visual input more than any one of the other two systems involved in balance. The patient with visual impairment may benefit from a substitution strategy as an alternative approach to replace vestibular loss. Although the COR is seldom mentioned, it may offer this alternative. COR is not to be confused with the OCR. The proprioceptive inputs of cervical muscles and joints result in a slow phase eye movement or COR. This reflex is complementary to the VOR when the head is moved in short, low frequencies. Exercises for VOR adaptation and enhancement of the COR are reviewed below.

In the event that the VOR is not available to stabilize the eyes during head movements, any decrease of visual input could leave the patient disabled from engaging in several activities (i.e., driving, sports). The therapist provides education about using night lights in the home and taking time to adjust before standing up from a chair or bed when in the dark. The patient is also advised that postural stability is rarely ever completely normal with bilateral vestibular loss. However, treatment should bring some improvement in most cases. The role of a therapist is to motivate and support the patient through the difficult initial phase of treatment.

In the case of bilateral vestibular loss, partial residual function may be present. The bithermal test or rotational chair test may be able to detect any residual vestibular function. If present, adaptation exercises may then strengthen that portion. Although exercises to enhance gaze stability are encouraged, any improvement will not fully compensate for VOR loss.

Exercises for Vestibulo-Ocular Reflex Adaptation

Assure that no distractions occur during these exercises.

1. While sitting, practice maintaining visual fixation on a small stationary target while moving the head horizontally (back and forth).

2. Visually fix on a target in the visual field while practicing vertical head movements (up and down).
3. The exercise can be varied by using different head positions.
4. Try to continue each exercise for up to 1 minute. As adaptation occurs, exercise duration is increased to 2 minutes and so on.
5. These exercises can be practiced while in the dark by imagining a target.

Exercises to Improve Gaze Stability

These exercises enhance the COR.

1. Eye/head movement with a single target.
   a. Attach a business card to a wall in front of you. Stand/sit within reading distance.
   b. Maintain visual focus on words while moving the head back and forth.
   c. Move the head at a faster pace while keeping words in focus up to 1–2 minutes.
   d. Repeat the exercises while moving the head up and down.
   e. Repeat the exercises using a large pattern (checkered) as a full visual field stimulus.
2. Eye/head movement between two targets. (Place the two targets close enough to allow the peripheral vision of one eye to see a target while keeping the eyes focused on the other target.)
   a. Horizontal targets. Rest eyes, as needed.
      (i) Look at one target. Keep head lined up with the target.
      (ii) Look at the other target by moving only the eyes to it. Then turn head to target keeping it in focus. A saccade should precede head movement.
      (iii) Repeat in the opposite direction.
      (iv) Vary speed of head movement but keep visual focus on target.
   b. Practice the above exercises with targets placed in vertical position.
   c. Imaginary targets. Practice each up to 5 minutes. Rest eyes, as needed.
      (i) Look at target directly in front of you.
      (ii) Close eyes, turn head slightly. Imagine that you are looking directly at the target.
      (iii) Open eyes to check if you have kept the eyes on the target.
      (iv) Repeat exercises in the opposite direction.
      (v) Vary speed of head movement.

MANAGEMENT OF CENTRAL VESTIBULAR DYSFUNCTION

Symptoms of central vestibular dysfunction are essentially the same as from peripheral vestibular dysfunction. One difference is that symptoms of central origin often have accompanying neurological symptoms related to diagnoses such as TBI, strokes, tumors, and/or vascular abnormalities. In some cases, dizziness, vomiting, poor balance, and gait abnormalities can originate from dysfunction in both peripheral and central vestibular systems. As previously discussed, most patients with peripheral vestibular dysfunction alone typically have successful outcomes from appropriate rehabilitation. However, when both peripheral and central dysfunctions are present, even the efforts of rehabilitation do not produce the same rate of success. Poorer outcomes are found in the patient with combined central vestibular and cerebellar dysfunction. However, in general, the possibility for improvement is best when a vestibular physical therapist provided treatment.[50]

Studies by Brown et al.[50] and Brown[90] set out to determine if vestibular physical therapy demonstrated functional improvement in patients with central vestibular dysfunction. Primary outcome measures included the following: (1) Activities-Specific Balance Confidence Scale (ABC),[91] (2) DHI,[56] (3) Dynamic Gait Index (DGI),[68] (4) timed up and go test (TUG),[69] and (5) five times sit-to-stand (FTSTS) Test.[70] Exercises used in the study included balance and gait training, general strengthening, flexibility exercises, and exercises for the somatosensory and visual systems. Vestibular adaptation exercises were added to subgroups with mixed peripheral and central disorders and substitution exercises for those with peripheral vestibular loss. The patients were also educated in safety awareness techniques to avoid falls. Chronic stages of dysfunction with symptom duration of about two or more years were represented. Treatment occurred for a mean of five visits over an average of 5 months. The mean age of the group was 64 ± 18 years of age. At each visit the patients completed the DHI and the ABC and performed the DGI, TUG, and FTSTS tests.

Study findings demonstrated postrehabilitation improvement on the ABC, DHI, TUG, and FTSTS over all groups tested. Patients with a diagnosis of central vestibular dysfunction showed significant improvements on the DHI, DGI, and TUG tests. Patients with posttraumatic etiology showed the greatest improvement in the DGI. Patients with cerebellar disorders did not fare as well. Some fall risks continued in the elderly patients with chronic vestibular dysfunction. Findings from this study underscore the importance of early, aggressive treatment to achieve more desirable outcomes.[60]

MANAGEMENT OF BENIGN PAROXYSMAL POSITIONAL VERTIGO

Bhattacharyya et al.[3] conducted an extensive study specific to chronic BPPV. This study involved a large group of clinicians in search of various components involved in the assessment and treatment of BPPV. The purpose of this work was to offer evidence-based recommendations to assist physicians and therapists in making treatment decisions for patients with BPPV. Their findings were published by the American Academy of Otolaryngology-Head and Neck Surgery Foundation (AAO-HNSF) in 2008.

The panel gave two "against" recommendations:

1. Radiographic imaging and/or vestibular testing after BPPV diagnosis has been made. The additional information offered "little to diagnostic accuracy." Exceptions would include cases of uncertain diagnosis or when other symptoms or signs unrelated to BPPV indicated a necessity for such testing.
2. Routine treatment of BPPV with vestibular suppressant medications was not recommended.

Earlier studies had also recognized that routine use of vestibular suppressants was not advised.[77,80,83,89] Instead, they found that vestibular rehabilitation was the most beneficial treatment with the best outcomes. Benefit of treatment was further enhanced with general conditioning exercises as the patient's tolerance for movement increased.

The AAO-HNSF panel recommended the following seven items for evaluations and treatment of BPPV:

1. If the history indicated BPPV, but the Dix-Hallpike test for posterior canal involvement was negative, a supine roll test should be performed to assess for horizontal (lateral) canal BPPV.
2. BPPV should be differentiated from other causes of imbalance, dizziness, and vertigo.
3. If BPPV has been identified, patients should be questioned about what factors seem to negatively impact management. This could include such factors as CNS disorders, inadequate supportive system in home/community, and/or greater risk for falls.
4. Treatment of patients with posterior canal BPPV should involve a particle repositioning maneuver (PRM).
5. Reassessment should occur within 1 month following an initial period of observation or treatment to confirm resolution of symptoms.
6. When BPPV was identified but the patient failed initial treatment, assessment should be performed to identify other possible causes. These include persistent BPPV and underlying peripheral vestibular or CNS disorders.
7. Patients should be counseled about the impact of BPPV on safety, potential for disease recurrence, and importance of follow up.

BPPV in the United States: A diagnosis of BPPV was found in 17%–42% of the 5.6 million annual clinic visits with primary complaints of dizziness. Of those, 86% without associated vestibular pathology reported complete resolution of symptoms following PRM. In patients with additional vestibular pathology, 37% reported complete resolution following repositioning treatment.[3,72,90–95]

Particle Repositioning Maneuver for Benign Paroxysmal Positional Vertigo

A displaced particle (otoconia) may be repositioned by one of three versions of a PRM, also called *canalith repositioning treatment (CRT)*: The *Liberatory maneuver* (Semont),[96] the *Epley maneuver,*[97] and the *Brandt-Daroff exercises.*[98] The most widely used maneuver for posterior canal BPPV is the Epley or Semont. Comparative studies found that repositioning treatment was more effective than Brandt-Daroff exercises or habituation exercises. Comparisons between PRM, vestibular rehabilitation exercises, and no treatment established that vestibular rehabilitation provided more effective resolution of symptoms than no treatment.[99] Another study compared outcomes of patients randomly assigned to the Brandt-Daroff habituation exercises, Semont maneuver, or Epley maneuver. Similar cure rates were found for the Semont (74%) and the Epley (71%) but much lower rates for the Brandt-Daroff (24%). Although Brandt-Daroff rates increased over a 3-month period, the rates continued to be less than results from the other PRMs.[100] One of the complaints of the Brandt-Daroff exercises was that patients had less tolerance to the repeated vertigo-induced positioning.[3]

Caution is given when treating patients with any spinal pathology or some vascular conditions, retinal detachment, or other restrictions. Before treatment, tolerance for the exercises should be evaluated.

MANAGEMENT OF POSTERIOR CANAL BENIGN PAROXYSMAL POSITIONAL VERTIGO

As mentioned, the Semont (Liberatory) maneuver and the Epley maneuver were both effective for posterior canal involvement.

Semont Maneuver

The patient is in a sitting position with legs hanging over the edge of a table or raised mat. The therapist turns the patient's head 45° toward the unaffected ear. While holding the patient's head, the therapist then rapidly moves the patient to a side-lying position. The position is held for about 30 sec. The patient is then rapidly moved to the opposite side-lying position without any pause in the sitting position and without changing head position relative to the shoulder. Hold the position for 30 sec and then gradually return to the upright sitting position.

Epley Maneuver

The patient is sitting on a table or raised mat with legs straight out (Figure 9.4): (a) the head is turned 45° toward the affected ear and the patient is rapidly laid back to the supine position with the head (at 45°) hanging over the table edge; (b) the position is held for 20–30 sec; (c) the head is turned 90° to the opposite side and held for 20 sec; (d) the head is turned another 90° (body moved from supine to lateral decubitus position with head almost face down) and the position is held for 20–30 sec; (e) the maneuver is completed by returning the patient to the upright sitting position. Complications most commonly experienced during the procedure include nausea, vomiting, fainting, and, rarely, a switch of the otoconia to another canal (6%–7%).[99–102]

MANAGEMENT OF HORIZONTAL CANAL BENIGN PAROXYSMAL POSITIONAL VERTIGO

Lempert Maneuver

If no response occurs from PRM treatment for posterior canal BPPV, it is possible that an otoconia was displaced into the horizontal canal into the posterior canal. The roll maneuver or Lempert[73] maneuver moves the otoconia from the horizontal canal into the vestibule by rolling the patient 360° in a series of steps to produce particle repositioning. Effectiveness with the Lempert maneuver is reported at about 75% with some studies reporting 50%–100% success.[73] Appiani et al.[103] found that the

Right ear anterior view

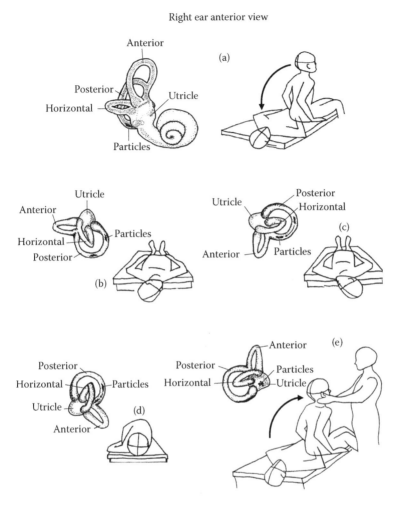

FIGURE 9.4 The Epley maneuver (particle repositioning) for BPPV. See text for explanation. (Adapted from Jones, H. R., (Ed.), *Netter's Neurology*, Icon Learning System, Teterboro, NJ, 2005, p. 131.)

liberatory maneuver was also effective for the treatment of horizontal canal BPPV. Studies have indicated that horizontal canal BPPV may spontaneously remit more quickly than other types of BPPV.[3,98]

BENEFIT OF EARLY COMPREHENSIVE TREATMENT

When PRM treatment for posterior canal BPPV is combined with a vestibular rehabilitation program, superior outcomes occur. This is particularly true when the program is focused on habituation exercises. This process also promotes adaptation and compensation for deficits related to several types of balance disorders. Additional exercises involve postural control, fall prevention training, conditioning exercises, and muscle relaxation techniques. Retraining for functional skills and education for the patient and family strengthens the recovery process.[3,74,103–105]

TREATMENT SUGGESTIONS

Findings from all tests performed during the initial evaluation provide a baseline. It is helpful to patient and therapist to have a system of feedback regarding progress or lack of it throughout the treatment program. At intervals, retest the patient's performance. Record the results in a serial format such as a graph. Many clinicians use video-tape to record the patient's performance during initial testing as well as interval testing. Whether graph or video-tape, visual feedback is stronger than just verbal feedback. If progress is not made from time to time the therapist can remind the patient that progress is not always a straight upward line. The patient will need encouragement to stay the course. On occasion, a "success sandwich" is helpful: the first and last exercises of the session are within the patient's comfort zone but exercises in the middle are the more challenging. The patient is more likely to return for the next session if some form of success has been achieved before leaving. However, lack of progress should always alert the therapist. The question to ask is "why?" Is the treatment protocol appropriate for the patient's dysfunction? Is something else going on? Has vision been tested for both acuity and ocular motor functions? By all means, do not ignore the problem. Be proactive. A reassessment by the therapist or referring physician may provide an answer. Care may need to be redirected.

SUMMARY

This chapter has been a brief review of the vestibular system and its many interactions with the somatosensory and visual systems. As their intricate structures, neural pathways, and complex neurochemistry are integrating in a cooperative manner, simple and elaborate movements of the human form are a sight to behold. The performances of many athletes provide evidence of this fact. Our uprightness in relation to gravity is sustained until the vestibular system is wounded in some way. In the case of posterior or horizontal canal BPPV, unpleasant symptoms are triggered with head movement. The patient prefers a dark, quiet room and avoids moving the head and eyes. Musculoskeletal stiffness sets in from restricted movement. Subtle changes in lifestyle become part of the disability. The significance of mTBI-related disabilities is compounded when dysfunctions in vestibular and ocular motor systems are present.

Vestibular pathology, evaluation, and treatment have been reviewed. It is evident that clinical expertise is required to understand the variations of symptoms. In that regard, early referral for appropriate evaluation should identify the "core cause" and, thus, designate an effective treatment protocol. In the process, evaluation should determine if dysfunction in the other two partners (vision/ocular motor and somatosensory) is contributing to the overall disability. Review of the patient's medications and other possible pathologies should be conducted. The choice of a treatment protocol will depend upon this survey. Most patients with vestibular pathology should not have to endure prolonged suffering. In the hands of a well-trained clinician, BPPV can be effectively treated. Vestibular rehabilitation in general has resulted in good outcomes and restored many patients to a productive lifestyle.

In review of the neurochemistry within the vestibular system it was evident that while much has been learned much is yet to be understood. Researchers are continuing to explore the vestibular system's own chemistry as well as the impact of introduced pharmaceutical agents. At present, the findings and advice from many studies is that use of vestibular suppressant medications is to be avoided. Suppression of central emetic centers simply addresses the symptoms but does not treat the "core cause," the underlying system dysfunction.

Many resources are available to inform, educate and direct both clinicians and patients. The Vestibular Disorders Association (VEDA) provides extensive information for the lay public. We are benefiting from studies performed by the National Institute on Deafness and Other Communication Disorders (NIDCD) in collaboration with the National Aeronautic and Space Administration (NASA). Findings have increased understanding the influences of gravity and weightlessness on the human body. Genetic and aging factors are being investigated. As previously mentioned, increased understanding of concussions and related vestibular and vision dysfunctions is emerging from media reports on sports medicine and the military actions in the Middle East. This recognition, in turn, is raising heads in the civilian world.

Prevention is always the ideal "cure" for any health issue. Until we attain that perfection, awareness and education continue to be key factors.

REFERENCES

1. Langlois, J. A., Rutland-Brown, W., & Thomas, K. E. (2006). *Traumatic brain injury in the United States: Emergency department visits, hospitalizations, and deaths*. Atlanta, GA: National Center for Injury Prevention and Control.
2. Healy, B. (1982). Hearing loss and vertigo secondary to head injury. *New England Journal of Medicine, 306,* 1029–1031.
3. Bhattacharyya, N., Baugh, R. F., Orvidas, L., Barrs, D., Bronston, L., Cass, S., & Haidari, J. (2008). Clinical practice guideline: benign paroxysmal positional vertigo. *Otolaryngology-Head and Neck Surgery, 139,* S47–S81.
4. Donohue, P. B. (n.d). The Sarah Jane brain project: Welcome. Retrieved from http://www.Thebrainproject.org. (Accessed February 09, 2010).
5. Nolte, J. (2001). *The human brain: An introduction to its functional anatomy* (5th ed., p. 358). St. Louis, MO: Mosby.
6. Eliot, L. (1999). Why babies love to be bounced: the precocious sense of balance and motion. In *What's going on in there? How the brain and mind develop in the first five years of life* (pp. 145–156). New York: Bantam Books.
7. Vestibular Disorders Association (VEDA). (2010, January 4). Vestibular disorders. Retrieved from http://vestibular.org/vestibular-disorders/balance/motor-output.php
8. Allison, L. K., & Fuller, K. (2007). Balance and vestibular disorders. In D. A. Umphred (Ed.), *Neurological rehabilitation* (5th ed., pp. 732–774). St. Louis, MO, Mosby.
9. Roland, P. S., Eaton, D., & Otto, E. (2004). Rehabilitation for posttraumatic vestibular dysfunction. In M. J. Ashley (Ed.), *Traumatic brain injury: Rehabilitative treatment and case management* (2nd ed., pp. 135–182). Boca Raton, FL: CRC Press.

10. Bermejo, J. (2004). Auditory function assessment in posttraumatic brain injury rehabilitation. In M. J. Ashley (Ed.), *Traumatic brain injury: Rehabilitative treatment and case management* (2nd ed., pp. 251–272). Baco Raton, FL: CRC Press.

11. Kandell, E. R., Schwartz, J. H., & Jessell, T. M. (2000). *Principles of neuroscience* (4th ed.). New York: McGraw-Hill.

12. Highstein, S. M. (1996). How does the vestibular part of the inner ear work? In R. W. Baloh, & C. M. Halmagyi (Eds.), *Disorders of the vestibular system* (pp. 3–11). New York: Oxford University Press.

13. Hillman, D. E., & McLaren, J. W. (1979). Displacement configuration of semicircular canal cupulae. *Neuroscience, 4,* 1989–2000.

14. Melnick, M. E. (2007). Clients with cerebellar dysfunction. In D. A. Umphred (Ed.), *Neurological rehabilitation* (5th ed., pp. 834–856). St. Louis, MO: Mosby.

15. Demer, J. L. (1996). How does the visual system interact with the vestibulo-ocular reflex? In R. W. Baloh, & C. M. Halmagyi (Eds.), *Disorders of the vestibular system* (pp. 73–84). New York: Oxford University Press.

16. Leigh, R. J. (1996). What is the vestibulo-ocular reflex and why do we need it? In R. W. Baloh, & C. M. Halmagyi (Eds.), *Disorders of the vestibular system* (pp. 12–19). New York, NY: Oxford University Press.

17. Suter, P. S. (2004). Visual dysfunction following traumatic brain injury. In M. J. Ashley (Ed.), *Traumatic brain injury: Rehabilitative treatment and case management* (2nd ed., pp. 209–250). Boca Raton, FL: CRC Press.

18. Fetter, M., & Dichgans, J. (1996). How do the vestibulo-spinal reflexes work? In R. W. Baloh, & C. M. Halmagyi (Eds.), *Disorders of the vestibular system* (pp. 105–112). New York: Oxford University Press.

19. Philbeck, J. W., Behrmann, M., Biega, T., & Levy, L. (2006). Asymmetrical perception of body rotation after unilateral injury to human vestibular cortex. *Neurophysiologia, 44*(10), 1878–1899.

20. Brandt, T., & Dieterich, M. (1999). The vestibular cortex. Its locations, functions, and disorders. *Annals of the New York Academy of Sciences, 871,* 293–312.

21. Bottini, G., Sterzi, R., Paulesu, E., Vallar, G., Cappa, S. F., Erminio, F., & Frackowiak, R. S. (1994). Identification of the central vestibular projections in man: positron emission tomography activation study. *Experimental Brain Research, 99*(1), 164–169.

22. Berthoz, A. (1996). How does the cerebral cortex process and utilize vestibular signals? In R. W. Baloh, & C. M. Halmagyi (Eds.), *Disorders of the vestibular system* (pp. 113–125). New York: Oxford University Press.

23. Bazarian, J., Boerman, H., Bolenbacher, R., Dalton, D., De Jong, M., & Doncevic, S., & Williams, C. (2008, July). *Acute management of concussion/mild traumatic brain injury in the deployed setting.* Presented at Defense and Veterans Brain Injury Center Consensus Conference, Washington, DC.

24. Terrio, H., Brenner, I., Ivins, B., Cho, J. M., Helmick, K., Schwab, K., & Warden, D. (2009). Traumatic brain injury screening: preliminary findings in a US Army brigade combat team. *Journal of Head Trauma Rehabilitation, 24*(1), 13–23.

25. Scherer, M. R., & Schubert, M. C. (2009). Traumatic brain injury and vestibular pathology as a comorbidity after blast exposure. *Physical Therapy Association, 89,* 980–992.

26. Seemungal, B. M., & Bronstein, A. M. (2008). A practical approach to acute vertigo. *Practical Neurology, 8*(4), 211–221.

27. Ernst, A., Basta, R. O., Seidl, I., Todt, I., Scherer, H., & Clarke, A. (2005). Management of post-traumatic vertigo. *Otolaryngol-Head and Neck Surgery, 132,* 554–558.

28. Brandt, T., & Daroff, R. B. (1980). The multisensory physiological and pathological vertigo syndromes. *Annals of Neurology, 7,* 195–203.

29. Luxon, L. M. (1996). Post-traumatic vertigo. In R. W. Baloh, & G. M. Halmagyi (Eds.), *Disorders of the vestibular system* (pp. 381–395). New York: Oxford University Press.

30. Gelber, D. A., & Callahan, C. D. (2004). The neurologic examination of the patient with traumatic brain injury. In M. J. Ashley (Ed.), *Traumatic brain injury: Rehabilitative treatment and case management* (pp. 3–26). Baco Raton, FL: CRC Press.
31. Parnes, L. S., Agrawal, S. K., & Atlas, J. (2003). Diagnosis and management of benign paroxysmal positional vertigo (BPPV). *Canadian Medical Association Journal, 169*(7), 681–693.
32. Parnes, L. S., & McClure, J. A. (1992). Free floating endolymph particles: a new operative finding during posterior semicircular canal occlusion. *Laryngoscope, 102,* 988–992.
33. Oghalai, J. S., Manolidis, S., Barth, J. L., Stewart, M. G., & Jenkins, H. A. (2000). Unrecognized benign paroxysmal positional vertigo in elderly patients. *Otolaryngology Head Neck Surgery, 122,* 630–634.
34. Gliddon, D. M., Darlington, C. L., & Smith, P. F. (2005). GABAergic systems in the vestibular nucleus and their contribution to vestibular compensation. *Progress in Neurobiology, 75*(1), 53–81.
35. Norrving, B., Magnusson, M., & Holtas, S. (1995). Isolated acute vertigo in the elderly, vestibular or vascular disease? Acta *Neurologica Scandinavica, 91*(1), 43–48.
36. Lee, H., Sohn, S. I., Cho, Y. W., Lee, S. R., Ahn, B. H., Park, B. R., & Baloh, R. W. (2006). Cerebellar infarction presenting isolated vertigo frequency and vascular topographical patterns. *Neurology, 67,* 1178–1183.
37. Cnyrim, C. D., Newman-Toker, D., Karch, C., Brandt, T., & Strupp, M. (2008). Bedside differentiation of vestibular neuritis from central "vestibular pseudoneuritis." *Journal of Neurology, Neurosurgery, and Psychiatry, 79*(4), 458–460.
38. Newman-Toker, D. E., Sharma, P., Chowdhury, M., Clemons, T. M., Zee, D. S., & Della Santina, C. C. (2009). Penlight-cover test: a new bedside method to unmark nystagmus. *Journal of Neurology Neurosurgery and Psychiatry, 80*(8), 900–903.
39. Treleaven, J., Jull, G., & Sterling, M. (2003). Dizziness and unsteadiness following whiplash injury: characteristic features and relationship with cervical joint position error. *Journal of Rehabilitative Medicine, 35*(1), 36–43.
40. Mallinson, A. I., & Longridge, N. S. (1998). Dizziness from whiplash and head injury: differences between whiplash and head Injury. *American Journal of Otology, 19,* 814–818.
41. Hamid, A. (2009). Ménière's disease. *Practical Neurology, 9,* 157–162.
42. Silverstein, H., Arruda, J., Rosenberg, S. I., Deems, D., & Hester, T. O. (1999). Direct round window membrane application of gentamicin in the treatment of Mènière's disease. *Otolaryngology-Head and Neck Surgery, 120*(50), 649–655.
43. Atlas, J. T., & Parnes, L. S. (1999). Intratympanic gentamicin titration therapy for intractable Ménière's disease. *American Journal of Otology, 20,* 357–363.
44. Minor, L. B. (1999). Intratympanic gentamicin for control of vertigo in Ménière's disease. *American Journal of Ontology, 20,* 209–219.
45. Fitzgerald, D. C. (1996). Head trauma: hearing loss and dizziness. *Journal of Trauma, Injury, Infection and Critical Care, 40*(3), 488–496.
46. Tangeman, P. T., & Wheeler, J. (1986). Inner ear concussion syndromes: vestibular implications and physical therapy treatment. *Topics in Acute Care Trauma Rehabilitation, 1,* 72–83.
47. Olsson, J. E. (1980). *Blunt Trauma of the temporal bone.* Houston, TX: American Academy of Otolaryngology- Head and Neck Surgery.
48. Longridge, N. S., & Mallinson, A. I. (1987). The dynamic illegible E (DIE) test: simple technique for assessing the ability of the vestibulo-ocular reflex to overcome vestibular pathology. *Canadian Journal of Otolaryngology, 16,* 97–103.
49. Reploeg, M. D., & Goebel, D. A. (2002). Migraine-associated dizziness: patient characteristics and management options. *Otology and Neurotology, 23,* 364–371.

50. Brown, K. E., Whitney, S. L., Marchetti, G. F., Wrisley, D. M., & Furman, J. M. (2006). Physical therapy for central vestibular dysfunction. *Arch Physical Medicine and Rehabilitation, 87*(1), 76–81.
51. Gurr, B., & Moffat, N. (2001). Psychological consequences of vertigo and the effectiveness of vestibular rehabilitation for brain injury patients. *Brain Injury, 15*(5), 387–400.
52. Thabet, E. (2008). Evaluation of patients with acute vestibular syndrome. *European Archives of Otorhinolaryngology, 265,* 341–349.
53. Shumway-Cook, A. (2000). Vestibular rehabilitation of the patient with traumatic brain injury. In S. J. Herdman (Ed.), *Vestibular Rehabilitation* (2nd ed., pp. 476–493). Philadelphia, PA: F.A. Davis Company.
54. Seemungal, B. M., Gresty, M. A., & Bronstein, A. M. (2001). The endocrine system, vertigo and balance. *Current Opinion in Neurology, 14,* 27–34.
55. Gresty, M. A., Bronstein, R., Brandt, M., & Dietrich, M. (1992). Neurology of otolith function: peripheral and central disorders. *Brain, 115,* 647–673.
56. Jacobson, G. P., & Newman, C. W. (1990). The development of the dizziness handicap inventory. *Archives of Otolaryngology-Head and Neck Surgery, 116,* 424–427.
57. Maskell, F., Chiarelli, F., & Isles, R. (2006). Dizziness after traumatic brain injury: overview and measurement in the clinical setting. *Brain Injury, 20*(3), 293–305.
58. Newton, R. (1989). Review of tests of standing balance abilities. *Brain Injury, 3*(4), 335–345.
59. Fitzgerald, D. C. (1995). Persistent dizziness following head trauma and perilymphatic fistula. *Archives of Physical Medicine and Rehabilitation, 76,* 1017–1020.
60. Gimse, R., Tjell, C., Bjørgen, I. A., & Saunte, C. (1996). Disturbed eye movement after whiplash due to injuries to the posture control system. *Journal of Clinical and Experimental Neuropsychology, 18*(2), 178–186.
61. Romberg, M. H. (1853). *Manual of nervous diseases of man* (pp. 385–401). London, UK: Sydenham Society.
62. Bohannon, R. W., & Leary, K. M. (1995). Standing balance and function over the course of acute rehabilitation. *Archives of Physical Medicine and Rehabilitation, 76,* 994–996.
63. Moffat, D. A., Harries, M. L., Baguley, D. M., & Hardy, D. G. (1989). Unterberger's stepping test in acoustic neuroma. *Journal of Laryngology Otology, 103,* 839.
64. Nashner, L. (1994). Evaluation of postural stability, movement, and control. In S. Hasson (Ed.), *Clinical Exercise Physiology.* Philadelphia, PA: Mosby.
65. Shumway-Cook, A., & Horak, F. (1986). Assessing the influence of sensory integration on balance. *Physical Therapy, 66,* 1548–1550.
66. Tinnetti, M. E. (1986). Performance-oriented assessment of mobility problems in elderly patients. *Journal of the American Geriatrics Society, 34,* 119–126.
67. Fukuda, T. (1959). The stepping test. *Acta Oto-Laryngologica, 50,* 95–108.
68. Shumway-Cook, A., & Woollacott, M. (1995). *Motor control theory and applications* (1st ed.). Baltimore, MD: Williams & Wilkins.
69. Podsiadlo, D., & Richardson, S. (1991). The Timed "Up & Go": a test of basic functional mobility for frail elderly persons. *Journal of American Geriatrics Society, 39,* 142–148.
70. Lord, S. R., Murray, S. M., Chapman, K., Munro, B., & Tiedemann, A. (2002). Sit-to-stand performance depends on sensation, speed balance, and psychological status in addition to strength in older people. *The journals of Gerontology. Series A, Biological Sciences and Medical Sciences, 57,* M539–M543.
71. Dix, M. R., & Hallpike, C. S. (1952). Pathosymptomatology and diagnosis of certain disorders of the vestibular system. *Proceedings of the Royal Society of Medicine, 45,* 341–354.
72. Hanley, K., O'Dowd, T., & Considine, T. (2001). A systematic review of vertigo in primary care. *The British Journal of General Practice, 51,* 666–671.

73. Lempert, T., & Tiel-Wilck, J. (1996). A positional maneuver for treatment of horizontal-canal benign positional vertigo. *Laryngoscope, 106,* 476–478.
74. Herdman, S. J., Tusa, R. J., Blatt, P., Suzuki, A., Venuto, P. J., & Roberts, D. (1998). Computerized dynamic visual acuity test in the assessment of vestibular deficits. *American Journal of Otology, 19*(6), 790–796.
75. Murphy, T. P. (1994). Vestibular autorotation and electronystagmography testing in patients with dizziness. *American Journal of Otology, 15,* 502–505.
76. Smith, P. F. (2000). Pharmacology of the vestibular system. *Current Opinion in Neurology, 13,* 31–37.
77. Yates, B., Miller, A. D., & Lucot, J. B. (1998). Physiological basis and pharmacology of motion sickness: an update. *Brain Research Bulletin, 47,* 395–406.
78. Leigh, R. J., & Ramat, S. (1999). Neuropharmacologic aspects of the ocular system and the treatment of abnormal eye movements. *Current Opinion in Neurology, 12,* 21–27.
79. Sulaiman, M. R., Niklasson, M., Tham, R., & Dutia, M. B. (1999). Modulation of vestibular function by nociceptin orphanin FQ: an in vivo and in vitro study. *Brain Research, 828*(1–2), 74–82.
80. Takeda, N., & Matsunaga, T. (1996). Neurochemical basis of motion sickness and its treatment and prevention. In R.W. Baloh, & G.M. Halmagyi (Eds.), *Disorders of the vestibular system* (pp. 529–537). New York: Oxford University Press.
81. Bronstein, A. M., & Hood, J. D. (1986). The cervico-ocular reflex in normal subjects and patients with absent vestibular function. *Brain Research, 373,* 399–408.
82. Paige, G. D. (1992). Senescence of human visual–0vestibular interactions. *Journal of Vestibular Research, 2*(2), 133–151.
83. Oman, C. M. (1990). Motion sickness: a synthesis and evaluation of the sensory conflict theory. *Canadian Journal of Physiology and Pharmacology, 68,* 294–303.
84. Hain, T. C., & Yacovino, D. (2005). Pharmacologic treatment of persons with dizziness. *Neurologic Clinics, 23,* 831–853.
85. Hain, T. C., & Uddin, M. (2003). Pharmacological treatment of vertigo. *CNS Drugs, 17,* 85–100.
86. Darlington, C. L., & Smith, P. F. (1996). What neurotransmitters are important in the vestibular system? In R.W. Baloh, & G.M. Halmagyi (Eds.), *Disorders of the vestibular system* (pp. 140–144). New York: Oxford University Press.
87. Horak, F. B., Jones-Rycewicz, C., Black, E., & Shumway-Cook, A. (1992). Effects of vestibular rehabilitation on dizziness and imbalance. *Otolaryngology—Head and Neck Surgery, 106,* 175–180.
88. Cawthorne, T. (1944). The physiologic basis for head exercises. *Journal of the Chartered Society of Physiotherapy, 30,* 106–107.
89. Herdman, S. J. (1996). Vestibular rehabilitation. In R.W. Baloh, & G.M. Halmagyi (Eds.), *Disorders of the vestibular system* (pp. 583–598). New York: Oxford University Press.
90. Brown, J. J. (1990). A systematic approach to the dizzy patient. *Diagnostic Neurotology, 8*(2), 209–224.
91. Powell, L. E., & Myers, A. M. (1995). Activities specific confidence (ABC) scale. *Journal of Gerontology, 50A,* M28–M34.
92. Carlow, T. J. (1986). Medical treatment of nystagmus and ocular motor disorders. *International Ophthalmology Clinics, 26,* 251–264.
93. Cesarani, A., Alpini, D., Monti, B., & Raponi, G. (2004). The treatment of acute vertigo. *Neurological Sciences, 25*(Suppl. 1), S26–S30.
94. Fujino, A.,Tokumasu, K., Yosio, S., Naganuma, H., Yoneda, S., & Nakamura, K. (1994). Vestibular training for benign paroxysmal positional vertigo. Its efficacy in comparison with anti-vertigo drugs. *Archives of Otolaryngology—Head and Neck Surgery, 120,* 497–504.

95. Pollack, L., Davies, R. A., & Luxon, L. L. (2002). Effectiveness of the particle repositioning maneuver in benign paroxysmal positional vertigo with and without additional vestibular pathology. *Otology and Neurotology, 23,* 79–83.
96. Semont, A., Freyss, G., & Vitte, E. (1998). Curing the BPPV with a liberatory maneuver. *Advances in Otorhinolaryngology, 42,* 290–293.
97. Epley, J. M. (1992). The canalith repositioning procedure: for treatment of benign paroxysmal positional vertigo. *Otolaryngology—Head and Neck Surgery, 107,* 399–404.
98. Brandt, T., & Daroff, R. B. (1980). Physical therapy for benign paroxysmal positional vertigo. *Archives of Otolaryngology, 106,* 484–485.
99. Cohen, H. S., & Kimball, K. T. (2005). Effectiveness of treatments for benign paroxysmal positional vertigo of the posterior canal. *Otology and Neurotology, 26,* 1034–1040.
100. Steenerson, R. L., & Cronin, G. W. (1996). Comparison of the canalith repositioning procedure and vestibular habituation training in forty patients with benign paroxysmal positional vertigo. *Otolaryngology—Head and Neck Surgery, 114,* 61–64.
101. Soto Varela, A., Bartual Magro, J., Santos Perez, S., Vélez Regueiro, M., Lechuga García, R., Pérez-Carro Ríos, A., & Caballero, L. (2001). Benign paroxysmal vertigo: a comparative prospective study of the efficacy of Brandt and Daroff, Semont and Epley maneuver. *Revue de Laryngologie—Otologie—Rhinologie (Bord), 122,* 179–183.
102. Herdman, S. J., & Tusa, R. J. (1996). Complications of the canalith repositioning procedure. *Archives of Otoloaryngology—Head and Neck Surgery, 122,* 281–286.
103. Appiani, G. C., Catania, G., & Gagliardi, M. A. (2001). Liberatory maneuver for the treatment of horizontal canal paroxysmal positional vertigo. *Otology & Neurotology, 22,* 66–69.
104. Hillier, S. L., & Hollohan, V. (2007). Vestibular rehabilitation for unilateral peripheral vestibular dysfunction. *Cochrane Database of Systematic Reviews 2007.* DOI: 10.1002/14651858.CD005397.pub2.
105. Kammerlind, A. S., Ledin, T. E., Odvist, L. M., & Skargren, E. I. (2005). Effects of home training and additional physical therapy on recovery after acute unilateral vestibular loss—a randomized study. *Clinical Rehabilitation, 19,* 54–62.

10 Evaluation and Treatment of Vision and Motor Dysfunction Following Acquired Brain Injury from Occupational Therapy and Neuro-Optometry Perspectives

Janet M. Powell and Nancy G. Torgerson

CONTENTS

We would like to thank Mary Pepping, Ph.D., ABPP-CN, for her invaluable insights and suggestions in reviewing this chapter.

INTRODUCTION

The fundamental importance of intact visual and visual-motor systems for ease of effective movement and efficient engagement in almost every aspect of daily life cannot be overstated. As one might expect from such a wide-ranging and multi-faceted process, the relationship between vision and motor behavior is complex. The actions that result from gathering and processing visual information are often motoric in nature with vision used for advance planning of motor actions. However, visual information is also used for feedback about and adaptation of motor actions during and after movement. Vision can also be used to compensate for dysfunction in other sensory systems that are impaired as a result of injury or disease. To complicate matters further, visual information often serves as the basis for posture and movement even when the visual information is degraded or inaccurate.

Dysfunction in the visual system has the potential to disrupt motor behavior in the absence of any motor system dysfunction. Furthermore, in persons with motor system dysfunction, visual system dysfunction can disrupt motor behavior over and above any direct consequences of the motor problem alone. At the same time, degraded or inaccurate visual input during gross and fine motor tasks can result in secondary problems such as headache, physical and/or cognitive fatigue, and even decreased cognitive functioning due to the resulting strain on cognitive resources as the person tries to compensate for less than optimal visual information. Problems can occur in the opposite direction as well, with motor dysfunction adversely affecting visual system function.

When one delves into the complexities of visual system dysfunction and its widespread and varied effects on human behaviors, it can feel like a Gordion knot with no clear "first string" to grasp in unraveling the key elements. This chapter is an attempt to unravel some of the important strings relating to the interplay between the visual and motor systems. We will begin by offering a historical perspective of the treatment of visual impairments following acquired brain injury in rehabilitation settings. Next, we will provide an overview of some of the research studies investigating the relationship between vision and motor behavior with a focus on findings that highlight the complex and often surprising nature of this relationship. We will then review the approaches used by occupational therapists (OTs) and neuro-optometrists in assessing and treating vision and motor dysfunction in adults following acquired brain injury as well as vision and motor screening protocols for referral to these disciplines. Finally, we will discuss the advantages we see of interdisciplinary collaboration between these two fields and close with suggestions for future directions.

A HISTORICAL PERSPECTIVE

Given the importance of vision in everyday performance and the potential for visual dysfunction to disrupt multiple systems, it is somewhat surprising, at first glance, to realize how little attention has been paid in typical medical rehabilitation settings to the basic visual function of people with acquired brain injuries. While the field of occupational therapy has had a long-standing interest in developing assessment and treatment approaches for visual perceptual and visually-based cognitive dysfunction, until recently, these treatment approaches have not typically included assessment of underlying visual functions. The few exceptions have been decreased visual fields following optic tract damage and diplopia resulting from cranial nerve palsies. In almost all instances, common rehabilitation practice has been to wait 6 months poststroke or traumatic brain injury (TBI) to address any deficits in visual functioning.

While there have been reports in the literature regarding the potential for vision impairments following acquired brain injury[1-5] and information about the evaluation and treatment of gross visual[6] and specific visual-perceptual deficits,[6-9] it was not until the early 1990s that OTs, and other rehabilitation professionals, began to realize more fully the importance of basic visual skills (e.g., visual acuity and ocular motor control) to everyday function and recovery following acquired brain injury.[10,11] Even then, the primary focus has been on the contribution of vision to cognitive skills such as attention and memory with little consideration paid to the contribution and influence of vision on motor behavior.

Clinical reasoning is dependent on (a) how one conceptualizes the system within which a problem occurs and (b) having the skills and tools to identify the cues that lead one to consider a particular problem.[12] Both of these factors have contributed to the typical treatment of visual dysfunction following brain injury in rehabilitation settings. The development of visual-perceptual and cognitive-perceptual treatment approaches that did not emphasize, or even sometimes include, the role of most basic visual abilities led rehabilitation personnel to view these systems as primarily perceptual and cognitive in nature. Furthermore, for many years, it was assumed that visual problems as a result of brain injury would only result from damage to the occipital lobe and the primary visual cortex and optic tracts. As a result of the perspective created by this limited view of visual systems, clinicians have been less likely to recognize the need to assess vision thoroughly following acquired brain injury. At the same time, without knowledge and training in the assessments needed to uncover the range of visual problems that can occur after acquired brain injury, it is difficult, if not impossible, for clinicians to find the cues leading to a visual-related hypothesis regarding the source of the problem.

The development of rehabilitation practice relating to visual dysfunction has also been influenced by the inclusion of ophthalmologists or neuro-ophthalmologists as the consulting vision provider for most hospital-based rehabilitation teams. As described above, discipline-specific characterizations of a system and typical assessment tools influence the understanding of the problem. The clinical focus of ophthalmology tends to be the integrity of the structures of the eye. As a result, some of the more functional visual problems, for example, sustained acuity over time, may not be recognized by the typical assessments in the field. Furthermore, interventions in ophthalmology tend to be primarily remedial in nature and surgically based. If the problems identified most frequently were visual field loss, where there was not a recognized remedial treatment, and diplopia, where surgery was the primary treatment option, then it makes sense to wait 6 months for an in-depth assessment to see if spontaneous recovery occurs in the meantime. Similarly, an impression that suppression of vision in one eye cannot occur in the adult visual system combined with a lack of assessment tools to identify suppression could lead to a conclusion that the elimination of patient-reported double vision indicates that a diplopia has resolved. More recent interest from rehabilitation clinicians in approaches from the field of behavioral or neuro-optometry has expanded this perspective somewhat. However, system delivery constraints have limited access to these providers in many facilities. In addition, differences in terminology, including different meanings assigned by different disciplines to the same terms, have introduced the possibility for communication barriers and misunderstandings.

Another critical influence on approaches to vision treatment relates to the nature of vision itself. As noted by Suter,[13] vision is primarily a covert process with little awareness and insight into our own visual processes. People probably have the most awareness of problems with visual acuity. Many adults, especially those over the age of 40, have firsthand experience with the impact of blurred vision on performing daily activities. This includes those who have had impaired distance vision since childhood as well as those with the impaired near vision associated with aging. Those without firsthand experience have often observed the consequences of decreased visual acuity in others. As a result, the importance of near visual acuity for motor tasks such as writing and distance visual acuity for tasks such as negotiating obstacles when walking should be fairly obvious. Even so, both authors have experienced situations where the glasses of elderly adults, who have needed corrective lenses for years to see clearly, have been found left behind in the nightstand hours or even days after admission to rehabilitation facilities while participating in evaluations and treatment activities.

At the same time, the importance of vision for many tasks is not obvious. The visual system involves many layers of interacting processes. For example, symptoms such as blurred near vision or double vision can result from different or even multiple causes within the system. At the same time, different vision problems can cause similar problems in functional performance. For example, fatigue with visually demanding near tasks can be due to convergence insufficiency or an accommodative dysfunction. Similarly, difficulty with maintaining an upright posture could be due to binocular dysfunction, visual midline shift, visual field defects, impaired depth perception, and/or problems with interaction between the central and peripheral visual systems. As a result, it can be difficult to identify the exact causes and consequences of visual dysfunction from observing the actions of clients in everyday activities or during paper/pencil tasks, two of the primary ways of obtaining clinical information in rehabilitation settings. To add to the complexity of the situation, many tasks can be done with at least some degree of degraded vision, making it even more difficult to recognize and characterize visual problems from observable motor performance.

It is somewhat easier for us to recognize the potential impact of degraded visual input on cognitive processes such as attention and memory. For example, we are not surprised if someone cannot remember something—a person's face, written information, the way to get somewhere—if they couldn't see it well in the first place. This may be due, in part, to more conscious awareness of these processes as compared to visually-based motor behavior. However, the impact of visual dysfunction on motor performance is also critical to brain injury recovery and better understanding of the relationships between vision and motor, and new approaches to integrating vision and motor assessment and treatment are needed.

RESEARCH OVERVIEW

Neurological Substrates of Visuomotor Behavior

In the past 40 years, there have been substantial gains in our understanding of the anatomical structures and neural processing systems that underlie the interaction of the vision and motor systems. It is useful to consider how this knowledge has been gained over time and how the techniques for gaining knowledge have influenced the types of questions that can be asked and, thereby, influenced the resulting knowledge. For example, more recent techniques such as functional magnetic resonance imagings (fMRIs) have given us some level of direct access to the working brains of normal persons. However, that access has not always been the norm.

Historically, one of the principal sources of knowledge about the organization and function of the brain has been observations of changes in the performance of individuals who have sustained brain damage through disease or injury. Observations of which task or tasks can and cannot be performed by an individual with a particular lesion give insight into the function of that area of the brain. Additional knowledge is gained when a person with a lesion in one part of the brain can do one task, but not another related task, and a second person, with a lesion in a different part of the brain, can do the second task, but not the first. Such double dissociations provide evidence that the neurological underpinnings of the two tasks are separate both anatomically and functionally. A similar approach has been taken with animal models of brain lesions. Animals have also been used for single and multiple neuron recordings to investigate brain functioning at the cellular level.

While this modular approach has given us information about the functioning of discrete brain structures, it has proven more difficult to determine how functional systems of multiple brain structures are organized. Current theories of visual processing suggest that there are multiple parallel pathways for visual processing in the brain with interconnections between and among those pathways at multiple levels. However, this multiplicity view has not always been the case. Up until the late 1960s, it was thought that the brain had one, unified system for vision. The system was thought to work in a hierarchical, stepwise fashion with each area of the brain adding a new layer of processing before information was passed on to the next area. For the past 40 years, there has been general agreement that there are two systems for processing visual information. However, there is still not full consensus on the names and features of the two systems (e.g., focal vs. ambient, cortical vs. midbrain, dorsal vs. ventral) as different possibilities for the anatomical and functional nature of the two systems have been proposed. Some of the suggested visual processing models have included motor function, while others have not.

Trevarthen[14] and colleagues[15] proposed one of the first models for two distinct visual processing systems. These ideas were based on work with monkeys and humans with split-brain lesions. This model consisted of two anatomically and functionally distinct systems: the focal system and the ambient system. The focal system was cortically based with a pathway from the lateral geniculate body of the thalamus to the primary visual (i.e., striate) cortex. The ambient system was based in the midbrain with input from the superior colliculus relayed through the pulvinar nucleus of the thalamus to association cortex. There were also anatomical differences in the input to the two systems. The focal system was described as receiving input primarily from the fovea. On the other hand, the ambient system was thought to receive input from the whole of the retina and, especially, the peripheral fields. The two systems were distinguished functionally by the type of motor action supported by each system. The focal system was thought to provide visual control of fine, precise movements through the ability to distinguish details and recognize objects. The ambient system was characterized as providing support for whole body movements, such as posture and locomotion, through visual information about the movement and position of objects in space and a person's movement through the environment.

The following year, Schneider[16] proposed a model with two visual systems that were anatomically similar to those of Trevarthen. However, the functional distinction between the two systems was different. Rather than being based on motor action as with Trevarthen's model, Schneider's distinction was based on how visual information was used to understand stimuli in the visual field. According to this model, the cortical system was used to identify a stimulus while the midbrain system was used to localize stimuli in visual space. This work laid the foundation for a subsequent distinction in visual processing between the "what" versus the "where" of an object that has remained highly influential for many years.

In 1982, Ungerleider and Mishkin,[17] using evidence primarily gained from brain lesions in monkeys, proposed a visual processing model with a similar functional dichotomy between the "what" and the "where" described by Schnieder. While the purpose of the two visual processing pathways remained the same, that is, to help identify and to locate objects in space, there were major differences in the anatomical location of the pathways. This model distinguished between two cortical visual processing streams, a ventral and a dorsal stream, both beginning in the striate cortex. From there, the ventral stream projects to the inferior temporal cortex while the dorsal stream projects to the posterior parietal cortex. They characterized the ventral stream as processing information regarding object qualities (the "what") and the dorsal stream as processing information regarding object location in space (the "where").

A few years later, Livingstone and Hubel[18,19] proposed an extension of the anatomical division of visual processing into a ventral "what" and a dorsal "where" system. In their model, the distinction between the two processing systems begins in the cells, which comprise the different layers of the dorsal lateral geniculate nucleus in the thalamus. They described the parvo system of cells (i.e., the parvocellular layers of the lateral geniculate nucleus) as providing visual information to the ventral stream for object identification. At the same time, the magno system of cells (i.e., the magnocellular layers) provides information to the dorsal stream for localization of objects in space.

In 1992, Goodale and Milner[20] presented a different explanation of the function of the ventral and dorsal streams. Rather than a distinction between the "what" and "where" functions in visual processing, they proposed a distinction between vision for perception and vision for action. In this model, the ventral stream is used for recognizing and identifying objects, persons, and events as needed for cognitive processes such as memory and decision making. This type of processing is done in allocentric space, meaning that objects are identified in relation to each other rather than to the individual viewing them. This processing for object identification purposes is not as dependent on precise details of object properties such as shape and size. In contrast, the dorsal stream is used for online visual control of motor action, that is, to guide movements. Processing in this stream is done in egocentric space (i.e., the objects in relation to the viewer), with many object details critical to accurate, efficient movements.

The initial evidence for this model came from Goodale and Milner's observations of DF, a woman with brain damage in the area of the ventral stream. DF could not recognize many objects or describe many object properties. However, she could use visual information to guide her movements in relation to those same objects. For example, while DF could not judge lines as being horizontal or vertical (or even match line orientation by holding up a card), she could quickly and accurately reach out with a card held in her hand, orient the card to a slot that was turned in different directions, and insert it into the slot. Those observations were in contrast to reports of individuals with brain lesions in the dorsal stream area who had the opposite problem (i.e., a double dissociation). These individuals could typically recognize, name, and point to objects, but had difficulty reaching and grasping effectively for those same objects.

Goodale and Milner concluded that the brain mechanisms underlying the more conscious perception of object qualities through vision were different from the less conscious mechanisms that underlie visually guided movement to objects. In their model, both the ventral and dorsal pathways carry spatial information, but it is used for different purposes. The spatial information needed to determine relationships between objects is different from that needed to guide eye, head, or limb movements toward objects. As a result, the precision of the spatial information in the two streams varies. For example, object orientation, motion, and location change need to be computed from the perspective of the individual every time action with the eyes, head, limbs, and/or body is taken. However, visual details such as color are typically not as important for movement.

Additional evidence for this model has come from primate studies that found neurons in the posterior parietal regions that are active only when there is visual stimulation along with motor action.[21] Evidence has also come from human behavioral studies. One line of research in this area uses visual illusions to compare perceptual judgments, such as size, with motor actions, such as reaching and/or grasping. Findings of increased difficulty with perceptual judgments with no effect on movement time for reaching or on size of grasp or a smaller effect on these motor actions than on the accuracy of perceptual judgment has been interpreted as support for a distinction between perception and action processing.[22]

Goodale and Milner point out the pitfalls of assuming that our introspective view of the visual experience is complete and true.[21,23] From their perspective, our conscious understanding of the visual system, which is based on ventral stream processing, makes it more difficult to determine how to study the role of the dorsal stream. They note that vision research has tended to focus on vision for conscious decision making and typically has not taken into account differences in the type of motor action that was required (or even possible, e.g., in studies where animals are anesthetized). Goodale and Milner argue that it is easier to think about what is under our conscious control (at least to some extent) and, because it is easier to think about, it is easier to think how best to study it.

At this time, there is general agreement that there are two anatomically distinct systems for processing visual information. However, the functional distinction between the two systems, that is, the precise nature of the information processed, is not completely understood and controversies remain.[24] Among the unresolved questions is the "binding problem" (i.e., how and where in the brain the information from the two streams is combined). Further research is needed before more definitive conclusions can be drawn.

VISION FOR ADVANCE PLANNING OF MOTOR ACTIONS

Another question of interest is how vision is used for advance planning of motor actions. In this section, we will review several studies relating to how vision is used in locomotion, making passability judgments, and in everyday tasks such as cooking.

Vision and Locomotion

The difficulties experienced in walking by those with vision impairments give us some insight about the importance of vision in planning motor actions relating to locomotion. While there is a great deal of individual variation, persons with moderate vision impairments tend to walk more slowly, bump into obstacles more often, stumble more frequently, and are more likely to fall, with some especially affected by lower light levels.[25–27] Studies of the relationship between visual abilities and fracture or risk of fall in older adults further highlight the importance of visual abilities in maintaining dynamic balance. One of the first reports in this area was based on over 2,500 older adults in the Framingham aging study.[28] This study investigated the incidence of hip fracture during the 10 years following the initial Framingham Eye Study exam. After adjustments for age, sex, weight, estrogen use (in women), and alcohol consumption, the participants with poor vision (i.e., 20/100 or worse) in at least one eye had over two times the risk of hip fracture as those with good vision (20/25 or better) in both eyes. Somewhat more surprising was the way an imbalance in visual acuity contributed to hip fracture risk. For example, those participants with moderately impaired visual acuity (i.e., 20/30–2/80) in one eye and good visual acuity in the other eye had a higher risk of fracture than those with moderately impaired vision in both eyes. Loss of vision in one eye increased the risk of hip fracture even if vision in the other eye was not impaired. On the basis of these findings, the researchers concluded that good stereoscopic vision that provides depth perception cues from the slightly disparate retinal images from the two eyes is important in preventing falls.

Some of the subsequent studies examining the relationship between visual impairments and falls have found poor binocular visual acuity to play less of a role than in the Framingham study. However, the role of reduced contrast sensitivity and the ability to judge distances accurately and perceive spatial relationships has been confirmed in multiple studies (see Lord[29] for review). Reduced visual fields have also been shown to be a key factor in falls in the elderly.[30]

Another question of interest is how visual information is used to walk safely and efficiently through an environment to a destination. Consider walking across a crowded central plaza where there are multiple crossing routes as people walk in different directions toward multiple destinations (e.g., the doorway to a specific building). Bumping into another person, even in a crowded setting, is an unusual event rather than the norm. This is a result of everyone effectively changing their speed and direction to negotiate the anticipated paths of the other people as they all move through space in slightly different directions.

The most obvious contribution of vision in this situation is the conscious location of the target destination with our central vision to establish our general route. However, less conscious peripheral vision is critical for moving through the environment without bumping into others. While the impact of the loss of central vision in conditions such as macular degeneration to everyday function is familiar to many in the general population, it is typically more difficult to compensate for the loss of peripheral vision. With peripheral visual field losses, it can be difficult to consciously decide where to look to get information that is typically provided outside of conscious awareness.

The importance of peripheral vision in goal-directed locomotion has been demonstrated in a study comparing gaze fixations during goal-directed walking for persons with normal vision and those with decreased peripheral vision as a result of retinitis pigmentosa.[31] The study task involved walking 6.4 m down an unfamiliar, obstacle-free, straight hallway with posters on the walls. Participants were instructed to walk down the hall and turn and go through the first door on the left. To record the eye and the scene simultaneously, participants viewed the environment through a virtual display from a head-mounted system. Eye fixations were classified into one of the following five categories: (a) on the goal (i.e., the target door or molding around the door); (b) on the layout (i.e., the boundaries between the floor or ceiling); (c) ahead (i.e., the wall or door at the end of the hall); (d) on objects (i.e., posters on the walls); and (e) down (i.e., at the floor).

On average, the gaze of the participants with decreased peripheral vision covered an area that was three times larger than that of the participants with normal vision. In addition, the two groups directed their gaze at different features in the environment. The participants with normal vision tended to look directly ahead or at the goal while walking. In contrast, the persons with impaired peripheral vision looked more frequently down at the floor, at the boundary between the wall and the floor, and at the posters on the wall (apparently in an effort to distinguish between the posters and the target doorway). This study demonstrates the amount and type of information gained by those with normal vision through peripheral vision without the need for direct gaze fixations. It appears that the people with normal vision were able to obtain the information needed to know where they were in space through their peripheral vision without having to look directly at their surroundings while those with impaired peripheral vision were working much harder to see and navigate. Interestingly, the one participant with normal vision who was familiar with the testing environment looked most often at the posters on the wall. Perhaps adequate information about the target from previous experience allowed for the possibility of looking for information that was not essential for achieving the goal.

Vision and Passability Judgments

Passability judgments provide another example of how we do not realize how we use vision for motor actions in everyday life. Most people take for granted the ability to pass through openings of various sizes without bumping into the sides or getting stuck part way through. It is only under relatively unusual circumstances, such as the rapidly expanding abdomen of late pregnancy, that we experience difficulty with such passability judgments. Similarly, we take for granted the ability to take steps of the appropriate height and length for stairs of varying sizes and to step successfully over objects of varying sizes.

One study identified a critical point that people use to distinguish passable openings from impassable ones.[32] Participants were instructed to walk through an opening turning their shoulders if they wished. The opening width was systematically increased or decreased without participant knowledge. Trials were run under normal and fast walking speed conditions. In both speed conditions, participants rotated their shoulders before entering the opening when the opening was approximately 1.3 times shoulder width. This ratio did not change as a function of body size.

However, when asked to estimate the maximum width of an impassable opening, participants predicted that they could not pass though openings smaller than 1.1 times shoulder width without shoulder rotation. The researchers speculated that the difference in this judgment from the actual width at which participants turned their shoulders when walking through the opening may have been because they were asked whether they *could* pass through the opening without shoulder rotation, not how they *would* do it. The greater width when moving certainly makes sense from an ecological standpoint as we would want to err on the side of caution to avoid collision or injury. We would also speculate that these results reflect the possibility of a difference between the perceptual-only judgment and the judgment made while moving in line with Goodale and Milner's model of the function of the dorsal and ventral processing streams.

Saccadic Eye Movements and Motor Actions in Everyday Tasks

Our ability to perceive visual images is dependent on eye movements that result in almost continual shifting of the visual image. These eye movements include the larger, rapid, jumping saccadic movements that serve to bring objects of interest onto the fovea and the minute drifting movements the eyes make during fixation. Indeed, in studies where the visual image is artificially stabilized on the retina, either by paralyzing the extraocular muscles or by using techniques where a scene is moved in synchrony with eye movements (e.g., with a scene projected on a mirror attached to the eye with a contact lens), the image disappears within a few seconds.[33]

Over 40 years ago, Yarbus[34] (first published in the Russian journal *Biofizika* in 1961) demonstrated that saccadic eye movements and fixations are used selectively to examine features of particular interest in a visual scene. He used suction devices on the eyes with small mirrors attached to show how the eyes move when inspecting a static image (e.g., a side view of a bust of the Egyptian queen Nefertiti). By recording the position of the reflected beam, Yarbus determined that the eyes spent much more time shifting toward and then looking intently at the eye, nose, mouth, and ear as compared to the cheek or neck. These results were the first to indicate that vision is an active, top-down process with the choice of focus based on the parts of an image that convey the most important information to the viewer.

In another classic study, Yarbus[34] monitored eye movements as subjects viewed a painting of a visitor coming into a room where people have been sitting at a table ("The Unexpected Visitor" by I. E. Repin). Before looking at the painting, subjects were instructed to do one of the following: (a) examine the picture without specific instructions; (b) estimate the material circumstances of the family in the picture; (c) give the ages of the people; (d) figure out what the family had been doing before the arrival of the visitor; (e) remember the clothing of the people in painting; (f) remember the position of the people and the objects; or (g) estimate how long the visitor had been away. Yarbus found that the eye movement patterns were highly dependent on the task. For example, when asked to estimate the ages of the people, eye movements were concentrated on the faces of the people in the painting. In contrast, when asked to estimate the material circumstances of the family, eye movements were concentrated on the furniture and objects in the room and on the walls, with some time spent on the clothing worn by the family.

The availability of head-mounted eye trackers in the 1980s made it possible to extend the study of eye movements from static images in the laboratory to active tasks performed in everyday life. Studies have investigated the relationship of eye movements and motor actions in such diverse tasks as making tea,[35] making sandwiches,[36] washing hands,[37] driving a car,[38] and crossing intersections.[39]

In a recent review of such studies, Land[40] concluded that saccadic eye movements guide active task performance in a proactive manner just as with static images. While there is some flexibility, different individuals use remarkably similar patterns of eye movements in completing everyday tasks. The eyes rarely look toward objects that are irrelevant to the motor action, even when the irrelevant objects are visually conspicuous. Rather, the gaze is typically directed toward objects that are relevant to the task at hand with the gaze shifted to each task object just before movement toward the object begins. The eyes often move on to the next task object before manipulation of the previous object is complete. Land concluded that this might indicate the existence of an information buffer for brief storage of task-related visual information. There are also occasional "look-ahead" fixations on task objects that appear to be used to determine object location for future use. During these dynamic tasks, the coordinated movement of the eyes, head, and trunk results in both movement flexibility and gaze stability.

Other studies have investigated the role of eye movements in learning motor tasks, including golf putting[41] and computer cursor control.[42] According to Land,[40] it appears that the eyes are used to provide feedback on motor performance while new tasks are being learned. However, after the learning phase, the eyes are used in a look-ahead manner as described above.

VISION FOR FEEDBACK AND ADAPTATION OF MOTOR ACTIONS

While vision is used for advance planning of motor actions, it is also used for ongoing feedback and adaptation of motor actions. In this section, we will highlight studies relating to these aspects of vision in two different situations: reaching toward stationary targets and intercepting moving targets.

Vision for Reaching toward Stationary Targets

Two of the earliest questions of interest to vision researchers were (a) Which parts of movements are under visual guidance? and (b) What is the speed at which visual processing can be used for online feedback and correction? Indeed, the initial work in studies of moving the hand to grasp a stationary target was done more than a century ago. In 1899, Woodworth[43] proposed that two distinct phases are involved in aiming movements of the arm and hand. The first phase of manual aiming consists of an initial impulse resulting in movement toward the target. Once movement is underway, feedback from the visual system is used to home in on the target. In this second phase, fine movements are made, as needed, to correct the aim and precisely reach the target.

Visually-based adjustments in the second phase can only be effective if there is sufficient time to process the error from the visual feedback, generate a signal to alter the movement, and complete the movement to the target. Numerous studies have investigated how much time is required for this online adjustment to occur. As noted by Schmidt and Lee,[44] the time needed appears to be dependent on the nature of the task, the predictability of the visual information, and the type of visual information available for feedback. For example, there are differences in speed if the movement is adjusted in response to changes in target position or to changes in target size. In general, however, the times are much faster than originally thought, with the fastest times in the 135–150 msec range (i.e., between 1/10 and 2/10 of a second).[44]

Vision for Intercepting Moving Targets

In contrast to reaching toward a stationary target from a stationary position, much of the visual information needed for motor action in everyday life is more dynamic in nature. In these situations, the nature and rate of the visual stimuli change as we move through the world. There is often simultaneous processing of multiple types and rates of information. Much of the research on the role of visual information in interacting with moving targets has focused on catching or striking a ball. In these situations, often called interceptive actions, two main types of information are needed. A person needs to know *when* the object will arrive, that is, a temporal prediction. One also needs to know *where* the object will be when it arrives, that is, a spatial prediction.

Many of the models for visually guided action are based on two primary assumptions: (a) error-nulling and (b) single-optical invariance.[45] According to the first assumption, the difference between the current state and where the person should strive to be at each moment in time (i.e., the ideal state) results in an error that must be corrected or nulled for a successful outcome. According to the second assumption, a single-optical variable (i.e., an optical invariant) can be used to guide action across a variety of conditions by giving the person information about the current state. One example is the optical variable *tau* defined by Lee[46] as the inverse of the relative rate of optical expansion on the retina of an approaching object. This optical invariant specifies the time-to-contact as the object size changes.

There is an extensive literature of studies based on these two assumptions. However, there is not complete agreement with other frameworks proposed that focus more on the role of knowledge (both of person and object qualities) and perceptual learning in visually guided actions.[45] At the same time, others have argued that the use of vision in real skill situations may differ from that found in more constrained laboratory tasks. In general, however, it seems clear that the time required to use and act on visual information changes in response to changes in the characteristics of the target and the goals of the movement as well as person characteristics such as age.

VISION AND OTHER SENSORY SYSTEMS

Vision is only one of the body's sensory systems. This section reviews studies that highlight the interaction of vision with the other sensory systems that contribute to balance as well as evidence of the predominance of visual input over that of other sensory systems.

Vision and Static Balance

The role of vision in postural control was first described by Romberg and other early nineteenth-century physicians, who noted a dramatic loss of balance in the dark or with the eyes closed for patients with severely impaired proprioception in the lower limbs.[47] Since that time, the effect of vision on postural control in quiet stance has been quantified in various ways, including changes in the center of pressure on the feet[48,49] and changes in the angular velocity of the body in space.[50]

Methods to investigate the contribution of various sensory and motor factors to the maintenance of static upright posture have also been developed (for further description, see Shumway-Cook and Woollacott).[51] One study of older adults[52] compared performance on sensory and motor measures with postural sway under four conditions: (a) standing on a firm surface with eyes open; (b) standing on a firm surface with eyes closed; (c) standing on foam rubber with eyes open; and (d) standing on foam rubber with eyes closed. They assessed two visual measures: visual acuity and contrast sensitivity. Poor visual acuity and contrast sensitivity were not associated with increased sway on the normal, firm surface. A different pattern was found, however, for standing with eyes open on the foam rubber. In this condition, the foam served to dampen proprioceptive and cutaneous inputs from the ankles and feet forcing participants to rely more on visual and vestibular cues. This simulates clinical conditions, such as diabetic neuropathy, that result in impairments in the proprioceptive and somatosensory input from the lower extremities. Under these circumstances, both reduced visual acuity and reduced contrast sensitivity (along with reduced vibration sense and decreased ankle dorsiflexion strength) were associated with more body sway.

Lord and Menz[53] investigated the relationship of a more comprehensive set of visual abilities to postural stability under similar conditions. In addition to visual acuity and contrast sensitivity, they looked at measures of depth perception using a Howard-Dohlman depth perception apparatus, stereopsis (i.e., the sensation of depth from the slight differences in the retinal image from the two eyes) using the Frisby stereotest, and visual fields. In this study, all of the visual measures (along with quadriceps strength and reaction time) were associated with increased sway in the foam condition. The most critical visual measures were contrast sensitivity and stereopsis. Lord and Menz noted that, while contrast sensitivity had been associated with decreased postural stability in previous studies, the importance of stereopsis had not previously been identified.

While the importance of vision in both dynamic and static balance is fairly clear, the exact nature and scope of vision's role are not so evident. A series of studies by Lee and colleagues in the 1970s led to some unexpected findings that gave further insight into our understanding of the relationship between vision and other sensory systems used in balance.[54,55] These studies used a specially designed room where the walls could be moved backward and forward without the floor moving. Participants, who were unaware that the walls could be moved, stood in the room looking forward.

Movements of the walls as small as 6 mm, resulted in marked postural sway in adults and more severe loss of balance in young children. Individuals interpreted the visual information as a loss of balance even though inputs from the vestibular and proprioceptive systems, the other sensory systems involved in balance, were in keeping with continued upright stance. Furthermore, the direction of the sway or fall was related to the direction of the moving walls. When the walls were moved backward, toward the standing person, adult participants swayed and child participants leaned or fell backward. When the walls were moved forward, away from the person, adult participants swayed and child participants leaned and stumbled or fell forward.

This unexpected reaction can be explained by normal responses to changes in optical flow. Optical flow refers to changes in the pattern of light rays entering the eye (i.e., the optical array) when the eye is moved from one location to another. Optical flow allows us to determine where our eyes, head, and body are in space and to distinguish between different types of movement within the body and the environment. As a result, we can determine if we are moving or not moving with respect to an object. If we are moving, optical flow allows us to determine if the movement is toward or away from the object and if the movement is toward the object's center or off to one side or the other (and how much to one side). Optical flow also contributes to our ability to determine if one object is further away than another.[44]

When the walls of the room were moved, the visual input from the optical flow was similar to the input if a person were, indeed, losing their balance in the opposite direction. Thus, the visual input from the wall moving back toward the person was interpreted as a loss of balance forward, and the person swayed backward to compensate. Similar postural adjustments (in the opposite direction) were made to optical array changes in the opposite direction. A subsequent study by Nashner and Berthoz[56] demonstrated that the visual information was processed quickly with changes in the electromyograms of the postural muscles seen within 100 msec (i.e., 1/10 of a second) of the change in the optical flow.

Predominance of Vision over Other Sensory Systems

Of particular interest in the study described above is the finding that the visual information was interpreted as loss of balance even though it was in conflict with input from the vestibular and proprioceptive/kinesthetic systems. The moving visual field resulted in a sense of self-motion that resulted in compensatory postural adjustments that were appropriate for the visual input, but inappropriate for input from the other sensory systems. These findings can be seen as evidence for the predominance of vision over the other sensory systems relating to balance (and perhaps to movement). This predominance may be due to two distinct advantages of the visual system in comparison to the other sensory systems. First of all, visual information is richly detailed and, second, vision gives advance information about what motor acts are needed. Vision is not only critical in situations where other sensory systems are not available. If visual information is not in keeping with input from other sensory systems even when the visual input is degraded or incorrect, the visual input takes precedence.

Yoked prisms can provide a dramatic illustration of how vision can take precedence over other body systems. Prisms are transparent optical devises that refract light. With yoked prisms, the prism is set so that the light going into each eye is bent in the same way. In this demonstration, a person is asked to feel the straight edge where two walls meet. They are instructed to look directly at their hand and feel if the edge of the wall is straight. When they do this, the edge looks, as well as feels, straight as would be expected. The person then puts on base right or base left yoked prisms (i.e., prisms that either bend the light to the right or to the left). The person is asked to look at the edge again and tell what it looks like now. The person reports that it looks bowed or curved. Then the person is asked to feel and look at the wall edge and hand simultaneously. The person is typically amazed to find that the edge also *feels* as if it were curved or bowed. They know intellectually that it is straight, but their eyes tell them it is curved and their touch agrees. The visual input (even when incorrect) can override tactile, proprioceptive, kinesthetic, and cognitive information.

This overview of research studies, while necessarily limited both in breadth and depth, highlights the importance of vision in motor actions as well as the complexity and frequently unconscious nature of that relationship. Owing to space limitations, we have focused on the role of vision in motor actions. However, we would like to point out that the role of motor actions in the use of vision, as well as the impact of impaired motor function on visual function, is as critical to the understanding of the interaction between the two systems and should not be overlooked.

OCCUPATIONAL AND OPTOMETRIC APPROACHES TO VISION AND MOTOR DYSFUNCTION

The following sections provide an overview of occupational therapy and optometric approaches to the treatment of vision and motor dysfunction following brain injury in adults with additional specifics of optometric evaluation and treatment. Advantages of collaboration between the two disciplines and strategies for effective collaboration will also be discussed. The reader should note that while occupational therapy is the focus of this chapter, physical therapists also play a key role in the rehabilitation of motor dysfunction following brain injury.

OCCUPATIONAL THERAPY APPROACHES

The overall purpose of occupational therapy interventions is to improve the ability of individuals to accomplish the everyday tasks (i.e., "occupations") they need and/ or want to do. Participation in meaningful occupations is seen as critical for physical and emotional well-being. For many years, OTs have worked from practice models that include three principal components: the person, the environment, and the task. While there are variations within these models, the person component typically includes the physical/sensorimotor, cognitive, and psychological/emotional abilities that are within the person. The environment component typically includes the physical environment, the social environment, and the socio/cultural environment. The task component is often divided into three main categories (again, with variations depending on the model): (a) activities of daily living (ADLs), both personal or basic self-care ADLs (i.e., PADLs or BADLs), and instrumental ADLs (IADLs) relating to household management tasks; (b) work (and school or other productive activity); and (c) play and leisure. Because OTs treat so many different types of problems, they often begin the evaluation process by identifying the domain(s) of the problem (i.e., physical/sensorimotor, cognitive, and/or psychological/emotional) and then selecting the appropriate treatment approach(es) to address that particular type of problem.

Remedial and Compensatory Approaches

In general, as with other rehabilitative disciplines, there are two main treatment approaches in occupational therapy: remediation (i.e., restoration) and compensation (i.e., adaptation). The goal of remediation is to improve (i.e., restore) an underlying impairment to allow for performance of the tasks a person needs and/or wants to do. OTs use remediation-focused treatment approaches when there is potential for the underlying impairment to change and there is sufficient time for that change to occur within the constraints of the service delivery situation. The goal of compensation, on the other hand, is to make up for the underlying deficit, that is, bridge the gap between the impaired abilities and the desired task. Compensation is used in several different situations: (a) while working on remediation; (b) while a short-term problem is expected to resolve on its own without direct remediation; (c) when a long-term problem is not amenable to remediation; (d) when the potential for remediation is met, but there are persisting underlying impairments limiting function; and (e) when the client does not have the time, resources, and/or desire to work on remediation. Compensatory approaches include substituting a task that can be accomplished more easily with the current limitations, changing the method of doing a task, using an adaptive/assistive device, changing the physical environment more permanently, and/or using social supports (i.e., assistance from others).

Bottom-Up and Top-Down Perspectives

Evaluation and treatment in occupational therapy can be performed from either a bottom-up or a top-down perspective. A bottom-up approach focuses on underlying impairments (e.g., spasticity, weakness, or decreased joint range of motion in the physical domain). Assessments of impairments lead to targeted interventions to remediate and/or compensate for specific deficits with the ultimate aim of improving performance of functional skills. For example, in remedial treatment for the motor impairment of decreased arm strength, a therapist using a bottom-up approach would use a progression of exercises or purposeful activities designed to improve the client's strength. In a pure bottom-up approach, the therapist extrapolates how the underlying deficits relate to everyday function and assumes that generalization will occur. However, the limitations of a pure bottom-up approach have become more evident, and a bottom-up approach in OT today typically includes engaging in and practicing functional activities to promote generalization.

On the other hand, a top-down approach focuses evaluation and treatment on the everyday tasks that an individual wants and/or needs to do in fulfilling their life roles. In a top-down approach, an OT assesses overall performance using techniques such as observation of functional tasks (e.g., dressing or cooking). Within the context of the task performance, the therapist assesses observable skills such as reaching or lifting and may hypothesize what the underlying deficits (such as decreased range of motion or strength) might be. Remedial treatment in a pure top-down approach typically provides graded practice with a meaningful, everyday activity (often the task that is impacted by the dysfunction) that requires the skills that need remediation, often in as naturalistic a setting as possible. A top-down approach gives an opportunity to see the interaction of various underlying components and the ability of the person to compensate in everyday life. The rationale for top-down approaches includes research showing that use of real objects and goal-related activities can impact movement patterns.[57] An OT may use a bottom-up or a top-down approach for the entire process of evaluation and treatment. In other situations, an OT may evaluate using a top-down approach and treat bottom-up or vice versa.

As noted by Kielhofner,[58] bottom-up approaches reflect a mechanistic paradigm that stems from the reductionist approach in medicine in the 1950s. From this perspective, function and dysfunction were characterized in terms of the underlying neurological and anatomical mechanisms with an emphasis on the part rather than the whole. These deficit-specific approaches were useful for clear identification and treatment of a specific problem, but did not facilitate understanding of how different problems might be interrelated. The more recent top-down approaches, which interestingly reflect the original perspectives of the OT field from the early 1900s, focus on systems that support function in occupation, that is, everyday activity. The focus of these approaches includes the interaction of impairments with conditions in the environment and the life of the individual person.

Bottom-Up Approaches to Motor Dysfunction

Typical bottom-up OT remediation approaches for motor impairments include sensorimotor and biomechanical approaches. Sensorimotor approaches were developed to treat abnormal muscle tone and abnormal movement patterns that occur following conditions such as cerebrovascular accident (i.e., stroke) or cerebral palsy that damage upper motor neurons in the brain. The key approaches of this type include the neurodevelopmental treatment (NDT) approach developed by Bobath[59,60]; proprioceptive neuromuscular facilitation (PNF) developed by Kabat, Knott, and Voss[61–63]; and approaches developed by Rood,[64–67] and Brunnstrom.[68] All of these approaches were developed by therapists (and physicians in some instances) in the 1950s and 1960s as a result of their clinical experiences along with the understanding of the workings of the nervous system at that time.

While all of these approaches were developed to treat similar impairments, there are some key differences. The NDT approach includes the modification of abnormal tone and inefficient postures and movement synergies in conjunction with therapeutic handling techniques to promote more normal movement patterns and functional abilities. As the client regains active control of movement, input from the therapist is reduced. The NDT approach was one of the first motor approaches to emphasize the importance of proximal control of trunk and pelvis in providing a stable base for movement of the upper and lower extremities. The PNF approach focuses on the facilitation of diagonal movement patterns, often in response to manual resistance to the desired movement by the therapist. The approach by Rood uses specific tactile, thermal, and proprioceptive stimuli to muscles and joints to modify abnormal tone. For example, techniques to inhibit abnormal tone include slow rocking and stroking, neutral warmth, light joint compression, and prolonged muscle stretch. Techniques to facilitate muscle activation include light touch or fast brushing of the skin, icing, and vibration. These techniques are used in conjunction with typical developmental motor sequences, for example, maintaining a position that requires proximal stabilization (such as prone on elbows), while engaging in distal movement of the limb(s). The Brunnstrom approach is based on working through a progression of movement patterns thought to be obligatory following central nervous system damage, from more abnormal reflexive patterns to more normal volitional movement. In this approach, abnormal movement patterns are sometimes used to facilitate active movement, especially in the early stages.

These sensorimotor approaches continue to evolve.[69,70] For example, the NDT approach now often incorporates increased practice with functional activities to improve performance and generalization. While Brunnstrom's treatment techniques are less widely used today, the Fugl-Meyer Assessment,[71] which evaluates the client's ability to move within and outside of abnormal movement synergy patterns and is based on Brunnstrom's approach to patient assessment, is frequently used as an outcome measure in research studies of motor recovery following stroke.[72] While these treatment approaches have been criticized by some for outdated theoretical explanations, others have provided explanations for how they can be understood and applied in light of more recent knowledge such as motor control theory.[69,70,73]

Biomechanical approaches focus on muscle strength, joint range, and endurance—the biomechanical capacities underlying movement. Treatment includes various techniques for progressive strengthening for muscle weakness and stretching for limitations in joint range. Electrical stimulation may be used to elicit active muscle contraction. Other physical agent modalities include thermal techniques such as heat and cold. While biomechanical techniques were not originally developed for use in clients with abnormal muscle tone, more recently, there has been increased awareness of the need for remediation of secondary weakness due to disuse of muscles in the presence of spasticity in opposing muscle groups. Biomechanical approaches can be used in conjunction with sensorimotor approaches to prepare the body for movement (e.g., soft tissue mobilization to give sufficient length in the muscles and connective tissue) or to treat secondary complications such as joint contractures. Biomechanical approaches are also used following acquired brain injury to treat co-occurring orthopedic injuries such as fractures.

Sensorimotor and biomechanical approaches are also used in addressing dysfunction in fine motor capacities. For example, a sensorimotor approach may include techniques to manage the abnormal tone in the wrist and fingers while improving grasp and release patterns. A biomechanical approach may include graded strengthening exercises for the hand to improve grasp and pinch strength. As grasp and release alone are not sufficient for functional use of the hand, OTs also use graded exercises and activities to improve in-hand manipulation—the ability to move objects within the hand to position them for use.

Top-Down Approaches to Motor Dysfunction

In contrast to the more bottom-up sensorimotor and biomechanical approaches, there are also top-down approaches used to improve motor function following acquired brain injury. These task-oriented approaches emphasize relearning motor skills through graded practice doing everyday activities.[73,74]

Constraint-induced movement therapy (CIMT) is another relatively new approach to upper limb motor recovery following stroke that emphasizes intense, repetitive practice with the involved limb. The original version of CIMT would be considered a top-down approach. It involved "forced use" of the involved upper limb in everyday activities by placing the nonaffected arm in a sling (or the hand in a mitten) for most waking hours for up to 2 weeks.[75] In addition to the use of the restraint of the nonaffected upper limb, the approach currently includes two additional elements: (a) intensive (e.g., several hours per day for 10–15 consecutive weekdays) arm movement training through clinician-structured and supervised graded task-oriented practice and (b) application of a set of behavioral strategies designed to promote transfer of gains made in the research or clinical setting to the patient's real-world environment[76,77] up to 6 hours a day for 2 weeks (e.g., Wolf et al.)[78] or less intensely over several weeks (e.g., Page et al.).[79] This approach could be considered a combination of top-down and bottom-up treatment. The "forced use" and CIMT approaches were developed from research in animal models followed by investigation of the application to humans. The research studies that provide evidence for the effectiveness of this approach have focused on individuals with chronic stroke (eligibility criteria range from 3 months to greater than 1 year post-stroke) with mild to moderate stroke and relatively good motor recovery (see Sirtori et al. for review[80]). Other approaches currently under investigation that emphasize training with high levels of repetitive movement include robotic systems such as the MIT-MANUS.[72]

Approaches to the Treatment of Vision Impairments in Occupational Therapy

At the present time, there is no clear consensus among occupational therapy clinicians on the role OTs should play in the evaluation and treatment of vision impairments following acquired brain injury. Current practice varies widely and includes OTs who do not evaluate and treat basic visual functions, those who focus on providing compensatory strategies for vision impairments, those who screen for vision impairments and refer to vision providers for further evaluation and treatment planning (with treatment provided in various degrees of collaboration between the OTs and the vision provider), and those who evaluate and treat vision impairments independently.

While OTs have assessed and treated visual-perceptual dysfunction for many years, until more recently the assessment and treatment of foundational visual abilities has not typically been covered in depth in entry-level occupational therapy curriculums. Therapists interested in gaining expertise in this area relied primarily on continuing education courses. While courses for practicing clinicians continue to be an important avenue for information, the current editions of the two most widely used textbooks for entry-level occupational therapy courses focusing on adult physical disability practice include specific assessment and treatment strategies for brain injury–related foundational vision impairments,[81,82] in addition to information related to low vision concerns. Similar information is covered in books focusing on visual and/or visual-perceptual impairments.[83–85] At the same time, most sources note the importance of collaboration between OTs and optometrists or ophthalmologists in assessing foundational visual impairments and the need for supervision in providing vision rehabilitation therapy.

Treatment approaches to basic visual dysfunction covered in these texts include remedial strategies such as eye exercises for muscle imbalance, activities to obtain fusion, and activities to improve saccadic eye movements. (**Editor's Note: It is critical that the OTs be aware of the importance of supervision and monitoring by a doctor specializing in vision care when working with "muscle imbalance," as it is possible to create strabismus or intractable diplopia where there was none prior, through inappropriate application of standard therapy techniques.**) In addition, compensatory strategies such as scanning training for visual field deficits, along with suggestions for lighting and magnification, are covered. In addition, there are more general cognitive-perceptual OT approaches that apply to this area. These include Toglia's multicontext approach, which emphasizes the use of compensatory cognitive processing and metacognitive strategies that can be generalized across environments.[86] Examples of processing strategies that might be used to address problems associated with visual dysfunction include teaching a client to use finger pointing to assist with scanning the environment to locate relevant objects.

OPTOMETRIC APPROACHES

For years, behavioral (i.e., functional or neuro) optometrists have been aware that motor function is an important component of vision. In the 1950s, the father of behavioral optometry, A. M. Skeffington, O.D.,[87] used a diagram with four over-lapping circles (Figure 10.1) to show how vision emerges from four subprocesses. One of the four subprocesses was termed antigravity ("A"). The antigravity subprocess included balance/vestibular function, bilateral coordination, and gross and fine motor skills. These motor functions were needed for a person to efficiently inter-act with their environment and to answer the question, "Where am I?" According to Skeffington, the antigravity subprocess interacts with three other subprocesses underlying vision: identification ("C"), centering ("B"), and the speech/audition subprocess and communication ("D"). The identification subprocess consists of eye movements, accommodation, and visual analysis, the skills needed to identify objects and answer the question, "What is it?" The centering subprocess consists of eye teaming, laterality, and directionality, the skills needed to perceive accurately where objects are in space and answer the question, "Where is it? Lastly, the speech/audition subprocess allows a person to label and communicate what is seen.

From the neuro-optometrist's perspective, one of the guiding questions when eval-uating and treating a person with acquired brain injury is whether vision is helping or interfering with the person's motor skills. For a person to navigate most effectively in the world, he/she must be guided by an efficient visual system. After brain injury, the

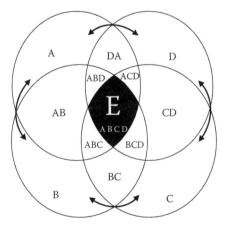

A: The Antigravity Process
B: The Centering Process
C: The Identification Process
D: The Speech-Audition Process
E: The Emergent: Vision

FIGURE 10.1   Skeffington's four circle model of vision modified by Schrock. (Courtesy of D. Press and E. Press.)

ability for vision to guide motor function may be impaired. An optometrist does not treat primary gross or fine motor problems. However, through probing (i.e., testing) the visual system, he/she ascertains whether the visual system could be creating a mismatch between vision and gross or fine motor systems.

For example, a person might be observed to have problems negotiating around furniture, pouring coffee, and losing their balance or even falling on stairs. The visual examination may uncover a binocular dysfunction such as convergence insufficiency with a high exophoria (i.e., the eyes deviating outward, but still working together) and inability to appreciate stereopsis (i.e., the sensation of depth from the slight differences in the retinal image from the two eyes). In this case, the visual system sends information to the brain that identifies objects as being further away than they actually are in space. Thus, the person bumps into furniture (because it is closer than expected), overshoots the rim of the cup, and oversteps on stairs. The visual information sent to the brain is a misrepresentation of the spatial world. As a result, gross and/or fine motor actions are inaccurate, even though the motor systems may be intact. This is a similar situation as seen in the yoked prism demonstration described above where vision overrides the other sensory systems.

Through the use of spectacles and/or vision rehabilitation therapy, the visual skills can be regained so that the visual message to the brain is no longer a misrepresentation of the spatial world. As described below, seemingly simple lenses can be used in treatment to impact visual-spatial perception beyond the ability to see clearly. Indeed, lenses are a powerful tool for modifying perception and visual function.[88] In vision rehabilitation therapy, lenses can impact posture, coordination, and thinking schemes. Lenses can make objects appear smaller and closer or larger and farther away and impact a person's motor response. (See Chapter 7 for further information.) As a result of such treatment, the match between visual and motor skills can be reestablished, and the person no longer has to wonder where the furniture, coffee cup, and stair step truly are in space.

There are two ways to approach optometric treatment of ocular motor or binocular dysfunction that impacts spatial perception and, thus, motor function. One approach has evolved from the ophthalmologic tradition of orthoptic vision therapy where ocular motor and binocular deficits are treated through techniques emphasizing eye muscle control systems.[89,90] However, for many patients, it can be more effective to emphasize improving spatial perception and/or cognitive interactions along with binocularity. This assists with guiding the locomotor and prehensile motor systems accurately and efficiently to the target object, that is, making good visual-motor matches (discussed at length in Chapter 4).

General Optometric Management Considerations

The overall goal of a neuro-optometric vision evaluation is to determine how well the person uses their visual system for functional tasks. The management of the case and duration of treatment should take into consideration: (a) the onset and duration of the problem, (b) the severity of symptoms, (c) other co-occurring visual conditions, (d) general health, (e) medications, (f) cognitive status, (g) current visual demands and those relating to future goals, (h) treatment adherence (i.e., compliance), and (i) prior interventions.

In examining people with acquired brain injury, care must be taken so that the person is able to respond to the best of their ability. The lighting of the room may need to be adapted. The speed of questions may need to be slowed and the complexity of the questions reduced. For those persons with reduced language abilities, it can be helpful if a family member, friend, or caregiver who is familiar with the client's communication needs is present to help the communication flow. Communication boards can be used for those with impaired expressive language. In some instances where receptive language is impaired, gestures can provide additional instructional cues. In other cases, gestures should be avoided as they may make it more difficult for the patient to concentrate on the task. Sessions may need to be shortened or breaks given for those people with decreased attention and/or irritability and low frustration tolerance.

In our opinion, optometric treatment priorities following acquired brain injury should be as follows: (a) management of ocular disease either directly or in collaboration with an ophthalmologist; (b) spectacles for distance and/or a separate pair or pairs of spectacles for near tasks such as reading and computers with or without tints for photophobia (i.e., light sensitivity); (c) fusional prism spectacles if needed to reduce double vision and encourage binocularity; (d) yoked prism spectacles for visual midline shift or visual-spatial hemi-inattention, with or without visual field defect, to provide more stable balance and movement; and (e) judicious occlusion to provide better function and comfort. In addition, vision rehabilitation therapy can be used to improve visual awareness; visual discrimination; visual thinking through the accommodative, binocular, and ocular motor systems; depth and stereopsis awareness; visual-motor and eye-hand coordination; and central-peripheral integration.

This is not a linear process. Sometimes things need to be done in combination. In our opinion, it is typically best to wait to assess the effect of spectacles before initiating vision rehabilitation therapy, and we will describe evaluation and treatment from that perspective. However, readers should note that some practitioners start vision rehabilitation therapy immediately after the evaluation. Further research needs to be done to determine the optimum timing to pursue vision rehabilitation therapy.

The optometrist consults with other professionals involved in the rehabilitation and health care of the patient on an ongoing basis and relates specific visual dysfunctions to the patient's symptoms and functional performance goals in providing treatment and guidance to the rehabilitation team. In some cases, depending on the severity of vision impairment after acquired brain injury, it may be beneficial to defer other types of rehabilitation activities, pending the stabilization of vision function to an appropriate level.

After lenses and/or prisms have been worn for several weeks, a progress visual evaluation is done. The follow-up evaluation starts with an updated case history to see what changes have occurred since the spectacles were prescribed. The patient, as well as caregiver, can give insight as to what has improved and what is still difficult or frustrating. The symptom checklist used at the initial visit (described below) is readministered and results compared with the first visit. At times, the person is unaware that things have changed, so it is helpful to have the initial checklist available to compare.

The full initial battery of tests is typically not given at follow up. Appropriate tests are selected on the basis of the current level of functioning. Are there still areas of impairment with binocularity, accommodative control, and/or ocular motor skills? Do these areas of impairment correlate with the patient's symptoms? If the person still has visual difficulty that is impacting their everyday life after a trial of lenses and/or prisms, vision rehabilitation therapy is often the most appropriate course of action.

Optometric Vision Rehabilitation Therapy

Vision therapy is "the art and science of arranging conditions so that an individual can acquire new relationships in his visual world and through these new relationships can learn to utilize processes that allow him to extract and act on a greater amount of information in a more efficient manner" (p. 29).[91] Goals in vision rehabilitation therapy for visual-motor control are individualized; however, typical global goals are to gain visual awareness and attention, good organization of central and peripheral vision, and effective integration of vision with the other sensory systems. Through vision rehabilitation therapy, the optometrist ascertains the level where the patient can achieve new visual skills and proceeds toward increasing the demands. In some instances, vision disorders that are not totally alleviated through vision rehabilitation therapy, for example gaze palsies, may still be ameliorated with significant improvement in visual function and quality of life.

The length of treatment is dependent on progress toward functional, measurable goals. A progressive and individualized program of vision procedures is performed under optometric supervision. Usually, vision rehabilitation therapy is conducted in office, in once or twice weekly sessions of 30 minutes to 1 hour. The procedures are typically supplemented with treatment activities done at home between office visits. If home activities are not possible, then three times weekly in-office therapy may be necessary. Typically, treatment is started monocularly (each eye alone), progresses biocularly (two eyes working at the same time, but each eye seeing a different part of what is being looked at), and then moves to binocular tasks (both eyes together as in normal vision). However, this sequence should be avoided if there is a possibility of breaking down a fragile binocular system by occlusion of an eye.

Neuro-Optometric Visual Evaluation and Treatment

In the following section, we will describe standard neuro-optometric evaluation procedures as they relate to adults with acquired brain injury, give examples of typical treatment strategies, and describe some of the connections between specific visual abilities and motor performance. Note that not all optometric or ophthalmologic evaluations look at visual skills in sufficient depth to determine how vision may be impacting motor or other functions.

Case History

A thorough case history is an essential first step in a visual evaluation. In taking a case history, symptom checklists can be helpful in guiding evaluation and determining changes over time. Such checklists typically include information regarding eye pain, fatigue, headache, or nausea when performing visually-based activities as well as difficulties with specific activities that require good visual abilities, such as reading, driving, and sports. Other critical information includes current and past medications and previous eye health history.

Ocular Health

The first priority following brain injury is to evaluate the health of a person's eyes. This is essential in determining if a person has any undiagnosed or inadequately treated medical conditions. Some of the more common medical conditions that may be found in both the general population and the patient with brain injury are glaucoma, diabetic retinopathy, macular degeneration, cataracts, and corneal opacities. While some of these conditions are more common in older adults, others (e.g., glaucoma) can begin as early as the forties. In addition, Rutner et al.[92] found markedly increased rates of superficial keratitis, traumatic cataract, vitreous degeneration, peripheral retinal degeneration, optic atrophy, and vitreous prolapse in patients with TBI as compared to the general population. They also found marked increases in ptosis, superficial epithelial keratitis, eyelid lesions, lagophthalmos, subconjunctival hemorrhage, vitreous degeneration, optic atrophy, and peripheral degeneration in patients with cerebrovascular accident. Early detection of those medical conditions that respond to treatment is critical in avoiding further damage and, where possible, irreversible vision loss.

An eye examination following acquired brain injury can also uncover some unexpected, but potentially serious, eye health findings. For example, in our practice, a client with a TBI was screened by OT several months after injury during outpatient rehabilitation and referred for a visual evaluation. The examination found that, unbeknownst to the client, her family, and health-care providers, one contact lens had been in place since the time of the injury. Fortunately, in this case, the lens was removed without causing lasting damage to the cornea. Others have not been so fortunate. Another client sustained damage to the cornea from a poorly fitting patch worn throughout her rehabilitation stay that resulted in long-term decrease of visual acuities.

In an optometric or ophthalmologic examination, medical conditions are evaluated and diagnosed through the use of (a) visual field instrumentation (i.e., perimetry) to investigate visual field loss, visual-spatial neglect, possible brain tumors, and other interruptions in the primary visual pathway; (b) tonometers to measure intraocular pressure for possible glaucoma; (c) biomicroscopes to ascertain the health of the cornea, iris, and anterior chamber, as well as ocular lens integrity and possible cataracts; and (d) binocular indirect ophthalmoscope to ascertain retinal health, including the optic nerve, retinal vessel integrity, and/or retinal tears. Standard treatments for eye-related medical conditions range from medications to surgery or may focus on compensatory strategies, depending on the specific diagnosis.

Accurate identification of medical conditions is complicated by the overlap of medical-related symptoms with those that result from brain injury. For example, rehabilitation clinicians may assume that a visual field loss is due to the brain injury (as is often the case). If a referral for an in-depth visual examination is not made, other medical possibilities that result in visual field loss, such as glaucoma, may not be investigated. Similarly, if a problem with an older adult distinguishing between blue and purple blocks in a block design task is assumed to be an unusual perceptual problem (as the first author is embarrassed to admit to doing early in her career), when an eye examination would have been likely to find that cataracts are the cause, expensive therapy time can be wasted. In these and other situations where the primary problem is one of ocular health rather than a brain injury, prompt diagnosis and appropriate treatment may either be delayed or not given. Furthermore, when vision symptoms are addressed without an ocular health examination (as is likely when treatment is provided by nonvision providers), it is possible to give a false sense of security that can result in further delay in scheduling a comprehensive visual evaluation. It is important for professionals to collaborate, or vision-threatening pathologies can be missed and long-term damage can result.

Refractive Status

In our opinion, the second priority in vision evaluation and treatment following brain injury should be refractive status. Addressing refractive status early on provides the person with the clearest and most comfortable vision possible in the greatest number of functional situations. Refractive status evaluation determines if the person is myopic (i.e., nearsighted), hyperopic (i.e., farsighted), astigmatic (unequal curvature in the cornea or lens), or presbyopic (i.e., difficulty seeing near due to age-related changes). On the basis of those findings, the vision provider determines the lens prescription that best compensates for the refractive status or presbyopia. The choice of lens prescription also takes into account the person's functional needs, that is, not only sight, but also focusing skills and the range, flexibility, and endurance of the eyes working together or "teaming." (Note that spectacles can also be prescribed for accommodative dysfunction as described below.)

What may seem to be a very small or insignificant amount of change in refractive status may be of great significance to a person following brain injury because they cannot compensate sufficiently to see clearly. An amount of refractive impairment that typically would not result in a decision for first-time corrective lenses or a change in lens prescription may cause visual symptoms for a person with an acquired brain injury. The opposite can also be found where the "just noticeable difference" is so vast that a large range of lenses could be given with no variation in the person's perception of visual clarity and/or visual comfort.

Refractive problems, as well as some of the management options, can impact motor abilities. Firstly, the blur that typically results from uncompensated refractive status can distort images making it more difficult to make spatial judgments (e.g., depth). Secondly, the type of spectacles used to compensate for refractive status can impact motor performance, especially for those who require one prescription for near and a different one for far. In the general population, a bifocal or progressive lens with distance and near prescriptions in one pair of spectacles is typically prescribed in this situation. However, following brain injury, a lined bifocal or progressive lens may interfere with mobility. For example, if a person wearing a bifocal does not move their head when looking down toward their feet, the near portion of the bifocal typically makes the floor and feet appear blurry. When looking at the floor through the lined portion, objects at floor level may appear to be double. Such visual distortions may cause difficulty judging stair location and height.[93,94] These problems may be further exacerbated if a person attempts to quickly look up and then down again as when greeting another person when walking on stairs.

The type of bifocal is also critical. People with brain injury can have more difficulty adapting to the distortion of a typical progressive or no-line bifocal. A lined bifocal may be better, or having two pairs may be the best choice with one prescription for distance and another for reading. The intermediate range of a trifocal may be needed for situations such as seeing a computer screen and reading prices of items on the shelf at the grocery store. This distance should not be forgotten and, in some instances, a third pair of spectacles is needed. In the general population, monovision in the form of one contact lens for distance and another for near (or just one contact lens for near if distance vision is not affected) has become a common solution for presbyopia to avoid wearing bifocals. However, with monovision, a person does not perceive stereopsis and does not have the visual cues for maximal depth perception. These challenges of monovision, along with the increased demand on the cognitive system to deal with the visual challenges, can cause unexpected problems for individuals with brain injury.

It is also possible that a person may require more than one set of spectacles if their vision status changes with recovery. While the cost of multiple pairs of spectacles cannot be ignored, not giving the appropriate lenses as the person goes through rehabilitation could actually be more costly. Visual clarity can impact performance on assessment and/or treatment in neuropsychology; occupational, physical, and speech and language therapy; and vocational counseling. Mobility and eye-hand coordination can be impacted along with training in basic self-care and home management skills, reading, computer use, and cognitive therapy. Without proper lenses, overall recovery may be diminished or slowed. A person may appear to be at a plateau when, in reality, their undiagnosed visual problems may be hindering their progress. The total cost of rehabilitation is high and not having the proper spectacles along the way may add to the expense. The amount of money spent on changes in lenses is miniscule compared to the overall cost of rehabilitation. In our opinion, spectacles should be considered one of the tools of rehabilitation. Just as clients may need a wheelchair initially and progress, in time, to a walker, four-pronged quad cane, and then to a single point cane, a person may need different spectacles along the way.

Accommodation

The simplest definition of accommodation is the ability to change focus from distance to near and vice versa. Accommodation requires flexibility of the lens, which is located behind the pupil. In the normal visual system, the lens is flat for distance viewing and curved for near-point activities. This is necessary to bend light coming into the eye the exact amount to come to a point of focus at the fovea. Accommodation supports the process of identifying form at various distances. Focusing skills diminish substantially with aging as a result of increasing inflexibility in the lens and related structures. However, after brain injury, accommodative ability may be impaired in addition to any age-related changes and in younger persons without age-related changes (reviewed by Leslie[95]). Accommodative dysfunction related to brain injury can impact the range, flexibility, and/or endurance of accommodation. It is important to note, however, that accommodation does not operate solo. It is tied closely to the vergence system, as discussed below.

The signs and symptoms associated with accommodative dysfunction are typically related to prolonged performance of visually demanding, near-centered tasks. The person may report difficulty sustaining near visual attention or shifting focus from one distance to another. There may be avoidance of or less time spent on tasks that produce visual stress. Visually demanding tasks may be performed with less accuracy, decreased quality, and/or take more time. Symptoms can include visual discomfort, such as pain in or around the eye, headache (usually frontal or temporal), and/or intermittent distance and/or near blur, including distance blur after performing near work. Patients may report illusory movement, such as, objects or print shifting or moving.

Optometric testing in this area includes positive and relative accommodation, binocular cross cylinder, near retinoscopy, and accommodative rock with and without suppression controls. Diagnostic findings include one or more of the following: (a) low accommodative amplitude relative to age; (b) reduced accommodative facility (monocular); (c) reduced accommodative flexibility; (d) reduced accommodative stability; (e) reduced ranges of relative accommodation; (f) abnormal lag of accommodation; (g) unstable accommodative, refractive, and retinoscopic findings; and (h) inconsistent vergence findings.

Treatment for accommodative dysfunction typically includes lenses. In addition, vision rehabilitation therapy is often needed to improve the range of accommodation, the ability to sustain accommodation, and the flexibility of accommodation. Therapy also focuses on improving the relationship between accommodative and vergence functions.

Vergence (Eye Teaming)

Vergence is the process of using both eyes together efficiently. Described in simple terms, vergence refers to the eyes aiming straight ahead when we look at a distant object and coming in toward each other when we look at a close object. This skill is necessary for good spatial localization. In Skeffington's terms,[87] eye teaming is included as part of the centering skills along with laterality and directionality. Skeffington described these as the skills needed to perceive accurately where objects are in space and answer the question, "Where is it?"

When vergence is not sufficient, we see double (diplopia). If both eyes cannot comfortably remain converged for a period of time, the ability to perform near activities, such as reading, writing, and needlework, may be limited and eye pain, eye fatigue, and headaches may result. The images from one of the eyes may be suppressed entirely or partially by the brain to give a single image. Abnormal postures may also be observed, especially in situations where diplopia results from a mismatch between the accommodative and binocular systems. In these instances, people often get one eye "out of the way" by tilting or turning the head. This serves to functionally eliminate the double vision from a horizontal or vertical misalignment while allowing the other eye to focus on the page. Interestingly, individuals often do not have conscious awareness of the posture change, another example of the effect of the dominance of vision over the other sensory systems.

Eye teaming is the basis for stereopsis, which allows us to see where objects are in relation to our own bodies. Stereopsis is a major contributor to our perception of depth. The variety of activities that rely on good depth perception for efficient performance is vast. Examples include driving or parking a car; throwing, catching, or hitting a ball; pouring something into a cup; threading a needle; shaking a person's hand; and walking up or down stairs. When binocular skills are poor, it is still possible to judge depth through monocular cues. These cues include the relative size of objects, overlap of objects, blurring of distant objects due to dust and moisture in the air, more distant objects appearing to have less detailed texture, apparent convergence of parallel lines in the distance, height cues, and relative motion parallax where more distant objects appear to move at a slower pace as a person moves through space. If someone never had stereopsis, the loss of the eyes teaming together may not be seen as a significant loss as they can still rely on overlap, size, and other cues to tell them about depth perception.[96] However, if a person had stereopsis before injury, the loss may be very difficult to deal with in their daily life as loss of stereopsis (e.g., from suppression, head posture, or patching one eye) can cause problems in eye-hand coordination, depth judgments, orientation in space, balance, and mobility in almost all, if not all, daily activities that involve gross and fine motor skills.

Optometric examination of eye teaming abilities following brain injury begins with a cover test to determine if there is strabismus. In strabismus, the eyes are aligning on different targets simultaneously. Strabismus may be constant, intermittent, and/or periodic (at one distance, but not another). It may be unilateral (only one eye turns) or alternating (either eye turns). The person perceives double when both eyes are being used or single if the images from one of the eyes are suppressed. It is possible for the visual images to change back and forth from single to double. It is also possible to suppress a portion of the information of each eye (such as with central suppression) versus the whole field. The misalignment may be horizontal and/or vertical and it may change with each angle of the gaze. The visual world may be perceived as double, jumping back or forth, or with objects not in the expected location when the hand reaches out to touch an object. As a result, a person's spatial representation of the world is in constant chaos and the visual guidance to the motor system is totally askew. If the misalignment were always the same, a person might be able to adapt to the resulting image, but, since the angle often changes with gaze, adaptation can be difficult, if not impossible. In addition to strabismus, diplopia may also be due to uncorrected refractive status that can manifest in blur, irregular vision, and double vision. In this case, a simple solution of prescriptive lenses may resolve the problem.

Patching has frequently been used in rehabilitation settings to eliminate diplopia. However, patching eliminates the use of stereopsis for depth perception and reduces the peripheral field of vision. It can also impair the subsequent recovery of stereopsis. Judicious use of patching may be necessary to provide better function and comfort of the person as well as for safety considerations. This can be in the form of sector or partial occlusion. An eye doctor with expertise in binocular vision and/or vision rehabilitation can provide assistance in evaluating the potential short-term gains and long-term consequences for each individual when making these decisions.

Correct identification of the reason for diplopia is essential in determining the appropriate compensatory or remedial treatment. In another example from our practice, a patient with diplopia following a cerebellar stroke had worn an eye patch during the hospital stay. After OT screening and referral during outpatient rehabilitation, the neuro-optometrist determined that the double vision was due to astigmatism.

In this case, the diplopia was a result of the patient wearing spectacles with an outdated prescription because she could not put in her more recently prescribed contacts due to ataxia. The diplopia resolved immediately with a new pair of spectacles with subsequent improvement in motor performance as well.

In further evaluating eye teaming, the optometrist conducts tests to determine if there is suppression or a lack of fusion. These measurements should be made at distance and near, as well as horizontally and vertically. The range of fusion, as well as the flexibility and endurance, are important to note as a person may be able to fuse for relatively short periods of time, but then suppress the information from one eye. Testing procedures, conducted at distance and near, may include the cover test, muscle imbalance measurement test, prism rock with and without suppression control, Worth Four Dot, and Randot stereopsis, along with measurement of convergence and divergence ranges.

Prisms, lenses, and/or vision rehabilitation therapy can many times help the patient achieve fusion and diminish the diplopia. (See Chapter 7 for specifics on the use of prisms and lenses in diplopia.) In optometric vision rehabilitation therapy, vergence activities that are done binocularly require a suppression check to make sure both eyes are functioning. In addition, the patient should attempt to be aware of any blurring, doubling, or suppression. This is accomplished through feedback mechanisms set up in therapy activities and practice with the procedures. Blurring indicates that the patient is at the threshold of his/her vergence ability and has recruited accommodative vergence to help hold the images together. Doubling means that the patient has exceeded his/her level of vergence ability and has lost fusion. Suppression means that the brain has exceeded its ability to fuse the two images and the image from one eye is being disregarded to avoid seeing double. In vision rehabilitation therapy, if the patient sees blurring, doubling, or is suppressing for a few seconds and then is able to fuse the images and see appropriately, the therapy activity can be continued. If the image remains blurry, double, or there is continued suppression, the activity level is too high. The activity should be discontinued until the patient has the foundational skills to perform at this level.

Accommodative-Vergence Interaction

The preceding information on accommodation and binocularity has been organized and somewhat simplified to assist with conceptual clarity. However, it does not represent the full range or complexity of the visual inefficiencies that can result from combined accommodative-vergence disorders. In accommodative-vergence disorders, an individual's visual system is not coping effectively with the load or stress placed on it. As there is no way to directly observe the interaction between the accommodative and vergence system, lenses and prisms are used as probes to gauge how well the patient copes when accommodative stress is put on the system. This knowledge is used to design the treatment to restore balance to the system. It is important to note that, as long as a patient is engaged in binocular therapy, any processing through the accommodative system will require a self-adjustment in the vergence system to maintain equilibrium between the two systems. Typically, when working with visually guided motor skills, only the binocular system is seen as important. However, it is limiting to view accommodative therapy only in terms of clarity of printed materials. A patient who does not perceive spatial or size differences through their accommodative system while using lenses must be made aware that he is ignoring important information that can help with motor skills.

Convergence Insufficiency

Convergence insufficiency is also associated with acquired brain injury.[97] Convergence insufficiency is the inability to adequately bring the eyes together, that is, to converge, and/or sustain convergence for near visual tasks. This condition is viewed by some practitioners as a form of an eye teaming problem,[98] while others see it as a central/peripheral problem.[99] The diagnosis of convergence insufficiency is based on one or more of the following findings: (a) higher than expected exophoria at near; (b) receded near point of convergence; and (c) low positive fusional vergence ranges, facility, and/or flexibility at near. The signs and symptoms of convergence insufficiency may include eye pain, eye strain, feelings of the eye "pulling," and/or diplopia during or after near tasks, especially visually demanding tasks that must be sustained over time. There may also be motion sickness in these situations. In addition, people may avoid or have diminished performance with visually demanding near tasks and experience difficulty sustaining near visual function. This can include difficulty reading with loss of place, repetition, and/or omission of words and/or lines of print; transpositions when copying; and inaccurate eye-hand coordination. People may report headaches, transient blurred vision, and illusory movement with near tasks, such as apparent movement of words on the page. In addition, people may have atypical postures or working distances with near tasks, spatial disorientation, photophobia, decreased visual attention and concentration, and fatigue.

Treatment includes supportive lenses, prisms, and vision rehabilitation therapy. Vision rehabilitation therapy should include treatment to improve fusional ranges and stability along with vergence flexibility, improve the relationship between accommodative and convergence abilities, and integrate binocular function with cognitive and motor tasks and other sensory skills to avoid training splinter skills that can only be used in isolation.

Ocular Motor Skills

Ocular motor dysfunction, that is, impairment in movement of the eyes, is a typical visual-motor problem following TBI.[100] The inability to perform accurate, effective saccadic and/or fixational eye movement patterns is a hallmark of problems in this area. Symptoms of ocular motor dysfunction are varied, as might be expected given the foundational importance of these skills to functional activity. They may include difficulty reading with loss of place, repetition, and/or omission of words and/or lines of print; incoordination or clumsiness with gross or fine motor activities; inconsistent visual attention or distractibility when performing visually demanding tasks; spatial disorientation with or without dizziness or motion sickness; and overall decreased speed and quality of task performance.

Optometrists assess the person's ability to fixate, track, and follow with the eyes through observation of eye movements on demand with tools such as the Northeastern State University College of Optometry Oculomotor Tests;[84] the Visagraph,[101] an eye movement recording system; and the Developmental Eye Movement test (DEM),[102] a visual–verbal test of saccadic eye movement in reading. It is vital to look not only at the scores on these tests, but also how the person functioned during the test. Indeed, as there are currently no norms for adult English speakers for the original single-digit version of the DEM,[103,104] results must be interpreted on the basis of clinical observations. Diagnostic findings may include the following: increased or decreased saccadic latency, decreased saccadic accuracy, difficulty separating head/body and eye movements, and difficulty sustaining adequate saccadic eye movements under cognitive demands. Findings are often compared to a symptom checklist to determine if there is a relationship between the testing and reports of difficulties with functional tasks.

Typically, if new lenses are prescribed, ocular motor performance is retested after the person has had time, typically four to six weeks, to use their new lenses and see if the use of the lenses resolves any of the ocular motor difficulties. Compensatory aids, such as using a window in a card for reading so that only one line a time is seen, can be used while the visual skills are remediated. If the ocular motor skills are still impaired with new spectacles and aids, vision rehabilitation therapy is advised. Vision rehabilitation therapy activities to improve ocular motor skills are typically done in monocular, biocular, and then binocular fashion. They include the use of prisms, filters, and different instrumentation to help give feedback as to how the person's fixations, smooth pursuits, and saccadic skills are functioning while the person is sitting, standing, or moving.

Ambient Vision

Dysfunction in the ambient or peripheral visual system can also occur following acquired brain injury. The signs and symptoms associated with unstable ambient vision result from loss of visual grounding in space. These include spatial disorientation; objects appearing to move; staring behavior; poor concentration and attention; and difficulties with balance, coordination, and posture.[99]

Functional assessment of the ambient visual system can be done by watching a person's visual-motor integration while attempting activities such as walking down a hallway, climbing steps or stairs, and attempting to put a cap on a pen held in various positions. Next, yoked prisms are worn in various positions (i.e., base up, down, right, or left) and the activity is repeated. Is there a change in the ability of the person to achieve the task? Is there a difference in the time taken to complete the task? Is the task done more confidentially? Are they more proficient at the task? If there is a marked improvement, yoked prisms may be prescribed. (For further information on yoked prism application see Chapters 6 and 7.)

Integration of Central and Peripheral Vision Systems

Integration of the central (i.e., focal) and peripheral (i.e., ambient) vision systems is vital to efficient everyday function. There is a delicate balancing act between these two systems in all that we do. The longer you look at a target, the more the focal attention decreases. However, if you are only aware of the periphery, you will miss the detail of the target. When central and peripheral integration is not efficient, the person may have difficulty walking straight, difficulty avoiding obstacles, balance and coordination problems, poor eye-hand coordination, slowed visuomotor performance, and decreased awareness of their surroundings.

Lenses and vision rehabilitation therapy can help create balance and integration between the systems. The functional effects of lenses and prisms exceed the conventional compensatory properties. As noted above, if there is a conflict between motor and vision, vision typically supersedes motor. By changing the visual input with prisms, it is possible to change motor performance as well as posture and sensation. Lenses can also change space perception as discussed in Chapter 7.

VISION REHABILITATION THERAPY EXAMPLE

In optometric vision rehabilitation therapy, the equipment used to help develop visual-motor skills includes septums (i.e., partitions between the two eyes), prisms, and lenses. In addition, polarized filters, red-green anaglyphic glasses, or overlays can be used to gain visual and suppression awareness. For example, in convergence insufficiency, the neuro-optometrist would use an array of instrumentation and materials to help one to develop "visual thinking" (i.e., awareness of how the eyes are working as a team as a method of improving function) through the binocular system. A hierarchy of activities would be used over a time period of weeks or months to gain visual awareness and control so that vision is more effective in leading motor actions.

Squinchel is one of the myriad of activities used in optometric vision rehabilitation therapy. This activity requires a high level of cognitive skill and may not be appropriate for all patients with acquired brain injury. However, it is a "high leverage" activity in that the patient can gain awareness and develop simultaneous perception, exploration of visual posture, visual dominance, visual manipulation, visual processing, and visual-motor coordination (unilateral and cross-lateral). A patient can learn to organize and process visual space more efficiently and to extend divergence/convergence ranges and endurance. Note that the possibility of visual inattention simulating suppression should be taken into consideration with patients with acquired brain injury. (See Chapter 5 for therapy activities that could be used specifically for visual inattention before working on Squinchel.)

High-powered base in and base down prisms are used to double the image. Patients are instructed to put their index finger on the table. They are instructed to look at their finger and are asked, "How many fingers do you see?" If the patient is having difficulty with simultaneous perception, one of several binocular abnormalities may be perceived. If there is cortical suppression of the image corresponding to the one eye, the patient perceives only one finger instead of the double image. If there is alternating cortical suppression between the images corresponding to one eye versus the other, the patient perceives one finger that jumps back and forth.

Next, the patient is asked, "Do the two fingers look equally real?" The goal is that, cortically, the image from each eye can be seen simultaneously and that the two images would look equally real. The person is then instructed to look at their right finger while rubbing it on the table and asked, "Does it feel the same as it looks?" We want to create a match between what is felt and what is seen and to assure that both the right and left eyes give equal information, such that the finger image that is being fixated at the time is perceived as the one that is feeling the table. Activities are repeated with the left finger with the person asked if the experience is different between the right and left fingers.

After the two eyes are simultaneously seeing the images as the same, a golf tee is placed vertically on the table. The patient looks at the golf tee and is asked how many golf tees they perceive and if the tee(s) are moving. The person will see two golf tees if both eyes are working simultaneously. It will take the person time to discover and gain awareness that the movement of the tees is actually the movement of their eyes. They are instructed to touch the right golf tee with their right finger. The kinesthetic feedback can be an effective cue to the object's actual location in space and an effective support to guide motor action. They should perceive two fingers and two tees. The optometrist will note the smoothness of the movement as well as any hesitation, redirection, or movement past the tee. Questions for the patient include, "Did both fingers look equally real? Did your finger tend to fade as you moved it?"

Through this type of probing, the patient can discover how their eyes align; if there is a vertical, exo, or eso component; and how the central and peripheral systems interact. A patient can learn to organize and process visual space more efficiently. If there is a residual vertical imbalance that the patient cannot overcome, the tees may be perceived as being on two different planes, one slightly higher than the other, so that the fingers/tees do not appear to be aligned at a single point in space. A slight head tilt may be needed to orient the finger/tees on the same plane.

Further exploration is done with the right finger on the left tee, the left finger on left tee, and the left finger on the right tee. A pick up stick is used to touch the top of the tee. "Is this easier or more difficult than all the activities above?" A loop is placed around the golf tee and the above activities are repeated. The patient is then asked to place the loop around the golf tee and move it up and down along the tee without touching it. The loop is made progressively smaller and the activities are repeated. An element of complexity with this activity is that we are asking the patient to simultaneously maintain awareness that is relatively focal in terms of the tee being fixated centrally on the visual axis and relatively ambient in terms of the loop being fixated peripherally. Patients with acquired brain injury who have difficulty simultaneously balancing focal and ambient vision will find it difficult initially to attain accurate spatial localization on the tee and the loop.

As the above tasks become easy, they are repeated using both hands simultaneously, so that the person perceives four fingers. Then the hands are crossed. Next, the person is asked to hold their right finger in front of them and look beyond their finger to a distance. They are asked, "What happened to your finger?" The fingers should change position in relation to each other. Now the person is asked to discover how to make the fingers move in the opposite direction. "What did you need to do with your eyes and vision to make this happen?"

Through these various activities over a series of weeks or months, a person can acquire visual thinking skills that help them learn to develop simultaneous perception and what they can do to help both eyes to work at the same time. They can learn how their eyes posture and what they can do visually to change the posture, how it feels to do that, and what it looks like. They can understand which of their eyes is more dominant and how to use information from both eyes simultaneously instead of relying on the more dominant eye. They are learning how to visually manipulate their eyes and process the visual information. They are learning to master visual-motor coordination. This can impact fine and gross motor function in everyday life as they can process visual space more efficiently. They can learn to extend divergence/convergence ranges and endurance so they do not visually fatigue in everyday life. Through hierarchical activities in the office and home practice, the visual skills are developed so that (a) a person is able to visually attend and not visually attend to information appropriately; (b) there is integration between the central and peripheral visual systems, as well as vision and the other sensory systems; and (c) vision guides motor function effectively. During the final stages of therapy, the patient's newly acquired visual skills are reinforced and made automatic through repetition and integration with motor and cognitive skills.

Readers should note that doubling prisms are a very powerful tool. They have as much power to do harm as to do good. A person can become very nauseated with the lenses and/or become disoriented. The impact often persists after the lenses are taken off. Prisms should be used only under the direction of an optometrist or ophthalmologist who has experience in this modality. Otherwise, it is very possible to exacerbate the person's vision and/or motor problems and put the patient at risk for injury from such things as falls and driving errors. *Worse, in a strabismic, or fragile binocular system, it is possible to create intractable diplopia where there was none prior by applying techniques such as Squinchel that work antisuppression.* Careful attention must be paid to the patient's behavior, orientation, and manner throughout these activities so that intractable diplopia is not induced.

COLLABORATION BETWEEN OCCUPATIONAL THERAPY AND OPTOMETRY

As described above, the vision and motor systems interact in complex ways in the performance of everyday tasks. Optimal functioning in both systems is needed for individuals to attain optimal efficiency, safety, and independence. This complexity is increased with the added complication of acquired brain injury. OTs and optometrists both have expert knowledge in evaluation and treatment techniques that address both of these systems. Note that this is also true for the evaluation and treatment of visual-perceptual dysfunction, a critical intermediary component between the visual and motor systems (see Chapters 4 and 11 for further discussion). While the knowledge of these two fields overlaps in some areas, each field also defines, evaluates, and treats the problems differently based on expertise that is not held by most practitioners in the other discipline. Perspectives from both disciplines can be beneficial in determining root causes and providing efficient and effective treatment. Involving both disciplines from the time of initial concerns can also minimize the potential for harm that could result from treating a problem (whether vision or motor) without a more complete understanding of the cause. As described above, in some instances what seems like a difficult problem may have a simple solution, as with the patient with diplopia caused by astigmatism. In others, what seems like a straightforward problem can have a potentially dangerous cause, as with visual field loss as a result of glaucoma.

Unfortunately, current rehabilitation systems often do not support collaboration with optometrists. Problems include decreased access to optometric providers, especially in hospital settings; limited availability of qualified providers; and payment restrictions. Increased awareness by rehabilitation personnel of the need to address vision concerns early on in a functional manner has led to increased frustration with the current systems. As a result, some rehabilitation providers have taken on the treatment of vision concerns without the guidance of a vision provider. In addition to the potential for less effective and efficient treatment when treating vision symptoms without an accurate diagnosis, this approach also has the potential to result in even slower system changes as it may lead to the belief on the part of other providers, payers, and clients that the vision concerns are being addressed adequately within the current system.

SCREENING FOR REFERRAL

In our opinion, persons with primary vision deficits following acquired brain injury should be referred to neuro-optometrists for in-depth assessment and treatment. Similarly, persons with primary motor deficits should be referred to occupational and physical therapists for assessment and treatment purposes. For this to occur, clinicians need good screening and referral protocols unless, of course, individuals with these difficulties are already referred to both disciplines by the physician or other provider managing the case.

Screening for Vision Impairments

The most comprehensive vision assessment battery designed for use by OTs working with adults with acquired brain injury is the commercially available Brain Injury Visual Assessment Battery for Adults (biVABA).[105] Equipment already available in some OT clinics for use in conducting driving evaluations can also be used for some aspects of vision screening, such as visual acuity and depth perception. Suggestions for assessment of specific visual abilities are also available.[84,85]

However, it is possible to perform a comprehensive brain injury focused vision screen quickly at very low cost using a minimal amount of materials. A vision screen of this type that we developed is presented in Appendix 10.1. This screen uses a limited amount of specialized materials, can be used in many settings, and is readily portable. For those with space issues, distance acuity can be tested at 10 or 5 feet and either reported as such or converted to the equivalent Snellen notation at 20 feet. We have used the following referral criteria in our practice (based on use of a Snellen chart and near vision card for acuity testing): (a) any one of the following major findings: (i) positive subjective complaint or objective observation, (ii) distance or near visual acuity equal to or less than 20/40, (iii) impaired visual fields; or (b) two or more of the following minor findings: (i) impaired tracking, (ii) impaired saccadic eye movement, (iii) binocular visual acuity worse than best monocular, (iv) impaired convergence, (v) impaired depth perception. If only one minor finding is present, the vision screen should be repeated in 1 month. Our purpose in setting these particular referral criteria was twofold: first, to be liberal in identifying those individuals where vision problems might be due to a medical condition so they could be referred and evaluated without delay and second, to be somewhat conservative in identifying those whose visual problems are likely to be solely related to a brain injury to minimize unneeded referrals. As a result, it is likely that these criteria will miss some individuals with brain injury–related impairments. If more liberal criteria to identify those with brain injury–related visual impairments are desired, patients with only one minor finding could be referred. However, this still may not be sufficient to rule out vision problems. Perhaps the best approach is that suggested by Gianutsos[106] who recommended that all patients with acquired brain injury have an optometric vision assessment from a qualified vision provider early on in the recovery process.

Screening for Motor Impairments

There are also screens for motor impairments that can be conducted by clinicians without specific expertise in the physical domain. A simple screen for motor impairments following acquired brain injury can start with a basic upper extremity placement test. This test screens for impairments in muscle strength and range of motion, as well as atypical movement patterns often seen after damage to the central nervous system, by having the client move the arms against gravity in a variety of movements used in functional activities. Clients are asked to move both hands over head, behind the neck, and behind the small of the back. They are instructed to hold the arms straight in front of the body and then bend the elbows to touch the hands to the shoulders. Next, they are asked to hold the hands in front of the body with elbows next to the trunk. In this position, they are asked to turn the palms up and down and to open and close the fingers. This motor screen can be concluded with a screen of hand strength by having the client squeeze the examiner's hand with each hand.

Observations should include: (a) asymmetry in the trunk and between the limbs on each side of the body, (b) atypical movement patterns as might be caused by abnormal muscle tone (either too high or too low), (c) fluidity of movement, (d) ease of movement, (e) speed of movement (especially slowed movement, i.e., bradykinesia), and (f) tremor. Additional observations include any near or complete loss of balance and atypical head, trunk, or limb postures.

Screening for cerebellar function[107] is often done through observation of quick alternating movements (diadochokinesia). Typical tests of this type include: (a) quickly moving the palms up/palms down (with the forearms in front of the body with the elbows bent next to the trunk) and (b) quickly touching each finger, in succession, to the thumb on the same hand. Another common test looking at control of muscle length (dysmetria) involves having the person alternately touch his/her own nose and the examiner's finger held in front of the person. This test, however, could be influenced by several different types of vision impairments (e.g., depth perception and acuity) so has less clinical usefulness in a motor screen where vision is already a concern.

Finding a Collaborator

With the wide range of approaches used in both occupational therapy and optometry, it can be difficult to identify an appropriate collaborator. In general, we recommend looking for clinicians who individualize treatment both in terms of what is done and for how long, who set functional, measurable goals with frequent reevaluation of progress toward those goals, and who modify treatment and discharge plans in response to progress.

Both occupational therapists and optometrists can begin by networking with colleagues for their recommendations. Faculty at curriculum programs and professional organizations such as the Neuro-developmental Treatment Association (www.ndta. org) and the College of Optometrists in Vision Development (www.covd.org) may have suggestions. Once a possible collaborator has been identified, an interview is important in determining if treatment philosophies and intervention priorities are compatible. Further discussions can include what referral criteria will be used and how outcomes will be evaluated, along with what information needs to be communicated, how that will be done, and how often.

CONCLUSIONS AND FUTURE DIRECTIONS

While much remains to be learned about the exact nature of the relationships within and between the visual and motor systems and how best to treat the impairments that can result from acquired brain injury, we do know enough about the significant potential downstream effects of damage or disruption in these systems to look early and more closely at patients reporting alterations in vision and/or complex motor functions. We can also view those problems with more sophistication. We should consider that alterations in reading may often not be due to changes in acuity or comprehension alone, but might result from problems with convergence. Similarly, significant reductions in the person's ability to tolerate complex natural environments may not be the result of anxiety or depression, but avoidance occasioned by a poorly identified visual disturbance that renders rapid motions of persons or objects in the surrounding environment into feelings of disorientation or nausea. Problems with higher level coordination may not be a primary motor or vestibular problem, or not that alone, but aggravated by mild impairments in visual-motor processing. Our day to day treatment approach to individuals with acquired brain injury and our conceptualizations of their difficulties both merit an expanded view that incorporates what we have learned from the research thus far.

One key component of that research is our evolving knowledge of the dual visual processing systems in the brain, for example the possibility of the ventral system for conscious perception of objects and their general features versus the dorsal system for somewhat less conscious, but more precise, processing of movement-related features. This is only one excellent example of the ongoing theory development and research that allows us, as clinicians and scientists, to begin devising more creative and effective treatments based on a more sophisticated and integrated view of visual and visual-motor systems.

It is also fair to say that, at this point in time, both clinicians and researchers have more knowledge of how vision relates to more conscious cognitive tasks than to more unconscious motor actions. Even less is known about how other systems, such as perception of emotional tone, facial expressions, or other neuropsychological disruptions or the person's own emotional state, may impact complex performance in visual and motor areas.

In addition, it is clear that it is not enough to evaluate and treat visual and motor impairments as if these systems worked independently of each other. Clinical approaches that recognize and address the interrelationship and complexities of these systems are needed to further the efficiency and effectiveness of differential diagnosis and treatment. For example, new approaches to the assessment and treatment of ambient/peripheral vision and saccadic eye movement dysfunctions as they relate to motor actions in everyday life are likely to be beneficial. Also promising are new ways to use visual input to promote motor recovery, such as the use of online visual feedback with the MIT-MANUS robotic systems[72] and visual distortion to facilitate movement.[108]

Continued interdisciplinary collaborations among all the fields involved are critical to gain the clinical and research knowledge needed to improve the treatment and ultimate recovery of individuals with acquired brain injury. In the meantime, increased understanding of the significant, yet sometimes relatively silent, role that disruptions in visual and visual-motor systems have upon higher level daily activities; upon features of neuropsychological functions; and upon physical, social, and leisure involvement should remain a part of our overall clinical awareness in evaluating and treating such individuals.

APPENDIX 10.1

1. **Vision history** (e.g., current corrective eyeglasses or contact lenses, mono-vision, previous eye surgery, medical conditions relating to eye health, date of last eye exam)
2. **a. Subjective report of vision-related symptoms** (e.g., eye strain/fatigue/pain, tearing, blurred vision, light or glare sensitivity, headache, perception of motion in stationary objects or print, impaired balance, dizziness, slow or inaccurate reading or fatigue with reading, double vision)
   b. Observation of vision-related symptoms (e.g., squinting, closing one eye, tilting/turning head, requesting additional lighting, difficulty recognizing familiar people, holding reading material close to face, skipping words when reading, reaching out for objects in an uncertain manner, missing objects when reaching, moving hesitantly, bumping into objects, seeming uncertain near stairs, falling)

   General instructions: Client seated comfortably and wearing current corrective lenses appropriate for task. Examiner seated directly opposite for #3, #4, #5, #8, #9, and #10.

3. **Range of motion**
   Instructions: "Look to the center. Now look to the right. Keeping your eyes to the right, look straight up, now straight down. Look back to the center. Look to the left. Keeping your eyes to the left, look straight up, now straight down."
   Expected findings: No restriction of eye motion.
4. **Tracking/Smooth Pursuits**
   Procedure: Pencil with colored ball (e.g., push pin) on top held vertically 14–16 inches from eyes. Move pencil slowly in the following directions:
   If client moves head on first attempt, repeat with instruction to keep head still.

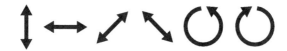

Instructions: "Follow the colored ball on the end of this pencil."

Expected findings: Smooth movement with both eyes maintaining gaze on target throughout all movements. No loss of target, jerkiness of motion, or under- or overshooting of target. No movement of head.

5. **Saccades**

   Procedure: Hold two pencils with colored balls (push pins) of two different colors vertically 14–16 inches from eyes and 8 inches apart from each other. Using an uneven rhythm, ask the client to look at one target and then the other for a total of 5 sets (10 total).

   Instructions: "Look at the (*one color*) ball. Now, the (*other color*) ball, etc."

   Expected findings: Quick, accurate eye movement to target for five sets. No under- or overshooting of target. No movement of head.

6. **Distance acuity** (use Snellen chart for more precise measurement, if available, or when examiner has less than 20/20 distance vision)

   Procedure: Using the smallest print on a poster that examiner can easily read at 20 feet, ask the client to read target print from that distance. Test each eye separately and then both eyes together using an index card or other occluder.

   Expected findings: Able to read without squinting or turning head. Monocular sight same for both eyes. Binocular sight ≥ monocular sight.

7. **Near acuity** (use near vision card for more precise measurement, if available)

   Procedure: Using newspaper or magazine held 14–16 inches from eyes. Test each eye separately and then both eyes together using an index card or other occluder. Point to six individual letters with a pen tip and ask client to identify each letter.

   Expected findings: Minimum 5/6 letters correct without squinting or turning head. Monocular sight same for both eyes. Binocular sight ≥ monocular sight.

8. **Peripheral visual fields**

   Procedure: Sit facing the client at eye level. Using a slow arc-like motion, bring a pencil, held horizontally, from above and below, and, held vertically, in from both sides, moving from the unseen field (behind the patient) around to the seen field. Next, bring the pencil in from halfway between each of the horizontal and vertical motions for a total of 8 test points.

   Instructions: "Keep looking at my nose. I am going to bring a pencil in from above (*below, behind*) you. Tell me when you first see the pencil."

   Expected findings: Identification of pencil (not colored ball) at 110° for side, 65° for above, 70° for below, with corresponding angles for the midpoint motions.

9. **Near point of convergence**[*]

Procedure: Hold a pencil vertically, 16 inches from eyes with ball (push pin) on top. Slowly move ball in at eye level (from below if wearing bifocals) and between the two eyes. After report of double and/or blur (or 2 inches from bridge of nose), bring the pencil back out.

Instructions: "I'm going to move the pencil toward you. Tell me when you see two balls or a blurry ball." Bringing the target back out, "Tell me when it looks single and clear again."

Expected findings: Both eyes looking directly at target throughout. Report of double or blur (break point) at 2–4 inches from bridge of nose. Recovery of single at 4–6 inches.

10. **Depth perception**

Procedure: Give the client a pencil to hold with the unsharpened end facing down. Hold a second unsharpened pencil vertically in front of the client with the unsharpened end facing up. One attempt only.

Instructions: "Hold this pencil at shoulder level. When I say, 'Go,' bring your pencil up and over as quickly as you can and touch the end of your pencil to the end of my pencil. Go."

Expected findings: Quick, direct motion resulting in contact of pencil ends.

Required materials: *Two unsharpened pencils with different colored, round push pins inserted in the erasers, Snellen chart or poster with print of varying sizes, near vision card, newspaper, or magazine, index card or other occluder, and string with knots 14–16 inches apart to measure test distances.*

REFERENCES

1. Bouska, M. J., & Gallaway, M. (1991). Primary visual deficits in adults with brain damage: management in occupational therapy. *Occupational therapy practice: Vision and performance, 3*(1), 1–11.
2. Gianutsos, R., Ramsey, G., & Perlin, R .R. (1988). Rehabilitative optometric services for survivors of acquired brain injury. *Archives of Physical Medicine and Rehabilitation, 69*, 573–578.
3. Mitchell, R., MacFarlane, A., & Cornell, E. (1983). Ocular motility disorders following head injury. *Australian Orthoptic Journal, 20*, 31–36.
4. Padula, W. V., Shapiro, J. B., & Jasin, P. (1988). Head injury causing post trauma vision syndrome. *New England Journal of Optometry, 41*(2), 16–21.
5. Sabates, N. R., Gonce, M. A., & Farris, B. K. (1991). Neuro-ophthalmological findings in closed head trauma. *Journal of Clinical Neuro-ophthalmology, 11*, 273–277.
6. Zoltan, B., Siev, E., & Freishtat, B. (1986). *The adult stroke patient: A manual for evaluation and treatment of perceptual and cognitive dysfunction* (revised 2nd ed.). Thorofare, NJ: Slack.
7. Bouska, M. J., Kauffman, N. A., & Marcus, S. E. (1985). Disorders of the visual perceptual system. In D. A. Umphred (Ed.), *Neurological rehabilitation* (Vol. 3, pp. 552–585). St. Louis, MO: Mosby.

---

[*] Editor's note. "Push-up" screenings for convergence insufficiency may be useful where justification for referral to a vision care practitioner is for some reason required, but this technique has been demonstrated to be insensitive, and will miss many convergence deficits.

8. Neistadt, M. E. (1990). A critical analysis of occupational therapy approaches for perceptual deficits in adults with brain injury. *American Journal of Occupational Therapy, 44,* 299–304.

9. Siev, E., & Freishtat, B. (1976). *Perceptual dysfunction in the adult stroke patient: A manual for evaluation and treatment.* Thorofare, NJ: Charles B. Slack.

10. Warren M. (1993a). A hierarchical model for evaluation and treatment of visual perceptual dysfunction in adult acquired brain injury, Part 1. *American Journal of Occupational Therapy, 47,* 42–54.

11. Warren M. (1993b). A hierarchical model for evaluation and treatment of visual perceptual dysfunction in adult acquired brain injury, Part 2. *American Journal of Occupational Therapy, 47,* 55–66.

12. Mattingly, C., & Fleming, M. H. (1994). *Clinical reasoning: Forms of inquiry in a therapeutic practice.* Philadelphia, PA: F. A. Davis.

13. Suter, P. S. (2004). Rehabilitation and management of visual dysfunction following traumatic brain injury. In M. J. Ashley (Ed.) *Traumatic brain injury: Rehabilitative treatment and case management* (2nd ed., pp. 209–249). Boca Raton, FL: CRC Press.

14. Trevarthen, C. (1968). Two mechanisms of vision in primates. *Psychologische Forschung, 31,* 299–337.

15. Trevarthen, C., & Sperry, R. W. (1973). Perceptual unity of the ambient visual field in human commissurotomy patients. *Brain, 96,* 547–570.

16. Schneider, G. E. (1969). Two visual systems: Brain mechanisms for localization and discrimination are dissociated by tectal and cortical lesions. *Science, 163,* 895–902.

17. Ungerleider, L.G., & Mishkin, M. (1982) Two cortical visual systems. In D. J. Ingle, M. A. Goodale, & R. J. W. Mansfield (Eds.), *Analysis of visual behavior* (pp. 549–586). Cambridge, MA: MIT Press.

18. Livingstone, M. S., & Hubel, D. H. (1987). Psychophysical evidence for separate channels for the perception of form, color, movement, and depth. *Journal of Neuroscience, 7,* 3416–3468.

19. Livingstone, M. S., & Hubel, D. H. (1988). Segregation of form, color, movement, and depth: anatomy, physiology, and perception. *Science, 240,* 740–749.

20. Goodale, M. A., & Milner, A. D. (1992). Separate visual pathways for perception and action. *Trends in Neurosciences, 15,* 20–25.

21. Milner, A. D., & Goodale, M. A. (2006). *The visual brain in action* (2nd ed.). Oxford: Oxford University Press.

22. Goodale, M. A., & Westwood, D. A. (2004). An evolving view of duplex vision: separate but interacting cortical pathways for perception and action. *Current Opinion in Neurobiology, 14,* 201–211.

23. Goodale, M. A., & Milner, A. D. (2004). *Sight unseen.* Oxford: Oxford University Press.

24. Jackson, S. R., & Husain, M. (2006). Visuomotor functions of the posterior parietal cortex [Special issue]. *Neuropsychologia, 44,* 2589–2593.

25. Friedman, D. S., Freeman, E., Munoz, B., Jampel, H. D., & West, S. K. (2007). Glaucoma and mobility performance: The Salisbury Eye Evaluation Project. *Ophthalmology, 114,* 2232–2237.

26. Geruschat, D. R., Turano, K. A., & Stahl, J. W. (1998). Traditional measures of mobility performance and retinitis pigmentosa. *Optometry and Vision Science, 75,* 525–537.

27. Wood, J. M., Lacherez, P. E., Black, A. A., Cole, M. H., Boon, M. Y., & Kerr, G. K. (2009). Postural stability and gait among older adults with age-related macular degeneration. *Investigative Ophthalmology & Visual Science, 50,* 482–487.

28. Felson, D. T., Anderson, J. J., Hannan, M. T., Milton, R. C., Wilson, P. W. F., & Kiel, D. P. (1989). Impaired vision and hip fracture: the Framingham study. *Journal of the American Geriatrics Society, 37,* 494–500.

29. Lord, S. R. (2006). Visual risk factors for falls in older people. *Age and Ageing, 35*(Suppl. 2), ii42–ii45.
30. Ivers, R. Q., Cumming, R. G., Mitchell, P., & Attebo, K. (1998). Visual impairment and falls in older adults: the Blue Mountains Eye Study. *Journal of the American Geriatrics Society, 46,* 58–64.
31. Turano, K. A., Geruschat, D. R., Baker, F. H., Stahl, J. W., & Shapiro, M. D. (2001). Direction of gaze while walking a simple route: persons with normal vision and persons with retinitis pigmentosa. *Optometry and Vision Science, 78,* 667–675.
32. Warren, W. H., & Whang, S. (1987). Visual guidance of walking through apertures: body-scaled information for affordances. *Journal of Experimental Psychology: Human Perception and Performance, 13,* 371–383.
33. Heckenmueller, E. G. (1965). Stabilization of the retinal image: a review of methods, effects, and theory. *Psychological Bulletin, 63,* 157–169.
34. Yarbus A. L. (1967). *Eye movements and vision.* New York: Plenum Press.
35. Land, M., Mennie, N., & Rusted, J. (1999). The roles of vision and eye movements in the control of activities of daily living. *Perception, 28,* 1311–1328.
36. Hayhoe, M. (2000). Vision using routines: a functional account of vision. *Visual Cognition, 7,* 43–64.
37. Pelz, J. B., & Canosa, R. (2001). Oculomotor behavior and perceptual strategies in complex tasks. *Vision Research, 41,* 3587–3596.
38. MacDougall, H. G., & Moore, S. T. (2005). Functional assessment of head-eye coordination during vehicle operation. *Optometry and Vision Science, 82,* 706–715.
39. Geruschat, D. R., Hassan, S. E., & Turano, K. A. (2003). Gaze behavior while crossing complex intersections. *Optometry and Vision Science, 80,* 515–528.
40. Land, M. F. (2006). Eye movements and the control of actions in everyday life. *Progress in Retinal and Eye Research, 25,* 296–324.
41. Naito, K., Kato, T., & Fukuda, T. (2004). Expertise and position of line of sight in golf putting. *Perceptual and Motor Skills, 99,* 163–170.
42. Sailer, U., Flanagan, J. R., & Johansson, R. S. (2005). Eye-hand coordination during learning of a novel visuomotor task. *Journal of Neuroscience, 25,* 8833–8842.
43. Woodworth, R. S. (1899). The accuracy of voluntary movement. *Psychological Review Monographs, 3* (Whole No. 13).
44. Schmidt, R. A., & Lee, T. D. (2005). *Motor control and learning: A behavioral emphasis* (4th ed.). Champaign, IL: Human Kinetics.
45. Fajen, B. R. (2005). Perceiving possibilities for action: on the necessity of calibration and perceptual learning for the visual guidance of action. *Perception, 34,* 717–740.
46. Lee, D. N. (1976). A theory of visual control of braking based on information about time-to-collision. *Perception, 5,* 437–459.
47. Lanska, D. J., & Goetz, C. G. (2000). Romberg's sign: development, adoption, and adaptation in the 19th century. *Historical Neurology, 55,* 1201–1206.
48. Colledge, N. R., Cantley, P., Peaston, I., Brash, H., Lewis, S., & Wilson, J. A. (1994). Ageing and balance: the measurement of spontaneous sway by posturography. *Gerontology, 40,* 273–278.
49. Lê, T., & Kapoula, Z. (2008). Role of ocular convergence in the Romberg quotient. *Gait & Posture, 27,* 493–500.
50. Gill, J., Allum, J. H. J., Carpenter, M. G., Held-Ziolkowska, M., Adkin, A. L., Honegger, F., & Pierchala, K. (2001). Trunk sway measures of postural stability during clinical balance tests: effects of age. *Journal of Gerontology: Medical Sciences, 56A,* M438–M447.
51. Shumway-Cook, A., & Woollacott, M. H. (2001). *Motor control: Theory and practical applications.* Philadelphia, PA: Lippincott Williams & Wilkins.

52. Lord, S. R., Clark, R. D., & Webster, I. W. (1991). Postural stability and associated physiological factors in a population of aged persons. *Journal of Gerontology, 46*(3), M69–M76.

53. Lord, S. R., & Menz, H. B. (2000). Visual contributions to postural stability in older adults. *Gerontology, 46,* 306–310.

54. Lee, D. N., & Aronson, E. (1974). Visual proprioceptive control of standing in human infants. *Perception & Psychophysics, 15,* 529–532.

55. Lee, D. N., & Lishman, J. R. (1975). Visual proprioceptive control of stance. *Journal of Movement Studies, 1,* 87–95.

56. Nashner, L., & Berthoz, A. (1978). Visual contribution to rapid motor responses during postural control. *Brain Research, 150,* 403–407.

57. Trombly, C. A., & Wu, C. Y. (1999). Effect of rehabilitation tasks on organization of movement after stroke. *American Journal of Occupational Therapy, 53,* 333–344.

58. Kielhofner, G. (2004). *Conceptual foundations of occupational therapy* (3rd ed.). Philadelphia, PA: F. A. Davis.

59. Bobath, B. (1969). The treatment of neuromuscular disorders by improving patterns of coordination. *Physiotherapy, 55,* 18–22.

60. Bobath, B. (1970). *Adult hemiplegia: Evaluation and treatment.* London, UK: William Heinemann.

61. Kabat, H., & Knott, M. (1953). Proprioceptive facilitation techniques for treatment of paralysis. *Physical Therapy Review, 33,* 53–64.

62. Knott, M., & Voss, D. E. (1968). *Proprioceptive neuromuscular techniques: Patterns and techniques* (2nd ed.). New York: Harper & Row.

63. Voss, D. E. (1967). Proprioceptive neuromuscular facilitation. *American Journal of Physical Medicine, 46,* 838–898.

64. Rood, M. S. (1954). Neurophysiological reactions as a basis for physical therapy. *Physical Therapy Review, 34,* 444–449.

65. Rood, M. S. (1956). Neurophysiological mechanisms utilized in the treatment of neuro-muscular dysfunction. *American Journal of Occupational Therapy, 10,* 220–225.

66. Rood, M. S. (1962). The use of sensory receptors to activate, facilitate and inhibit motor response, autonomic and somatic, in developmental sequence. In C. Sattely (Ed.), *Approaches to the treatment of patients with neuromuscular dysfunction* (Study Course VI, 3rd International Congress World Federation of Occupational Therapy, pp. 26–37). Dubuque, IA: W. C. Brown.

67. Stockmeyer, S. A. (1967). An interpretation of the approach of Rood to the treatment of neuromuscular dysfunction. *American Journal of Physical Medicine, 46,* 900–956.

68. Brunnstrom, S. (1970). Movement therapy in hemiplegia: a neurophysiological approach. Hagerstown, MD: Harper & Row.

69. Howle, J. (2002). *Neuro-Developmental treatment approach: Theoretical foundations and principles of clinical practice.* Laguna Beach, CA: Neuro-Developmental Treatment Association.

70. Royeen, C. G., & McCormack, G. (2006). Traditional sensorimotor approaches to intervention: section 1: the rood approach: a reconstruction. In H. M. Pendleton, & W. Schultz-Krohn (Eds.), *Pedretti's occupational therapy: Practice skills for physical dysfunction* (6th ed., pp. 735–747). St. Louis, MO: Mosby.

71. Fugl-Meyer, A. R., Jääsko, L., Leyman, I., Olsson, S., & Steglind, S. (1975). The post-stroke hemiplegic patient. I. A method for evaluation of physical performance. *Scandinavian Journal of Rehabilitation Medicine, 7,* 13–31.

72. Lo, A. C., Guarino, P., Krebs, H. I., Volpe, B. T., Bever, C. T., Duncan, P. W., Peduzzi, P. (2009). Multicenter randomized trial of robot-assisted rehabilitation for chronic stroke: methods and entry characteristics for VA ROBOTICS. *Neurorehabilitation and Neural Repair, 23,* 775–783.

73. Bertoti, D. B. (2004). *Functional neurorehabilitation through the life span*. Philadelphia, PA: F. A. Davis.

74. Bass-Haugen, J., Mathiowetz, V., & Flinn, N. (2008). Optimizing motor behavior using the occupational therapy task-oriented approach. In M. V. Radomski & C. A. Trombly Latham (Eds.), *Occupational therapy for physical dysfunction* (6th ed., pp. 598–617). Baltimore, MD: Lippincott Williams & Wilkins.

75. Wolf, S. L., Lecraw, D. E., Barton, L. A., & Jann, B. B. (1989). Forced use of hemiplegic upper extremities to reverse the effect of learned nonuse among chronic stroke and head-injured patients. *Experimental Neurology, 104*, 104–132.

76. Morris, D. M., Taub, E., & Mark, V. W. (2006). Constraint-induced movement therapy: characterizing the intervention protocol. *Europa Medicophysica, 42*, 257–268.

77. Winstein, C. J., Miller, J. P., Blanton, S., Taub, E., Uswatte, G., Morris, D., Nichols, D., & Wolf, S. (2003). Methods for a multisite randomized trial to investigate the effect of constraint-induced movement therapy in improving upper extremity function among adults recovering from a cerebrovascular stroke. *Neurorehabilitation and Neural Repair, 17*, 137–152.

78. Wolf, S. L., Winstein, C. J., Miller, J. P., Taub, E., Uswatte, G., Morris, D., & Nichols-Larsen. (2006). Effect of constraint-induced movement therapy on upper extremity function 3 to 9 months after stroke: the EXCITE randomized clinical trial. *Journal of the American Medical Association, 296*, 2095–2104.

79. Page, S. J., Sisto, S., Levine, P., & McGrath, R. E. (2004). Efficacy of modified constraint-induced movement therapy in chronic stroke: a single-blinded randomized controlled trial. *Archives of Physical Medicine and Rehabilitation, 85*, 14–18.

80. Sirtori, V., Corbetta, D., Moja, L., & Gatti, R. (2009). Constraint-induced movement therapy for upper extremities in stroke patients. *Cochrane Database of Systematic Reviews, (4)*, Art. No.: CD004433. doi: 10.1002/14651858.CD004433.pub2.

81. Quintana, L. A. (2008). Optimizing vision, visual perception, and praxia abilities. In M. V. Radomski, & C. A. Trombly Latham (Eds.), *Occupational therapy for physical dysfunction* (6th ed., pp. 728–747). Philadelphia, PA: Lippincott Williams & Wilkins.

82. Warren, M. (2006). Evaluation and treatment of visual deficits following brain injury. In H. M. Pendelton, & W. Schultz-Krohn (Eds.), *Pedretti's occupational therapy: Practice skills for physical dysfunction* (6th ed., pp. 532–572). St. Louis, MO: Mosby Elsevier.

83. Gentile, M. (2005). *Functional visual behavior in adults: An occupational therapy guide to evaluation and treatment options* (2nd ed.). Bethesda, MD: American Occupational Therapy Association.

84. Scheiman, M. (1997). *Understanding and managing vision deficits: A guide for occupational therapists*. Thorofare, NJ: Slack.

85. Zoltan, B. (2007). *Vision, perception, and cognition: A manual for the evaluation and treatment of the adult with acquired brain injury* (4th ed.). Thorofare, NJ: Slack.

86. Toglia, J. P. (2005). A dynamic interactional approach to cognitive rehabilitation. In N. Katz (Ed.), *Cognition and occupation across the life span: Models for intervention in occupational therapy* (2nd ed., pp. 29–72). Bethesda, MD: American Occupational Therapy Association.

87. Skeffington, A. M. (1988). *Introduction to clinical optometry* (revised edition). Santa Ana, CA: Optometric Extension Program.

88. Press, L. J. (2008). *Foundations of vision therapy*. Santa Ana, CA: Optometric Extension Program.

89. Han, Y., Ciuffreda, K. J., & Kapoor, N. (2004). Reading-related testing and training protocols for acquired brain injury in humans. *Brain Research, Brain Research Protocols, 14*(1), 1–12.

90. Schor, C. (2009) Neuromuscular plasticity and rehabilitation of the ocular near response. *Optometry and Vision Science, 86*, E788–E802.

91. Schrock, R. E, Heinsen, A. C. (1966). *Schur-Mark out-of-office training system.* Meadville PA: Keystone View Co.

92. Rutner, D., Kapoor, N., Ciuffreda, K. J., Suchoff, I. B., Craig, S., & Han, M. E. (2007). Frequency of occurrence and treatment of ocular disease in symptomatic individuals with acquired brain injury: a clinical management perspective. *Journal of Behavioral Optometry, 18*(2), 31–36.

93. Buckley, J. G., Heasley, K., Scally A., & Elliott, D. B. (2005). The effects of blurring vsion on medio-lateral balance during stepping up or down to a new level in the elderly. *Gait & Posture, 22*(2), 146–153.

94. Lord, S. R., Dayhew, J., & Howland, A. (2002). Multifocal glasses impair edge-contrast sensitivity and depth perception and increse the risk of falls in older people. *Journal of the American Geriatrics Society, 50,* 1760–1766.

95. Leslie, S. (2001). Accommodation in acquired brain injury. In I. B. Suchoff, K. J. Ciuffreda, & N. Kapoor (Eds.), *Visual and vestibular consequences of acquired brain injury* (pp. 56–76). Santa Ana, CA: Optometric Extension Program.

96. Barry, S. (2009). *Fixing my gaze: A scientist's journey into seeing in three dimensions.* New York: Basic Books.

97. Cohen, A. H., & Rein, L. D. (1992). The effect of head trauma on the visual system: the doctor of optometry as a member of the rehabilitation team. *Journal of the American Optometric Association, 63,* 530–536.

98. Scheiman, M., & Gallaway, M. (2001). Vision therapy to treat binocular vision disorders after acquired brain injury; factors affecting prognosis. In I. B. Suchoff, K. J. Ciuffreda, & N. Kapoor (Eds.), *Visual and vestibular consequences of acquired brain injury* (pp. 89–113). Santa Ana, CA: Optometric Extension Program.

99. Padula, W. V., Argyris, S., & Ray, J. (1994). Visual evoked potentials (VEP) evaluating treatment for post-trauma vision syndrome (PTVS) in patients with traumatic brain injuries (TBI). *Brain Injury, 8*(2), 125–133.

100. Ciuffreda, K. J., Kapoor, N., Rutner, D., Suchoff, I. B., Han, M. E., & Craig, S. (2007). Occurrence of oculomotor dysfunctions in acquired brain injury: A retrospective analysis. *Optometry, 78*(4), 155–161.

101. Colby, D., Laukkanen, H. R., & Yolton, R. (1998). Use of the Taylor Visagraph II system to evaluate eye movements made during reading. *Journal of the American Optometric Association, 69,* 22–32.

102. Garzia, R. P., Richman, J. E., Nicholson, S. B., & Gaines, C. S. (1990). A new visual-verbal saccade test: The Developmental Eye Movement Test (DEM). *Journal of the American Optometric Association, 61*(2), 124–135.

103. Powell, J. M., Birk, K., Cummings, E. H., & Ciol, M. (2005). The need for adult norms on the Developmental Eye Movement Test (DEM). *Journal of Behavioral Optometry, 16*(2), 38–41.

104. Powell, J. M., Fan, M., Kiltz, P. J., Bergman, A. T., & Richman, J. (2006). A comparison of the Developmental Eye Movement Test (DEM) and a modified version of the Adult Developmental Eye Movement Test (A-DEM) with older adults. *Journal of Behavioral Optometry, 17,* 59–64.

105. Warren M. (1998). *The biVABA: Brain injury visual assessment battery for adults.* Birmingham, AL: visAbilitiies Rehab Services.

106. Gianutsos, R. (1997). Vision rehabilitation following acquired brain injury. In M. Gentile (Ed.), *Functional visual behavior: A therapist's guide to evaluation and treatment options* (pp. 267–295). Bethesda, MD: American Occupational Therapy Association.

107. Neistadt, M. E. (2000). *Occupational therapy evaluation for adults: A pocket guide.* Baltimore, MD: Lippincott Williams & Wilkins.

108. Brewer, B. R., Klatzky, R., & Matsuoka, Y. (2008). Visual feedback distortion in a robotic environment for hand rehabilitation. *Brain Research Bulletin, 75,* 804–813.

11 Acquired Brain Injury and Visual Information Processing Deficits

Sidney Groffman

CONTENTS

Not only our pleasure, our joy and our laughter but also our sorrow, pain, grief and tears arise from the brain. With it we think and understand, see and hear, and we discriminate between the ugly and the beautiful, between what is pleasant and what is unpleasant and between good and evil. Within the head's spherical body is the divinest part of us and lord over all the rest.

Hippocrates

INTRODUCTION

Acquired brain injury (ABI) includes a number of insults to the brain, including traumatic brain injury (TBI), cerebral vascular accident (CVA)/stroke, substance abuse, disease (e.g., Parkinson's disease, multiple sclerosis), and surgical mishaps.[1] The ABI patient often exhibits a multitude of physical and neurological disabilities and symptoms that may be apparent to even untrained observers. Less obvious perceptuo-cognitive impairments are often overlooked during the rehabilitation process. It is obviously necessary that the focus of treatment in the early stage of an injury be directed toward life-threatening conditions and physical injuries. However, all too often hidden information processing, emotional, and social issues are ignored or overlooked even in the later stages of rehabilitation.[2] Unfortunately, these issues may be the determinants of placement, return to work, school, and subsequent adjustment to daily living.

Traumatic brain injury is the most frequent cause of admission to a neurology ward.[3] Epidemiological research on TBI indicates that TBI is a leading cause of morbidity, mortality, disability, and economic loss in the world. In the United States, approximately 2 million TBIs are estimated to occur each year.[4]

Mild traumatic brain injury (mTBI), commonly known as concussion, is one of the commonest neurological disorders. Seventy-five percent of all brain-injured patients sustain mTBI. Early mTBI symptoms may appear mild, but they can lead to significant, life-long impairment in an individual's ability to function physically, cognitively, and psychologically with a substantial number of them experiencing persistent disabling problems.

VISUAL INFORMATION PROCESSING

Among the many sequelae of ABI are impairments in visual information processing. Visual information processing is the active process of locating, extracting, and interpreting visual information from the environment. The terms visual information processing and visual perception processing can be used interchangeably. Deficits in visual perception are common and persistent in ABI and can be academically, socially, and vocationally disabling. They are characterized by difficulties in attention, memory, speed of processing, spatial orientation, spatial relations, perceptual organization, and fine motor skills. They affect learning ability, thinking, creativity, and other aspects of cognition and motor function. Perception is the core process in acquisition of knowledge. Forgus[5] conceptualized perception "as the superset, with learning and thinking as subsets subsumed under the perceptual process." Information processing can be viewed as a process of interacting with the external environment by means of a myriad of skills.[6] These skills require a high degree of integration and analysis of the environment, particularly when the environment involves abstract, unfamiliar, and detailed visual information or conditions under which distinctive visual features are partially obscured.[7] Perception steers us through our lives, and acts as a guide. Perceptual knowledge is pervasive in our daily lives. As Bolles[8] put it,

> It is foremost in our dreams, our attentive examinations, our associations, and our creative musings. Perception keeps us oriented, evaluates experiences, engages us with the day...When we do turn to symbolic reasoning—be it verbal, scientific, or mathematical—we still have not done with perception, for reason's details and form comes through perceptions. (pp. xxii–xxiii)

VISUAL PERCEPTION DEFICITS FOLLOWING TRAUMATIC BRAIN INJURY

Traumatic brain injury is a universal public health problem. An incidence of 235 hospitalized cases per 100,000 populations has been reported in Europe. In the United States, the incidence is estimated at 150 per 100,000 population. These incidence rates do not include individuals who are not hospitalized. The actual incidence may be 3–4 times larger than the number reported.[9] In recent years the number for the United States has undoubtedly increased substantially because "TBI has been tagged the signature injury of the Global War on Terror."[10] A number of studies indicate that moderate to severe TBI result in visual information processing deficits.[11–15]

SPEED OF INFORMATION PROCESSING

> If speed deserves any weight in determining the measures of intellect it is by virtue of the principle that other things being equal, the more quickly a person produces the correct response, the greater is his intelligence
>
> **Edward Thorndike**

Processing speed is a fundamental mechanism of cognitive development.[16] It is a common observation that many TBI patients can successfully complete various perceptuo-cognitive tasks if given prolonged time, but they do poorly if time limits are imposed.

Disorders in speed of information processing refer to difficulty in the following:

1. Quickly registering incoming information,
2. Rapid cognitive processing of the material, and/or
3. Rapid output[13]

Consequently these individuals often miss pertinent information, and misperceive the essence of incoming stimuli. They may be slow in the simplest tasks and in most learning, avocational, and vocational situations. Problems with speed of processing represent a common long-term symptom following TBI.[14] Processing speed is analogous to the operating speed of the central processing unit (CPU) of a microcomputer. This speed is for all practical purposes, fixed for a given CPU, and consequently is to be considered a part of the architecture of the computer in which it is installed. Differences in rate of processing are explained in terms of the complexities of the electronic circuitry. Similarly, processing speed can be linked to the complexities of neural development, function, and health. Neurological changes have been linked to changes in processing speed.

Evidence that mild to moderate to severe ABI results in slowed speed of information processing spans several decades.[15] It is associated with normal aging,[17] TBI,[18] and several neurological diseases.[19] The more severe the ABI the more severe is the deficit in speed of processing.[20] Converging evidence in nonclinical and clinical samples suggests slower processing speed may mediate some higher-order cognitive deficits.[21] In a study by Ponsford and Kinsella,[22] a TBI group was significantly slower on all speeded tasks, compared with healthy normal controls. The authors concluded that following TBI, there was a tradeoff between speed and accuracy in performance, where quality of performance could improve by slowing down speed. Likewise, Madigan and her associates[23] assessed speed of information processing in TBI, and found that speed of information processing is a major impairment in those with TBI when not confounded by performance accuracy. By manipulating information at a pace customized for an individual through compensatory strategies and environmental modifications, they concluded that the performance could be enhanced significantly. They also examined speed of processing in a dual modality format (auditory-visual) that resulted in greater impairment in the TBI group. Battistone[24] and her associates conducted another speed-accuracy experiment. These studies have significance for vision rehabilitation therapy (VRT). In devising a therapy program for processing speed we must consider the presentation speed of stimuli, size of targets, number of targets, and other factors. We should also use auditory-visual integration and other intermodal therapy for these patients.

Felmingham, Baguley, and Green[25] tested the hypothesis that slowed information processing in TBI is related to diffuse axonal injury (DAI). The authors compared 10 severe TBI patients with predominant DAI with 10 severe TBI patients with minimal DAI on the Symbol Digits Modalities Test, Reaction Time, Trailmaking Tests A&B, and the Stroop Neuropsychological Screening Test. The predominant DAI group was slower than the minimal and control groups on these tests of speed of information processing. This study confirms the importance of speed of processing following TBI and suggests that slower speed of processing mediates more complex cognitive deficits in TBI.

Reaction time (RT) tests have been utilized often to evaluate speed of information processing. Stuss[26] and his associates compared three groups of patients who had suffered severe head injury with matched control groups on RT tests. The findings indicate that TBI causes slower information processing, deficits in divided attention, an impairment of focused attention, and inconsistency of performance. An interesting multisensory experiment by a German group[27] studied RT between pairings of vision, touch, and audition. Since almost all events stimulate several senses simultaneously, any appropriate behavioral responses relies upon the ability to integrate the information in each sensory channel. They compared 35 patients with severe TBI to a normal group on RT with four attentional and sensory combinations:

1. Visual-visual task
2. Visual-auditory task
3. Visual-tactile task
4. Auditory-tactile task

The following conclusions can be drawn from this study. RTs were prolonged in TBI patients. The fastest reactions were in response to auditory stimuli followed by visual and tactile stimuli. The TBI group showed a significantly larger intraindividual variability than the control group. Such variability in performance is considered as a very good parameter of attention deficits after TBI. RTs in TBI patients are strongly influenced by the physical features of the stimuli. This study also has implications for VRT. Malojcic et al.[28] explored the impact of mTBI upon short-term memory (STM) or working memory (WM) and attention. The performance of 37 individuals with mTBI was compared with that of 53 age-, sex-, and education-matched controls. A battery of computerized tests measured sustained visual attention, STM, simple RT, and decision time. Subjects with mTBI showed performance deficits at sustained visual attention, STM, scanning, and a trend toward slowing in decision making. These changes in the cognitive performance of persons with mTBI were hypothesized to be a consequence of impaired central information processing. The authors feel that their results support several premises. The first is that individuals who have suffered mTBI may still show symptoms more than 6 weeks postinjury. A second conclusion is that complaints of cognitive deficit, while not often supported by standard imaging or neuropsychological examinations, represent real cognitive deficits. Finally, their data suggest that the nature of these deficits lies almost wholly in controlled, not automatic cognitive processes,[29] which indicates that some central measure of resource or decision making is being disrupted in individuals who experience residual visual information processing deficits. This supports optometric management with VRT for these patients.

MEMORY DEFICITS

The true art of memory is attention.

Samuel Johnson

Disturbances in memory functioning are among the most marked and persistent effects of TBI. The effects of this impairment on individuals have been found to be long term, debilitating, and a major obstacle to rehabilitation.[30] Many researchers will point to memory as being the most common symptom after mild, moderate, and severe brain injury.[31] Memory deficits due to TBI have been reported to occur in 69%–80% of victims.[32] The severity of TBI, which is typically determined at the time of injury with the Glasgow Coma Scale (see Chapter 12, Appendix 12.1), is related to both the degree and persistence of the resulting memory deficit, with more severe injuries resulting in greater deficits.[33] In a large proportion of people with severe TBI, these memory impairments will be permanent. Longitudinal studies do not demonstrate significant decreases in complaints of memory deficits following severe TBI, even at 7 years postinjury.[34]

Memory deficits can profoundly impact a person's day-to-day functioning, often preventing them from returning to work, or impacting their capacity to engage in independent living.[35] The impairment affects the encoding and retrieval of both verbal and visual materials equally, because TBI typically affects both the right and left temporal lobes.[36] The importance of visual memory impairment should not be underestimated for a number of reasons. The ability to remember visual patterns and spatial positions is essential in a number of occupations such as graphic design, architecture, drafting, painting, sculpture, clothes designing, chauffeuring, and piloting a plane. Visual memory impairment in individuals engaged in these and similar occupations can significantly affect their chances of returning to work. Indeed, it has been reported[37] that visual memory is an important predictor of general employability in people with ABI. The ability to remember visual patterns and spatial relations is also important for everyday activities such as remembering where one has placed an object or finding one's way around in a new environment. Difficulty with these activities can lead to frustration, embarrassment, or even risk. A number of investigators have found significant visual memory deficits following mild to severe TBI.[38] For these reasons, the assessment of memory abilities should include a comprehensive and accurate assessment of visual as well as verbal memory. A concussive or mTBI can result in deficits in the early period following the trauma, including reduced processing speed, visual attention, spatial problems, and memory, However, some reviews indicate that a single uncomplicated mTBI is inconsequential and without residual impairment in the long term. Bernstein,[39] however, claims that subtle, long lasting cognitive changes may be present, and can prevent a complete return to preinjury levels. Blakely and Harrington[40] examined the concept that mTBI involves an essentially reversible physiological process and found it to be largely invalid. They concluded that long-term impairment is fairly common and that the degree of impairment can be assessed clinically.

Other studies,[41,42] have reported that memory span for locations and visual-spatial short-term memory were discernible effects of head injury. Chuah et al.[43] investigated the long-term effects of mTBI on visual, spatial, and visual-spatial STM on 16 well-functioning university students. In other words, they compared memory for polygon shapes (visual), locations (spatial), and polygon shapes in their locations (visual spatial). The study demonstrated that spatial STM tasks may be more sensitive compared to visual STM tasks, in the subtle long-term cognitive deficits related to mTBI.

Working memory refers to the ability to hold and manipulate information in the mind over short periods of time. WM is a kind of mental workspace that is used to store information in the course of everyday activities. A good example of an activity that uses WM is mental arithmetic. Solving the arithmetic problem $45 \times 63 = ?$ presented to you verbally, without being able to use a calculator or pencil and paper, is an example of WM. Baddeley[44] introduced and made popular the multicomponent model of WM. This theory proposes that two "slave systems" are responsible for the short-term maintenance of information and a "central executive" is responsible for information integration and for coordinating the slave systems. One slave system, the phonological loop, stores phonological information and prevents its decay by continually articulating its contents. The other slave system, the visuospatial sketch pad, stores visual and spatial information. It can be used for constructing and manipulating visual images and for the representation of mental maps. The sketch pad can be further broken down into a visual subsystem dealing with a "what" visual component (pattern, shape, color, texture, and so on) and a spatial subsystem dealing with a "where" component (location, movement, and orientation). WM is one of our most crucial perceptuo-cognitive capabilities, essential for countless daily tasks such as following directions, remembering information momentarily, complex reasoning, or staying focused on a project. WM deficits are common sequelae of TBI. Finke et al.[45] found that damage to the left parietal lobe resulted in "What" WM impairment, while right parietal injury was associated with both "What" and "Where" deficits. Nonparietal injury was not associated with comparable deficits. These results suggest that spatial WM depends critically on right parietal areas; in contrast, visual WM depends on both left and right parietal areas. VRT can be helpful in ameliorating WM.

Spatial Deficits/Perceptual Organization

> Pooh looked at his two paws. He knew that one of them was the right, and he knew that when you had decided which one of them was the right, then the other was the left, but he could never remember where to begin.
>
> **A.A. Milne**

Spatial problems are often reported after TBI. Visual-spatial skills are necessary for internal and external spatial concepts and are used to interact with and organize the environment. They allow us to make judgments about location of objects in visual space, in reference to other objects and to the individuals own body space.[46]

Spatial disturbances are apparent on perceptual testing. The individual may experience difficulty with figure-ground discrimination, visual closure, form perception, spatial orientation, right-left discrimination, analysis of visual information, spatial manipulation, and visualization. These deficits tend to compound the inability to perceive information accurately in everyday situations or in a social context. Visuospatial deficits are often reported after TBI but few studies have documented the presence of complex visuospatial information processing deficits in children after a mTBI. Brosseau-Lachaine et al.[47] felt it was important to assess children's visual perception after mTBI to ensure a safer return to their activities and sports. In their study, they compared the sensitivity to complex visual information processing of children who have sustained a mTBI to that of noninjured children matched for age. Sensitivity to static and dynamic forms of simple and complex stimuli were assessed at 1-week postinjury for 12 injured children and controls, aged 8–16 years of age. Results indicate that the sensitivity to all complex stimuli was significantly reduced for the mTBI children while sensitivity to simple information remained within the normal range.

Perceptual organization is a basic component of visual processing in which individual components of a visual scene are resolved into a series of unified forms.[48] Perceptual organization is an essential process that serves to organize stimuli in preparation for high-order visual functions. It is the process by which the bits and pieces of visual information that are available in the retinal image are structured into the larger units of perceived objects and their interrelations.[49] Figure-ground perception, a fundamental aspect of perceptual organization, entails segregating and identifying visual input into shaped figures presented against blank or confusing backgrounds.[50] Find the hidden picture is a classic illustration of figure-ground visual perception. Perceptual organization is how we process sensory information in context[51] and disruption at the level of perceptual organization can interfere with the subsequent processing of object recognition or exacerbate deficits in other cognitive processes such as memory.[52] Perceptual organization is established from a variety of spatial and temporal relationships. Spatial relationships include proximity and regularity in position, as well as similarity in luminance, shape, or color.[53] A specific index of Perceptual Organization can be obtained from three subtests of the Wechsler Adult Intelligence Scale-R: Picture Completion, Block Design, and Matrix Reasoning. These three tests require extensive spatial abilities that respond to VRT. Disruption of perceptual organization skills resulting from TBI have been associated with reduced performance on the Hooper Visual Organization Test, used to assess visuospatial abilities.[54]

Kurylo et al.[55] completed a study examining perceptual organization following TBI. They compared the perceptual organization characteristics of a TBI group with a control group. Participants viewed stimuli that could be perceptually grouped as either vertical or horizontal lines. There were four tests that were based on either spatial proximity or temporal contrast (flicker). The stimuli were briefly presented on a computer monitor. The results identified impairment at the level of perceptual organization that resulted from TBI. Deficits were evident as elevated grouping thresholds, as well as reduction in information processing speed. These findings are clinically significant because perceptual organization occurs at an early or intermediate level of visual processing. Impairment is likely to degrade performance on other perceptual and cognitive functions that occur at any stage of processing. High-order visual processing, including spatial relationships and the identification of common objects and familiar faces, may be impaired. Similarly, perceptual organization can impact performance on visual STM, visual search, and selective attention.

The influence of factors such as TBI, education, perceptual organization, and speed of information processing on performance on the Rey Complex Figure Test (RCF) was examined by Ashton et al.[56] The RCF is a task that involves the copying and subsequent reproduction from memory of a complex geometric design. As is the case with many other tests designed to measure visual memory, performance on a test like the RCF that requires visual-motor skill can potentially be confounded by perceptual organization and other abilities.[57] Meyers and Meyers[58] concluded that RCF variables are associated with perceptual organization skills, visual scanning, and attention, but not language or verbal fluency abilities. The objective of this study was to determine which variables predicted performance on the RCF. Higher levels of perceptual organization skills, as assessed by the WAIS-III, and to a lesser extent the absence of a diffuse injury were both predictive of better performance on the recall and recognition trials of the RCF. These factors were not strongly correlated suggesting they contributed independently to RCF performance. Level of education did not impact performance on the RCF above and beyond perceptual organization skills. They concluded that RCF performance of persons with TBI is affected primarily by premorbid levels of perceptual organization and to a relatively lesser effect by injury severity characteristics.

REHABILITATION INTERVENTIONS AFTER BRAIN INJURY

Ponsford[59] reviewed a variety of interventions including the following:

- Educational information about mTBI symptoms and reassurance that these are likely to recover. There is some weak evidence for the effectiveness of early education, reassurance, and encouragement to return to activities gradually.
- Treatment with medication or homeopathy. Evidence regarding effectiveness of pharmacological treatment is weak with only one study showing a positive impact of a selective serotonin reuptake inhibitor, sertraline, on depressive symptoms and cognitive functions. One other study showed a positive effect of a range of homeopathic remedies.
- Psychological therapy, particularly for the "miserable minority" who experience protracted symptoms. This therapy aims to demonstrate to the patients that their symptoms are common following mTBI and that their inner dialogue may be increasing stress levels and to equip them with strategies to manage and have a sense of mastery over symptoms and take control of their lifestyle. Cognitive remedial intervention may also be offered to assist in overcoming or managing cognitive difficulties. Although there are some case examples of success, there is as yet limited empirical evidence to demonstrate the impact of these therapies.
- Ponsford also reviewed the optometric work of Kapoor et al.[60] citing their success in improving versional oculomotor accuracy, reading ability, and visual scanning. She also called for the replication of this research.

Carter and colleagues[61] examined whether a cognitive skills remediation program could help acute stroke patients regain important thinking skills. Therapy consisting of workbooks, simple cuing procedures, positive reinforcement, and immediate feedback, were administered for visual scanning, visual-spatial orientation, and time judgment for 30 minutes a day for 3 weeks. Patients receiving treatment had overall and separate skill improvement scores that were significantly higher than those for control patients.

Subitizing is the immediate visual-perceptual apprehension and enumeration of a small set of items. Subitizing deficits are correlated with difficulty in mathematics at all age levels. Subitizing therapy is vision therapy for subitizing and math deficits.[62] Recent research in subitizing using computerized programs shows great promise. Wilson et al.[63] describe the design of software for training tasks involving subitizing for small quantities of items and a combination of subitizing and counting for larger quantities of items. The results of a limited clinical research project showed significant ($p = .0003$) improvement RTs and accuracy of subitizing between the pre- and post-tests. Fischer and his associates[64] completed a study in which visual stimuli were flashed on a computer at fast exposures. Subjects were selected on the basis of their poor performance in subitizing and arithmetic basic skills. The test group contained 74 subjects in the age range of 7–14 years. After training, the number of children who reached the subitizing range of the normal control children was estimated at 85%. Improvement in certain arithmetic skills was highly significant ($p = .0001$).

Cognitive remediation is a behavioral intervention utilized by some psychologists and other therapists, as a treatment, in part, for the decline in visual information processing following ABI. Thickpenny-Davis and Barker-Coles[65] examined the efficacy of a structured memory rehabilitation group (MRG) for adults following brain injury. Participants were 12 individuals with TBI and 2 with CVA whose caregivers reported presence of memory deficits for a period of at least 12 months. A battery of standardized tests and two questionnaires was employed. The memory group consists of eight learning modules held as 60-minute sessions twice a week over 4 weeks. In each session, material was presented using a combination of didactic teaching about memory and memory strategies, small group activities, and both problem solving and practice implementing memory strategies. The study indicates that the MRG is a viable format for memory rehabilitation. Participation significantly increased the use of memory aids and strategies, increased the knowledge of memory and memory strategies, and significantly reduced self-rated behaviors indicative of memory impairment.

A widely used cognitive training program is the Amsterdam Memory and Attention Training for Children (AMAT-C) developed at the Karolinska Institute in Stockholm, Sweden. It consists of structured exercises in specific attention and memory techniques for half an hour a day in school or a private office for a period of 17–20 weeks. In one study,[66] an experimental group of 18 children with ABI, working with a cognitive training program, was compared on measures of memory and attention with a group of 20 control subjects who were involved with supportive adults in interactive activity of equal length and intensity, but no directed remediation . Statistically significant improvement within the experimental group was demonstrated on sustained and short-term attention tests and a delayed word memory test, compared to no changes in the control group. Significant changes were not seen in both groups on a measure of RT and immediate recall of words.

Edwards et al.[67] trained older adults with speed of processing therapy and concluded that it may enhance the speed at which older adults can perform instrumental activities of daily living. Another paper[68] combined data from six studies using the same speed of processing training program; results indicated that training produces immediate improvements across all subtests of the Useful Field of View test as well as activities of daily living. Participants maintained benefits of training for at least 2 years.

Ball et al.[69] used a randomized, controlled, single-blind trial with a sample of 2,832 persons aged 65–94 years, in six metropolitan areas, to evaluate whether three training interventions improve mental activities and daily functioning. There was a 2-year follow up. Participants were randomly assigned to one of four groups: 10-session group training for memory, or reasoning, or speed of processing, or a no-contact control group. Results showed that each intervention improved the targeted cognitive ability compared with baseline, durable to 2 years ($p < .001$ for all). Most (87% of speed trained, 74% of reasoning trained, and 26% of memory trained) participants demonstrated reliable improvement immediately after the therapy period. Booster training enhanced gains in speed and reasoning, which were maintained at 2-year follow up. *While this study did not use ABI patients, the basic principles utilized apply for ABI patients. The size and procedures of the study are exemplary and provide evidence that VRT can improve visual memory, reasoning, and speed of processing.*

EVALUATION FOR VISION PERCEPTION DEFICITS IN ACQUIRED BRAIN INJURY

Perception is the core process in acquisition of knowledge. Perceptual knowledge and skills are pervasive in our daily lives. Perception is a mosaic of many different ability areas. It is not a simple unitary process but is, in fact, an amalgam of many different skill sets. ABI may affect none, some, or all of these skills and our evaluation should determine the pattern of perceptual strengths and weaknesses of each patient. Even though the most common deficits in ABI patients are speed of information processing, visual memory, and spatial deficits/perceptual organization, a detailed pattern of the patient's visual information processing must be obtained before optimum management of the patient can be decided. The perceptual abilities to be evaluated, when possible, include the following:

- Visual form perception (visual closure, figure-ground, visual organization)
- Spatial relations (spatial reasoning, visual imagery, spatial perception
- Spatial orientation (laterality, directionality)
- Visual cognition (visual thinking, visual manipulation)
- Visual-motor integration (visual stimulus motor response)
- Information processing speed (perceptual speed, automaticity, motor speed, rapid automatized naming)
- Visual memory (visual-spatial memory, visual sequential memory, WM)
- Auditory memory (digit span, word sequences)
- Auditory-visual integration (auditory stimulus-visual response)
- Eye-hand coordination (fine motor skills)

A complete perceptual evaluation is necessary to determine the management strategies for patients with ABI. The information obtained is useful for the following:

- Planning specific therapy regimens
- Obtaining baseline measurements
- Indicating additional testing
- Deciding need for referral to other professionals
- Aiding referral sources in their management of the patient
- Judging outcome efficacy of the VRT
- Assessing outcomes of other therapies as they relate to visual information processing
- Evaluating progress and reexamining patient
- Research

Types of Evaluation

Two types of evaluation are commonly used to assess perceptual skills: a formal standardized assessment and an informal observational assessment. "A psychological measurement, even though it is based on observable responses, would have little meaning or usefulness unless it could be interpreted in light of an underlying theoretical construct" (Crocker and Algina, p. 7).[70] Formal assessment utilizes a fixed battery of standardized tests, based on a valid theory of modern thinking, to collect data, and employs specified established analytical procedures for analysis, conclusions, and recommendations. Formal assessment is a deductive process in which the clinician specifies the ability to be evaluated and then selects a valid instrument that will yield information about the ability of interest. The process can be replicated with other patients or by other examiners. The obtained results are quantitative and allow comparison with established norms.

> "Observe what a man does: listen to what he says. How then can you not know what he is?"
>
> **Confucius**

Informal assessment allows for much variation in procedure. It involves a range of inductive reasoning strategies, but the distinguishing factor is the absence of standardized mechanisms as a means of data collection. Most of the perceptual tasks that we ask our patients to do can be solved in a variety of ways. Standardized tests yield scores that reflect the level of performance. The clinician must also determine the nature of the problem. What is the quality of the performance as opposed to the quantity of the performance? An observational assessment does not lend itself to formal standardized procedures but typically relies on a binary decision process. We are essentially interested in the following:

- Does the patient have the relevant skill and knowledge to complete the task?
- Can the patient demonstrate it in an appropriately organized and automatic fashion?
- What is the working style the patient uses to approach the task?
- What is the problem-solving strategy by which a solution is reached?
- What are the behavioral aspects exhibited when the patient is under stress?

The process of testing individuals places them under stress by the very nature of the task. The behavioral controls (often dependent on the extent of the head injury and other factors) exhibited by the patient provides us with relevant information. During both formal and informal testing, a clinician should observe the following:

- Head position and head activity
- Paper position and paper rotations
- Pencil grasp
- Speed of working
- Effort expended
- Attention span, concentration, and distractibility
- Reflectivity versus impulsivity
- Verbalization
- Ability to follow directions
- Flexibility
- Frustration level
- Fatigue

- Cooperation
- Physical impediments to performance
- Emotional lability
- Hyper or hypoactivity
- Visual disabilities

While flexibility on the part of the clinician during the assessment process is important for all patients, it may even be more vital for ABI patients. Any of the above factors may affect the choice of tests, the length of the battery, and the validity of the results. Flexibility in administering the evaluation will improve the ability to collect meaningful data. It is necessary that we distinguish between testing and assessment. Although test results contribute significantly to the ultimate diagnosis, patient management decisions rely on careful consideration of presenting problems, symptoms, prior history, psychological and social problems, physical status, and impressions gleaned from observations during the evaluation. Functional vision diagnosis is both a science and an art. Clinical acumen may modify, or even in some situations, supersede testing. *Tests do not diagnose, people do!*

Prognosis
The prognosis for recovery of brain-injured patients depends on three factors:

1. Severity of the brain injury—The more damage to the brain, the less optimistic is the degree of improvement. This information may be obtained from the neurological records. Pertinent information including the length of unconsciousness, how long was required for the patient's physical recovery. the extent of other bodily injuries, the amount and nature of drugs the patient is taking, can aid in assessing prognosis.
2. Premorbidity—Patient's preinjury intelligence, skills, and abilities in damaged areas are important. This information may be obtained from academic records, family and friends, occupation, interests, and hobbies.
3. Motivation—The motivation of the patient to improve is a key factor in determining a prognosis. Will the patient keep appointments in a timely and regular manner? Will he or she cooperate in the prescribed office or out of office therapy procedures? Is attitude upbeat or morbid?

Questions to Help Evaluate Perceptual Tests
Following are the questions that are used to help evaluate perceptual tests:[71]

1. Does the test fit into a battery of tests based on a valid underlying theoretical construct?
2. Is the test observational or standardized?
3. Is the test reliable?
4. Is the test valid?
5. Is the test age appropriate for the patient we are evaluating?
6. Does the test aid us in prescribing therapeutic procedures?

TABLE 11.1
Comparison of Informal and Formal Assessment Procedures

Informal Assessment	Formal Assessment
Inductive	Deductive
Standardized	Nonstandardized
Observational	Testable
Qualitative	Quantitative
Standards may be subjective	Standards are objective
Patients judged against self	Patients judged against group

Comparison of Informal and Formal Assessment Procedures

Refer Table 11.1 for comparison of informal and formal assessment procedures.[72]

Specific Perceptual Tests for Acquired Brain Injury

1. Spatial relations/perceptual organization
2. Hooper Visual Organization (WPS)
3. Developmental Test of Visual-Motor Integration-5 (Pearson)
4. Southern California Test of Visual Figure-Ground (WPS)
5. DTLA-4 Symbolic Relations (Pro-ed)
6. Minnesota Spatial Relations Test (American Guidance)

Speed of Information Processing

1. Symbol Digit Modalities Test (WPS)
2. Rapid Automatized Naming (Pro-ed)
3. Grooved Pegboard (Lafayette)
4. Tachistoscope (HTS)

Memory

1. DTLA-4 Design Sequences (Pro-ed)
2. TOMAL-2 Memory for Location (WPS)
3. TOMAL-2 Visual Sequential Memory (WPS)
4. TOMAL-2 Manual Imitation (WPS)
5. WRAML-2 Symbolic Working Memory (WPS)

See Appendix 11.1 for publisher information.

THERAPY FOR VISUAL PERCEPTION DEFICITS FOLLOWING ACQUIRED BRAIN INJURY

Optometric Vision Rehabilitation Therapy

Behavioral optometrists have been involved in treating ABI for 50 years, but in recent years optometric interest has multiplied at a rapid pace. Suter[73] terms it an evolving subspecialty in optometry. In 2000, the College of Optometrists in Vision Development requested its Committee on Rehabilitative Optometry, to draft a paper providing information specific to vision and TBI. In conjunction with the executive members of the Neuro-Optometric Rehabilitation Association (NORA) the committee started a 2-year project and resulted in an excellent paper published in 2003.[74] Cohen and Rein[75] contend that optometrists are uniquely qualified to diagnose and treat visual and functional deficits of the brain-injured population and call for optometric participation in the rehabilitation of head trauma and stroke patients. Gianutos and Suchoff[76] write that optometrists are sometimes the first health-care professional to encounter the patient who has undiagnosed ABI. The implication of this is that we have a responsibility to help the patient, and Gianutos and Suchoff detail procedures to follow in the work up. There are a variety of modalities that optometrists employ in managing the visual problems associated with ABI.[77] Glasses to correct refractive errors, prism glasses for fusional problems, yoked prisms for spatial inattention or visual field defect, tinted glasses for photosensitivity, vision therapy for all varieties of binocular problems, referral for patients with complex diplopia, and vision therapy for information processing deficits. Suter[78] describes specific vision therapy and four illustrative case reports for perceptual deficits following ABI.

Occupational Visual-Perceptual Therapy

When patients are seen in both acute and postacute rehabilitation centers, the occupational therapist is often the first rehabilitation personnel to screen for visual-perceptual disorders (see Chapter 2). Occupational therapists are in-house staff at most rehabilitation centers, and have a tradition of working with patients with ABI on remediation of visual-perceptual deficits. Thus, it is most efficient, when a patient is in a rehabilitation center setting, for the occupational therapist to administer visual-perceptual remediation. While it is certainly true that some progress can be made for most patients by an occupational therapist trained in this area, many occupational therapists, rehabilitation centers, and case managers are realizing that this treatment should be performed in collaboration with an optometrist who has specialized training in VRT. While some occupational therapists have special training in visual perception and most have training in visual-motor integration (particularly from the motor aspects of visual-motor integration), the neuro-optometrist (or functional or behavioral optometrist) has access to important information about the patient's visual sensory, binocular, and spatial perception status, which will affect the vision rehabilitation applied. Optometrists who are involved in vision therapy or VRT also have experience in applying a broad knowledge base on vision to the rehabilitation therapy.

KEYS TO SUCCESSFUL THERAPY

The improvement of perceptual disabilities through VRT involves active participation in what are often long, tedious, and repetitive activities. It soon becomes evident to patients, and their families, that a significant amount of effort and cooperation is required of them. Motivation is a key factor, and it is essential to maintain a high rate of success in therapeutic activities.[79] It is important that therapists provide success reinforcement, employ cognitive and metacognitive techniques, encourage patients and their families, avoid frustrating the patient, and use perceptual vision therapy materials that are rewarding, pleasurable, and within the patient's capability.

If a patient fails at a VRT procedure, it is not his or her fault, it is our fault for not programming correctly.[80]

> Alice came to a crossroads and was thinking about which way to go. She asked the Cheshire cat who was in a nearby tree, "Which road should I take?" The cat asked, "Where are you going?" Alice replied, "I don't know," "Well, then," said the cat, "Any road will get you there."

Lewis Carroll

A variety of techniques should be used to improve motivation and cooperation, since no one individual modality or procedure is a panacea. There is no magical effectiveness in any given technique and the context in which it is used is as important as the instrument itself. This context consists of the manner in which patients work with their training material, their understanding of its purpose, and the interaction that develops with the patient. VRT should be a shared experience between patient and therapist that evolves over time. Therapy should be prescribed on the basis of the diagnostic battery. Objectives should be created for each procedure for maximum efficiency. There should be specific short-term and long-range objectives, or like Alice we won't know where were going and we might be stumped when someone asks, *"If you don't know where you are going, how do you know when you get there?"*

Bottom-Up/Top-Down Information Processing

Broadbent[81] proposed that most cognitive processing proceeds in a staged sequence. On the presentation of a stimulus, perceptual processes act on the input, then attentional processes transfer some of the perceptual information to a short-term, transitory memory store, then if the material is rehearsed it could be transferred into a more permanent long-term memory.

A sequence of processing stages that proceeds from analysis of sensory data upward to the higher, more cognitive levels is bottom-up processing. It is stimulus driven because it is based on the properties of the stimulus. When we observe an object (e.g., a cup) the visual system extracts simple low-level features like lines and shapes. These simple features are then combined into more complex, complete shapes and we finally perceive a set of integrated shapes, which we recognize as a pair of glasses.

Top-down processing is used to describe the higher, more cognitive influences on perception. It is based on the idea that sensory information from the retina is insufficient to explain how we interpret visual information. We also need to use our stored knowledge about the world to make sense of the visual input. This higher level input of stored mental concepts works downward from the top to influence the way in which we interpret sensory inputs. To recognize a pair of glasses we must have prior knowledge of a pair of glasses. Very often, there is an overlap, an interaction between top-up and bottom-down processing.

Theeuwes et al.,[82] in a discussion of attentional capture uses the following example. When watching a football game, a particular event (e.g., the sudden change of a billboard advertisement) may grab your attention. Does this event grab your attention because you were set for it (i.e., keeping track of things that change), or did it grab your attention automatically even though your top-down processing goal was to watch the game. Goal-directed or top-down control of selection refers to those abilities to select those areas, objects, features, and events needed for our current tasks. Stimulus-driven or bottom-up selection refers to the capacity of certain stimulus attributes to attract our attention irrespective of our goals and beliefs. Attentional capture is a bottom-up process.

Julesz[83] writes that computer-generated random dot stereograms, devoid of all familiarity cues, when briefly presented followed by a mask, yield vivid depth. He says that these are bottom-up processes and are independent of top-down processes based on semantic memory.

A child attempting to complete a new jigsaw puzzle will initially use bottom-up processing by trying to match individual pieces, but when the puzzle begins to take shape the child will use top-down processing because intelligent and productive guesses can now be used. This is also apparent when solving the widely used developmental vision test, the Divided Form Board. This interactive process is valuable with many of the manipulatives that are used in vision therapy, such as Tangrams.

Lauritzen et al.[84] employed fMRI and coherency analysis in a study of sustained visual-spatial attention without visual stimulation. Their findings imply a top-down flow of information. Malcolm and Henderson[85] write that successful visual search for a target object in a real-world scene involves selecting and extracting relevant information from a noisy environment. This task involves eye movements that direct the region of highest resolution, the fovea, toward an informative part of the environment. Since the fovea makes up only a tiny portion of the visual field, our visual system must integrate low-resolution information in the visual periphery, to efficiently direct our eye movements. Their research indicates that the visual system will actively use multiple sources of top-down information processing to facilitate a search process. The following excerpt from "The Adventure of the Blanched Soldier" is a Sherlock Holmes story written by A. Conan Doyle:

> I find from my notebook that it was in January, 1903 just after the conclusion of the Boer war, that I had my visit from Mr. James M Dodd, a big, fresh, sunburned, upstanding Briton. The good Watson had at that time deserted me for a wife, the only selfish action which I can recall in our association. I was alone.
>
> It is my habit to sit with my back to the window and to place my visitors in the opposite chair, where the full light falls upon them. Mr. James M. Dodd seemed somewhat at a loss how to begin the interview. I did not attempt to help him, for his silence gave me more time for observation. I have found it wise to impress clients with a sense of power, and so I gave him some of my conclusions.

> 'From South Africa, sir, I perceive,'
> 'Yes sir,' he answered with some surprise.
> 'Imperial Yeomanry, I fancy.'
> 'Exactly.'
> 'Middlesex Corps, no doubt,'
> 'That is so. Mr. Holmes, you are a wizard.'
> I smiled at his bewildered expression.

> 'When a gentleman of virile appearance enters my room with such tan upon his face as an English sun could never give, and with his handkerchief in his sleeve instead of his pocket, it is not difficult to place him. You wear a short beard, which shows that

you were not a regular. You have the cut of a riding man. As to Middlesex, your card has already shown me that you are a stockbroker from Throgmorton Street. What other regiment would you join?'

'You see everything.'

'I see no more than you, but I have trained myself to notice what I see. However, Mr. Dodd, it was not to discuss the science of observation that you called upon me this morning.'

Sherlock Holmes devotees are rarely surprised by his remarkable reasoning powers. This excerpt teaches us that his deductive ability is based on remarkable visual observational skills that he combines with his stored mental information. In addition, his speed of information processing is unusually rapid, so that the visitor is truly amazed at the quickness of Holmes conclusions. These paragraphs provide an elegant illustration of top-down information processing at its best.

Therapy Modalities

A variety of modalities can be adapted for any of the basic processes we are interested in treating.[86] Therapy should be directed at the deficit processing areas identified by our assessment. The basic VT modalities that are available include the following.

Motoric Activities

Chalkboard exercises, gross and small motor activities (when the patient is able) are used to improve deficient motor skills (in conjunction with physical and occupational therapy treatment), rhythm, automaticity, processing speed, spatial relations, spatial orientation, eye-hand coordination, and visual-motor integration.

Manipulatives

These are table-top activities that engage the senses. They can be touched, moved about, rearranged, stacked, and otherwise handled. Typical manipulatives are Tangram, Perceptual Puzzle Blocks, Rush Hour, Labyrinth, Connect Four, Katimino, Pentomino, Parquetry, Pegboards, Attribute Blocks, and many more. Manipulatives are basic therapy for ABI patients.

Why use manipulatives? Piaget[87] believed that all learning must proceed from the concrete to the abstract. Physical materials are helpful for patients learning the simplest, most basic skills as well as more complex ones. The more that patients involve themselves in manipulation, the clearer the images they form that support an abstract concept. Everyone who is introduced to a new idea benefits from "seeing" the idea. Manipulatives help us visualize, discover patterns and relationships, provide problem-solving experiences, promote creativity, and build concepts. Manipulatives are available for many information processing skills, including form perception, spatial orientation, visual memory, eye-hand coordination, spatial relations, perceptual speed, visual sequencing, and visual cognition. Manipulatives may stimulate top-down, bottom-up, or interactive information processing. Manipulatives can be found in toy stores, educational supplies stores, or on the Internet at many sites.

Neistadt[88] described how treatment protocols derived from research literature can help provide more rigorous treatment and more systematic assessment of patient progress.

Research findings about the influence of task, subject, and feedback parameters on adult performance with block designs was applied to a treatment protocol for parquetry block assembly—a widely used manipulative task. Task parameter research suggests that parquetry tasks can be graded according to the features of the design cards, with cards having all block boundaries drawn in being easier than those with some block boundaries omitted. Subject parameter findings suggested that location of brain injury and initial competence at the task can influence their approach to parquetry.

Tangram, an old Chinese puzzle game, is one of the most popular and useful manipulatives. The origin of Tangram is hazy and a number of legends have developed over time.

> One such story holds that thousands of years ago a sage was asked to transport a large, perfectly square pane of glass that was to be used in his royal palace. The sage wrapped it in several layers of various materials, but unfortunately he tripped while descending a steep hill and the package tumbled all the way down. When the sage opened the package he was amazed that it had not shattered into a thousand pieces. Instead, it had broken into seven perfect geometric shapes. When he tried to put the pieces back in their original form, he realized that they could make many other designs. When the sage told his tale, the king was amazed at the shapes and he and his people quickly embraced them. And so the art of Tangram was born.

Tangram is valuable in vision therapy because it is fun, interesting, and meaningful in developing spatial/perceptual organization skills. The use of Tangram puzzles in teaching mathematics[89] is common because it helps develop spatial relations, which is basic to many math concepts, including fractions, geometry, area, and perimeter. Tangrams are physical objects that require physical manipulation. Flipping pieces, moving them around, and discerning the whole from its randomly scattered parts help patients develop spatial pattern recognition, problem solving, and divergent thinking. Most patients find it an interesting hands-on technique that they find enjoyable as well as challenging. Like jigsaw puzzles and visual closure tasks, Tangram is a bottom-up process until enough progress in solving the problem is attained, and then it becomes a top-down process.

Necessary Tangram materials include seven puzzle pieces:

- One small square
- Two small congruent triangles
- Two large congruent triangles
- One medium size triangle
- One parallelogram

These seven pieces can be assembled into a perfect square. Also necessary are the Tangram puzzles that the patient must solve (Figure 11.1). As in all VT procedures it is necessary to use materials at the patient's level of competency. If the task is too difficult, the patient will become frustrated and uncooperative. Remember—*if the patient cannot succeed, it is not his or her fault, it is our fault*. If the task is too easy the patient will become bored. Age, or verbal ability, is generally not a good criterion for determining competence with Tangram puzzles. Scores on spatial perception/ perceptual organization tests is a better guide. If uncertain where to start, begin

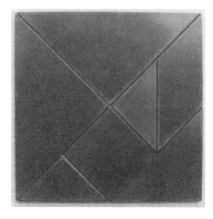

FIGURE 11.1 (See color insert following page 270.) On the left, is a Tangram puzzle to be solved by placing the Tangram pieces, shown on the right, to create the puzzle figure.

with easy puzzles or procedures. Use the following Tangram procedures to help your patients get acquainted with Tangram and to estimate their level of skill.

1. Create a triangle using two shapes
2. Create a square using one shape
3. Create a square using three triangles
4. Create a rectangle using three shapes
5. How many shapes can be made using just the two large triangles, placing them edge to edge? (Answer: three)
6. Create a triangle using four shapes
7. Create squares using two shapes, three shapes, and so on all the way up to seven. One arrangement is not possible. Which is it? (Answer: six shapes)
8. Create a rectangle using all seven shapes

Patients who have great difficulty solving Tangram puzzles with its varying angles, often find Pentominoes, available from wrightgroup.com, easier to use.

There are many sources for Tangram material. A wonderful set of Tangram Puzzles was an outgrowth many years ago of a project called *Elementary Science Study* (ESS). The set consisted of three sections, easy, medium, and difficult. Unfortunately, it is no longer in print but some copies, along with other Tangram books are available on the Internet. For patients who need simpler puzzles, Matching Activities* with Tangrams and Tangram Pattern Cards as well as Tan-tastic Tangrams† are good beginning programs. Tangrammables, published by Learning Resources, Inc.,‡ contains 75 puzzles

---

* Therapro, Inc., 225 Arlington Street, Framingham, MA, 01702–8723, 1–800–257–5376, www.therapro.com
† MindWare, 2100 County Rd C W, Roseville, MN, 55113-2501, 1-800-999-0398, www.mindwareonline.com
‡ Learning Resources, Inc., 380 N. Fairway Drive, Vernon Hills, IL, 60061, 1–800–333–8281, www.learningresources.com

organized by level of difficulty. A full rage of Tangram products, from elementary to extremely difficult challenge levels, can be found under the rubric Tangoes.

Lens Therapy

There is not any direct relationship between refractive error and visual information processing in particular; an accurate refractive correction is basic to all therapy. Plus lenses have the capacity in some patients to alter visual-spatial skills, near vision posture, and visual information processing. They should be prescribed when appropriate. Yoked prisms may change body posture, spatial relations, and vestibular abilities (see Chapters 4 and 7).

Workbooks

Workbooks are available for almost all areas of visual information processing. They may be utilized extensively for either in-office or out of office therapy. An excellent source for workbooks from many publishers is the Therapro catalog. (therapro.com).

Computers

Computers are a very useful modality for treating perceptual dysfunction.[90] They are as popular with therapists as with patients and their use is expanding rapidly. Computer therapy programs have many desirable features:

1. *Patient acceptance*: it is stimulated by the ubiquitousness of computers in all aspects of society and the feeling that computers do things more rapidly and efficiently. Patients expect to use and benefit from complex electronic devices. Therapy is more effective when patients believe in the mystique of the modality.
2. *Flexibility*: computers are not limited to one function or level of difficulty. With appropriate software, it is possible to utilize computers for a large number of VT procedures. Almost all visual information processing abilities can be trained using a computer. They are particularly useful for speed of information processing, visual memory, and spatial relations/perceptual organization. They are available for both office and home use.
3. *Proven learning principles*: vision therapy is subject to the principles of educational therapy and the laws of learning. The general procedure in rehabilitation is to raise the individual processes, abilities, and components to higher levels of performance. This requires a thorough and well-structured protocol consisting of a sequence of programmed steps.
4. *Adaptable Programming*: computers are uniquely adaptable to the needs of VT because of the following:
   - Programs are user friendly and self-instructional.
   - The primary interaction is between the patient and the program rather than between the patient and the therapist.
   - The stimuli are divided into small, discrete units.
   - Computer programs can provide a large number of stimuli for many activities and an infinite number for others.

- The stimuli can be programmed in sequences raging from simple to complex.
- Each stimulus demands an overt response from the patient.
- Each response is recorded by the computer and immediate feedback can be provided.
- The computer stores information during each session and can furnish a visual, auditory, or printed summary of the patient's activities. Some programs permanently store results and others are connected to the Internet.
- Computer programs can feature bottom-up information processing, top-down information processing, or interactive information processing. All three should be included in vision therapy programs.

There are a number of computer programs on the market designed to improve visual-perceptual skills. Two examples are discussed here. The Posit Science Corporation InSight[§] program, has been demonstrated to create significant changes in activities of daily living, such as driving safety, in elderly program users. It includes five programs designed to increase visual processing speed, expand useful field of view, exercise divided attention, and improve visual WM.

The *computerized perceptual therapy* series, available from Home Therapy Inc.[**] includes 18 modules, which can be purchased separately. The modules address multiple areas of visual processing, with various models emphasizing top-down, bottom-up, or integrated visual processing. The modules are designed to address visual processing deficits, including processing speed, directionality, visual-spatial relations, visual closure, visual discrimination, figure-ground perception, visual imagery, visual sequential memory, visual-spatial memory, and visual span. A number of the programs also include exercises that work ocular motility, visual planning, and visual attention skills. In addition, there is also a visual thinking module, two, or three attributes. Tests for tachistoscopic speed and visual coding are also available. The programs can be categorized into speed of processing modules, visual memory modules, and spatial relations/perceptual organization. Examples of each are presented here.

Perceptual speed: The Perceptual Speed program displays an array of a varying number of columns consisting of a varying number of rows of stimuli (Figure 11.2). A target stimulus is displayed at the top of the array. The patient is required to follow one of three instructions to rapidly identify one of the stimuli that is like the target, two of the stimuli that are like the target, or one of the stimuli that is different from the rest. In addition to speed of processing, this program also stimulates RT and saccadic fixation. It is bottom-up information processing. A perceptual speed test is included in the program.

Visual memory: The Visual Memory program provides therapy for two distinct, necessary types of visual memory: visual sequential memory and visual-spatial memory. The visual sequential memory program requires patients to identify, recall, and indicate the correct order of a sequence of colored stimuli that are briefly displayed individually

---

[§] **Posit Science Corporation**, 225 Bush Street, Seventh Floor, San Francisco, CA, 94104; from within the US: 1–866–599–6463; outside the US: +1–415–373–5685, www.positscience.com

[**] HTS, Inc. 5301 S. Superstition Mtn Dr., PMB 483, Ste. 104, Gold Canyon, AZ, 85218, 1–800–346–4925, www.visiontherapysolutions.net

Perceptual Speed   00.33

Choose 1 that is like: 7 Q U X N

→ 7 X N U Q   7 U N X Q   7 U Q X N   7 Q U X N
  A X 6 H 3   H X 6 A 3   H 6 X A 3   H 6 3 A X
  N M P I 9   I M P N 9   I 9 P N M   I 9 M N P
  T Z B E R   T R B E Z   T R B Z E   B R T Z E
  N 9 5 P V   N P 5 9 V   N P V 9 5   N V P 9 5
  N K Z 2 G   N K Z G 2   G K Z 2 N   G K Z N 2
  P R 3 4 X   X R 3 4 P   X R P 4 3   4 R P X 3
  1 U I 9 K   1 I U 9 K   I U I 9 K   K U 1 9 I
  Q Y 0 5 S   Y Q O 5 S   Y 5 0 Q S   Y 5 Q 0 S
  J R K Y C   R J K Y C   R Y K J C   R K Y J C
  9 E V D M   W E V D 9   W D V E 9   E W V D 9
  M 3 B T 1   B 3 M T 1   3 B M T 1   3 1 M T B
  L A N 4 V   L A V 4 N   V A L 4 N   A L V 4 N
  4 W K 9 Y   4 Y K 9 W   W Y K 9 4   W Y 9 K 4
  8 M J X C   8 X J M C   8 X J C M   X 8 J C M

1 of 5

FIGURE 11.2 (**See color insert following page 270.**) Perceptual speed module from *Computerized Perceptual Therapy*. (Home Therapy, Inc.)

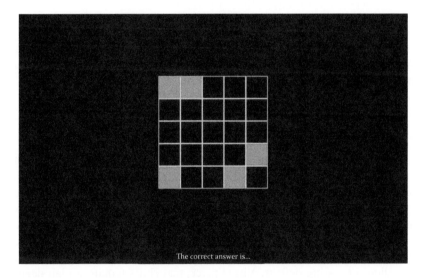

The correct answer is...

FIGURE 11.3 (**See color insert following page 270.**) Visual memory module from *Computerized Perceptual Therapy*. (Home Therapy, Inc.)

in the cells of a matrix grid. Following the presentation, the entire grid, with the stimulus cells indicated is displayed, and the patient must click on the cells in order of presentation (Figure 11.3). The visual-spatial memory program requires patients to identify, recall, and indicate the spatial location of an array of colored stimuli that are briefly displayed all at once in the cells of a matrix grid. In addition to visual-spatial and visual-sequential memory, this program also stimulates speed of information processing, visual attention, and spatial visualization. It is bottom-up information processing.

Visual thinking: This program requires the patient to complete various sized grids with stimuli that differ from each other in one, two, or three attributes (Figure 11.4). The stimuli may be geometric forms, numbers, colors, or pictures. When using geometric forms, the attributes are four shapes, two sizes, and four colors. The patient

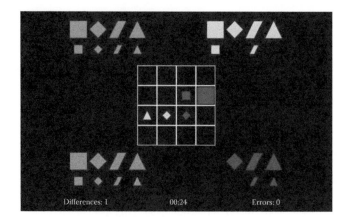

FIGURE 11.4 (See color insert following page 270.) Visual thinking module from *Computerized Perceptual Therapy.* (Home Therapy, Inc.)

places the forms adjacent to each other, but the forms must differ from all sides by the chosen amount of difference. It has been particularly used for patients with ABI. In addition to visual thinking, this program stimulates visual planning, spatial relations, visual discrimination, visual conceptualization, and visualization. It is top-down information processing.

SUMMARY

Visual information processing deficits are common in ABI, and can cause problems in attention, memory, learning ability, thinking, creativity, and other aspects of cognition and motor function. Among the various deficits of visual information processing following ABI, speed of information processing, memory deficits, and spatial relations/perceptual organization are the most common. Visual information processing deficits must be considered in light of the entire visual system, as focusing, ocular motor, binocular, and other visual system dysfunction can cause or exacerbate visual information processing deficits. Visual-perceptual skills require a high degree of integration and analysis, which begins with the sensory input.

While normative testing is useful and helpful, the clinician must be flexible when working with patients with ABI. Both formal (normed) and informal (observational) testing is necessary and appropriate with any population, but more so with ABI patients. It is important for the clinician to make good observations and synthesize all of the information, as the clinician, not the test, makes the diagnosis.

Vision rehabilitation therapy is effective in treating many aspects of visual information processing deficits. It is important to use multiple therapeutic modalities that are engaging to the patient, as discussed in this chapter. These must be carefully programmed to the level of the patient. If the patient has tried, and leaves the therapy feeling unsuccessful, then the clinician has made a programming error. It is especially critical, when doctors are prescribing therapy programs to be carried out by occupational therapists at a rehabilitation center, for the therapists to communicate quickly and effectively if the patient is unable to carry out some part of the program prescribed, so that it can be modified.

Rehabilitation of visual information processing deficits is critical to the patient being able to understand the world around them as they move through daily life. Following ABI, every patient should be evaluated for visual information processing deficits and treatment should be a routine part of an integrated rehabilitation plan.

APPENDIX 11.1

Test publisher contact information:

AMERICAN GUIDANCE SERVICE

4201 Woodland Road
Circle Pines, MN, 55014
763–786–4343
http://www.agsnet.com

LAFAYETTE INSTRUMENT COMPANY

3700 Sagamore Parkway N
Lafayette, IN, 47904
800–428 7545
http://www.lafayetteinstrument.com

PEARSON ASSESSMENT

19500 Bulverde Road
San Antonio, TX, 78259
800–328–5999
http://www.pearsonassessments.com

PRO-ED

8700 Shoal Creek Blvd.
Austin, TX, 78757
800–897–3202
http://www.proedinc.com

WESTERN PSYCHOLOGICAL SERVICES

12031 Wilshire Blvd.
Los Angeles, CA, 90025
800–648–8867
http://portal.wpspublish.com

REFERENCES

1. Suchoff, I. B., Kapoor, N., Waxman, R., & Ference, W. (1999). The occurrence of ocular and visual dysfunctions in an acquired brain-injured patient sample. *Journal of the American Optometric Association, 70,* 301–309.

2. Gordon, W. A., Brown, M., Sliwinski, M., Hibbard, M. R., Weiss, M. J., Kalinsky, R., & Sheerer, M. (1988). The enigma of "hidden" traumatic brain injury. *Journal of Head Trauma Rehabilitation, 13*(6), 39–56.

3. Gazzaniga, M. S., Ivry, B. B., & Mangum, G. R. (2002). *Cognitive neuroscience: The biology of the mind* (2nd ed.). New York: Norton.

4. Thatcher, R. W., North, D. M., Curtin, R. T., Walker, R. A., Biven, C. I., Gomez, J. F., & Salazar, A. M. (2001). An EEG severity index of traumatic brain injury. *Journal of Neuropsychiatry and Clinical Sciences, 13*, 77–87.

5. Forgus, R. H. (1966). *Perception the basic process in cognitive development.* New York: McGraw Hill.

6. Su, C. Y., Chang, J. J., Chen, H. M., Su, C. J., Chien, T. H., & Huang, M. H. (2000). Perceptual differences between stroke patents with cerebral infarction and intracerebral hemorrhage. *Archives of Physical Medicine and Rehabilitation, 81*, 706–714.

7. McKenna, K., Cooke, D. M., Fleming, J., Jefferson, A., & Ogden, S. (2006). The incidence of visual perceptual impairment in patients with severe traumatic brain injury. *Brain Injury, 20*(5), 507–518.

8. Bolles, E. B. (1991). *A second way of knowing: The riddle of human perception.* New York: Prentice Hall.

9. McAllister, T. W. (2008). Neurobehavioral sequelae of traumatic brain injury: evaluation and management. *World Psychiatry, 7*, 3–10.

10. Young, J., & Ari, A. (2009). Traumatic brain injury-induced anomalous head posture and vertical diplopia. *Journal of the American Optometric Association, 80*(6), 286.

11. Gianutsos, R., & Suchoff, I. B. (1998). Neuropsychological consequences of mild brain injury and optometric implications. *Journal of Behavioral Optometry, 9*(1), 3–6.

12. Cohen, A. H., & Rein, L. D. (1992). The effect of head trauma on the visual system. The doctor of optometry as a member of the rehabilitation team. *Journal of the American Optometric Association, 63*, 530–536.

13. Schapiro, S. R., & Swersky-Sacchetti, T. (1993). Neuropsychological sequelae of minor head trauma. In S. Mandel, R. T. Stataloff, & S. R. Schapiro (Eds.), *Minor head trauma: Assessment management and rehabilitation.* New York: Springer.

14. Gronwall, D., & Wrightson, P. (1974). Delayed recovery of intellectual function after minor head injury. *Lancet, 2*(7881), 605–609.

15. Battistone, M., Woltz, D., & Clark, E. (2008). Processing speed deficits associated with traumatic brain injury: Processing inefficiency or cautiousness? *Applied Neuropsychology, 15*(1), 69–78.

16. Kail, R. (1992). Processing speed, naming speed, and reading. *Developmental Psychology, 28*, 899–904.

17. Salthouse, T. A. (2000). The processing speed theory of cognitive aging. *Psychology Review, 103*, 403–428.

18. Zahn, T. R., & Mirsky, A. F. (1999). Reaction time indicators of attention deficits in closed head injury. *Clinical and Experimental Neuropsychology, 21*, 352–367.

19. Archbald, C. J., & Fisk, J. D. (2000). Information processing efficiency in patients with multiple sclerosis. *Clinical and Experimental Neuropsychology, 22*, 686–701.

20. Tombaugh, T. N., Stormer, P., Rees, L., Irving, S., & Francis, M. (2006). The effects of mild and severe traumatic injury on the auditory and visual versions of the Adjusting-Paced Serial Addition Test. *Archives of Clinical Neuropsychology, 21*, 753–761.

21. Salthouse, T. A. (1999). The aging of working memory. *Neuropsychology, 8*, 535–543.

22. Ponsford, J., & Kinsella, G. (1992). Attentional deficits following closed head injury. *Clinical and Experimental Neuropsychology, 14*, 822–838.

23. Madigan, N. K., DeLuca, J., Diamond, B. J., Tramontano, G., & Averill, A. (2000). Speed of information processing in traumatic brain injury: modality specific factors. *Journal of Head Trauma Rehabilitation, 15*(3), 943–956.
24. Battistone, M., Woltz, D., & Clark, E. (2008). Processing speed deficits associated with traumatic brain injury. *Applied Neuropsychology, 15*(1), 69–78.
25. Felmingham, K. L., Baguley, I. J., & Green, A. M. (2004). Effects of diffuse axonal injury on speed of information processing following severe traumatic brain injury. *Neuropsychology, 18*(3), 564–571.
26. Stuss, D. T., Stethem, L. L., Hugenholtz, H., Picton, T., Pivik, J., & Richard, M. T. (1989). Reaction time after head injury: fatigue, divided and focused attention, and consistency of performance. *Journal of Neurology, Neurosurgery, and Psychiatry, 52*(6), 742–748.
27. Sarrno, S., Erasmus, L-P., Lipp, B., & Schlaegel, W. (2003). Multisensory integration after tr28aumatic brain injury: a reaction time study between pairings of vision, touch and audition. *Brain Injury, 17*(5), 413–426.
28. Malojcic, B., Mubrin, C., Coric, B., Susnic, M., & Spilich, G. J. (2008). Consequences of mild traumatic brain injury on information processing assessed with attention and short term memory tasks. *Journal of Neurotrauma, 25*(1), 30–37.
29. Shiffrin, R. M., & Schnider, W. (1977). Controlled and automatic human information processing II: perceptual learning, automatic attending and a general theory. *Psychology Review, 84*, 127–190.
30. Williamson, D. J. G., Scott, J. G., & Adams, R. L. (1996). Traumatic brain injury. In R. L. Adams, O. A. Parsons, & S. J. Nixon (Eds.), *Neuropsychology for clinical practice: Etiology, assessment and treatment of common neurological disorders* (pp. 9–64). Washington DC: American Psychological Press.
31. Mild Traumatic Head Injury Committee of the American Congress of Rehabilitation Medicine. (1993). Definition of mild traumatic brain injury. *Journal of Head Trauma Rehabilitation, 8*(3), 86–87.
32. Brooks, N., Campsie, Li., & Symington, C. (1986). The five year outcome of severe blunt head injury: a relative's view. *Journal of Neurology, Neurosurgery and Psychiatry, 49*(7), 764–770.
33. Levin, H. S. (1990). Memory deficit after closed head injury. *Journal of Clinical and Experimental Neuropsychology, 12*(1), 129–153.
34. Oddy, M., Coughlan, T., Tyerman, A., & Jenkins, D. (1985). Social adjustment after closed head injury: a further follow-up seven years after injury. *Journal of Neurology, Neurosurgery and Psychiatry, 48*(6), 564–568.
35. Tate, R. I. (1997). Beyond one-bun, two-shoe: recent advances in the psychological rehabilitation of memory disorders after acquired brain injury. *Brain Injury, 11*(12), 907–918.
36. Mapou, R. L. (1992). Neuropathology and neuropsychology of behavioral disturbances following traumatic brain injury. In C. J. Long, & L. F. Ross (Eds.), *Handbook of head trauma—Acute care to recovery* (pp. 75–122). New York: Plenum Press.
37. Lam, C. S., Priddy, D. A., & Johnson, P. (1991). Neuropsychological indicators of employability following traumatic brain injury. *Rehabilitation Counseling Bulletin, 35*, 68–74.
38. Shum, D. H. K., Harris, D., & O'Gorman, J. G. (2000). Effects of severe traumatic bran injury on visual memory. *Journal of Clinical and Experimental Neuropsychology, 22*(1), 25–39.
39. Bernstein, D. M. (1999). Recovery from mild head injury. *Brain Injury, 13*, 151–172.
40. Blakely, T. A. Jr., & Harrington, D. E. (1993). Mild head injury is not always mild; implications for damage litigation. *Medicine, Science, and the Law, 33*(3), 231–242.

41. Wilson, J. T. L., Wiedmann, K. D., Hadley, D. M., & Brooks, D. N. (1989). The relationship between visual memory function and lesions detected by magnetic resonance imaging after closed head injury. *Neuropsychology, 3,* 255–265.
42. Fox, G. A., & Fox, A. M. (1991). A neuropsychological test for diffuse brain damage. In W. R. Levick, B. G. Frost, M. Watson, & H. P. Pfister (Eds.), *Brain impairment advances in applied research* (pp. 165–172). Newcastle, Australia: University of Newcastle.
43. Chuah, Y. M., Mayberry, M. T., & Fox, A. M. (2004). The long-term effects of mild head injury on short term memory for visual form, spatial location, and their conjunction in well-functioning university students. *Brain and Cognition, 56*(3), 304–312.
44. Baddeley, A. D. (2003). Working memory: looking back and looking forward. *Nature Reviews. Neuroscience, 4*(10), 829–839.
45. Finke, H., Bubiak, P., & Zihl, J. (2008). Visual spatial and visual pattern working memory: neuropsychological evidence for a differential role of left and right dorsal visual brain. *Neuropsychologia, 44*(4), 649–661.
46. Scheiman, M. M., & Gallaway, M. (2006). Optometric assessment: visual information processing problems. In M. M. Schieman, & M. W. Rouse (Eds.) *Optometric management of learning-related vision problems* (2nd ed., pp. 369–414). St.Louis, MO: Mosby Elseiver.
47. Brosseau-Lachaine, O., Gagnon, I., Forget, R., & Faubert, J. (2006, May). *Complex visual information processing in children after mild traumatic brain injury.* Presented at the Vision Sciences Society Meeting, Sarasota, FL.
48. Uttal, W. R. (1988). *On seeing forms.* Hillsdale, NJ: Lawrence Erlbaum.
49. Palmer, S. E., Brooks, J. L., & Nelson, R. (2003). When does perceptual grouping happen? *Acta Psychologia, 114,* 311–330.
50. Trujillo, L. T., Allen, J. J. B., Schnyer, D. M., & Peterson, M. A. (2010). Neurophysiological evidence for the influence of past experience on figure-ground perception. *Journal of Vision, 10*(2), 1–21.
51. Pomerantz, M. J., & Kubouy, M. (1981). Evolution of the visual cortex and the emergence of symmetry. In M. Kubouy, & J. Pomerantz (Eds), *Perceptual organization* (pp. 27–54). Hillsdale, NJ: Lawrence Erlbaum.
52. Humphrey, D. G., & Kramer, A. F. (1999). Age—related differences in perceptual organization and selective attention: implications for display segmentation and recall performance. *Experimental Aging Research, 25,* 1–26.
53. Kurylo, D. D., Allan, W. C., Collins, T. E., & Barron, J. (2003). Perceptual organization based upon spatial relationships in Alzheimer's disease. *Journal of Behavioral Neurology, 14,* 19–28.
54. Nadler, J. D., Grace, J., White, D. A., Butters, M. A., & Malloy, P. F. (1996). Laterality differences in quantitative and qualitative Hooper performance. *Archives of Clinical Neuropsychology, 11,* 223–229.
55. Kurylo, D. D., Waxman, R., & Kezin, O. (2006). Spatial-Temporal characteristics of perceptual organization following acquired brain injury. *Brain Injury, 20*(3), 237–244.
56. Ashton, V. L., Donders, J., & Hoffman, N. M. (2005). Rey Complex Figure Test performance after traumatic brain injury. *Journal of Clinical and Experimental Neuropsychology, 27,* 55–64.
57. Kixmiller, J. S., Verfaellie, M., Mather, M. M., & Cermak, L. S. (2000). Role of perceptual and organizational factors in amnesiac's recall of the Rey Osterrieth Complex Figure: a comparison of three amnesic groups. *Journal of Clinical and Experimental Neuropsychology, 22,* 196–207.
58. Meyers, J. E., & Meyers, K. R. (1995). *Rey complex figure test and recognition trial.* Odessa, FL: Psychological Assessment Resources.

59. Ponsford, J. (2005). Rehabilitation interventions after mild head injury. *Current Opinion in Neurology, 18*, 692–697.
60. Kapoor, N., Ciuffreda, K. J., & Han, J. (2004). Oculomotor rehabilitation in acquired brain injury. A case series. *Archives of Physical Medicine and Rehabilitation, 85*, 1667–1676.
61. Carter, L. T., Howard, B. E., & O'Neil, W. A. (1983). Effectiveness of cognitive skill remediation in acute stroke patients. *American Journal of Occupational Therapy, 37*(5), 320–326.
62. Groffman S. (2009). Subitizing: vision therapy for math deficits. *Optometry & Vision Development, 40*(4), 229–238.
63. Wilson, A. J., Revkin, S. K., Cohen, D., Cohen, L., & Dehaene, S. (2006). An open trial assessment of "The Number Race," an adaptive computer game for remediation of dyscalculia. Retrieved from http//www.behavioralandbrainfunctions.com/contents2/1/20 (Accessed September 28, 2009).
64. Fischer, B., Kongeter, A., & Hartnegg, K. (2008). Effects of daily practice on subitizing, visual counting, and basic counting skills. *Optometry & Vision Development, 39*(1), 30–34.
65. Thickpenny-Davis, K. L., & Barker-Coles, S. L. (2007). Evaluation of a structured group format memory rehabilitation program for adults following brain injury. *Journal of Head Trauma Rehabilitation, 22*(5), 303–313.
66. Hooft, I. V., Andersson, K., Bergman, B., Sejersen, T., Von Wendt, L., & Bartfai, A. (2005). Beneficial effect from a cognitive training programme on children with acquired brain injures demonstrated in a controlled study. *Brain Injury, 19*(7), 511–518.
67. Edwards, J. D., Wadley, V. G., Myers, R. S., Roenker, D. L., Cissell, G. M., & Ball, K. K. (2002). Transfer of a speed of processing interventions to near and far cognitive functions. *Gerontology, 48*(5), 329–340.
68. Ball, K., Edwards, J. D., & Rose, L. A. (2007). The impact of speed of processing training on cognitive and everyday functions. *Journal of Gerontology. Series B, Psychological Sciences and Social Sciences, 62*(Spec No. 1), 19–31.
69. Advanced Cognitive Training for Independent and Vital Elderly Study Group. (2002). Effects of cognitive training interventions with older adults: a randomized controlled study. *Journal of the American Medical Association, 288*(18), 2271–2281.
70. Crocker, L., & Algina, C. (1986). *Introduction to classical and modern test theory.* New York: Holt, Rinehart, and Winston.
71. Groffman, S. (2003). Perceptual testing—where are you going? *Optometry & Vision Development, 34*(2), 57–60.
72. Depoy, E. (1992). A comparison of standardized and observational measurement. *Journal of Cognitive Rehabilitation, 10*(1), 30–33.
73. Suter, P. S. (1999). A quick start in post-acute vision rehabilitation following brain injury. *Optometry & Vision Development, 30*, 73–82.
74. Valenti, C. (2003). Rehabilitation of persons with visual sequelae resulting from traumatic brain injury. *Optometry & Vision Development, 34*, 105–110.
75. Cohen, A. H., &Rein, L. D. (1992). The effect of head trauma on the visual system: the doctor of optometry as a member of the rehabilitation team. *Journal of the American Optometric Association, 63*(8), 530–536.
76. Gianutsos, R., & Suchoff, I. B. (1998).Neuropsychological consequences of mild brain injury and optometric implications. *Journal of Behavioral Optometry, 9*(1), 3–6.
77. Kapoor, N., & Ciuffreda, K. J. (2002). Vision disturbances following traumatic brain injury. *Current Treatment Options in Neurology, 4*(4), 271–280.
78. Suter, P. S. (2004). Rehabilitation and management of visual dysfunction following traumatic brain injury. In M. J. Ashley (Ed.), *Traumatic brain injury* (2nd ed., pp. 209–249). Boca Raton, FL: CRC Press.

79. Groffman, S. (1993). Motivational factors in visual therapy: comparison of computerized vs. manipulative techniques. *Journal of the American Optometric Association, 67*(6), 344–349.

80. Groffman, S. (1997). Consideration of individual characteristics and learning theory in vision therapy. In L. J. Press (Ed.), *Applied concepts in vision therapy* (pp. 21–32). St. Louis, MO: Mosby.

81. Broadbent, D. (1958). *Perception and communication.* London, UK: Pergamon Press.

82. Theeuwes, J., Kramer, J. F., & Kingstone, A. (2004). Attentional capture modulates perceptual sensitivity. *Psychonomic Bulletin & Review, 11*(3), 551–554.

83. Julesz, B. (1990). Early vision is bottom-up, except for focal attention. *Quantitative Biology, 55*, 973–978.

84. Lauritzen, T. Z., D'Esposito, M., Heeger, D., & Silver, M. A. (2009). Top-down flow of visual spatial attention signals from parietal to occipital cortex. *Journal of Vision, 9*(13), 1–14.

85. Malcolm, G. J., & Henderson, J. M. (2010). Combining top-down processes to guide eye movements during real-world scene search. *Journal of Vision, 10*(2), 1–11.

86. Groffman, S. (1993). Treatment of visual perception disorders. *Practical Optometry, 4*, 76–83.

87. Piaget, J. (1952). *The origins of intelligence in children.* New York: International Universities Press.

88. Neistadt, M. E. (1994). Using research literature to develop a perceptual retraining treatment protocol. *American Journal of Occupational Therapy, 48*(1), 62–72.

89. Rigdon, D., Raleigh, J., & Goodman, S. (2000). Math by the months: tackling Tangrams. *Teaching Children Mathematics, 6*(5), 304–305.

90. Groffman, S., & Press, L. J. (1992). Computerized perceptual therapy programs, parts 1 and 2. In L. J. Press (Ed.), *Computers and visual therapy programs* (pp. 21–32). Santa Ana, CA: Optometric Extension Program.

12 Vision Examination of Patients with Neurological Disease and Injury

Thomas Politzer and Penelope S. Suter

CONTENTS

INTRODUCTION

As discussed in Chapter 2, patients with brain injury frequently need acute intervention for vision problems, while they are still hospitalized followed by postacute
vision intervention after their discharge. In both cases, the patient will typically have
a rehabilitation team working with them, and the functional rehabilitation vision
care doctor (frequently an optometrist) should be one of the members of that team.
In this chapter, diagnosis and intervention in both the acute and postacute settings
are discussed, as they are quite different in scope.

VISION EXAMINATION OF PATIENTS IN AN ACUTE
CARE NEUROREHABILITATION HOSPITAL

INTRODUCTION

Historically, optometry has not been part of the medical team in a hospital setting.
Then, beginning in the early 1980s, a general awareness started to increase regarding the impact of vision problems in patients who had suffered strokes, cerebral

aneurysms, brain injuries, and other neurological diseases (NDs) and injuries. Following that, a few optometrists around the United States were contacted by members of various neurorehabilitation teams and asked about ways to potentially examine and treat patients with vision problems. The result was that optometrists began seeing neurological patients in rehabilitation hospitals and became part of the medical neurorehabilitation team.

Examining and caring for patients in an acute care hospital setting can be a very rewarding experience. The scope of problems encountered is extensive, as is the responsibility for treating them. It is not good enough to have good clinical skills. The optometrist wanting to pursue this must also possess a good understanding of neuro-anatomy, physiology, neurology, and rehabilitation. He or she must be able to put ego aside and be a committed member of a team. One must be able to see and appreciate the "big picture" of how to achieve desired future outcomes with an understanding that vision is just one piece of the puzzle.

Patients requiring care can generally be placed in two broad categories: acquired neurological injury (ANI) and neurological disease (ND). Patients with vision problems from ANI include, in general, the subgroups of traumatic brain injury (TBI), cerebral vascular accident (CVA), cerebral aneurysm, and spinal cord injury. Patients with vision problems from ND include, in general, the subgroups of tumor, movement disorders, such as Parkinson's disease, Huntington's disease, and multiple sclerosis.

In acute care rehabilitation hospitals, the medical team is comprised of several disciplines and consultants. The primary team typically includes the attending physician, who specializes in physical medicine and rehabilitation (physiatrist), neurologist, neuropsychologist, occupational therapist (OT), physical therapist (PT), and speech and language therapist (SLP). There is a broad array of consultants including anesthesiology, cardiology, dentistry and oral surgery, dermatology, electrophysiology, general surgery, internal medicine, neuro-ophthalmology, neuro-otology, neurosurgery, neuroradiology, optometry, ophthalmology, orthopedics, surgery, psychiatry, podiatry, rheumatology, and urology.

The vision team is comprised of specialists in optometry and ophthalmology. A good example of the vision team is based on that of Craig Hospital in Englewood, Colorado. Craig Hospital is designated by the National Institute on Disability Rehabilitation and Research (NIDRR) as a Model System Center for both spinal cord injury and TBI.

At Craig Hospital, the optometrist serves as the primary gatekeeper for evaluation and management of vision problems. Subspecialties consulted include the following: neuro-ophthalmology, cornea, oculoplastics, retinal specialists, and general ophthalmology.

Patients are selected to go to the vision clinic based on the nature of their injury/disease, symptoms, and observations. Given the extensive representation that vision has in the brain, both anatomically and functionally, patients maybe referred to evaluate and rule out problems based on the neuro-anatomy involved.

Among the more common reasons for referral to the vision clinic are the following:

- Strabismus
- Double vision

- Disorder of eye movements
- Nystagmus
- Ptosis, lagophthalmos, or other lid abnormality
- Gaze preference, hemineglect, or inattention
- Suspect visual field loss
- Ocular disease or injury
- Pupil abnormality
- Suspect Terson's syndrome
- Dizziness or imbalance
- Blurred vision

Once a patient has been identified for the vision clinic, an order is written in the hospital chart for the consult. A pretest screening may be performed by the attending OT, but is not required. If done, this will list observations and concerns. Visual acuity, basic eye alignment, fixations, eye movements, and confrontation visual field are screened. The OT may accompany the patient to the exam, or provide the findings.

EQUIPMENT

Some hospitals have a lane of equipment, but most do not. A lot of good portable equipment is available and can be carried in a small mobile case.

The list of recommended equipment includes the following:

- Portable biomicroscope with fundus lens
- Portable tonometer
- Ophthalmoscope
- Retinoscope with retinoscopy lenses
- Transilluminator or penlight
- Trial lens kit with loose prisms and trial frame
- Spectacle magnifiers (for external examination without slit lamp)
- Portable lensometer
- Occluder with Maddox rod on one end
- Distance and near acuity charts

A small bag can hold dilation drops, anesthetic, temporary lid weights, and bandage contact lenses. A supply of Fresnel prisms can be carried, or left at the hospital.

EXAMINATION

The basic examination begins with an introduction to the patient and a general observation of them. If the OT has accompanied the patient to the examination, they will facilitate this and review their observations and concerns. If a screening has been performed it will be reviewed and discussed. For the examination, objective testing is preferred to as much of a degree as possible.

Review of Records

Review of the records is absolutely necessary if at all possible. In the hospital chart there are sections for medications, history and physical (H&P), orders, progress notes, consultant reports, transfer records, and admissions. The H&P, medications, and appropriate consultant reports are reviewed. In the H&P particular attention is given to sections describing the nature and extent of the injury/disease, neurological findings, HEENT (head, eyes, ears, nose, and throat), neurologic exam, assessment, and plan. It is helpful to be familiar with the Glasgow Coma Score (Appendix 12.1) as in acute injury, this scale is frequently used to describe the patient's general status.

> PEARL: This is the time when one begins thinking about the involved neuro-anatomy and how it might affect vision.

History

A detailed visual history is conducted to the extent the patient is able to comply. Sometimes patients have expressive, and/or receptive aphasia making their input difficult. A patient may also be at a lower level of function and be minimally able to cooperate in the examination. History is assisted with input from the family, OT, PT, and SLP.

Observation

One should look critically at facial symmetry, or asymmetry, eye alignment, gaze preference, posture, general appearance of the eyes, and positioning if in a wheel chair. Take note of interaction with others in the room, visual, or other perseveration, and general and visual attention. For example, a head tilt might indicate a CN IV injury, a gaze preference may indicate neglect, and/or CN III or CN VI involvement, and a lagophthalmos may indicate a CN VII with possible CN V involvement.

Visual Acuity

Acuities are measured using standard techniques with modification as needed. Distance acuity is usually measured at 10 feet. Snellen letters or shapes may need to be individually masked to assist with impaired attention. If there is indication of possible neglect, or visual field loss, begin by pointing to letters on the side of the chart to the expected intact side.

Ocular Alignment

Ocular alignment can be determined by performing the Hirschberg test, cover test, and Maddox rod. With the exception of strabismus from a Trochlear nerve involvement, which is usually a fairly small angle deviation, most strabismus deviations in these groups of patients will have a large angle of deviation that is easily seen with observation. When a strabismus is present the examiner should evaluate it both at distance and near, and in all nine fields of gaze. If the strabismus is noncomitant, it is important to do a Park three-step test. The Park three-step test is used in evaluation of vertical diplopia caused by a paretic cyclovertical muscle.[1] Each step reduces by half the number of possible affected muscles until only one remains.

After testing eye movements (below), if there is a limitation of gaze caused by a paretic, or paralytic muscle, the strabismus should be reevaluated with that in mind.

Fixations

Fixations are evaluated with standard tests. Patients may be photophobic, so the use of a nonilluminated fixation target is indicated. The patient is instructed to look at a steady target (e.g., the examiners' finger) held in front of them and at a distance of about 16 inches from them. The examiner is observing for signs of steady gaze, unsteadiness, loss of fixation, and nystagmus. For lower level functioning patients one can consider using mirrors for fixation, and/or supplementing with proprioceptive, kinesthetic, and auditory cuing.

Nystagmus and other uncontrolled rapid eye movements are ocular signs of an underlying neurologic deficit. They can have the following presentations:

a. Rhythmic involuntary eye movements with a slow phase and fast recovery that are usually binocular are indicative of nystagmus from inner ear dysfunction.
b. Fast downward jerk with a slow upward return to midposition is referred to as ocular bobbing and indicative of extensive pontine injury.
c. Gaze overshoot followed by several oscillations is referred to as ocular dysmetria and indicative of cerebellar disorders.
d. Rapid horizontal oscillations around a fixation point is referred to as ocular flutter and indicative of a potential wide range of disorders including anoxic/hypoxic encephalopathy, neoplasm, encephalitis, and drug toxicity.
e. Rapid, conjugate, multidirectional irregular movements is referred to as opsoclonus and indicative of a potential wide range of disorders including anoxic/hypoxic encephalopathy, neoplasm, encephalitis, and drug toxicity.

Nuclear/Infranuclear Eye Movements

Ductions are the eye movements that test nuclear and infranuclear eye movements. When testing eye movements, keep in mind their neuro-anatomic basis (discussed later), the neuro-anatomy of the injury or disease, and the findings observed.

Ductions refer to the movement of each eye by itself. These are monocular eye movements and include the range of up, down, right, left, and on the diagonals.

Ductions are tested by covering one of the patient's eyes and instructing them to fixate on a small light, or fixation target held approximately 16 inches from them. The target is then moved slowly at a speed of well less than 40 degrees/sec through the above noted ranges. Repeat for the other eye. Look for signs of apraxia (deficits in initiation of movement), ataxia (impaired quality of movement), nystagmus, loss of fixation, and limitation in range of movement. Limitations in the range of motion in one eye is generally due to a nuclear or infranuclear muscle palsy or cranial nerve palsy (as opposed to a gaze palsy, which is a supranuclear defect).

Supranuclear Eye Movements

There are four types of supranuclear ocular movements to evaluate. These classes of eye movements require coordinated movements of multiple extraocular muscles to stabilize retinal images. They are versions, saccades, vestibular-optokinetic movements, and vergences.

Versions are binocular pursuit eye movements. They are evaluated to the nine cardinal positions of gaze. They are tested as above, except done binocularly. The nine positions of gaze are measured by testing to the patient's right and left, up and down, and on the diagonals. Look for signs of apraxia, ability to cross midline, nystagmus, dysconjugate gaze, and limitation of gaze.

Smooth pursuits are a type of duction or version. They are smooth tracking movements designed to maintain foveal fixation when viewing a moving object. The stimulus to initiate and maintain pursuits is movement of the object near the fovea. They have a relatively slow maximum velocity of (generally) less than 40 degrees/sec.

The pursuit nerve pathway originates in the peristriate cortex of the occipital motor area. From there nerve fibers descend and terminate in the ipsilateral horizontal gaze center in the pontine paramedian reticular formation (PPRF). The right occipital lobe controls pursuit movements to the right and vice versa.

Saccadic Movements

Saccadic eye movements serve to rapidly place an object of regard on the fovea or to move the eyes quickly from one object to another. These movements are both voluntary and reflexive. They are very fast eye movements, occurring at a velocity of between 400 and 700 degrees/sec.

The saccadic eye movement pathway originates in the premotor cortex of the frontal motor area. Nerve fibers then travel to the contralateral horizontal gaze center that is located in the PPRF. The right frontal lobe controls saccadic movement to the left and vice versa.

Saccades are evaluated by standard methods. During evaluation, consider the impact of potential visual field loss, and/or neglect on test results. Fixation targets should be separated by 3–4 inches and at a distance of 16–20 inches from the patient. Instruct the patient to look back and forth between the objects. Verbal, tactile, auditory, and/or visual cuing may be needed. Look for signs of apraxia, hypometria (undershooting), hypermetria (overshooting), dysmetria, inaccuracy, and dysconjugate gaze. Saccades may be different in right and left gaze and should be tested in both directions.

> PEARL: The control and innervations of saccadic and pursuit eye movements are mediated both at the cerebral and brainstem levels. The cerebral or supranuclear gaze palsies (as opposed to brainstem, or nuclear involvement) are characterized by the absence of diplopia (except in vergence deficits) and the preservation of normal vestibulo-ocular reflexes (VOR).

Optokinetic Nystagmus

Optokinetic nystagmus (OKN) is a normal physiologic set of eye movements that are a combination of smooth pursuit and rapid saccadic refixation. OKN is tested by moving a black and white striped piece of tape, or fabric, or rotating an OKN drum horizontally, or vertically, in front of the patient. It is a reflex set of movements. Absence of the fast saccadic refixation component is characteristic of lesions of the frontopontine tract, and absence of the slow phase indicates lesions of the occipitopontine tract.

Vestibulo-Ocular Reflex and Nonvisual Eye Movements

There are reflexive eye movements that are triggered by vestibular and certain proprioceptive stimuli. Their function is to hold and stabilize eye fixation on a target when the head moves by causing eye movements of an equal speed and opposite direction.

The VOR is mediated by the vestibular system. It can be triggered by nonvisual stimulus such as with caloric stimulus testing. The VOR is evaluated by having the patient fixate a steady object and then instructing them to move their head side to side, and up and down while maintaining fixation. Assess steadiness of gaze and assess for any symptoms of dizziness or imbalance.

The oculocephalic reflex (OCR and also known as "Doll's Eyes") is an eye movement in response to proprioceptive changes in head and neck movement. This test is of importance in the unconscious patient or when voluntary or pursuit movements are impaired. The examiner physically rotates the patient's head in a horizontal plane to one side and looks for an ocular turn to the opposite side. The examiner should also test by pushing the patient's chin down looking for an upward movement, and elevating their chin looking for a downward movement. In the lower level patient there is typically a short delay in the eye movement response. Full movements indicate an intact brainstem, ocular motor nuclei, and efferent motor nerves. Absence of this reflex is indicative of significant brainstem injury.

Vergence Movements

Vergence eye movements refer to binocular movements where the two eyes (are supposed to) move in a synchronous and symmetrical, but opposite, direction. The vergence movements are convergence and divergence.

Testing is done in the following manner. Begin by holding a small fixation target on midline, in front of the patient and at a distance of about 24 inches from them. Instruct the patient to look at the target. Slowly move the target toward the bridge of the patient's nose. Take note of when one or both eyes stop tracking. That eye will typically diverge out. This distance from the patient is the near point of convergence. Next, begin moving the target back out away from the patient. Take note of when both eyes fixate back on the target. This is the recovery point of divergence. Next, continue to move the target away from the patient out to about 3 feet and then back toward the patient, but stay beyond their near point of convergence. Observe for smoothness, or ataxia of vergence, degree of synchronicity, and symmetry of movements.

Common Disorders of Ocular Motility

Paresis of horizontal gaze in one direction is referred to as a conjugate horizontal gaze palsy and indicative of a lesion in the ipsilateral pontine horizontal gaze center, or contralateral frontal cortex.

Paresis of horizontal gaze in both directions is referred to as a complete bilateral horizontal gaze palsy and indicative of Wernicke's encephalopathy, or a large bilateral pontine lesion that affects both horizontal gaze centers.

Bilateral paresis of all horizontal eye movements except for abduction of the eye contralateral to the lesion and with convergence spared is referred to as a "One-and-a-half syndrome" and indicative of a lesion in medial longitudinal fasciculus (MLF) and ipsilateral horizontal gaze center.

Unilateral or bilateral paresis of an eye adduction in attempted horizontal, but not in convergence is referred as an internuclear ophthalmoplegia and indicative of a lesion in the MLF.

Bilateral paresis of upgaze with a downgaze preference and downbeating nystagmus is referred as Parinaud's syndrome and indicative of a Pineal tumor, or midbrain infarct.

Bilateral paresis of downgaze is referred to as a conjugate downgaze palsy and is indicative of progressive supranuclear palsy.

Visual Field

A careful and extended confrontation visual field test can pick up even subtle defects. Understanding the neuro-anatomy and pathophysiology of the injury will give clues as to what type of loss, if any, can be expected. The examiner should evaluate monocular and binocular visual fields. The more common types of visual field losses encountered are as follows:

Hemianopia from occipital lobe involvement
Quadrantanopia from injury to the optic radiations
Monocular from prechiasmal involvement
Diffuse from hypoxic or anoxic brain injury. This is a diffuse and scattered vision loss. Presentation is analogous to a "Swiss Cheese" appearance with islands of vision that are intact, islands that are lost, and some areas of partial sparing.

Visual Inattention/Neglect

Visual inattention is a term used to describe a perceptual loss of vision (discussed in detail in Chapter 5). It most often arises from a parietal lobe injury and is most typically a left neglect from a right parietal lobe injury. It can mimic a hemianopic visual field loss, but is actually a perceptual loss of vision with actual vision still intact. When the inattention is quite dense, the patient will present with a strong right gaze preference and virtual inability to cross midline tracking to their left. It can also be as mild as to manifest in only extremely stimulating and demanding environments.

One way of understanding visual neglect is as follows. The parietal lobe is in part, visual association cortex. It attaches relevance to what is seen. When it is damaged the speed of visual processing will be slowed and incomplete. Subsequently, when visual stimulation is presented bilaterally to the patient, the information from the right is processed more quickly and completely than that from the left. This then masks, to varying degrees, visual information coming from the left.

Evaluating for visual inattention is done in a number of ways. It frequently is not a clear-cut diagnosis because of the varying depth of involvement. While performing a confrontation visual field one can test for neglect with double simultaneous stimulation (DSS). DSS is performed by presenting a different number of fingers to the patient's right and left peripheral vision simultaneously while they fixate on the examiner. If the patient has a visual neglect, the typical response is to have full monocular and binocular fields, but on DSS the neglect side will be extinguished and they will only accurately report the fingers seen on the intact side. Additional tests are done by OT, PT, and SLP. Tests include, for example, line bisection and drawing a clock.

Scanning

Scanning can be thought of as wide field saccades. Two objects are presented to the patient. Hold the objects between 12 and 24 inches apart and at a distance of 16–24 inches from the patient. The patient is instructed to look back and forth between the objects. They may need additional cuing. Vary the separation between the targets and their location in the patient's visual field throughout the test.

Pupil Reflexes

Pupil responses are carefully evaluated. The examiner should look for signs of anisocoria, sluggish pupils, minimally reactive pupils, Adie's pupil, miosis, afferent pupil defect (complete, partial, unilateral, or bilateral), and fixed and dilated pupil (CN III). Anisocoria of up to 1.5 mm can be considered physiologic in the absence of other abnormalities. Less commonly seen is a random episodic dilation, or miosis that can arise from dysautonomia. Consider the effect of medications on pupil responses. In patients who have suffered cervical spinal cord injury one should look for signs of Horner's syndrome with ipsilateral miosis, anhydrosis, and ptosis.

Health Evaluation

External examination is evaluated by observation, slit lamp examination, and sensory testing. Test for corneal sensitivity (corneal branch of CN V). Look for signs of ptosis (CN III, Horner's syndrome), dry eye, lagophthalmos (CN VII), blepharitis, conjunctivitis, diffuse keratitis, filamentary keratitis, neurotrophic cornea, hyphema, iris tears, and cataract.

A dilated fundus examination is preferable. Pay special attention for signs of vitreous hemorrhage (Terson's syndrome), papilledema, optic nerve pallor, and retinal detachment.

Tonometry can be performed with a portable contact tonometer.

Medical eye conditions are frequently found in the neurologically affected population of patients. Some of the conditions are fairly mild and not sight threatening, but are uncomfortable for the patient. Some are quite serious and sight threatening. Effective therapy is available for many of these conditions.

Specific Conditions

Dry Eye

Dry eye can arise from a slower than normal blink rate, which is encountered in patients with TBI. It may also be secondary to systemic medications (e.g., muscle relaxants, Opioids, Gabapentin, Lyrica) or be a premorbid condition. In general, this is not sight or health threatening, but it can make the patient uncomfortable and become a distraction for them.

Evaluation Perhaps the easiest way to evaluate for dry eye is by assessing the tear breakup time. Fluorescein is placed in the eye. Using a Burton lamp, slit lamp, or other ultraviolet light, one observes the quality of the tears. Instruct the patient to blink and then hold their eyes open. Count the length of time it takes the smooth green appearance of the tear film to begin to develop some open patches. This is the tear breakup time. Less than 5 sec s is considered evidence of a dry eye.

Treatment If the condition is mild, then virtually any of the commercial over-the-counter (OTC) products for "Artificial Tears" should be sufficient. If it is more moderate or long term, then any of the OTC preservative free eye drops should be used. If symptomatic relief can be achieved with one to two drops four to six times daily, then most likely no more aggressive intervention is indicated. If this is not satisfactory, then punctal plugs and/or Restasis (cyclosporine) can be used.

Filamentary Keratitis

When a dry eye condition progresses, it can evolve into an ocular surface disease. The most common next phase is filamentary keratitis. This presents with symptoms of moderate to severe pain, red eye, foreign body sensation, and photophobia. On examination there are mucoepithelial strands that are attached to the cornea on one or both ends.

Evaluation Inspection of the cornea with a magnifying lens or slit lamp will show thin filaments that usually attached at one end. The filaments may be as small as 1–2 mm in length, or 6–8 mm in length.

Treatment Strands can be debrided under local anesthetic. Easier, however, is the use of a bandage contact lens. Topical use of compounded acetylcysteine 10% given QID is an effective mucolytic agent. Preservative free drops are indicated. If persistent, Restasis BID can be considered.

Lagophthalmos with Exposure Keratitis

Following facial nerve palsy there will be a partial to complete inability to close the eyelid. Lagophthalmos exposes the cornea to excess drying, which can progress to ocular surface disease and loss of vision if not treated. This is compounded by the common accompaniment of CN V involvement causing reduced or complete loss of corneal sensitivity (addressed below).

Evaluation Observation of the patient shows they are not able to close their eye completely with a normal casual blink. If prompted to do a forced blink, they will usually be able to close their eye further.

Initial Treatment Placing a temporary lid weight (Blinkeze available from MedDev*) can assist the amount of corneal coverage with blinking. These are made from hypoallergenic metal, shaped to conform to the outside of the upper eyelid, and held in place

* MedDev Corporation, 730 N. Pastoria Ave., Sunnyvale, CA, 94085, www.meddev-corp.com/1%20product/Eyelid%20Closure%20Products/External%20Weights-FAQ.htm

with double stick tape. Aggressive use of preservative free eye drops up to every hour and nighttime ointment is indicated. The lid(s) can be taped shut at bedtime. A bandage contact lens may be indicated to help protect the cornea.

Surgical Management   In refractory conditions where the corneal integrity is compromised, a partial, complete, or Botox tarsorraphy may be needed.

Neurotrophic Cornea

Patients who have suffered a traumatic CN VII injury may also have a CN V injury. This causes a decrease, or complete loss of corneal sensation. The combination of an anesthetic cornea with exposure from lagophthalmos is termed a *neurotrophic cornea*. This condition is sight threatening because the cornea can scar and result in a permanent loss of vision.

Evaluation   On observation the eye is quite inflamed. There may be discharge. On slit lamp examination there will be areas of corneal epithelial defects. Using a thread from a cotton swab to touch the cornea will reveal decrease, or absence of corneal sensation.

Treatment   All of the treatments discussed above for lagophthalmos are also options. If an ulcer is present appropriate antibiosis is indicated.

Patients with nonhealing/neurotrophic corneal ulcers or exposure keratitis due to cicatricial lagophthalmos or facial nerve palsy may be treated with a tarsoconjunctival flap.

Terson's Syndrome

Terson's syndrome refers to the occurrence of a vitreous hemorrhage associated with an intracranial hemorrhage.[2] It usually results from a subarachnoid hemorrhage. In TBI patients it is often found in one eye, but may be bilateral. The vitreous hemorrhage is usually so dense and large so as to effectively eliminate vision for the affected eye other than some surrounding peripheral vision.

The exact pathogenesis of Terson's syndrome remains unsettled. Initially it was believed that the subarachnoid hemorrhage traveled from the brain to the eye along the optic nerve sheath.[1] This mechanism, however, is unlikely since there is no direct communication between the subarachnoid space and the vitreous cavity. Another more current theory suggests that the acute rise in intracranial pressure from the injury and brain hemorrhage leads to intraorbital venous stasis. This in turn causes a rapid rise in intraocular venous pressure, causing rupture of peripapillary and retinal vessels.

Evaluation   Ophthalmoscopic examination of the eye will show appearance of the hemorrhage and absence of the normal red reflex except to the far periphery. An ultrasound of the eye is confirmatory.

Treatment   Previously, initial treatment would include just observation since the hemorrhage occasionally clears spontaneously with a return of vision. While many vitreous hemorrhages will reabsorb, for example, from diabetic retinopathy, vitreous hemorrhage from Terson's syndrome is less likely to, and if so, is over a long period of time. A vitrectomy can be performed with a high degree of success.

While the final visual outcome depends on concurrent ocular or central nervous system damage from the initial injury, early intervention is helpful in hastening systemic and vision rehabilitation. From a rehabilitation perspective early intervention is beneficial. Some patients have been mistakenly diagnosed as "cortically blind," when they actually have bilateral Terson's syndrome. Recovery of vision allows for faster and more appropriate rehabilitation with better outcomes. Even patients with unilateral Terson's syndrome benefit from early treatment. This allows for the reestablishment of binocular vision, stereopsis, and expansion of the binocular versus monocular visual field.

Refraction

Patients may be either unable, or unreliable in their refractive responses. Objective refraction by retinoscopy is a preferred method and performed by standard methods using loose lenses, and/or a lens rack. As a general rule, 20/40 acuity is considered adequate functional vision for normal daily activities.

TREATMENT PLANNING

Medical management of disease and trauma should be initiated as soon as possible and coordinated with the attending physician and if indicated an ophthalmology specialist. Functional vision treatment should logically follow from the diagnoses found and be in agreement and coordination with the goals as determined by the entire team. Many times these decisions are straight forward, but not always. For example, consider the patient with a left hemianopic visual field loss and with a left exotropia from a CN III paresis. Treating the strabismus reduces the effective visual field, but if the patient has diplopia it may be bothersome. In this case it would be recommended to not treat the strabismus. The rationale is that reducing the useable visual field by eliminating the strabismus is a less desirable functional outcome for the patient than teaching them to manage their diplopia.

CONCLUSION

Caring for neurologic patients in a hospital setting can be a rewarding experience. To be successful in the medical team approach and in good patient care several things are required. The clinician must be able to work with a team; have superb observation, diagnostic and therapy skills; think quickly and "on their feet," and be able to view achieving good outcomes from a function based approach. The clinician must also have a thorough grasp of the sensory and motor aspects of vision, medical aspects of vision, and functional aspects of vision. Finally, all of this must be combined with a good understanding of neurology, neuro-anatomy, physiology, occupational therapy, physical therapy, and speech therapy.

VISION EXAMINATION OF PATIENTS IN
A POSTACUTE CARE SETTING

INTRODUCTION

As the patient progresses to the medically stable state, the emphasis changes from acute intervention, to functional vision rehabilitation for a lifetime. As patients recover from the trauma of the ANI, or, more frequently, acquired brain injury (ABI), their functional level begins to rise, uncovering higher-level deficits that impact their quality of life. When working with these patients, it is helpful to regard their examination and treatment as a spiral process where multiple therapies such as vision rehabilitation therapy (VRT), OT, PT, and SLP work in concert to bring the patient to successively higher levels, where previously adequate skills are no longer adequate. For instance, on intake, the patient may be uninterested in reading, as simple activities of daily living such as eating, bathing, moving from here to there, and dressing are difficult and exhausting. However, as the patient recovers function and has time and energy beyond these "simple" daily tasks, his rehabilitation goals may expand to other, more complex activities such as cooking, reading, and/or driving.

Frequently, these patients are changing status quickly, due to ongoing recovery and medication changes. Be aware that health crises and medications may cause the patients to lose abilities charted by the prior vision doctor. However, in general, what is seen in the postacute stage is forward progression—sometimes surprisingly fast progression—of vision and other functional abilities.

Vision evaluation of patients following discharge from the acute rehabilitation phase may occur in the postacute rehabilitation center or in the neuro-optometrist's (or sometimes neuro-ophthalmologist's) office. It is possible to consult for a postacute care facility, with the doctor commuting in to evaluate patients at the rehabilitation center. In these situations, the care is similar to that presented above in the hospital setting. However, if the patient can be examined in the neuro-optometrist's office, testing can be extended and refined to prescribe treatments to further enhance visual and visual-motor function.

HISTORY

If the individual makes an appointment with your office for a vision rehabilitation evaluation, it is important to gather history information to indicate which other doctors and therapists are still involved in his rehabilitation so that you can coordinate care with those other professionals. In general, the patient will have filled out an extensive history form before arriving at your office (Appendix 12.2). However, it is important to ask the patient to tell you everything that is different since his injury. Many times the patient will respond that the old glasses are fine and that nothing has changed, assuming that eye examinations are about visual acuity. So questions must be pursued to get the patient to talk about his residual deficits so that the doctor can decide which residuals may have a visual etiology. Perhaps the two most important areas to pursue are reading and mobility. The doctor will get more meaningful information by asking the patient whether he has been doing any extended reading since the injury rather than just if he is able to read. For example, a patient will generally respond with a quick "yes" when asked if he can read. However, if the doctor then asks whether the patient has done any extended reading since his injury, the answer is often a considered "no," or "I cannot read for more than a paragraph before my eyes water and I get a headache." How much time and what sort of reading was done before the ABI should be documented. Mobility problems, such as leaning, veering, or imbalance also need to be discussed, as patients do not think of these as visual problems, and will not generally volunteer this information.

EXAMINATION

The confrontation portions of the examination are the same as described in the hospital setting above, or as in a standard eye examination if possible. However, the in-office setting allows for more thorough evaluation of areas of visual processing of both, form and motion, as well as visual integration skills, binocularity, and eye movements. A full evaluation for a patient with TBI may require up to 4 hours, which should be split into at least two sessions. Surprisingly, most patients are able to complete the bulk of testing in one 3-hour session, as the tasks are varied and there are small breaks between tasks. The higher the functional level of the patient, the more testing they are able to complete, and the longer it takes. There are a myriad of areas to be assessed, and it is the clinician's responsibility to prioritize. Sometimes, rather than a normed test, a simple qualitative test gives information that is just as useful in terms of determining the pattern of deficits and the immediate treatment plan and goals. However, particularly in a TBI case, where the entire brain may be involved, it is important to have as much data as is practical, because the goal is return to maximal function, and if the clinician's test battery fails to include major functional areas, then an incorrect impression may be formed, resulting in wasted time and insufficient treatment efforts. Fewer tests are required in patients with limited neurological injury, such as a mild CVA. In such cases, the patient's radiologic and other medical reports can be very helpful in deciding which portions of the test battery to administer.

Refraction and Accommodation

If the patient does not have the cognitive, communicative, or motor skills necessary for a routine phorometric refraction, then retinoscopy, typically with lens racks should be performed for both distance and nearpoint. Occasionally, TBI may cause significant shifts in refractive error, most often in a myopic direction.[3] Many patients with ANI or ND have accommodative dysfunction. Most commonly you will encounter accommodative insufficiency, or presbyopia, but accommodative spasm or short lags of accommodation, which may indicate convergence insufficiency, are also observed on nearpoint retinoscopy such as monocular estimate method (MEM) retinoscopy or dynamic retinoscopy.[4] Further, presbyopia should not be assumed to follow the normal progression for the patient's age, as it may be exacerbated by accommodative insufficiency related to neurologic compromise. Therefore, nearpoint refraction or retinoscopy should be performed on every patient. It is important to be aware of alignment of the visual axis on the eye on which you are performing retinoscopy, as the patient may not be able to fixate as instructed. Using the Hirschberg reflexes to maintain alignment while scoping the patient is frequently helpful. In patients with low response levels, it is sometimes easiest to get them to fixate the retinoscopic light, or to judge nearpoint accommodation by having them fixate a compelling target at a distance of approximately 8–18 inches, dependent on the patient's "normal nearpoint working distance" and simply backing up, estimating the dioptric distance between the fixated target and the retinoscope when a neutral reflex is obtained. For example, if the target is held at 40 cm from the patient's eyes, and the retinoscopic reflex turns neutral at 67 cm, the dioptric difference (accommodative lag)—in this case the difference between the 2.5 diopter accommodative demand and the 1.5 diopter accommodative response is 1 diopter of accommodative lag.

Contrast Sensitivity
There are numerous commercially available charts for testing contrast sensitivity. Decreased contrast sensitivity can create the subjective complaint of not seeing well, in the absence of a visual acuity or visual field loss. Sensitivity loss to low to mid spatial frequencies is commonly seen in patients with TBI, perhaps due to magnocellular dysfunction.

Binocular Vision
Frequently patients with ANI and ND can be examined behind the phoropter as with routine vision patients. However, these patients *must* also be tested outside of the phoropter in various fields of gaze (discussed in Chapter 4) with sensitive measures of binocularity, such as Maddox rod; they will frequently have subtle vertical phorias, particularly in downgaze (due to CN IV palsy), or variations in lateral phoria that can make them symptomatic due to subtle CN VI innervation defects, which will not be observed in the phoropter. Phorias that vary with direction of gaze may cause visual midline shift-like symptoms of disorientation and imbalance (discussed in Chapter 6).

Visual-Spatial Perception
Testing and treatment for shifts in perceived straight ahead (also known as egocentric visual midline shift) are discussed in Chapters 6 and 7. In the postacute setting, various methods of testing for spatial perception are available, including the Padula test for egocentric visual midline as well as space board testing, although space board testing requires good range of motion with the upper extremities. In yoked prism testing, one may choose to neutralize the egocentric visual midline with yoked prism (described in Chapter 6) or normalize space board responses (described in Chapter 6 and 7). Perhaps most commonly, the patient's posture, standing balance, and gait are observed for abnormalities, including stability, leaning, veering, head tilts, and postural rotations.

If abnormalities in posture, balance, and gait are noted, then yoked prisms are placed on the patient and behavioral changes are observed as the patient is able, during sitting, standing, and mobility. Unless the observed abnormality is fairly subtle, it is generally useful to start with a five or six prism diopter pair of yoked prisms, and test with bases in upward, downward, rightward, and leftward positions. If the patient is very symptomatic, but the observed postural or gait abnormalities are subtle, then it is important to begin with a lesser amount of prism, such as two prism diopters. If there is an apparent affect of prism, one should usually see a worsening of the abnormalities in the direction opposite the direction that provides effective relief of symptoms. If the prism is applied in the correct direction, but is too strong, then the signs will switch to the opposite direction; for instance, if the patient had been veering leftward, they will begin to veer rightward. If two directions of prism are helpful, then the prism is rotated between them and power and direction are manipulated empirically to achieve the best balance, posture, and gait attainable. The goal is the least amount of prism that provides the maximum benefit. Sometimes, yoked prism must be combined with compensatory prism or base in prism for post trauma vision syndrome (PTVS) (Chapter 6). This can be a time-consuming and fatiguing process for the patient, and care must be taken to be ready to support the patient to

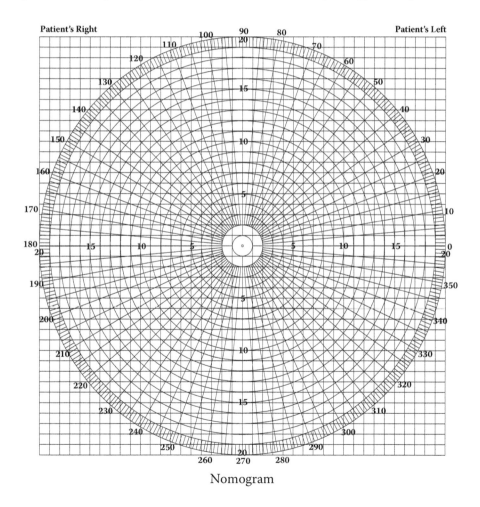

Nomogram

FIGURE 12.1 Nomogram for prescribing oblique yoked prism.

guard against falls during testing. If there is primary vestibular dysfunction, yoked prism may be helpful, but will not be absolutely effective; the vestibular dysfunction may drive the eyes more in one direction than another, creating an egocentric visual midline shift, but the primary deficit is vestibular and there will be other vestibular symptoms in balance and orientation, If there is a significant spatial perception distortion, properly prescribed yoked prisms can normalize balance and gait immediately. At that point, prism may either be prescribed for wear in the patient's glasses, or VRT may be prescribed for a month to see whether the patient can normalize perception of space. Prisms as low as 1–2 prism diopters and as high as 15 prism diopters may be necessary. It is uncommon to prescribe more than 10 prism diopters in glasses for routine wear. The nomogram commonly used for Fresnel prism may be used to measure and prescribe the direction of the base of the prism in degrees when it falls on an oblique axis (Figure 12.1). It is typical that the doctor will need to train your opticians and optical laboratory on how to interpret and properly execute a yoked prism prescription.

Visual Fields/Neglect
Visual fields should be tested to the maximum capabilities of the patient (Chapter 5). Neglect must be carefully tested for, as it is extremely common following both CVA and TBI. As discussed in Chapter 5 there is no single test that is sensitive to all forms of the neglect phenomenon, and neglect is a predictor of reinjury and poor functional outcome when left untreated. Thus a battery of tests including line bisection, distance line bisection, a cross-out task, figure copying, and perhaps tests for visual extinction should be administered.[5]

Object Perception/Perceptual Organization
As with all testing, tests of object perception or perceptual organization are limited by functional level. At a low functional level, qualitative testing, such as shape identification, matching, and construction may be the limits of the assessment. Some of the normed tests are discussed in Chapter 11. Other commonly used tests, which do not rely on verbal or fine visual-motor tasks (such as copying), are the Motor Free Test of Visual Perception (MVPT)[6] and the *Test of Visual Perceptual Skills*, third edition.[7] Both of these tests are simple to respond to, as they are designed with a test figure and a limited number of answer figures so that the correct answer may be pointed to or designated verbally. The MVPT also comes in a format where the answer figures are arranged vertically so that the test is less affected by visual-spatial neglect.[8] Normed perceptual tests may also be administered by the occupational therapy department of the outpatient rehabilitation center, and forwarded to the doctor to use in formulating the treatment plan.

Visual Memory
The *Test of Visual Perceptual Skills* discussed above has short-term recognition memory subtests for visual memory (abstract line figures) and visual sequential memory. An enhancement on this is the Continuous Visual Memory Test (CVMT),[9] which has subtests for recognition memory, delayed recognition memory (after a 30-minute delay), and a visual discrimination test. The advantage of the CVMT

is that it gives some idea whether the patient is able to consolidate information into long-term memory stores. The CVMT has been demonstrated to have good criterion validity in patients with moderate to severe TBI.[10] However, CVMT total score was mediated by visuospatial ability, and so this must be taken into account and appropriate additional testing must be performed in using the CVMT to determine whether there is a visual memory loss. Visual memory is further discussed in Chapter 13.

Visual-Perceptual Speed

Traditionally in optometric practices, tachistoscopes have been used for perceptual speed testing and training. Considering the neurology of the dorsal and ventral processing streams (see Chapter 3), two types of visual-perceptual speed should be taken into consideration, those for stationary flashed and for moving targets. Targets may be flashed at various speeds by specialized instrumentation, tachistoscopes, and computer tachistoscopes. It is important to remember that with flashed targets, visual memory interacts with performance. Observation in the clinic demonstrates that visual-perceptual speed for moving targets (appears to be dissociated from perceptual speed for flashed targets). Unfortunately, stimuli to measure magnocellular or dorsal stream processing speed through coherent motion or other techniques for measuring perceptual speed of moving targets have not yet reached clinical application. It is possible to use a dynamic acuity tester, or a tachistoscope with the Wayne's variable speed rotating prism mount to get an internally normed measure of perceptual speed for moving targets.

Visual-Motor Accuracy

Visual-motor accuracy is simple, and important to evaluate, as it frequently will give clues as to which eye has the muscle or innervation deficit and where much of the patient's frustration with visual-motor tasks arises. Although there are established protocols for isolating the involved muscle or cranial nerve causing an ocular motor problem, in real life practice, with more subtle deficits, skew deviations, or compensatory muscle actions already in place, a simple monocular visual-motor test can be illuminating. The task is simply to hold a straw or pen cap horizontally, with the opening facing the patient. The patient holds a pointer in their better hand (this may be either their dominant hand or the hand on the side with better range of motion in the arm). They fixate the straw, and make a ballistic motion with the stick to place it in the straw. It is important that the motion be speeded, rather than a gradual approach, as the patient will correct as they approach the target if they are allowed to approach gradually. The task is performed monocularly with each eye, and then with both eyes together in all four quadrants of gaze if the patient is able. Frequently, the performance for one eye is significantly impaired, particularly in the field of gaze of the affected muscle. The binocular finding can be affected by monocular input or by binocular dysfunction.

Visual-Motor Speed

Visual-motor speed tasks are often described as speed of visual processing tests. Tests such as Dynavision, Acuvision, Vision Coach, or sometimes copying tasks such as the Wold Visual Motor Test may be used to assess visual-motor speed. One must keep in mind that these tasks are all impacted directly by motor deficits, and it is important to chart how much impact the clinician judges the motor system to be contributing to performance deficits so that deficits recorded on paper are not interpreted as strictly visual or visual-motor integration problems.

Useful Field of View

Useful field of view refers to the extent of periphery that one can process information from while engaged in a central task, as in driving. Posit Sciences Corporation has taken the programmatic research in this field,[11–13] and developed a useful field of view training program, which also has an assessment at the beginning of the training program that gives scores for how well one keeps track of multiple peripheral stimuli with distracters introduced, as well as speed of processing when the task demands attending to both central and peripheral targets. This assessment and training may be useful in patients who find themselves overwhelmed by peripheral visual stimuli when the standard interventions do not alleviate symptoms.

Cerium Tints

The cerium intuitive colorimeter may be used to determine if there is a specific wavelength filter, or tint, that improves visual comfort, decreases photophobia, or increases reading speed. Specific wavelength filters may also decrease sensations of visual overload in visually busy surroundings, decrease headaches, and in some cases decrease seizures (see Chapter 8 for further details).

Ocular Health

Although many hospital and acute rehabilitation settings realize the need for speedy ophthalmologic or optometric examination, there will frequently be patients who have not yet had a thorough ocular health evaluation since their brain injury. The in-office setting allows for thorough evaluation of ocular health with standard in-office instruments, provided that the patient can achieve an upright, seated position. Patients with CVA should have dilated retinal evaluations to examine retinal vessels on at least a yearly basis. Patients with TBI should be dilated on at least a yearly basis for a minimum 10 years postinjury to rule out retinal tears related to the inertia changes that caused the original TBI, and, if cognizant enough, should be advised of the signs, symptoms, and emergency nature of a retinal tear.

Visually Evoked Potential

The visually evoked potential (VEP) is not usually performed at the initial evaluation. However, if there are questions regarding what sort of detail the patient is capable of resolving, if the patient is noncommunicative and it is unclear from the patient's responses, then the VEP can be useful in establishing that the primary visual pathway is intact, and the approximate visual acuity. It can also be used as an objective determination of PTVS, by following the published PTVS protocol.[14]

REPORTS

If the patient is being evaluated in the rehabilitation vision doctor's office, communication is key; rather than charting in a communal chart where all of the rehabilitation professionals have access to the patient's information, one must generate reports that communicate effectively with other members of the rehabilitation community, which still includes most of the specialists referred to in the hospital setting, as well as insurance adjusters and case managers who ultimately determine, for many patients, what diagnostic and therapeutic avenues may be pursued.

Report generating in a specialty setting such as neuro-optometry is frequently a time-consuming job, for which some insurance companies are no longer reimbursing. Dictation (e.g., Appendix 12.3), as well as report templates that can be partially completed by staff (e.g., Appendix 12.4) are helpful. Sometimes, the report may be a simple handwritten form to fill out (e.g., Appendix 12.5). However, copies of chart notes are seldom sufficient to assist the physiatrist, OT, case manager, or other rehabilitation professional in understanding your findings, impressions, and recommendations.

TREATMENT PLANNING

Frequently, patients with ANI have multiple, complex visual (and other) deficits; the clinician must be able to step back and look at the entire individual when formulating a plan of treatment. The plan of treatment is, in many cases, dictated by the setting in which one sees the patient. If the patient is in the hospital, temporary frames to which patches or Fresnel prisms can be applied may be necessary. VRT is often started as soon as possible if the patient is able to respond to ocular motor, scanning, or visual attentional therapy, generally prescribed by the neuro-optometrist and performed by the staffing OT. If the patient is in a postacute rehabilitation facility, again, therapy is applied as quickly as possible, as insurance coverage frequently limits the length of stay, and maximal progress is desirable while the patient is in the intensive rehabilitation setting. Lenses and prisms may be ordered at the initial visit, or after a month of therapy to see how the patient responds. In general, if prior authorization is required before providing the glasses, depending on the insurance company, there may be up to a month delay before the glasses are received—particularly if specialty tints such as cerium intuitive colorimeter tints are required. If the patient is at home, and pursuing therapy individually, one may apply lenses and prisms initially, and wait to see those results, as this may save some therapy visits in the end. Therapy for specific diagnoses is further discussed in the relevant chapters in this text. As the patient's functional level rises, deficits that were left untreated initially, become more important and the clinician must constantly reorient to the new functional demands and what sorts of therapies are appropriate. It is helpful, at the end of each progress evaluation, to list the testing that the doctor and staff will be performing at the next visit. This prevents the doctor from having to review the chart again before that progress visit.

SUMMARY

Working with patients who have neurological impairment is the most complex and multifaceted specialty in vision practice. It requires knowledge of every aspect of the field of vision care, from optical and refractive corrections, to ocular motor, binocular, spatial and object perception, and integration with other senses, as well as a broad familiarity with related disciplines so that appropriate communication and referral can take place. Organization of the clinical practice to accommodate this type of work (Chapter 13) is critical to maximize patient outcome and help the clinician succeed in this challenging specialty area.

APPENDIX 12.1

GLASGOW COMA SCALE

The Glasgow Coma Scale (GCS) is comprised of three types of tests: eyes (E), verbal responses (V), and motor responses (M). Points are given for various levels of performance in each of the three areas. The three values are considered separately, as well as their sum. The lowest sum of scores possible (deep coma) is 3. The highest score (fully awake) is 15. Frequently, only the sum of scores is reported. If individual scores are reported as well, the score is expressed in the form "GCS 8 = E2 V3 M3 at 12.16."

Generally, brain injury is classified as Severe if the GCS is ≤8, Moderate if the GCS = 9–12, and Minor if the GCS is ≥13.

EYES

1 point: Does not open eyes
2 points: Opens eyes in response to painful stimuli
3 points: Opens eyes to voice
4 points: Opens eyes spontaneously

VERBAL

1 point: Makes no sounds
2 points: Makes incomprehensible sounds
3 points: Utters inappropriate words
4 points: Confused, disoriented speech
5 points: Oriented, converses normally

MOTOR

1 point: Makes no movements
2 points: Extension to painful stimuli (decerebrate response)
3 points: Abnormal flexion to painful stimuli (decorticate response)
4 points: Flexion/withdrawal to painful stimuli
5 points: Localizes painful stimuli
6 points: Obeys commands

APPENDIX 12.2

VISION REHABILITATION QUESTIONNAIRE
Please fill out this questionnaire <u>carefully</u> prior to your appointment time.
THANK YOU.
We understand that it is long, but it will help us provide the best care for your
vision needs.

Appointment: Day _____ Date _____ Time _____

Were you referred to our office? ☐ Yes   ☐ No

    If yes, whom may we thank for this referral? _____ Phone: _____

GENERAL INFORMATION

Patient Name: _____ ☐ Male ☐ Female

Birth Date: _____ Age: _____

Marital status: ☐ Single ☐ Married ☐ Divorced ☐ Widowed

Home Address: _____

Home Phone: _____ Work Phone: _____

Social Security Number: _____ Driver's License No.: _____

What is your occupation? _____ Employer: _____

Business Address: _____

Spouse's Name: _____ Occupation: _____

Spouse's Employer: _____ Phone #: _____

Business Address: _____

Responsible Party: _____

MEDICAL HISTORY

Please list all medications or supplements you are currently taking:

_____

_____

Allergies to Medications: _____

Other Allergies: _____

List all other major injuries, surgeries and/or hospitalizations you have had:

_____

REVIEW OF SYSTEMS Do you, or have you ever had any problems in the following areas? Circle, or explain.

Eyes: Blurred vision, Loss of vision, Flashes/floaters, Distorted vision/halos, Blind spots, Double vision, Discharge, Burning, Tearing, Itching, Eye pain, Dryness, Redness, Foreign body sensation, Light sensitivity, Chronic eyelid infection, Sties, NONE_____

_____

Ears/Nose/Mouth/Throat: Allergies/Hay fever, Runny nose, Post-nasal drip, Chronic cough, Sinus congestion, Dry throat/mouth, NONE _____

Lymphatic/Hematologic: Anemia, Bleeding problem, NONE _____

Psychiatric: NONE _____

Allergic/Immunologic: NONE _____

Constitutional: Fever, Weight Gain/Loss, NONE _____

Neurological: Headache, Migraines, Seizures, NONE _____
_____

Endocrine: Thyroid/other glands, NONE _____

Respiratory: Asthma, Emphysema, Chronic bronchitis, NONE _____

Vascular/Cardiovascular: Diabetes, High blood pressure, Heart pain, Vascular disease, NONE _____
_____

Gastrointestinal: Genital, Kidneys, Bladder, NONE _____

Bones/Joints/Muscles: Rheumatoid arthritis, Joint pain, Muscle pain, NONE
_____

Social

Do you drink Alcohol, Smoke, Use any recreational drugs? (Please circle any yes answers.)

How often/much? _____

Any other health or developmental issues, please explain: _____
_____
_____

Any history of prior injuries, including head other than one we may be examining you for today, please explain: _____
_____

HISTORY OF CURRENT INJURY

Please complete this section (a) if there was an incident or multiple incidents that resulted in the neurological impairment and (b) you do not have copies of reports that explain the detailed history of the injury. OTHERWISE, skip to:
SUBSEQUENT/OTHER PROFESSIONAL CARE

Date of injury/accident (if applies): _____
Brief description of injury: _____
_____

Was the injury OPEN HEAD (skull fracture) or CLOSED HEAD (no skull fracture)? (Please circle one.)

Did you lose consciousness? ☐ Yes ☐ No   If yes, for how long? _____
Were you in a coma?   ☐ Yes ☐ No   If yes, for how long? _____

SYMPTOMS IMMEDIATELY FOLLOWING ACCIDENT/INJURY (check all that apply):

☐ Double vision   ☐ Blurred vision   ☐ Flashes of light   ☐ Pain in or around eyes

☐ Headache   ☐ Memory loss   ☐ Disorientation   ☐ Restricted field of view

☐ Vomiting   ☐ Dizziness   ☐ Loss of balance   ☐ Neckpain/whiplash

Other: _____

INITIAL TREATMENT

When did you first see a doctor regarding your accident/injury? _____

Name of Doctor: _____ Specialty: _____

Were you hospitalized?   ☐ Yes ☐ No   How long? _____

What were your diagnoses?_____

_____

What prognosis/recommendations were you given? _____

_____

SUBSEQUENT/OTHER PROFESSIONAL CARE

Has a neurological evaluation been performed?   ☐ Yes ☐ No

    If yes, by whom? _____ Date: _____

    Recommendations: _____

Has a psychological evaluation been performed?   ☐ Yes ☐ No

    If yes, by whom? _____ Date: _____

    Recommendations: _____

Has a vision/eye evaluation been performed?   ☐ Yes ☐ No

    If yes, by whom? _____Date: _____

    Recommendations: _____

PLEASE LIST any other professionals that have evaluated or are currently working with you or your child such as a: Physician, Physiatrist, Neurologist, Neuropsychologist, Psychologist/Psychiatrist, Physical Therapist, Speech/ Language Therapist, Occupational Therapist, Osteopathic Physician, Tutor or others, Please list:

Name	Profession	Recommendations	Date(s)

LIFESTYLE

Do you feel your vision interferes with activities of daily living?   ☐ Yes   ☐ No

If yes, please explain (please include effects involving home, work, hobbies social and personal relationships): _____

_____
_____

What activities comprise the majority of your daily life since your accident/injury?
_____
_____
_____

What activities can you no longer engage in due to your visual or other difficulties? _____
_____
_____

What other changes/limitations in your daily life do you attribute to your accident/injury? _____
_____
_____

What do you hope a Visual Rehabilitation Program can do for you? _____
_____
_____

EMPLOYMENT/EDUCATION INFORMATION (IF APPLICABLE)

What was your employment position prior to your injury? _____

What is current employment position? _____

What is the highest grade you completed in school? _____

How were your grades? _____

If a student, what is the major course of study? _____

How many hours daily are spent working at near distance? _____

How many hours daily are spent reading/studying? _____

How many hours daily are spent with a computer? _____

PLEASE CHECK IF YOU CURRENTLY EXPERIENCE OR EXPERIENCED PRIOR TO YOUR INJURY (IF APPLIES) ANY OF THE FOLLOWING:

	Current		Prior to Injury	
	Yes	No	Yes	No
Headaches	☐	☐	☐	☐
Blurred vision	☐	☐	☐	☐
Double vision	☐	☐	☐	☐
Flashes of light	☐	☐	☐	☐
Pain with movement of eyes	☐	☐	☐	☐
Pain in or around eyes	☐	☐	☐	☐
One eye turns in, out, up or down	☐	☐	☐	☐
Difficulty moving or turning eyes	☐	☐	☐	☐
Reduced depth perception	☐	☐	☐	☐
Squinting, covering or closing one eye	☐	☐	☐	☐

	Current		Prior to Injury	
	Yes	No	Yes	No
Difficulty with peripheral vision	☐	☐	☐	☐
Objects jump in and out of field of view	☐	☐	☐	☐
Eye redness	☐	☐	☐	☐
Eye burning	☐	☐	☐	☐
Eye itching	☐	☐	☐	☐
Eye watering	☐	☐	☐	☐
Brightness is bothersome	☐	☐	☐	☐
Fluorescent light is bothersome	☐	☐	☐	☐
Difficulty seeing in dim lighting	☐	☐	☐	☐
Patterned wallpaper or carpets are bothersome	☐	☐	☐	☐
Movement of objects in the environment is bothersome	☐	☐	☐	☐
Motion sickness/car sickness	☐	☐	☐	☐
Lose place/skip words often when reading	☐	☐	☐	☐
Words jump or move around when reading	☐	☐	☐	☐
Difficulty understanding what is read	☐	☐	☐	☐
Hold books too close	☐	☐	☐	☐
Discomfort/fatigue when reading	☐	☐	☐	☐
Short attention span for close work	☐	☐	☐	☐
Orient writing/drawing poorly on page	☐	☐	☐	☐
Dislike heights	☐	☐	☐	☐
Awkward, poor balance	☐	☐	☐	☐
Dizziness	☐	☐	☐	☐
Confusion/disorientation	☐	☐	☐	☐
Get lost often	☐	☐	☐	☐
Difficulty dressing/bathing/personal hygiene	☐	☐	☐	☐
Difficulty following a series of directions	☐	☐	☐	☐
Difficulty using both sides of the body together	☐	☐	☐	☐
Bothered by noises	☐	☐	☐	☐
Bothered by touch	☐	☐	☐	☐
Difficulty remembering things heard	☐	☐	☐	☐
Difficulty remembering things seen	☐	☐	☐	☐
Difficulty remembering name of objects	☐	☐	☐	☐
Difficulty remembering people's names	☐	☐	☐	☐
Difficulty recalling recent information	☐	☐	☐	☐
Difficulty recalling information from the past	☐	☐	☐	☐
Difficulty remembering formerly familiar people/objects	☐	☐	☐	☐
Difficulty with time management	☐	☐	☐	☐
Difficulty with numbers	☐	☐	☐	☐
Difficulty counting money	☐	☐	☐	☐

Release Of Information and Insurance Filing:

It is often beneficial for us to discuss examination results and to exchange information with other professionals involved in your care. Please sign below to authorize this exchange of information.

I authorize the release of medical information to other health care providers or insurance carriers upon their written request, or upon the recommendation of Dr. Vision Rehab when it is necessary for the treatment of my visual condition or for the processing of insurance claims. This authorization shall be considered valid for the duration of my treatment.

_____   _____
Signature of patient or authorized representative   Date

Thank you for carefully completing this questionnaire. The information supplied will allow for a more efficient use of time and will enable us to perform a more comprehensive evaluation and to better meet your specific visual needs.

If at any time you have any questions or concerns regarding your vision or treatment, please do not hesitate to contact us.

We request a minimum of 24 hours notice if you are unable to keep this appointment.

Please be on time for your evaluation so that we may have the maximum opportunity to evaluate your visual status.

Thank you.

APPENDIX 12.3

February 10

Re: R.S.

Dear Dr. W.

Thank you for asking me to see R. I examined him earlier today. I did review your record and discuss history with him, his therapist, and his parents who were present for the exam.

R. is a 22 year old male who was injured snow boarding in a half pipe competition on January 22nd. He suffered a severe traumatic brain injury with subdural hematoma, subarachnoid hemorrhage, bifrontal contusions, and a left orbital floor fracture with entrapment of the inferior rectus muscle. He had a craniotomy for the hematoma and surgery to release the inferior rectus and repair the orbital floor. The Trauma Center diagnosed a suspect left Third Nerve injury. R. is complaining of blurred and double vision.

Uncorrected distance visual acuities are 10/40 right eye and 10/15 left eye. Uncorrected near visual acuities are 20/200 right eye and 20/40 left eye. Cover test shows a small angle left exotropia distance and near. Fixations are intact with no nystagmus. Ductions are full for the right eye, but limited in upgaze of the left eye to 10 degrees. Versions are likewise. Pursuits are 2+ ataxic. Saccades are slow and inaccurate. Convergence is absent per the exotropia. Pupil reflexes are abnormal. Each pupil is minimally reactive to direct light, consensual, and accommodative reflex and there is no afferent defect. There is anisocoria with the right pupil at 4mm and the left 3mm. Each is quite sluggish. Slit lamp exam is negative. Corneas are clear, lids and lashes unremarkable and there are no cataracts. Dilated fundus exam is negative with no sign of hemorrhage and the discs are pink flat and sharp. Pressures are normal. Visual field is full monocular, binocular and to simultaneous perception. Refraction is hyperopic astigmatism right eye greater than left. Accommodation is reduced right eye.

Dr. W., R. is exhibiting a left exotropia, bilateral Adies pupil with ciliary body involvement on the right, ocular motor dysfunction s/p inferior rectus muscle entrapment and repair, and an uncorrected refractive error. These combine to explain his signs and symptoms. I do not believe he has a LCN3.

I have consulted with Dr. H. of oculo-plastics who is treating and following R. for the muscle entrapment. He and I discussed the neuro-ocular findings and he agrees.

I would recommend OTC reading glasses (+1.50) with the left lens removed for distance acuity. Initially a Spot Patch for the diplopia from the exotropia. Also, ocular motor therapy combined with OT and PT. I believe the prognosis is good and will follow to monitor.

Thank you for including me in his care,

Sincerely,

APPENDIX 12.4

NEURO-OPTOMETRIC REHABILITATION REPORT

Date

Re: NAME1 NAME2

DOB:

To Whom It May Concern:

NAME1 was seen for post-brain injury vision evaluation on DATE1, in my CITY, CA office. The patient was referred by XXX and was accompanied to the appointment by XXX. NAME1's records from XXX were reviewed prior to the initial appointment.

TESTING PROCEDURES

The evaluation took 3.5 hours to complete.

Following is a list of the testing procedures that were performed during this evaluation.

1) General history (functional problems)
2) Ocular history
3) Visual fields-automated
4) Visual acuity-distance and near
5) Retinoscopy (objective determination of refractive error for distance and nearpoint)
6) Refraction (subjective determination of refractive error for distance and nearpoint)
7) Ocular motility (eye movements)
8) Binocularity (eye coordination)
9) Sensory-motor testing
10) Visual perceptual speed for flashed targets
11) Contrast Sensitivity
12) Color naming/Color testing
13) External ocular health examination
14) Goldmann tonometry
15) Internal ocular health evaluation

RELEVANT HISTORY

NAME1 was involved in a work related accident on DOI, where XXX, which resulted in a traumatic brain injury.

NAME1's primary and secondary diagnoses from his prior records are:

(1) XXX
(2) XXX

CHIEF VISUAL COMPLAINTS

Complaints that are, or may be, related to NAME1's vision include:

(1) XXX

OBSERVATIONS AND FINDINGS

NAME1 displayed good attention and effort at the initial evaluation appointment. He had prescription glasses prior to his injury, which he wore for XXX.

Visual Acuity

NAME1's visual acuity is as follows:

		Unaided	With Correction
Distance Visual Acuity:			
	Right eye:	20/	20/
	Left eye:	20/	20/

Near Visual Acuity:

Right eye:	20/	20/
Left eye:	20/	20/

Refractive Status

Using retinoscopy and refraction, NAME1 was XXX in his right eye, and XXX in the left eye. He is presbyopic appropriate to his age.

Ocular Motor Evaluation

Pursuits were XXX. NAME1 demonstrated a mild saccadic dysfunction.

Binocular Evaluation

NAME1 demonstrated

Visual Perceptual Analysis

Visual-motor accuracy was XXX with the right eye, and XXX with the left eye, or both together.

Visual-perceptual speed for flashed targets was XXX. Visual perceptual speed for moving targets was XXX.

The Test of Visual-Perceptual Skills-3rd edition (TVPS-3) was administered by the occupational therapy department at the XXX rehabilitation center and is included here for completeness. Based on the test ceiling age of 18 years 11 months, His scores are as follows:

Subtest	Percentile Rank
Visual Discrimination	
Visual Memory	
Visual-Spatial Relations	
Visual Form Constancy	
Visual Sequential Memory	
Visual Figure-Ground	
Visual Closure	

Drawing tasks were administered by the Occupational Therapy department at the XXX rehabilitation center, and demonstrated XXX.

Egocentric Visual Midline Shift

The Padula Visual Midline Shift test was performed. NAME1 indicated his egocentric visual midline to be XXX.

On casual observation of gait, NAME1 veered/leaned/rotated XXX, with a XXX head tilt.

Visual Field Evaluation

NAME1 was able to respond appropriately to automated visual field testing and demonstrated full fields to 60 degrees XXX with either eye.

Contrast Sensitivity

Contrast sensitivity testing demonstrated a XXX with the right eye, and XXX with the left.

Color Vision

Color naming was XXX. Color vision testing was XXX.

Ocular Health

XXX

CLINICAL IMPRESSIONS

The following conditions are present:

(1) Astigmatism
(2) Presbyopia

NAME1's refractive conditions are not due to his injury of DOI. However, it is well within medical probability that the following ocularmotor, binocular, visual perception, and spatial perception deficits are due to his injury of DOI.

(3) EXAMPLE
(4) Ocularmotor dysfunction in Saccades
(5) Left hyperphoria increasing in left gaze
(6) Decreased visual motor accuracy
(7) XXX deficits in visual form perception (if present)
(8) XXX deficits in spatial perception (if present)
(9) XXX deficits in visual memory (if present)

TREATMENT PLAN

(1) EXAMPLE
(2) NAME1 should wear reading glasses for all nearpoint therapies and detailed tasks.
(3) Vision rehabilitation therapy to be carried out by the occupational therapy department at XXX rehabilitation center in order to remediate NAME1's ocularmotor, binocular, visual-spatial, and visual perceptual deficits. The initial exercises should include:

   a. XXX
   b. XXX
   c. XXX
   d. XXX

I would like to follow-up with NAME1's progress in one month. If you have questions, please feel free to call.

Sincerely,

DOCTOR

Distribution list:

APPENDIX 12.5

VISION EVALUATION REPORT

Date:_____

Patient: _____DOB:_____

Purpose of Visit:_____Accompanied by:_____

Chief Complaints:_____
_____
_____
_____

Findings:_____
_____
_____
_____
_____

Recommendations:_____
_____
_____
_____
_____
_____
_____

Follow-up Visit 1/2/3/4/5/6 Weeks/Months Other_____

_____   _____

   Dr. Vision Rehab   DATE

Distribution List:

Name: _____   Title:_____

              _____   _____
              _____   _____
              _____   _____

REFERENCES

1. Knapp, P. (1974). Classification and treatment of superior oblique palsy. *American Orthoptic Journal, 24*, 8–22.
2. Joondeph, B. C., Nguyen, H., Politzer, T., & Weintraub, A. (2007, December). Terson's syndrome managed with 25-gauge vitrectomy. Poster presented at The American Society of Retinal Specialists, Palm Springs, CA.
3. Leslie, S. (2009). Myopia and accommodative insufficiency associated with moderate head trauma. *Optometry and Vision Development, 40*(1), 25–31.
4. Guyton, D. L., Miller, J. M., & West, C. (1995). Optical pearls and pitfalls: tricks and traps in strabismus. In K. W. Wright, & P. H. Spiegel (Eds.), *Pediatric ophthalmology and strabismus* (pp. 243–248). St. Louis, MO: Mosby-Year Book, Inc.
5. Proto, D., Pella, R. D., Hill, B. D., & Drew Gouvier, W. (2009). Assessment and rehabilitation of acquired visuospatial and proprioceptive deficits associated with visuospatial neglect. *NeuroRehabilitation, 24*, 145–157.
6. Colarusso, R. P., & Hammill, D. D. (2003). *MVPT-3: Motor-free visual perception test* (3rd ed.). Novato, CA: Academic Therapy Publications.
7. Martin, N. A. (2006). *Test of visual perceptual skills* (3rd ed.). Novato, CA: Academic Therapy Publications.
8. Mercier, L., Hebert, R., Colarusso, R., & Hammill, D. (1997). *Motor-free visual perception test-Vertical format manual*. Novato, CA: Academic Therapy Publications.
9. Trahan, D. E., & Larabee, G. J. (1988). *Continuous visual memory test*. Lutz, FL: Psychological Assessment Resources.
10. Strong, C. A. H., & Donders, J. (2008). Validity of the continuous visual memory test (CVMT) after traumatic brain injury. *Journal of Clinical and Experimental Neuropsychology, 30*(8), 885–891.
11. Novack, T. A., Baños, J. H., Alderson, A. L., Schneider, J. J., Weed, W., Blankenship, J., & Salisbury, D. (2006). UFOV performance and driving ability following traumatic brain injury. *Brain Injury, 20*(5), 455–461.
12. Edwards, J. D., Ross, L. A., Wadley, V. G., Clay, O. J., Crowe, M., Roenker, D. L., & Ball, K. K. (2006). The useful field of view test: Normative data for older adults. *Archives of Clinical Neuropsychology, 21*(4), 275–286.
13. Edwards, J. D., Vance, D. E., Wadley, V. G., Cissell, G. M., Roenker, D. L., & Ball, K. K. (2005). Reliability and validity of useful field of view test scores as administered by personal computer. *Journal of Clinical and Experimental Neuropsychology, 27*(5), 529–543.
14. Padula, W. V., Argyris, S., & Ray, J. (1994). Visual evoked potentials (VEP) evaluating treatment for post-trauma vision syndrome (PTVS) in patients with traumatic brain injuries (TBI). *Brain Injury, 8*(2), 125–133.

13 Successfully Incorporating Vision Rehabilitation into the Primary Care Vision Practice

Allen H. Cohen

CONTENTS

INTRODUCTION

The management of virtually all health-care practices has increasingly become a major challenge. This has occurred, certainly in part, because of the gradual decline of the fee-for-service model and the emergence of, and patient and doctor dependence on, the managed care model, particularly over the past two decades.[1] While the fee-for-service method remained relatively unchanged for many years, managed care has been the opposite; its overall health-care and reimbursement policies are subject to change because of federal and state governmental mandates, and health-care marketplace conditions. This challenge becomes more complex when specialty services, such as vision therapy (VT) or vision rehabilitation therapy (VRT), often referred to as neuro-optometric rehabilitation, are involved.

In terms of ophthalmic care, there are basically two types of plans. One is the optical (or vision plan), which usually only provides for routine eye examinations, refractions, and optical corrections. These plans most frequently do not cover the diagnosis and treatment of nonoptical problems. There is a myriad of plans that fit under the umbrella of the second type, that is, managed care, or, as it is sometimes termed, "medical insurance." These provide reimbursement for the diagnosis and treatment of illness, sickness, accident, or disease and they usually exclude optical care. A basic tenet of these plans is that covered diagnostic and treatment services must be "medical necessary." In most cases, the International Classification of Diseases (ICD-9-CM)[2] codes are sufficient to document the medical necessity. The Physician's Current Procedural Terminology (CPT) or Evaluation and Management (E/M)[3] codes are acceptable for representing the treatment services. Many of the treatment codes have established treatment protocols and fee reimbursement schedules. The practitioner is responsible to provide support documentation for the diagnosis as well as the treatment for which payment is requested. In many of these plans, VT or VRT services are included to various degrees, especially for patients who have acquired brain injury. Those practitioners who provide specialty services for acquired brain injury, vestibular problems, and visual problems associated with systemic disease may be seeing patients who are covered under no-fault insurance and Worker's Compensation and are, by necessity, obliged to participate in third-party reimbursement.

The goal of this chapter is to provide a comprehensive method and guide to facilitate the inclusion of vision rehabilitative services into an optometric practice, within the managed care model that is in accord with the most common rules and policies of these plans, in a manner that is honest and financially feasible for the patient and optometrist. Thus, a key requirement for patients enrolled in managed care plans is to make absolutely certain they understand, before any optometric services are initiated, that some or all of these services might not be reimbursed by the plan. The proposed method includes first a discussion of a written fee policy and the diagnostic services that are usually included. This is followed by an office sequence that proceeds from making the initial appointment to additional required diagnostic services and finally to the provision of VRT.

OFFICE BASICS

A FEE POLICY DOCUMENT

First and foremost the practitioner should develop a written policy of how the practice's fees for all VRT services and necessary equipment were derived. This must be consistent for all patients, be the fee-for-service, covered by indemnity plans, or members of a plan where the practitioner is a panel provider. The policy serves to establish a sense of rational planning and organization for the office staff who are involved with billing; it is an informational document for medical insurance administrators who are sometimes unaware of the optometric management aspects of VRT. A reader of the policy should be able to follow the management plan from the initial visit to the case completion.

BASICS FOR DIAGNOSTIC EXAMINATIONS

The following codes may be applicable to the vision evaluation:

1. Consultation examination (CPT 99241–99245).
2. A consultation examination is defined, by most insurance companies, as a referral to an optometrist by another health-care provider. Its purpose is to obtain additional information that can be incorporated into the patient's existing management plan. The levels of coding of this examination (99241–99245) are based on the same criteria for other E/M services and a report to the referring practitioner is required. That provider's National Provider Identification number (NPI) must be indicated when billing for this service.
3. The consultation examination is reimbursed at a higher rate than a comprehensive exam. Since the majority of patients who are seeking rehabilitative services will be referred for consultation and management, it is important to understand and utilize the consultation services when appropriate.
4. Refractive analysis (CPT 92015): This service is almost never covered by medical insurance plans. Most optometrists directly charge the patient for this service.
5. Comprehensive exam (CPT 92004): This is a level of care that is reimbursed on the basis of the complexity of the diagnosis and the examining sequences performed to reach a management decision. The thorough understanding of the coding of this service is important, and I recommend that the reader contact the insurance companies for their guidelines. This

service level is usually the billing level for a new patient who is not referred for consultation by another health-care professional.

6. Sensory-motor examination (CPT 92060): This code covers the evaluation of classical ocular motor and binocular vision dysfunction. However, it is a very limited code and does not account for the complexity and time required for the standard optometric evaluation of, for example, an acquired brain injured patient.[4,5] The sensory-motor exam is the measurement of angles of deviation and the quantification of ocular motor skills and requires interpretation, decision making, and the generation of a treatment plan by the optometrist. The optometrist will further evaluate the patient using the information from the sensory-motor examination to develop a treatment/management plan. This procedure is usually billed with either CPT 92012, or an appropriate E/M level or an appropriate consultation level.

7. Neural Behavioral Testing (CPT 96116): This code describes a systematic approach to evaluate the intactness of higher cerebral functioning and best describes the neuro-optometric assessment of the intactness of higher level visual processing especially related to brain injury. In 2005 the description of this service was redefined and made more specific as to testing procedures and which providers are covered. Often, insurance plans will limit this service to neuropsychologists and neurologists although many states specifically include optometrists as covered providers.[6] It is recommended that the optometrist check with the State Board of Optometry and each individual insurance plan. If this service is covered, the optometrist may bill the patient but should advise the patient of this charge prior to the visit.

8. Intermediate level and E/M levels: It is appropriate to use either an intermediate exam code or the appropriate E/M code including the appropriate level for the consultation code to bill for optometric services associated with evaluating the data from the sensory-motor or assessment of higher cerebral functioning exams as well as any additional evaluations that you may do to determine a diagnosis and management plan. With most medical plans it is acceptable to bill for both the procedure codes as well as the cognitive codes on the same day. It is important that the optometrist is knowledgeable about which insurance plans allow for this and which ones deny payment for both codes on the same visit.

9. Unlisted codes: The unlisted codes CPT 99199 are used for services that do not have a specific CPT code, which specifically defines your services. When using these codes for billing, they should be designated as "unlisted" and be accompanied by an appropriate description. My perception is that these codes are not utilized to the extent they might be in billing for VRT diagnostic and therapeutic services. The most common VRT-related diagnostic services that I feel fall under this category are
   a. Developmental vision evaluation
   b. Visual perception evaluation
   c. Learning disability evaluation
   d. Sports vision evaluation
   e. Conferences and reports

    f. Review of reports by other health-care providers
    g. Visual therapy equipment and software
    h. Demonstration of out-of-office therapy
    i. Development of out-of-office therapy program

A PROPOSED OFFICE MANAGEMENT SEQUENCE

What follows is the sequence and policies used in my group practice. There are three other optometrists, and we offer full scope optometric care. Two of us specialize in all aspects of rehabilitative optometry. This includes providing care for patients with acquired brain injury, vestibular dysfunction, neuromuscular disease, strabismus and nonstrabismic anomalies of binocular vision, low vision, and children with learning-related vision disorders. We utilize certified vision therapists and VT assistants in the diagnosis and therapy of these conditions. These ancillary personnel always work under the supervision of an optometrist.

THE INITIAL APPOINTMENT

The front office staff determines the reason for the requested appointment. Basically, the callers have been referred for a consultation by another health-care provider, or for the evaluation of self-determined visual problems. The staff determines the patient's health-care insurance status and informs the callers of fees for which they will be responsible.

For patients enrolled in plans in which the optometrist participates, this includes applicable copayment and the refraction fee. Fee-for-service patients are informed that they are responsible for all fees. To ensure that there is no misunderstanding about fees, both groups of patients are sent a package that includes a cover letter, case history form, brochure, summary of fees, directions to my office, and other business paper work (see Appendix 13.1A and B). Since this chapter is geared to the population that have acquired brain injury, it is important that the protocol is discussed when dealing with patients who are injured while working and for whom optometric services are covered by Worker's Compensation, and for those patients who are injured during a motor vehicle accident and are covered by No Fault insurance. In general, the patient will bring to the office a form from their insurance company with all the necessary information required to file a claim, including the policy number, name and address of the responsible insurance company, and the name and telephone number of the case manager. Since each state may have specific requirements regarding No Fault and Worker's Compensation coverage, it is important that the optometrist and staff familiarize themselves with the specific regulations regarding optometric care in their state. The following examples represent the No Fault regulations in New York State and some general Worker's Compensation guidelines.

No Fault

In NY State no-fault carriers cannot discriminate between the services of an optometrist and a physician if your services are within your scope of licensure. However, the carrier does have the right to request an independent medical examination (IME) to determine if the visual problems are related to the motor vehicle accident. If they determine that the visual problems are not related to the accident, they can deny payment and you may then submit charges for your services to the patient's medical insurance for reimbursement. For this reason, it is important that the office also has the information regarding the patient's medical insurance and that the patient signs a form that makes them responsible for charges if No Fault denies the claim. In NY State a provider does not have to accept assignment from No Fault. The provider may elect to receive payment from the patient and the patient is responsible to submit to his insurance agency for reimbursements. In my practice, I generally accept payment from No Fault. It is my experience that these patients have so many financial and other problems associated with their injury that it is in their best interest and my best interest to accept direct reimbursement from No Fault.

Worker's Compensation

Worker's Compensation is a different issue. In NY State, if a patient is injured during work, the provider may not charge the patient for covered expense, even if the patient requests that they are willing to pay for your services. It is imperative that before scheduling the patient for consultation, they provide written documentation that vision care services are included as approved care by the Worker's Compensation board. Without this document the optometrist may find themselves in a catch 22.

Knowing how to work within the Worker's Compensation system is vital if one is going to care for traumatic brain injury patients. The first step is to contact the patient's case manager before the scheduled appointment. Authorization for the appointment should include the procedure codes (CPT or E/M) that potentially will be used during the examination. It is a good practice to submit a list of the procedures and fax those to the case manager for preapproval. The potential codes would include a consultation (99244 and 99243) or comprehensive examination (99204 or 92004), visual field test (92082 or 92083), sensory-motor evaluation (92060), refraction (92015), and a medical conference (99361). A neurobehavioral status evaluation (96116) to evaluate visual thinking, visual memory, and visual-spatial abilities may also be included. Each one of these procedures should be done and billed for separately. The medical conference code is reserved for comanagement with therapists or doctors to communicate diagnosis and treatment protocols and is usually not reimbursed by insurance companies and Workers Compensation.

After the examination a comprehensive report (99080) is prepared that covers the following items:

1. History (medical and ocular)
2. Objective findings
3. Impression/diagnosis
4. Recommendations
5. Plan

The plan should include what needs to be done next. It may be additional testing, medical treatment, coordination for therapy program, and prescribing lenses and/or prisms.

A second evaluation will cover additional testing. This may include visual information processing, visual evoked potential, additional sensory-motor testing, and possibly a low-vision evaluation. Special testing such as fundus photography (92250), anterior segment photography (92285), contrast sensitivity testing, or color testing could be done, as well.

When these extra tests are requested, the case manager may question what they are for and a written or verbal explanation would be required. After the second evaluation an additional report (99081) is generated. This is not as extensive as the first report.

After the evaluations are complete the next step is to request authorization for neuro-optometric rehabilitation. The format that I recommend is billing (92012 associated with 92065) as discussed later in this chapter. Be sure to get authorization before using any of the above codes.

Negotiating Fees

It is possible to negotiate fees with Worker's Compensation carriers. Each code that is billed generates a specific reimbursement. Usually the case manager cannot override the designated reimbursements. When there are special situations, exceptions can be made. An example would be that justification for extra expertise would be needed for a special procedure.

Prescription Glasses

Patients with brain injury often need multiple prescriptions. Authorization requests for glasses may include prisms, tint, high-index, impact-resistant lenses, and field-expansion prisms. This authorization is usually available with proper documentation. The request should include the proper V-code for each specific item. When billing these items it is important to differentiate each individual prescription, so the adjustor will understand that there is more than one prescription.

Stay on Top of Worker's Compensation Claims

It is important that each office has a designated person who requests authorization and bills Worker's Compensation. Each month the accounts receivables should be reviewed to see what is being paid and what is being denied. It is interesting to note that even though authorization is given by the case manager for the codes that you submitted, often times the case adjustor will not allow certain codes. In some cases the adjustor will down-code a consultation code to an office visit. Be on the alert for this. When Worker's Compensation does not pay for the services that were authorized, the biller needs to resubmit the claim for reconsideration. This will involve sending a letter along with the claim. It can be a time-consuming process.

COMPLETING THE INITIAL APPOINTMENT

At the completion of the initial consultation allow time to discuss impressions and the next sequence of the recommended diagnostic testing. Document which of the recommended services are covered and which are not covered by the patient's insurance and provide the patient with a form that summarizes this information. The responsible party is required to read, understand, and sign the form before appointments are made for subsequent services (see Appendix 13.2A, B, and C).

Once the form is signed, the patient is scheduled for the appropriate appointments, which may include any of the following:

1. A sensory-motor examination with an optometric vision therapist when appropriate.
2. A visual-perceptual examination with an optometric vision therapist when appropriate.
3. Extended medical diagnostic testing such as extended ophthalmoscopy, visual fields, and so on. Extended ophthalmoscopy is frequently performed at the initial evaluation if the patient has not had prior dilated retinal evaluation, particularly with a patient who has suffered traumatic brain injury— dependent on the patient's ability and fatigue level.
4. A visit with the optometrist to evaluate the data from the above tests and to perform additional appropriate testing procedures.
5. A conference appointment with the patient and responsible family attending. In my opinion, this visit is a key factor in determining the success of the treatment program. It is during this time that the patient and significant others have the opportunity to fully understand the nature of the vision problems and how and why the proposed rehabilitative program is a reasonable and feasible way to solve it. The optometrist's communication style should be clear, concise, and respectful of all who attend. It is recommended that the following are important points to be considered:
   a. Schedule this appointment after all diagnostic data have been fully reviewed and organized.
   b. Allow appropriate time during the case presentation to answer questions from the patient and extended family.
   c. Strongly encourage both parents to attend if the patient is a minor, because the family will have to make both time and financial commitments, and the attendance of both parents is conducive to these commitments.
   d. Encourage other professionals who are involved in the patients care to attend this conference with the patient.
   e. Relate the presentation of clinical findings to the patient's overall problems, chief complaints, and when appropriate relate to the assessments of other involved professionals. Diagnostic information and recommendations should be expressed in layman's terms; technical terms should be avoided. For example, I use the model of how a computer processes information as an analogy to describe visual information processing. I use the keyboard to represent functional visual skills, the software and ram to represent the brain and visual perception, and the printer to represent visuomotor performance.
   f. Discuss the goals of the management/treatment plan and fully discuss the responsibilities of the patient, family, and others in carrying out the prescribed out-of-office treatment program.

g. Do not denigrate other health-care professionals whose recommendations are different than yours; rather, support your recommendations with logic, scientific data, and confidence.
h. Control any discussion, but don't dictate. Allow enough time to cover all of the recommendations; however, it is recommended that the conference last 1 hour or less.

DISCUSSION OF FEES

It is important to allow ample time to review fees and office policies. It is my experience that patients and/or their responsible family members often are more comfortable discussing the financial aspects with the optometrist rather than with ancillary personnel. I try to respond to their concerns and I assure them that my staff will be helpful and supportive in arranging for their insurance and financial needs. There are special considerations for patients with and without medical insurance.

Be very knowledgeable about the policies on allowable services for those plans in which you participate. For patients who are members of these plans enumerate the services that are covered and those not covered. When questions are raised about non-covered services that, in your professional judgment, are deemed necessary, emphasize that it is the plan that has made this decision and not your office. The patient and responsible parties must understand that they are responsible for noncovered services. Further, do not inappropriately change or modify the diagnosis or treatment plan so that these services are covered. This can constitute fraud as well as patient management problems. For example, the time to develop and demonstrate a comprehensive out-of-office therapy program (home therapy or a program that is incorporated into their overall rehabilitation program) is usually not a covered service by insurance companies, and the unlisted code should be documented when billing for this service. Your patient must be made aware of the fact that they are responsible to pay for this service and sign a waiver. This service is not appropriate for E/M billing. Use the diagnostic code that most truly reflects the optometric assessment. The development of an out-of-office therapy program is quite time consuming and I charge a fee for this service that is commensurate with the time allotted in the schedule to do the program. Likewise, when my vision therapist demonstrates each phase of this program to the patient, extended family member, or rehabilitation specialist, this visit is billed on the basis of the time required for the demonstration. As previously stated, in these instances, the unlisted code should be used. In most instances, the fees for these services will be the responsibility of the patient and this must be understood before therapy is initiated and the patient must sign a waiver that documents that they accept this provision.

For patients not enrolled in a plan in which I participate, several options for payment are offered. They can pay at each therapy visit. A second method is to make a per case payment; the number of visits that will be required is estimated and a 10% discount is offered if the entire fee is paid in advance. Finally, if the patient elects to use a commercial finance plan accepted in my office, I agree to absorb the 1-year finance charge. The rationale for giving the discount and/or paying the finance charge is that in these cases the total fee is received when therapy is initiated, which eliminates billing and costly administrative overhead costs.

A special case is those patients whose visual problems are the result of accidents, and who have no insurance, and cannot afford VRT. These patients are in the process of litigation. In these cases I accept a legal lien, with the caveat that they are still responsible for eventual payment.

SCHEDULING THERAPY SESSIONS

1. At the conclusion of the conference the responsible parties are informed that the staff will request preauthorization of VRT when the plan requires this. Once authorization is completed, the responsible parties are sent an information packet including forms to sign (see Appendix 13.3A, B, C, and D). The information packet clearly documents the patient's treatment responsibilities, type of visits, equipment and materials required, and their payment responsibilities. There are also legal and waiver forms for the patient to sign. When the completed forms are received, the vision therapist arranges the schedule of therapy appointments. It is my experience that this procedure helps to reduce many of the misunderstandings that I experienced in the past, and confirms the commitment of the patient and family to the VRT program.

2. In the event that preauthorization is not provided, unless I perceive a blatant error, the family and patient are informed that it is their responsibility to pursue the issue with their insurance company. Our office will provide them with the diagnosis and treatment plan, as well as some appropriate references, but will not become directly involved in the issue.

3. Special issues:

   a. In NY State, No Fault will not preauthorize treatment services. Fee for services are submitted for payment and No Fault will determine if the injuries are associated with the accident or not. In my office, we will provide two sessions of therapy and then bill No Fault to determine if the services will be covered. Once we are reimbursed, we will then continue the therapy. The patient signs a document acknowledging that they are responsible for payment if No Fault denies the claim. It is recommended that the case manager be contacted to determine if the case is open and if funds are available.

   b. For patients that are being treated under Worker's Compensation, the procedure requires a narrative report and the case manager will determine and approve if the treatment services are appropriate.

CODING VISION REHABILITATION THERAPY TREATMENT SERVICES

Most insurance companies, including Medicare, Worker's Compensation, and No Fault insurance, recognize CPT 92065 (orthoptic treatment) as the code that represents office-based VT/VRT. It is defined as an independent procedure with ongoing medical supervision. In my practice, we schedule visual therapy appointments of 30 minutes and bill with the code 92065.

By definition, the therapy requires ongoing medical supervision and it is customary at each session for the doctor to evaluate the overall progress and the patient's response to, and the effectiveness of, the procedures prescribed for prior sessions as well as the effectiveness of the out-of-office program. New procedures are pre-scribed when appropriate. The most appropriate code for this service is CPT 92012 (Intermediate Examination). In my office, we allow about 15 minutes for this service. This procedure code can only be billed for face-to-face patient encounters.

Some patients require extensive supplemental home-based therapy procedures. I develop a comprehensive plan for this and there is a one time, global fee that is based on the time spent in crafting the plan. An additional fee is charged for the services of the vision therapist to demonstrate the prescribed procedures. This is usually sched-uled in phases approximately 4–6 weeks apart or as progress is made. For both of these services I use the unlisted code CPT 99199, with the description: Development of out-of office procedures and demonstration of out-of-office procedures. Neither of these services is usually covered by medical insurance plans, and therefore they are the responsibility of the patient.

The billing of rehabilitation codes (CPT 97530–97537) is a special issue. Recently Medicare has broadened certain rehabilitation codes to cover treatment services for visually impaired patients. Most of the codes are specific for the rehabilitation of low-vision patients; however, several codes could be appropriate for patients with acquired brain injury. I don't recommend using these codes if the patient's diagnoses are reimbursed under CPT 92065 for the following reasons:

1. They allow for only a limited number of sessions.
   a. Usually a maximum of 10 sessions within 90 days.
   b. Detailed documentation is required if more sessions are required.
   c. A very well documented treatment plan with defined goals and objec-tives, which result in the patient performing more independently is required. Since most of the accepted diagnosis codes except for visual field loss are related to low vision, the required treatment plan is very specific. It must address how therapy and procedures performed will enable the patient to be more independent in daily living activities.
2. They require constant reevaluation of progress with documentation.
3. The supporting diagnoses are limited.
   a. Except for visual field loss, most of the diagnosis codes related to the rehabilitation codes are specific to low vision.
   b. Each session must demonstrate a process that incorporates an assess-ment of progress related to goals and objectives and a modified treat-ment plan. Each code billed must represent a minimum of 15 minutes of face-to-face therapy between the doctor and the patient.

If VRT is billed appropriately as described in this chapter, the difference between fees reimbursed under most insurance companies will be very close in amount to the rehabilitation fees without the significant auditing and intensity of documentation and restrictions that are required with the rehabilitation codes.

DOCUMENTATION OF VISION REHABILITATION THERAPY SERVICES

Careful and complete documentation for all optometric services is essential in dealing with managed care plans and medical insurance companies, and this is particularly true for VRT. It is not unusual for plan administrators and workers to be unfamiliar with this diagnostic and therapeutic regimen. Consequently, it is recommended that the SOAP (Subjective, Objective, Assessment, Plan) model of documentation be used, which is the generally accepted format. It is specifically important when treating patients who sustained their injuries during a motor vehicle accident or during a work-related accident because often there is a litigation process involved with the case. This usually results in your records being requested by the parties involved and possibly, a request that you be a witness if this case goes to trial.

The documentation for the VRT visits (CPT 92065) is recorded by whoever is providing the therapy procedures. The notes should clearly document that the procedures used during the treatment session are in accord with the doctor's treatment plan; the patient's performance on each technique should be recorded. The visits must be dated and initialed by the prescribing optometrist.

It is recommended that the documentation for the doctor's intermediate examination (CPT 92012) be recorded on a dated progress note, separate from the recording of the therapy visit. It should include the evaluation of progress during prior VRT sessions, the home supplemental procedures, and any appropriate modifications to the treatment plan. There should also be preprogramming of the techniques for the next VRT session.

Both levels of documentation should have the date of service, patient's name, provider of services' name, and should be clearly signed by the provider.

CODING EXAMPLES FOR BILLING

The following are examples of cases that are common in VRT practices. The fee for each service is that which is consistent with the written office policy.

1. Basic Binocular Vision Dysfunction Evaluation.
    a. Consultation Exam (CPT 99244) or comprehensive exam (CPT 92004).
    b. Refractive analysis (CPT 92015).
    c. Sensory-motor examination (CPT 92060).
    d. Intermediate examination (CPT 92012) or appropriate E/M or consultation level.
    e. Conference and report (Unlisted Code).
2. Complicated injuries with visual processing deficits.
    a. Consultation Exam (CPT 99244) or comprehensive exam (CPT 92004).
    b. Refractive analysis (CPT 92015).
    c. Sensory-motor examination (92060).
    d. Intermediate examination (CPT 92012) or E/M or consultation level. For assessment of visual-perceptual processing skills, review of testing by other health-care providers, and educational testing, conference with family and reports use CPT 96116. If the insurance company does not cover this service, use the unlisted service to bill for the noncovered aspects of your evaluation.

3. Treatment.
   a. Out-of-office therapy planning fee and demonstration of procedures use unlisted codes.
   b. In-office VRT (orthoptic therapy) use 92065.
   c. Ongoing evaluation of in-office therapy progress and the prescribing of additional treatment procedures use 92012.
   d. Reevaluations as appropriate use 92012.

THE SUCCESSFUL VISION REHABILITATION PRACTICE

There are basically two aspects that are key for all optometric services, and particularly for VRT. There should be a blending of the provision of high-quality services with office policies and administration in a manner that assures the doctor a fair measure of fiscal feasibility. Thus, fees should be set that are commensurate with the doctor's training, experience, responsibility, along with the importance and complexity of the services that are provided. Further consideration must be given to the office overhead costs that include wear and tear on equipment and materials loaned or dispensed for supplemental home-based therapy procedures. The overall financial goal is that the "net flow income" from VRT services (the income per hour which considers all pertinent factors) should, at a minimum, equal the per-hour income the office generates when providing optometric primary care examination and treatment services. The VRT practice requires special training and expertise, as well as increased paperwork, and therefore should generate a greater per-hour income than the primary care portion of the practice. This is more easily accomplished with fee-for-service patients, but this can also be achieved for those patients enrolled in a medical plan when there are clearly defined and consistently used office policies and procedures The development and ability to grow a specialty practice in optometric rehabilitation is easier than most other optometric specialties because of the nature of the population served. The rehabilitation professionals involved in the care of these patients are dedicated professionals who usually will do what is necessary to help their patients. The optometric rehabilitation model and the model that other rehabilitation specialists base their treatment on are similar and share the same goals: help the patient to perform more efficiently and improve their quality of life. Furthermore, there are several optometric groups that represent optometric VRT that share information and educational programs with related rehabilitation groups such as occupational therapists, physiatrists, physical therapists, chiropractors, and so on. It is my experience that optometry is invisible to other rehabilitation specialists and the key to increasing referrals is networking. The following are some of the recommended methods that help to increase a referral base:

1. Join optometric professional organizations that represent visual therapy (e.g., the Neuro-Optometric Rehabilitation Association, College of Optometrists in Vision Development, and the Optometric Extension Program).
2. Achieve certification and or additional competency in visual therapy and neuro-optometric rehabilitation therapy.

3. Develop an office pamphlet that explains what rehabilitative services are provided and the staff's qualifications. Have these pamphlets available in the waiting rooms, examination rooms, and mail them with reports.
4. Mail a report and pamphlet to the referring professional, the rehabilitation team, the patient, and the patient's neurologist and primary care physician.
5. Provide in-service education to rehabilitation centers, support organizations for patients with acquired brain injury, and most importantly to optometric organizations to encourage referrals.
6. Make the office user friendly for this population. This means wide hallways, handicapped accessible rest rooms, and appropriate equipment to examine this population.
7. Educate the staff about the necessary care and attitude to appropriately register the patient and guide the patient through the examination; The staff must be knowledgeable about optometric vision rehabilitation services.
8. Modify the scheduling of patients so that enough time is allowed for this special patient population. My recommendation is to allow 1 hour for the consultation visit, 1 hour for each diagnostic visit, and 30 minutes for the consultation.
9. Develop or register with a web site and link your web site to related rehabilitation web sites.
10. Networking and making yourself visible to rehabilitation specialists is important.

SUMMARY

The basic components of conducting a successful VRT practice have been discussed in this chapter:

1. Create an office policy document that provides the rationale for diagnostic and treatment fees for all services. The fees must be consistent for all patients.
2. Establish fees to cover materials dispensed to patients that are associated with the treatment plan.
3. Allow adequate time to explain to the responsible parties the reason for the fees for which they will be responsible. Have the responsible parties sign a letter that summarizes these services and fees before any services are provided.
4. Be thoroughly familiar with the policies and procedures of plans in which you participate.
5. Understand and appropriately utilize the Unlisted CPT codes.
6. Use the most appropriate diagnostic codes when billing plans. Do not inappropriately modify the diagnosis or treatment plan to have the services covered by the patient's medical plan.

7. Make certain that all services are fully and properly documented and are signed by the provider.

CONCLUSION

I have presented the basics of what some 38 years of experience has indicated, and are needed to conduct a successful VRT practice for all patients. The rules and regulations for managed care have changed from year to year, and the optometrist must be alert to be informed and understand these changes. The interested reader is referred to a chapter by Wright[7] for further information about coding for VT, another by Sanet[8] for developing fees, and an article by Press[9] that presents templates for various letters and reports.

Optometry fought to have its services included in medical care plans, first at the state, and then at the federal levels. At this time participation in one or more of these groups is the rule, rather than exception in all types of optometric practices. Indeed, these plans have enhanced the profession and its practitioners. The key to flourish in this environment is the ability to be knowledgeable of the rules and regulations of these plans. With a willingness to be flexible, the practitioner can then maximize the opportunities, and honestly and intelligently address the challenges that are part of every plan.

This chapter contains some information presented in an article that I authored in 2004 in the *Journal of Behavioral Optometry*, *15*(4), 100–105.

APPENDIX 13.1A

SAMPLE

Out of Network Healthcare Disclosure/Financial Release

I hereby attest that I fully understand my financial responsibility for the charges resulting from my decision to do the following:

Your Insurance Carrier has issued a pre-determination approval for orthoptic/vision/vision rehabilitation therapy. The fee for each session is: $_____.

According to your Plan, all reimbursements will be made DIRECTLY to YOU. Therefore, you are financially responsible for all fees. As a courtesy we will submit claims on your behalf for reimbursement.
Payment is expected At the Time of Service. If two payments are missed, Vision Therapy will be SUSPENDED UNTIL YOUR ACCOUNT IS UP TO DATE.

I understand my financial responsibility.

Member/Guardian signature: _____ Date:_____

SAMPLE

In Network Healthcare Disclosure/Financial Release

Based on the information that your insurance provided us, Vision Therapy will be considered a covered service. You are eligible for_____visits per year.

**Considering Dr. V. Rehab accepting assignment of your insurance payment from your insurance company _____to cover services rendered, the following additional terms are agreed to:

1. In the event the insurance carrier pays YOU the sum directly, you agree to immediately pay the said amount received to this office.
2. By signing this agreement you represent that to the best of you knowledge the above insurance coverage is in full force and effect and you believe that the insurance covers the treatments performed by this office.
3. Co-Pays for each therapy session are due At the Time of Service. For your convenience, payment can be made weekly or monthly: but each month they must be up to date. IF NOT PAID UP TO DATE, THERAPY WILL BE SUSPENDED UNTIL PAID.
4. **In the event your insurance carrier DOES NOT pay the claim submitted, or in the event that the insurance carrier disclaims coverage for any reason, then YOU agree to pay this office Privately, Out of Pocket, the Vision Therapy fee of $, less any sums paid by the insurance carrier. Said payment is due immediately upon notification to you by this office.**

I understand that the provisions of my coverage plan will determine my financial liability.
Member/Guardian signature: _____   Date:_____

SAMPLE

No Fault Healthcare Disclosure/Financial Release

I, hereby attest that I fully understand my financial responsibility for the charges resulting from my decision to do the following:

I choose to see a provider WITHOUT an authorization from No Fault Insurance. I am aware that No Fault Insurance DOES NOT pre-authorize services for Vision Rehabilitation Therapy. The OUT-OF-NETWORK provider I elect to see is Vision Rehab, OD/MD. The fee for each session is: $_____.

I understand that the provisions of my coverage plan will determine my financial liability.
Member/Guardian signature: _____   Date:_____

NOTE: You have two options that we can offer you at this time:

1. **Come to the office for 2 vision therapy sessions (for which you are financially responsible if your insurance does not cover these services) and we will bill your insurance for these visits. Therapy is then suspended until we hear from your insurance. If you choose to continue and not wait for your insurance's decision you will be responsible for all fees until we receive payment.**

2. **Pay Privately for all Vision Rehabilitation Therapy sessions and you can bill No-Fault for these services.**

THANK YOU

SAMPLE

Private Pay Healthcare Disclosure/Financial Release

I, hereby attest that I fully understand my financial responsibility for the charges resulting from my decision to do the following:

Unfortunately, your insurance carrier does not cover orthoptic/vision therapy.

I choose to have a service/procedure performed that is NOT covered by my plan. The service/procedure I am having is: _____

THE FEE IS $ PER SESSION.

Payment is expected At the Time of Service. If two payments are missed, Vision Therapy will be SUSPENDED UNTIL YOUR ACCOUNT IS UP TO DATE.
I understand my financial responsibility.
Member/Guardian signature: _____   Date:_____

APPENDIX 13.1B

TBI/ABI VISUAL SYMPTOMS REQUIRING OPTOMETRIC REFERRAL

Please consider each symptom and place a check under 0 if the symptom is not present, 1 if the symptom is minimally present, under 2 if the symptom is moderately present, or 3 if the symptom is severely present.

SYMPTOMS	DEGREE OF PRESENCE			
Emergent Visual Conditions	**0**	**1**	**2**	**3**
Floaters in field of vision	—	—	—	—
Restricted field of vision	—	—	—	—
"Curtain" billowing into field of vision	—	—	—	—
Urgent Visual Conditions	—	—	—	—
Inability to completely close eyes	—	—	—	—
Difficulty moving or turning eyes	—	—	—	—
Pain with movement of eyes	—	—	—	—
Pain in or around the eyes	—	—	—	—
Wandering eyes	—	—	—	—
Double vision	—	—	—	—
TBI/ABI Optometric Vision Rehabilitation Conditions				
Blurred vision, Distance viewing	—	—	—	—
Blurred vision, Near viewing	—	—	—	—
Slow to shift focus, near to far to near	—	—	—	—
Difficulty taking notes	—	—	—	—
Pulling or tugging sensation around eyes	—	—	—	—

Face or head turn	—	—	—	—
Head tilt	—	—	—	—
Covering, closing one eye	—	—	—	—
Disorientation	—	—	—	—
Bothered by movement in spatial world	—	—	—	—
Bothered by noises in environment	—	—	—	—
Light sensitivity	—	—	—	—
Discomfort while reading	—	—	—	—
Unable to sustain near work/reading for adequate periods				
General fatigue while reading	—	—	—	—
Loss of place while reading	—	—	—	—
Eyes get tired while reading	—	—	—	—
Headaches	—	—	—	—
Easily distracted	—	—	—	—
Decreased attention span	—	—	—	—
Reduced concentration ability	—	—	—	—
Difficulty understanding what has been read	—	—	—	—
Loss of balance	—	—	—	—
Poor eye-hand coordination	—	—	—	—
Poor handwriting	—	—	—	—
Poor posture	—	—	—	—
Dizziness	—	—	—	—
Poor coordination	—	—	—	—
Clumsiness	—	—	—	—

APPENDIX 13.2A
DATE:

PATIENT NAME:

During your last visit to this office Dr. Vision Rehab indicated that you or your child needed additional testing relating to an eye muscle problem. Dr. Vision Rehab. specializes in this area and will coordinate and provide all the testing and if appropriate, vision therapy.

Unfortunately, Dr. Rehab. is **NOT** a participating provider under you plan so therefore you will be financially responsible for all the testing fees. Our office will provide the necessary documents for you to submit to your insurance for **YOU** to be reimbursed.

TYPE OF TESTING:

Eye Muscle Testing:

92060 Sensory-Motor Exam $
92012 Finish Testing w/ Doctor $
92012 Conference w/ Doctor $
TOTAL $

I understand that I am financially responsible for all of the above fees. In the event that the insurance reimburses Dr. V. Rehab, the insurance checks will be signed over to me, given that my account is current.

Member/Guardian signature: _____   Date:_____

APPENDIX 13.2B

Vision Therapy Acceptance / Declination Statement

Once you have reviewed the information provided in this letter, please read and select from the options below:

[__] Please call me to set up my vision therapy schedule
[__] Please call me to set up my demonstration of my home therapy program (check this if no "in office" therapy)
[__] I am not interested in receiving vision therapy at this time. Please let us know why you decided not to take the therapy.
Thank you.

Once we have received this notice of your desire to initiate vision therapy treatment, we will make every effort to accommodate your scheduling needs. Thank you for your time and cooperation.

Name _____   Date _____

APPENDIX 13.2C

To Whom It May Concern:
Re: Patient Name:
Policy Holder:
Policy Number:
EMPLOYER

The above patient was recently examined in this office. The diagnostic examination revealed the following diagnoses and the appropriate ICD-9 CODES:

The treatment for the above problem(s) is ORTHOPTIC/VISION THERAPY (CPT CODE 92065). This treatment is specific for the diagnosed neuromuscular anomaly(ies), and IS NOT for routine eye care or glasses. This therapy consists of in-office treatment sessions and it is anticipated that sessions are needed to ameliorate the above-diagnosed problem(s). The fee for each session is $.

My patient has requested that I pre-authorize benefits for my services. Please provide me with the following information:

1. Is this treatment a covered service?
2. What is the insured's annual deductible?
3. Has deductible been met?
4. If not, what is remaining balance?

A prompt reply would be greatly appreciated.
Very truly yours,
Doctor
I grant permission to company to release the above information to
Insured Signature _____ Date _____

APPENDIX 13.3A

TO ALL VISION THERAPY PATIENTS:

The forms checked below MUST be signed and returned back to our office before any appointments for Therapy/Homework can be made.

————Healthcare Disclosure

————Insurance Assignment Letter

————Equipment Fee Letter

————Developmental Fee Letter

————Referral Request Form for Primary Care Physician]

————Therapy Acceptance Letter

————Care Credit Application (Optional)**

THANK YOU.

**Care Credit is the Office's only accepted payment plan.

APPENDIX 13.3B

Date:

The complexity of visual problems require a very structured and sequential out-of-office therapy program which must be followed and repeated several times per week. Dr. must schedule a block of time to plan and develop a goal-oriented program, which will be refined and adjusted as progress is made. The fee for the developing this program is *$* Unfortunately, this is *not covered by your medical insurance and must be paid in advance by you prior to your first vision therapy appointment.*

Each month, based on _____ progress, a homework appointment will be set up to demonstrate new home therapy procedures. The fee for this service is $_____. Unfortunately this is NOT covered by insurance and must be paid by you.

Please sign below that you acknowledge the above was presented to you and that you agree to accept payment responsibility. Upon receipt of the program fee a homework appointment & Vision Therapy appointment will be scheduled with you.

Thank you.

Signed

Date

APPENDIX 13.3C

Durable Medical Equipment For Orthoptic Vision Therapy.

In most instances, Optometric Visual Therapy is more effective when reinforced by a specifically prescribed home therapy program. Many of the home therapy sequences require medical equipment specifically designed for your diagnosed problems.

There is a ONE time fee of $ for use of this equipment. You must make payment for this equipment at the *start* of your vision therapy program.

**There may be other diagnosed conditions that require additional durable medical equipment. In these instances it may be necessary that you purchase this equipment. The equipment will be used beyond the duration of the active in-office treatment as recommended by the doctor.

APPENDIX 13.3D

Vision Therapy Information (Weekly)

VISION THERAPY: Vision therapy is a specialized field of optometry that develops the visual performance of children and adults. Vision therapy is a means of improving visual conditions, which cannot be adequately treated by glasses or contact lenses alone. Because vision therapy is a learning process, the patient must be motivated and actively involved. Vision therapy is something the patient does, not something that is done to the patient. **Initial:** _____

DURATION OF THERAPY: Your doctor has recommended vision therapy on a weekly basis, as indicated by her findings. If paying weekly, the payment of $XXX for each therapy session is due at the time of patient sign-in. A re-evaluation will be conducted at the completion of one unit (12 sessions) of therapy. Re-evaluations require comprehensive re-testing by the doctor to determine the progress of therapy. The fee for reevaluation is $XXX. **Initial:** _____

HOMEWORK: Homework is always a crucial element of vision therapy, making the difference in your success. You should do at least 30 minutes of homework at least 5 days a week. The more therapy you do, the faster you will finish. If you feel that you are not motivated enough to keep up on the homework we advise that you not pursue therapy at this time. Each week a homework sheet will be sent home with the exercises to be done and a brief explanation of how to do them. This sheet must be returned at each therapy visit with parent comments and/or notes. Any improvements in, or difficulties with, any of the exercises should be noted on the homework sheet. **Initial:** _____

RE-EVALUATION: A progress examination will be scheduled with the doctor after each unit of therapy to assess the patient's vision and to make any necessary alterations in the program. Patients make progress at varying rates depending upon the severity of the problem, the patient's motivation, the cooperation of the patient and/or parents in carrying out the homework assignments. **Initial:** _____

MISSED APPOINTMENTS: When a patient is too sick to go to work or attend school, the patient is also too sick to attend therapy and benefit from it. Please be sure to notify us as soon as possible if you will be unable to make it to your regular appointment. You are allowed to miss **ONE** session at no charge during each unit of therapy. In addition, you have ONE allotted appointment that you may reschedule to a different day, at no charge in case of illness or an emergency. The further in advance we know of your absence the greater the chance an appointment may be available. We advise that you reserve this session for a day you may miss due to an unexpected illness or emergency. Otherwise, your therapy slot is reserved for you and **any further missed sessions will be charged at the regular fee. Initial:** _____

VISION THERAPY EQUIPMENT: To do vision therapy homework, equipment is needed. Vision therapy equipment will be checked out to each patient. At the time of equipment check-out or equipment return, the patient/parent and therapist will initial the equipment inventory sheet. This will keep any misunderstanding and equipment fees to a minimum. A non-refundable, $XX.00

equipment fee is due at the first visit of each unit of vision therapy. This equipment fee is for rental and any wear and tear that is put on the equipment during each 12 week unit of therapy. A $XXX.00 equipment deposit fee will also be required at the beginning of therapy. The deposit will be held until the vision therapy unit has been completed. This deposit will only be kept in the event of loss, breakage or non-returned equipment. Vision therapy equipment is expensive and should be handled with care. At the beginning of each new therapy unit you will be asked to reissue a replacement check for the $XXX equipment deposit. If all equipment has been returned in good order, your previous check will be returned to you. If equipment has been returned damaged, the cost of replacement will be deducted from your deposit check.

REMEMBER: If you are planning on therapy, remember your success is dependent on you being able to come into the office once a week. You must do vision therapy homework five times weekly and keep accurate notations about it. If for any reason your lifestyle does not permit you to meet these specific requirements, you should not commit to therapy at this time. Great results in vision therapy are only seen when time, effort, and patience are given to it. **Initial:** _____

REFERENCES

1. Coddington, D. C., Fischer, E. L., Moore, K. D., & Clarke, P. L. (2000). *Beyond managed care: How consumers and technology are changing the future of health care.* San Francisco, CA: Josey-Bass.
2. American Medical Association. (2010). *ICD-9-CM Code Book 2010.* Chicago, IL: Author.
3. American Medical Association. (2010). *CPT 2010 Code Book.* Chicago, IL: Author.
4. Suchoff, I. B., Kapoor, N., Waxman, R., & Ference, W. (1999). The occurrence of ocular and visual dysfunctions in an acquired brain injury sample. *Journal of the American Optometric Association, 70*(5), 301–308.
5. Scheiman, M., & Wick, B. (2002). *Clinical management of binocular vision: Heterophoric, accommodative, and eye movement disorders* (2nd ed.). Philadelphia, PA: Lippincott Williams & Wilkins.
6. Blue Cross Blue Shield of Kansas. (2005). Sensorimotor and neurobehavioral status exams for optometric providers. Retrieved from http://www.bcbsks.com/CustomerService/Providers/MedicalPolicies/professional/policies/010106SensorimotorNeurobahavioral.pdf
7. Wright, M. R. (1998). Third party rules and regulations. In W. B. Bleything (Ed.), *Developing the dynamic vision therapy practice* (pp. 107–112). Santa Ana, CA: Optometric Extension Program.
8. Sanet, R.B. (1998). Rational for fee structures. In W. B. Bleything (Ed.), *Developing the dynamic vision therapy practice* (pp. 85–92). Santa Ana, CA: Optometric Extension Program.
9. Press, L. J. (1998). Vision therapy services agreement. *Journal of Optometry and Vision Development, 29*(4), 214–20.

14 Advocating for Your Patient in the Legal System

Joseph Kiel

CONTENTS

INTRODUCTION

So here you are, a little confused. Did you think that becoming an accomplished expert witness would follow naturally from being a conscientious, competent medical provider? Did you somehow miss the classes in school that would have taught you how to be an effective expert witness? Are you apprehensive about what will be expected of you at trial? Are you puzzled why lawyers don't understand a thing you say about your patient's condition? This chapter is written to explain the rudiments of litigation and what will be expected of you in the litigation process.

RECOGNIZE THE POTENTIAL FOR LITIGATION AT INITIAL INTAKE

The first step in becoming a confident participant in the litigation process is to recognize the potential for litigation in your initial patient contact. Principally, you should be concerned with the nature of the presenting condition and the possibility of a claim being asserted by your patient. That which involves the greatest potential for litigation is the circumstance in which your patient has sustained an injury to the visual system that gives rise to a claim for damages. This is called a *tort*, that is, a negligent or intentional civil wrong—as opposed to a criminal act—not arising out of a breach of contract that injures someone. A tort may be intentional such as a deliberate assault and battery or, more likely, a negligent act such as careless driving, defective equipment resulting in a carbon monoxide exposure, or allowing a dangerous condition to exist on property, which results in a slip and fall. Once you recognize the potential for a claim, you need to shift away from your usual procedures and start thinking of what you have to do to become an effective advocate on behalf of your injured patient.

RECORD KEEPING

No doubt your customary practice is to inquire of your patient what condition has brought her into your office. You will then conduct an appropriate visual examination, make chart notes of your findings, and prescribe appropriate treatment. These practices are no different in the context of litigation, but everything you do must be done in exquisite detail and be thoroughly and intelligently documented. Every note you make, every procedure you undertake, every prescription you write has the potential to be scrutinized and inquired into by lawyers in the case. The history taken from your patient must document in detail the circumstances of the event that brought her into your office. It is not enough to state, "Patient involved in motor vehicle accident." You must detail the nature of the collision, speeds involved, occupant positioning on impact, whether the patient struck anything inside the vehicle, immediate sensations following the impact, the nature and time of the onset of the visual disturbances, and how her condition has progressed down to the time of her seeing you. In short, you want to document the mechanism of injury in great detail so that if called upon, you will have an adequate basis to render an opinion as to the cause of your patient's visual disturbances.

As part of the patient's history, you will also want to obtain information from your patient as to her pre- and postincident visual care, so that you will be able to determine whether any of the complained of conditions were preexisting and whether there has been consistency in the nature of her visual complaints. Obtain copies of any prior records.

It is more likely than not that your present style of charting your patient's condition will be of no value to anyone but you, should you become involved in litigation. Incidentally, more often than not, you do not have a choice of whether to become involved in the litigation process. If your patient actively pursues a claim and you have information that will be of value in the presentation of her claim for damages, you will become involved, like it or not.

Your present chart, replete with symbols, measurements, ocular diagrams, and the use of terminology peculiar to the visual system most likely will be unintelligible to all but fellow visual providers. To be of any value in the world of litigation, your chart will have to convey in an understandable fashion the nature of your patient's condition and your actions. Most medical providers utilize the SOAP note format, that is, a recordation of the patient's Subjective complaints, the Objective findings on examination, the diagnostic Assessment of the patient's condition, and the Plan for future care or treatment. Most attorneys are comfortable with this style of reporting, and utilization of this format will facilitate an understanding of the nature of your patient's problem. Speaking of communicating in understandable terms, the field of optometry uses terminology that is foreign to most attorneys and certainly to most jurors. When using terms peculiar to the visual system, it is most helpful to define the term in brackets. For example, binocularity (eye teaming ability), convergence insufficiency (inability to sustain eye alignment when viewing at a near range of distance), ocular motilities (eye movement efficiency), accommodation (focusing ability), and so on.

Finally, I have found it helpful for the treating doctor to prepare a brief narrative report setting forth the circumstances of injury, patient complaints, examination findings, assessment, cause of the injury, and treatment measures. Keep in mind that it is the job of the attorney representing your patient to effectively communicate the nature and the impact of the injury suffered by your patient. A narrative report from you can greatly facilitate such an understanding.

THE INITIATION OF LITIGATION

Litigation is commenced by the injured party, the plaintiff, filing suit. Suit is commenced by filing a Complaint, which sets forth the circumstances of the event, the acts of negligence of the defendant, the nature of the injuries sustained, and what relief your patient seeks—usually money damages. A copy of the Complaint is served upon the defendant who then has a short period of time within which to file an Answer. In most instances, the defendant denies the allegations contained in the Complaint, which simply means that the plaintiff is then required to go forward and prove her allegations. Usually a trial date will be set, which establishes a number of deadlines by which a number of pretrial procedures will need to be completed.

PRETRIAL DISCLOSURE AND DISCOVERY

Pretrial disclosure and discovery then commence in which each side seeks to learn all of the relevant facts regarding the plaintiff's claims. Written discovery requests are customarily exchanged by both sides that include answering Interrogatories (written questions), requesting that certain documents be produced, and requesting that a party admit that certain facts are undisputed. Of importance to you is that your patient will need to disclose the nature of the injuries she sustained, all medical providers with whom she has treated, and the impact that such injuries have had in terms of the pain and suffering that she has experienced, whether any of her injuries are permanent in nature, the economic consequences of the injuries such as lost earnings or incurred medical bills, and how the injuries have impacted her ability to engage in her usual pursuits such as employment, family, and recreational activities. Detailed SOAP notes or a narrative report from you will assist your patient's attorney in responding to these information requests.

TESTIMONY

At some point, your patient's attorney will be required to disclose the identity of all of the expert witnesses who have knowledge about your patient's injuries. As a treating doctor, you are regarded as an expert witness. An expert witness is a person who by knowledge, skill, experience, training, or education is permitted to express an opinion at trial regarding scientific, technical, or medical knowledge that will assist the jury in understanding the evidence or in determining facts that are in dispute. Whereas a fact witness may only testify regarding facts actually seen, heard, or perceived by that witness, an expert can testify not only to such observed facts but also render an opinion on the meaning of such facts. For example, an expert can testify not only to his or her perceived findings on examination, but can also render opinions based upon education, training, and experience that the patient sustained an injury such as a post trauma vision syndrome, that the injury was caused by a certain event—the trauma of an automobile collision—and that the post trauma vision syndrome is permanent in nature, that is, it is not likely to resolve in the foreseeable future. These facts and opinions are necessary for your patient to prove her claim, and the more the information, which is plainly set forth in your medical records, the easier it will be for your patient's attorney to develop a clear understanding of the injuries sustained by your patient. As an expert witness, oftentimes you will be asked to furnish a curriculum vitae, a list of previous cases in which you have given testimony, and a list of any articles, books, or publications you have authored. Once you have put together such a set of documents, it is easy to periodically update them.

PRODUCTION OF RECORDS

Once you have been identified as an expert in the case, you can expect to receive requests from the attorneys for both sides for copies of your entire file. Such requests may come in the form of a written request, accompanied by a release signed by your patient, or a subpoena to produce the records. Such requests include not only your medical notes, but also intake forms prepared by you and/or your patient, all items of correspondence, records from other medical providers, and copies of all invoices for your services. You are permitted to bill for the cost of copying such records. Knowing that every scrap of paper in your file will be scrutinized by the attorneys for both sides, it is imperative that your file contain only relevant, detailed information about the nature of your interaction with your patient. Carelessness or inaccuracies in record keeping will quickly be exposed.

DEPOSITION

Once the attorneys for both sides have obtained copies of the relevant medical records and have exchanged certain basic facts about the occurrence, depositions of both fact and expert witnesses may be taken. A deposition is testimony given under oath for the purpose of discovering the facts and opinions held by the expert witness. The deposition of an expert witness is usually taken in the office of the expert, but can also be taken in the office of one of the attorneys or in a conference center.

Customarily, your deposition as a treating expert would be taken by the attorney for the defendant. In scheduling your deposition, the attorney should indicate how much time he or she requires for your deposition. It is appropriate for you to request prepayment for your time and to terminate the deposition at the end of the scheduled time if you have other commitments. It is ethically improper for the attorney for the defendant to have unilateral discussions with you about the case.

The purpose of such a deposition is to discover all relevant facts of which you are aware and to ascertain your diagnosis, the cause of the condition, the nature and effectiveness of your treatment, any functional limitations your patient experiences as a result of the injuries, whether your patient's condition is permanent in nature, what you foresee in terms of the need for future care, and the cost of past and future treatment. Also, the attorney will seek to discover any possible defenses to the claim brought by your patient such as whether her condition was preexisting, whether there were causes other than the negligence of the defendant that could account for your patient's condition such as other traumatic events, whether your patient is exaggerating her symptoms, and so on.

At the deposition, you probably will be asked to produce a current curriculum vita. You should be prepared to explain in detail the exact nature of the condition you have diagnosed, the pathophysiology of such condition, and the etiology of such condition. You should also have at your command any treatise authorities or journal articles that describe the nature of the diagnosed condition and whether it can be caused by trauma. The attorney may ask you to identify any literature upon which you relied in formulating your opinions. If you refer to notes, the attorney may ask to inspect and copy such notes. Keep in mind that the deposition is the opportunity of the defendant's attorney to discover the facts and opinions he or she wishes to obtain. As such, you need to be responsive to the questions asked. Since the attorney controls the subject matter of the questioning, you need not feel frustrated if such questioning did not elicit all relevant information. The attorney for your patient will have ample opportunity to fully present your testimony at trial.

Speaking of causation, you surely will be called upon to render an opinion on whether the condition, for example, post trauma vision syndrome, was caused by the trauma of the event. Utilizing epidemiological principles, this is not a difficult determination. There is a three-step analysis in determining causation:

(1) There must be a biologically plausible link between the event and the outcome. Is it possible that the post trauma vision syndrome could have resulted from the collision?

(2) There must be a temporal relationship between the event and the outcome. The outcome (post trauma vision syndrome) may have preexisted the event (the collision) in a less severe form and be worsened by the event. The outcome cannot post date the event by a time period that is clinically considered to be too long or too short to relate the two.

(3) There must not be any likely alternative explanation for the symptoms or condition. The term "likely" is of the greatest importance. For an alternative etiologic explanation to be considered more likely than the event, it must be both biologically plausible and have a stronger temporal relationship to the onset of symptoms than the alleged event.[1]

On the subject of rendering opinions, any opinion you express must be stated to "a reasonable degree of medical probability" or "a reasonable degree of medical certainty." This is legal jargon, which must be utilized by the attorney to admit your opinion into evidence. Expressing an opinion to a reasonable degree of medical probability means nothing more than it is more probably true than not; that is, there is more than a 50/50 probability that your opinion is more true than not. The manner in which you will be asked to express your opinion will be, "Doctor, do you have an opinion based upon a reasonable degree of medical probability whether the post trauma vision syndrome you diagnosed was caused by the motor vehicle collision?" Your response will be, "Yes, I do." To which the attorney will then ask, "What is that opinion?" And you will respond, "The post trauma vision syndrome was caused by the motor vehicle collision." It's just that simple.

With respect to giving a deposition, you should charge your usual and customary hourly rate for preparing for the deposition and for the time of giving your testimony, including travel to and from the deposition site. Usually, the attorney for your patient pays for your preparation time; the attorney for the Defendant pays for your deposition and travel time. As an expert witness, you are entitled to be paid for your time even where you are testifying pursuant to a subpoena.

Before the deposition, it is usually a good idea to meet with the attorney for your patient to review your anticipated testimony. This is especially true where the attorney may not be intimately familiar with the conditions you have diagnosed. In this prep meeting, you and the attorney will have the opportunity to discuss your opinions, to discuss any potential weaknesses in your position, and to discuss what the attorney anticipates will be the focus of the deposition from the standpoint of the other side. It also gives you the opportunity to discuss with the attorney the findings of other providers who have seen your patient so that you have a better sense of where you fit in the overall scheme of injuries and treatment. Your time for this conference should be billed to your patient's attorney. Some attorneys like to have such a conference; some do not. A lot depends on your level of testimonial expertise, the presence or absence of problems in the case, the relationship between you and the attorney, and the cost considerations. You will need to follow the lead of the attorney; however, there is nothing that says that you cannot call the attorney and suggest a predeposition conference if you think it would be helpful.

You should bring to the deposition your entire file, which you may consult in responding to questions. Be prepared to have the opposing attorney ask to review your file and to make copies of any documents he or she may not already have received. You should be sufficiently familiar with your file to be able to testify without reading from your notes or narrative report. Your deposition will be much more effective and persuasive if you are able to discuss knowledgeably all aspects of the case without resorting to the file for anything other than a memory prompt.

METHODS OF PRETRIAL RESOLUTION

There are three principal ways in which litigation can be resolved short of trial: (1) informal settlement where the parties agree to settle the plaintiff's claim, usually by payment of money damages; (2) mediation, an out-of-court claim resolution process that is overseen by an impartial, third-party mediator who endeavors to assist the parties in reaching a mutually agreeable settlement; and (3) arbitration, an out-of-court proceeding where an impartial adjudicator considers evidence and makes a decision that is legally binding on the parties.

TRIAL

A trial is a formal judicial proceeding in which evidence is presented and a decision is made by either a judge or a jury that results in a binding resolution of the claim. In the case of a claim for injuries, there are four elements that the injured party must prove: (1) liability—legal responsibility, that is, the defendant was negligent and that such negligence was a cause of plaintiff's injuries; (2) the nature and extent of the injuries sustained by the plaintiff; (3) the impact that such injuries have had on the plaintiff; and (4) the amount of monetary damages that will fairly and adequately compensate the plaintiff for her injuries. The elements to be considered in determining the amount of monetary damages are the pain and suffering and mental anguish that the plaintiff has experienced in the past and will likely experience in the future; whether the plaintiff has a permanent impairment; that is, some loss of function that will persist into the foreseeable future; economic losses that include medical treatment expenses and loss of past and future earnings; and loss of enjoyment of life; that is, the diminished pleasure one experiences in activities such as family or recreational pursuits as a consequence of the injuries.

Preparation is the be all and end all of a successful trial outcome. As an expert witness, you should be prepared to respond to questions regarding every aspect of your patient's injuries and care. It is essential that you meet with your patient's attorney to review the scope of your expected testimony, to review any weaknesses in the case, and to anticipate your cross examination by opposing counsel.

At trial, your testimony will begin by your being asked questions by your patient's attorney. This is referred to as your direct examination.

When you appear in court, you should have your entire chart with you and any authoritative references you feel are appropriate. Some witnesses find it helpful to prepare a brief outline from data in the chart, which eliminates the need to thumb through the chart. You can have with you any notes that will help you testify effectively. You can refer to your chart or your notes if necessary to answer questions; however, opposing counsel is entitled to see any documents to which you refer. In responding to questions, do not read from your chart. Jurors will tune out as soon as you start reading. Use your chart only as a memory prompt. Allow your patient's attorney to fully complete his or her question before you begin your response, even though you know where the question is going. Make certain you understand exactly what the attorney is asking. If there is any doubt, simply ask the attorney to repeat or to clarify the question. Answer the question completely and then stop. Allow the attorney to ask the next question. Do not try to encapsulate the entire case in one stream-of-consciousness answer. Let the attorney guide you question-by-question through your testimony. Effective testimony is nothing more than an exercise in good communication between you and the attorney.

Generally, jurors will not be familiar with medical terminology, anatomy, or the visual system. Therefore, your answers should be in lay terms, easily understandable. Whenever you use a medical term, define it in lay terms. Anecdotes involving your patient's difficulties are particularly effective in bringing your testimony to life. Consider using anatomical illustrations or demonstrations to explain your testimony. For example, an anatomical illustration showing the occipital lobe may assist jurors in understanding your testimony. Having the jurors try on a pair of prism glasses may help them understand the concept of visual midline shift. Remember, jurors are accustomed to getting their information in sound bites and pictures. Your objective is to be an instructor—to make certain that the jury understands the thoughts and concepts you wish to convey.

When answering questions, the natural tendency is to direct your response to the questioner. However, you need to engage the jury—bring them into the dialogue. Make eye contact and direct your responses to the jury. Your testimony should be natural and unforced, as if you are having a conversation with the jury. Your demeanor should be respectful. Even though you want to help your patient, you should not become a blatant advocate. You want to convey to the jury that you are a knowledgeable and skilled clinician who is there to assist them in understanding the issues in the case. On cross examination, do not become adversarial or argumentative with opposing counsel. An effective expert is one who exudes intelligence and mastery of his subject matter without evident bias or partisanship.

Generally speaking, the following topics will be covered in your direct examination:

(1) Your background and qualifications—your educational background, any specialized training you have had in your area of practice, your clinical experience, and the nature of your practice.

This qualification is necessary to have you accepted by the court as an expert in the field of optometry, which will then allow you to express opinions regarding the injuries, causation, permanency, and so on.

(2) The circumstances of how your patient came to see you.

(3) The history—the circumstances of the event that caused the injury, your patient's immediate complaints, the problems she was experiencing at the time of your initial encounter, how her complaints have affected her ability to function, any relevant past medical history, and the nature of any treatment she has already received.

(4) The examination—a review of your clinical examination, including the results of all tests performed. There may be components of your examination that are just part of your normal, thorough evaluation but which have no bearing on the issues in the case. Don't bring up irrelevant matters—you'll lose the jury.

(5) The diagnosis—your impression or assessment of your patient's condition on the basis of the history given to you and the results of your clinical evaluation. Enumerate in serial fashion your diagnostic findings that are relevant to the issues in the case. In a trauma case, findings of astigmatism and myopia are probably irrelevant and will obscure your pertinent findings. After you have enumerated your diagnoses, the attorney will then ask you to explain each diagnosis. Do so in understandable terms as if you were explaining your findings to your patient for the first

time. In discussing your diagnoses, it is appropriate to discuss the visual difficulties and functional limitations experienced by your patient as a result of her condition, for example, her photophobia causes her discomfort in bright light and she has to wear sunglasses all of the time, her peripheral hallucinations cause her to see things in her peripheral vision that aren't there, she has trouble reading because the words move on the page, and so on.

Your diagnostic findings must be limited to your area of expertise. As an optometrist, it is probably beyond the scope of your expertise to render a diagnosis of mild traumatic brain injury. However, you can testify that you have reviewed the reports of the treating neurologist or the neuropsychologist, and it is your understanding that your patient has been diagnosed with a mild traumatic brain injury by such providers. This will open the door to allow you to testify that you have treated a number of patients who have been diagnosed with a mild traumatic brain injury and that in your experience, the condition that you diagnosed—post trauma vision syndrome—is associated with a mild traumatic brain injury.

(6) Causation—your opinion, on the basis of a reasonable degree of medical probability that the conditions you have diagnosed were caused by the motor vehicle collision.

(7) Treatment—a full discussion of the treatment you have rendered, how such treatment improves or resolves the conditions that you have diagnosed, and the results of such treatment measures.

(8) Permanency—your opinion, based upon a reasonable degree of medical probability, whether the conditions that you have diagnosed are going to be permanent in nature.

(9) Prognosis—how you expect your patient to progress in the future, including the need for further or ongoing treatment.

(10) Treatment expenses—a statement of the total amount of charges incurred by your patient; this is part of your patient's proof of an economic loss she has sustained. To be admissible, your charges must be reasonable in dollar amount and your optometric services must have been necessitated by the injuries your patient received in the motor vehicle collision. Here you are concerned only with the actual expenses for treatment. Your bills for trial preparation or trial testimony are not included.

(11) Cross examination—at the conclusion of your direct examination, the opposing attorney will have the opportunity to ask you questions. The objective of the opposing attorney will be to elicit admissions from you that are helpful to the defense of the case. For example, your patient had similar symptoms before the trauma, your patient did not complain of visual symptoms until months after the occurrence, the conditions that you diagnosed have resolved, your patient was inconsistent in her reporting of her symptoms, your patient exaggerates her symptoms, your patient has not been compliant with your treatment recommendations, the medical literature does not recognize the condition that you have diagnosed, and so on. Be aware that on cross examination, the attorney is permitted to ask a leading question, that is, a question that seeks an acknowledgment of a stated fact or suggests the answer, the answer to which is a "yes" or "no." For example, "When first seen by you, your patient made no complaint of blurry vision, did she?" The nonleading formulation would be, "What complaints did your patient make when you first saw her?" Leading

questions are designed to elicit information helpful to the defense without giving you the opportunity to elaborate or explain your answer. Before answering "yes," be certain that you are in full agreement with the stated fact. You can always ask to explain your answer; however, skillful counsel will deflect that question by stating, "Your attorney will have the opportunity to have you explain your answer." By asking to explain your answer, you are signaling your patient's attorney to follow up on redirect examination and give you the opportunity to fully explain the "yes" or "no" answer that you previously gave. Leading questions can be couched in innocuous terms, but be absolutely certain you agree with the statement before answering "yes." For example, "Would it be fair to say that your patient wasn't as diligent in performing her home exercises as you would have liked her to have been?" "Would you agree with me that it would be very difficult to apportion how much of your patient's problems were caused by the motor vehicle collision as opposed to the tumble she took down the stairs shortly after the collision?"

CONCLUSION

Becoming a skilled and effective expert witness is not difficult once the nature of the litigation process has been demystified and you know what will be expected of you. It does, however, require extra attention to detail and the ability to adapt the manner in which you practice to meet the demands of the litigation process. Of one thing I am certain: Being involved in the litigation process will raise your level of competence. The demands of litigation will make you a better record keeper, you will become more analytical in your assessment of your patient's problems, you will be more sensitive to doing everything you can to improve your patient's condition, and you will improve your ability to effectively explain little understood aspects of the practice of optometry.

REFERENCE

1. Freeman, M. D., & Rossignol, A. C. (2008). Forensic epidemiology: a systematic approach to probabilistic determinations in disputed matters. *Journal of Forensic and Legal Medicine, 15*(5), 281–290.

Glossary

Accommodation: The act of focusing the eyes to provide a clear image.

Accommodative lens flippers: A vision therapy procedure using lenses that alternately stimulate and relax accommodation so as to produce flexibility in the system.

AC/A ratio: The amount of reflex accommodative-convergence stimulated during accommodation. Expressed as a ratio of accommodative-convergence/accommodation.

Activities of daily living (ADL): Activities of daily living are divided into various categories: personal and basic self-care, relating to household management tasks, school or other productive activity, and play or leisure.

Aniseikonia: A condition where there is a significant difference in the perceived size of visual images. It can occur as an overall difference between the eyes, or only in one meridian.

Anomalous correspondence (AC): Observed in strabismus, the condition in which an area other than the fovea of the strabismic eye "corresponds" to the fovea of the other eye. This avoids double vision and may provide for some degree of stereopsis.

Astigmatism: When the refractive power of the eye is not uniform in all directions (meridians) making it more difficult to form sharp images on the retina.

Aphasia: Difficulty producing and/or comprehending spoken or written language.

Apraxia: A disorder of motor planning causing an inability to execute or carry out learned purposeful movements, without a loss of the physical ability to perform the movements. Some may include ideational—difficulty planning a specific movement; verbal—difficulty with oral-motor movements; constructional—difficulty drawing figures or constructing objects; oculomotor—difficulty with eye movements, especially saccades.

Asthenopia: Eye fatigue which may be accompanied by headache or eyestrain (pain).

Ataxia: A broad term signifying a lack of coordination in a physiological process. Optic ataxia is a lack of coordination between visual processing and hand movement, resulting in difficulty reaching for and grabbing objects.

Attention: The cognitive process of allocation of processing resources, or selectively concentrating on one aspect of the environment. Overt attention is the act of directing sensory organs toward a stimulus. Covert attention refers to the act of mentally focusing on one stimulus, or enhancing the signal from a particular part of the sensory panorama, while appearing to have the sense organ directed at another stimulus. Divided attention refers to the ability to mentally focus simultaneously to multiple tasks or demands.

Bifoveal fixation: In normal eyes, the condition in which the fovea of one eye "corresponds" to the fovea of the other eye, and the image of the target object is fixated so that the image of the target falls on both foveas. This provides the basis for fusion of the images and stereopsis.

Binocular: Refers to the organized simultaneous perception of information from the right eye and the left eye.

CA/C ratio: The amount of reflex convergence-accommodation stimulated during convergence. Expressed as a ratio of convergence-accommodation/convergence.

Cheiroscopic tracing: A drawing made in a stereoscope that can give information about binocular alignment, suppression, visual stability, aniseikonia, and visual-spatial projection.

Comitant: Also known as concomitant. In strabismus, when the angle of deviation is the same in all positions of gaze. Noncomitant, also known as nonconcomitant, in strabismus, or phoria, when the angle of deviation varies as the eyes are moved to different positions of gaze.

Compensatory lens: *See* Lens.

Constructional apraxia: *See* Apraxia.

Convergence: *See* Vergence.

Cover test: A test that provides an objective determination of the presence, type (phoria or tropia, eso, exo, hyper, or hypo), and amount of an ocular deviation.

Covert attention: *See* Attention.

Cranial nerves: Twelve pairs of nerves that emanate directly from the nervous tissue of the brain. This is in contrast to spinal nerves that emerge from segments of the spinal cord. Six of the twelve pairs are involved with the eyes and vision.

Cyclotorsion: Rotation of the eye around its visual axis. It occurs normally. However, it may also be pathological after an eye injury, surgery, or ABI and, if large in magnitude, it will interfere with or prevent binocular alignment of the eyes and fusion of visual images.

Divided attention: *See* Attention.

Decision tree: A decision support tool for calculating conditional probabilities to help to identify a strategy most likely to reach an outcome or goal.

Decompensated phoria: *See* Phoria.

Diplopia: Double vision. The condition in which a single object is perceived as two objects instead of one.

Divergence: *See* Vergence.

Duane's Retraction Syndrome: A congenital eye condition characterized by a limitation of abduction (outward movement) of the affected eye, retraction of the eyeball on adduction (inward movement), with an associated narrowing of the palpebral fissure (closing of the eye).

Duction: The movement of only one eye.

Eso: A prefix indicating that the eyes are deviated inward, or pointing closer than the object of regard.

Esophoria: *See* Phoria.

Exo: A prefix indicating that the eyes are deviated outward, or pointing farther than the object of regard.

Exophoria: *See* Phoria.

Egocentric localization: The localization of objects in space in reference to one's own body.

Fixation: The maintenance of visual gaze on a single location.

Fixation disparity: A small misalignment or instability in eye alignment under binocular viewing conditions.

Gaze palsy: A limitation of the movement of one eye or of both eyes to move in the same direction at the same time.

Graded occlusion: *See* Occlusion.

Guidance lens: *See* Lens.

Hemiparesis: *See* Paralysis.

Homonymous hemianopia: Loss of vision in the same visual field of each eye resulting in a loss of vision in the right or left visual field.

Homolateral: Pertaining to one side of the body.

Hyper: A prefix indicating that one of the eyes is deviated upward, or pointing higher than the object of regard. Also, greater or more, as in hypermetric saccades.

Hypo: A prefix indicating that one of the eyes is deviated downward, or pointing lower than the object of regard. Also, insufficient or less, as in hypometric saccades.

Hypermetric saccade: *See* Saccade.

Hypometric saccade: *See* Saccade.

Hyperopia (farsightedness): Light rays coming from a distant object strike the retina before coming to sharp focus. Causes the individual to use additional accommodative effort to keep objects clear.

Ideational apraxia: *See* Apraxia.

Lens: Optical device that causes light to bend or become focused in a different point in space. Minus lenses (concave) are used for myopia and make objects appear smaller and closer in space. Plus lenses (convex) are used for hyperopia and make objects appear larger and further in space. Astigmatic lenses have different powers in one meridian than another causing light to be focused at different places in space. A compensatory lens is one that allows the person to function better with their existing visual anatomy and physiology. A guidance lens is one prescribed with the desire of shifting the posture of either eyes or the body to some different status in the future

Minus lens: *See* Lens.

Monocular: Having only one eye, or when each eye is used separately, for example, when one eye is covered, as during a vision therapy procedure.

Myopia (nearsightedness): Light rays coming from a distant object are brought to focus in front of the retina interfering with the formation of a clear image of objects viewed in the distance.

Nearpoint retinoscopy: *See* Retinoscopy.

Neglect: (Also called *visual neglect, hemispatial agnosia, visual-spatial inattention*, or *hemi-imperception*)—a passive unconscious decreased awareness of one side of the body, visual field, or other stimuli.

Neuro-ophthalmologist: A physician concerned with the neurological aspects of diseases affecting the visual system.

Neuro-optometrist: A doctor of optometry who delivers care related to visual function, or visual habilitation and rehabilitation for the neurologically challenged patient.

Noncomitant: *See* Comitant.

Nystagmus: Rapid involuntary movements of the eyes in a rhythmic pattern.

Occlusion: The partial or total covering of one eye. Various forms include a patch placed directly over the eye, an opaque contact lens, or translucent or opaque spectacle lenses. Total occlusion means that no image or light reaches any part of the eye. Sectoral occlusion is the covering of only part, so that only one area of the visual field is obscured. Spot occlusion is the placing of a spot, usually centrally, so that only the central part of the visual field is occluded, allowing for normal peripheral awareness. Graded occlusion is a translucent occlusion where form is degraded but light and movement can still be detected.

Ocular motor: Pertaining to eye movements, such as pursuits or saccades, or the muscle system controlling the eyes.

Oculocentric localization: The localization of objects in space with reference to the eye.

Oculomotor: Having to do with ocular motor movements, or pertaining to CN III.

Oculomotor apraxia: *See* Apraxia.

Optokinetic nystagmus (OKN): Subcortically mediated function based on the principle that the eyes tend to follow or track the motion of one element at a time in a steadily moving display, and make a rapid refixations to continue the pursuit.

Optic ataxia: *See* Ataxia.

Optic flow: Movement of image information across the retina caused when objects move in the world, or we move through the environment, used in determining one's visual direction or heading.

Overconvergence: *See* Vergence.

Overt attention: *See* Attention.

Parallax: The apparent movement in the position of an object viewed along two different lines of sight. Used to judge distances.

Paralysis (hemiplegia): Total paralysis of the arm, leg, and trunk on the same side of the body. Hemiparesis is weakness on one side of the body.

Phoria (heterophoria): The neuromuscular "resting position" of the eyes. An esophoria is a spatial mismatch where the neuromuscular posturing of the eyes is closer than the actual object of regard. An exophoria is a spatial mismatch where the neuromuscular posturing of the eyes is farther than the actual object of regard. When a heterophoria cannot be compensated by fusional vergence, strabismus ensues.

Phoropter: A refractive instrument containing lenses and prisms used to determine the amount of nearsightedness, farsightedness, and astigmatism; phoric posture and vergence; and accommodative measurements.

Photoreceptors: Sensory structures (rods and cones) that receive light stimuli.

Physiological diplopia: A normally occurring event under binocular conditions, where objects in front of and behind the object of regard are perceived as being double.

Plus lens: *See* Lens.

Prism: A wedge of refractive material that shifts light 1 cm per prism diopter at a distance of 1 m. The greater the power of the prism or the distance, the greater the shift in apparent movement of the object viewed through the prism. Prisms are said to be yoked when the bases in front of both eyes point in the same direction and the prism amounts are the same.

Presbyopia: A loss of elasticity of the lens of the eye, normally occurring in middle age. It causes deficiencies in accommodation resulting in an inability to focus clearly for near vision.

Pursuit: Ocular movement that holds the image of a target on the fovea, when either self, the target, or both are moving, to keep the dynamic image from blurring.

Refraction (refractive measurements): Test used to determine which lenses will provide the sharpest, clearest, and most comfortable sight, for example, with a phoropter and retinoscopy.

Retinoscopy: A technique using an instrument called a *retinoscope* to obtain an objective measurement of the refractive condition of the eyes, that is, determination of nearsightedness, farsightedness, and/or astigmatism. Nearpoint retinoscopy is an objective method to evaluate the focusing accuracy of the eyes relative to a target within arms length, and gives a direct measure of the accuracy and stability of focusing.

Saccade: A relatively rapid jump movement of the eyes from one place in space to another to bring images of objects of interest onto the fovea. A hypermetric saccade is one where the saccadic movement is longer or overestimates the amount of jump needed to go from one point to another. A hypometric saccade is one where the saccade is shorter, or an underestimation.

Sectoral occlusion: *See* Occlusion.

Spatial map: A neurological or mental representation, which may be a tactile, proprioceptive, or visual map of the body, or an auditory or visual map of the body or space. The maps may be two or three dimensional, have one or multiple frames of reference and be static or dynamic.

Spot occlusion: *See* Occlusion.

Stereopsis: The binocular appreciation of depth due to the retinal disparity of objects viewed from a slightly different perspective in each eye.

Strabismus: Also called "tropia" refers to the visual condition in which the visual axes of the eyes are not directed toward the same object at the same time and binocular (bifoveal) fixation is not present.

Subitize: The ability to, in a glance, make rapid, accurate, and confident judgements of number for small numbers of items. This ability appears to be innate in human, infants. The limit for adults is approximately seven objects.

Suppression: The condition where all or part of the visual field is not perceived by one eye due to inhibition of the image, rather than visual field loss. The main purpose of suppression is to secure binocular single vision where it would not be attainable otherwise.

Supranuclear: Situated or occurring superior or cortical to a nucleus in the brain.

Transilluminator: A light source used to evaluate external eye health and pupillary reflexes.

Tropia: Strabismus, a suffix indicating a misalignment of the eyes. Usually combined with prefixes such as eso, exo, hyper, hypo, or cyclo.

Underconvergence: *See* Vergence.

Vectogram: A vision training instrument using polarized targets that is designed to develop binocularity, expand fusional ranges, increase flexibility between the accommodative and binocular systems and match sensory systems.

Verbal apraxia: *See* Apraxia.

Vergence: Eye movements involving both eyes in which each eye moves in opposite directions. Vergence movements help to attain and maintain fusion at various distances. Convergence is the turning inward of the lines of sight to attain or maintain single vision while viewing objects or print at nearpoint. Divergence is the relaxation of convergence, allowing the two lines of sight to become more parallel as an object moves away. Overconvergence pertains to the posturing of the eyes closer than the actual object. Underconvergence pertains to the posturing of the eyes further away than the actual object of regard.

Version: The movement of both eyes in a coordinated and conjunctive manner. Sometimes used synonymously with pursuit and visual tracking.

Vertical imbalance: A phoric or tropic vertical misalignment of the eyes.

Vestibulo-ocular reflex (VOR): A reflex eye movement in the direction opposite to head movement to stabilize an image on the retina during a head movement.

Visual confusion: The condition in strabismus where each of the two foveas receives an image of a different object and the brain perceives the two objects as superimposed and in the same spatial location.

Visual midline: The perceived visual-spatial perception of straight ahead.

Visual neglect: *See* Neglect.

Visual inattention: *See* Neglect.

Wolff wand: A testing instrument that is used as a target during the testing of pursuits, saccades, and convergence.

X, Y, and Z axes: Refers to meridians or axes in reference to the eyes or body. The X axis refers to a movement along the horizontal, the Y axis along the vertical, and the Z axis perpendicular to or closer or further away from the eyes or body.

Yoked prism: *See* Prism.

Zone of proximal development (ZPD): The difference between what a learner can do without help and what he or she can do with help. The distance between the actual developmental level as determined by independent problem solving and the level of potential development as determined by problem solving under guidance.

Index

*For Product Safety Concerns and Information please contact
our EU representative GPSR@taylorandfrancis.com Taylor & Francis
Verlag GmbH, Kaufingerstraße 24, 80331 München, Germany*

T - #0007 - 160425 - C12 - 234/156/29 [31] - CB - 9781439836552 - Gloss Lamination